Pediatric PET Imaging

Pediatric PET Imaging

Martin Charron, MD, FRCP(C)

Professor, Department of Radiology, University of Toronto, Division Head of Nuclear Medicine, Head of Research for Diagnostic Imaging, Senior Associate Scientist, Research Institute, The Hospital for Sick Children, Toronto, Canada

Editor

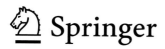 Springer

Martin Charron, MD, FRCP(C)
Professor, Department of Radiology
University of Toronto
Division Head of Nuclear Medicine
Head of Research for Diagnostic Imaging
Senior Associate Scientist
Research Institute
The Hospital for Sick Children
Toronto M5G 1X8
Canada

Library of Congress Control Number: 2005932082

ISBN-10: 0-387-28836-8
ISBN-13: 978-0387-28836-9

Printed on acid-free paper.

Printed in the United States of America.   (BS/MVY)

9 8 7 6 5 4 3 2 1

springer.com

*To my wife Teran, without whose love and support
this book would not be possible and who is the better
part of me,
To my children Sophie, Claire, George, Annie, and
Mimi for providing meaning to my life,
To the memory of my dad who taught me what is
important,
To my mother who made me what I am and gave me
the necessary patience to deal with the aforementioned kids!*

Foreword I

Positron emission tomography (PET) has been at the forefront of functional and molecular imaging for a number of years. The future of diagnostic imaging depends upon the ability to change from imaging anatomy to examining the processes at work in the body. The fact that there are now monographs examining particular aspects of PET, such as this book on the examination of children, speaks to the newly won maturity of PET. The authors are to be congratulated for the timely appearance of this volume.

In recent years, PET has transformed the contributions of nuclear medicine to the diagnosis, staging, and follow-up of patients with cancer. Children with cancer deserve the very best and most compassionate care that society can provide. Ultimately the greatest compassion we can offer as physicians is to provide the best possible care. Those charged with creating public policy in the context of diagnostic medicine must make common cause with physicians and other scientists to ensure that that best possible care is realized at the bedside. All of the evidence suggests that PET is central to such optimal cancer care.

In addition to the distinguished cast of physicians and researchers who contributed to this book, I welcome the contributions from technologists who are a key part of the interaction between the diagnostic process and the sick or potentially sick child. Good care is contingent upon putting parents and child at ease, and the technologist has a lead role in this.

Scientists, working alongside physicians and physician-scientists, have done much to ensure that PET continues to evolve in at least two directions. One direction is the technical development of imaging devices, particularly in the form of hybrid detector systems to image both biochemistry and morphology simultaneously; combined positron emission and x-ray computed tomography (PET-CT) is an example of this. In another direction, new radio-labeled molecular probes are emerging that will take PET beyond the mapping of regional glucose metabolism. PET will continue to evolve in ways we can now see but dimly. The inherent power of PET is represented for me by the fact that it has been the first technology in diagnostic imaging to serve not only in the diagnosis of individual patients but also to address the wider issue of our understanding of disease mechanisms and the localization of biochemical events in the living body.

Pediatric PET Imaging clearly represents the importance of PET. The reader will be enriched with useful clinical information for daily practice and alerted to recent developments so as to be in a position to anticipate and benefit from evolution in a field that is in a constant process of change.

It has been said that developments in molecular biology and genomics will cause medicine to change more in the next few decades than it has over the past several centuries. I have no doubt that PET will have an important role to play at the "bedside" in realizing the benefits of our growing understanding of the molecular basis of disease and its treatment. I am sure my colleagues will join me in welcoming *Pediatric PET Imaging* as a timely synthesis of our current knowledge in pediatric PET, coming as it does at the cusp of so much progress in diagnostic methods and in our ability to image disease.

Brian Lentle, MD
Emeritus Professor of Radiology
University of British Columbia

Foreword II

While the importance of PET in the understanding of physiologic and pathological conditions in adults has been well described, this is the first book to be published concerning the importance of PET imaging in pediatric patients.

The use of PET in medicine is a relatively recent development. In 1968 Kuhl and Edwards at the University of Pennsylvania introduced the concept of emission tomography and built a device to measure the regional distribution of single gamma emitters. In 1975 Ter-Pogossian and colleagues at Washington University described the first instrument designed to image positron emitting radioligands. Interest in using short-lived positron emitters for the study of biologic functions in humans was greatly enhanced by the development of the ^{14}C-deoxyglucose method for measuring region cerebral glucose metabolism (rCMRgl) autoradiographically in animals by Sokoloff and colleagues at the National Institute of Mental Health and Reivich at the University of Pennsylvania in 1977. It was clear that adapting this method to studies in humans offered great potential, and in late 1973 Reivich, Kuhl, and Alavi discussed the possibility of labeling deoxyglucose with a gamma-emitting radionuclide for measuring rCMRgl in humans. We contacted Alfred Wolf at Brookhaven National Laboratory, and at a joint meeting in December 1973 Wolf suggested using ^{18}F to label the glucose analogue fluorodeoxyglucose (FDG) because of its relatively long half-life and its low positron energy. By 1975, ^{18}F-FDG was successfully synthesized by Ido in Wolf's laboratory in sufficient quantity to be shipped to the University of Pennsylvania for human studies. In preparation for these studies, the Mark IV scanner at the University of Pennsylvania was equipped with high-energy collimators to image the ^{511}Kev gamma rays emitted by ^{18}F-FDG. In August of 1976, the first study of rCMRgl in humans was performed at the University of Pennsylvania. The development of the ^{18}F-FDG method for the measurement of regional cerebral glucose metabolism in humans, together with the method for the measurement of regional cerebral blood flow using ^{15}O labeled water pioneered by Herscovitch, Raichle and co-investigators in 1983 gave birth to functional imaging of the human brain. Since then, hundreds of tracers labeled with positron-emitting radionuclides have been developed to measure various physiologic and biochemical processes in the human body. In recognition of the stimulus provided to this field, FDG was nominated as the "molecule of the century" by Henry Wagner in 1996 at the meeting of the Society of Nuclear Medicine. FDG continues to be the most widely used PET tracer.

Pediatric PET Imaging amply documents the great importance that these developments have had in the field of pediatrics. The application of PET methodology to pediatric patients has expanded our understanding of disorders ranging from attention deficit hyperactivity disorder, learning disorders, and neuropsychiatric disorders to epilepsy, central nervous system tumors, cardiac disorders, and infectious processes, among others. This book is extremely informative for health care professionals caring for children with these conditions including nuclear medicine technologists performing the PET scan, researchers preparing a proposal utilizing PET in the pediatric population, nuclear medicine physicians interpreting the PET scan, and clinicians treating the patients.

Martin Reivich, MD
Emeritus Professor
University of Pennsylvania

Preface

Positron emission tomography (PET), a powerful research tool 20 years ago, has recently gained widespread application in oncology and is now a procedure clinically available on each continent. Despite the fact only a few PET centers are dedicated to children, data from Children's Oncology Group indicate that virtually all children in North America have easy access to a PET center. As the table of contents of this book indicates, clinical and research applications of PET for children with cancer represent only a fraction of the current pediatric uses for PET technology. Small animal PET scanners are now available commercially as there has been tremendous interest in applying PET technology to in vivo imaging of animal models.

PET can dynamically image trace amounts of radiopharmaceuticals in vivo. By applying appropriate tracer kinetic models, tracer concentrations can be determined quantitatively. In addition to superior spatial resolution and quantitative potential, PET also offers much greater sensitivity (i.e., number of y-rays detected per unit injected dose) than single photon emission computed tomography (SPECT). Furthermore, the biologic ubiquity of the elements that are positron emitters gives PET unprecedented power to image the distribution and kinetics of natural and analog biologic tracers. Because of the exquisite sensitivity of detection systems to y-ray emission, these biologic probes can be introduced in trace amounts (nano- or even picomolar concentrations) that do not disturb the biologic process under investigation. By combining a tracer that is selective for a specific biochemical pathway, an accurate tracer kinetic model, and a dynamic sequence of quantitative images from the PET scanner, it is possible to estimate the absolute rates of biologic processes in that pathway. Examples of such processes that have been successfully measured with PET include regional cerebral and myocardial blood flow, rates of glucose utilization, rates of protein synthesis, cerebral and myocardial oxygen consumption, synthesis of neurotransmitters, enzyme assays, and receptor assays. In summary, some of the distinctive advantages of PET are its exquisite sensitivity, the flexible chemistry, and the better imaging characteristics of PET isotopes. Thus PET provides access to biological processes that is well beyond the scope of current MR technology.

Although FDG has been successfully and widely employed in oncology, it has not demonstrated significant uptake in some tumors in adults. Some other positron emitter tracers seem to be more promising. Among the many radiopharmaceuticals that show great potential is the serotonin precursor 5-hydroxytryptophan (5-HTP) labeled with 11C, which shows increased uptake in carcinoids. Another radiopharmaceutical in development for PET is 11C L-DOPA, which seems to be useful in visualizing endocrine pancreatic tumors such as Hyperinsulinism (Chapter 26).

PET is now widely used in children in most health care institutions in North America, Europe, and Asia. When an imaging modality is used routinely in children, it usually implies that it has reached a certain maturity, that the modality in question has achieved widespread recognition in the clinical field by peers. Yet there are no PET books available to pediatricians that offer a comprehensive review of diseases and/or issues specific to children. Often those diseases are not reviewed in sufficient details in "adult textbooks," and issues specific to children not discussed at all (e.g., sedation, dosage). The goal of this text is to fill those gaps. We did a comprehensive review of all clinical and research applications of PET in children and gathered a distinguished cast of authorities from the Americas, Europe, and Australia to summarize their experience with PET and to perform exhaustive reviews of the literature in their areas of interest. Although this book focuses on practical applications, it includes detailed reviews of current and future research applications.

Pediatric PET Imaging offers a comprehensive review of practical issues specific to the pediatric population such as sedation, radiopharmaceutical dosage, approach to imaging children, and "tips" for technologists. For those interested in the research applications of PET, the book also offers practical reviews of regulations, IRB requirements, ethical issues, and biological effects of low level radiation exposure.

The scope of the pathologies reviewed in this work is much wider than what is seen in the typical "adult textbook." The physiopathology and the imaging findings of the most common cancers afflicting children are scrutinized. Many chapters of this book review non-oncological applications such as neurological and psychiatric diseases, some unique to children, some affecting both children and adults. Some chapters are thorough reviews of inflammation, or variants of it (FUO, IBD, and infection). New applications that appear to have the potential to offer great clinical usefulness, such as imaging of hyperinsulinism, are included. Because the biodistribution of FDG and the "normal variants" are different in children, two imaging atlases are included to allow readers to become familiar with those idiosyncrasies.

The book also reviews principles of operations and instrumentation challenges specific to children. A chapter is dedicated to coincidence imaging, as some of us do not have access to dedicated PET imaging. (One could also foresee similar imaging findings with coincidence imaging and Tc99 –glucose scanning, which may become a viable alternative to PET imaging in some precise clinical applications.) Finally, there are also expert reviews of multimodality imaging such as PET/CT and PET/MR.

Pediatric PET Imaging addresses typical concerns about imaging children and will be useful to the nuclear medicine physician who sees an occasional pediatric patient in his/her clinical practice. This book may also become a bedside reference for nuclear physicians and radiologists who practice only pediatric imaging. The book is also designed to be useful to all pediatricians, especially oncologists and radiation therapists, clinicians, or researchers looking to learn how the many recent imaging innovations in PET can influence their own areas of interests. Finally, this book offers a comprehensive review of research issues valuable to scientists.

PET will offer many new solutions to current and future problems of medicine. As a scientific community, we need to ensure that the current or proposed uses of PET are evaluated with the greatest accuracy, rigor, and appropriateness within the inherent limits of our current economic infrastructure. One of our many ethical challenges is to choose which pathology should first be scrutinized.

As PET technology continues to mature, we are seeing the beginning of a powerful merger among biology, pharmacology, and imaging, and with it the true birth of in vivo biologic imaging. Because of the flexible chemistry inherent to positron emitting isotopes, PET is vested with tremendous potential to evaluate the physiopathology of pediatric diseases.

Martin Charron, MD, FRCP(C)
Toronto, Canada

Contents

Section 1   Basic Science and Practical Issues

Section 4   Other Applications

Section 5   Imaging Atlas

Contributors

Roberto Accorsi, PhD
Research Scientist, Nuclear Medicine, Children's Hospital of Philadelphia, Philadelphia, PA 19104, USA

Jean-Louis Alberini, MD
Nuclear Medicine Department, Cancer Research Center R. Huguenin, 92210 Saint-Cloud, France

Rajendra D. Badgaiyan, PhD, MD
Assistant Professor, Department of Radiology, Harvard University, Department of Radiology, Massachusetts General Hospital, Boston, MA 02114, USA

Girish Bal, PhD
Post-Doctorial Fellow, Nuclear Medicine, Department of Radiology, Children's Hospital of Philadelphia, Philadelphia, PA 19104, USA

Peeyush Bhargava, MD
Assistant Professor, Department of Radiology, Columbia University College of Physicians and Surgeons, Attending in Nuclear Medicine, St. Luke's Roosevelt Hospital Center, New York, NY 10019, USA

Nathalie Boddaert, MD, PhD
Service de Radiologie Pédiatrique, Hôpital Necker-Enfants Malades, 75015 Paris, France

Nicolaas I. Bohnen, MD, PhD
Associate Professor, Departments of Radiology and Neurology, Division of Nuclear Medicine, University of Michigan, Ann Arbor, MI 48109, USA

Francis Brunelle, MD
Professor and Chairman, Department of Radiology, Service de Radiologie Pédiatrique, Hôpital Necker-Enfants Malades, 75015 Paris, France

Martin Charron, MD, FRCP(C)
Professor, Department of Radiology, University of Toronto, Division Head of Nuclear Medicine, Head of Research for Diagnostic Imaging, Senior Associate Scientist, Research Institute, The Hospital for Sick Children, Toronto M5G 1X8, Canada

David K. Chung, BSc (Med), MB BS, FRACP, DDU, DCH
Physician, Department of Nuclear Medicine, The Children's Hospital at Westmead, Sydney, Australia

Pascale De Lonlay, MD, PhD
Département de Métabolisme et Pédiatrie, Hôpital Necker-Enfants Malades, 75015 Paris, France

Jeffrey S. Dome, MD
Associate Member, Department of Hematology-Oncology, St. Jude Faculty, St. Jude Children's Research Hospital, Memphis, TN 38105, USA

Ghassan El-Haddad, MD
Chief Fellow, Nuclear Medicine Training Program, Hospital of the University of Pennsylvania, Philadelphia, PA 19104, USA

Josephine Elia, MD
Assistant Professor, Department of Psychiatry, University of Pennsylvania, Medical Co-Director of the ADHD Center, Children's Hospital of Philadelphia, Philadelphia, PA 19104, USA

Monique Ernst, MD, PhD
Staff Clinician, National Institute of Mental Health, Section of Developmental and Affective Neuroscience, Bethesda, MD 20892, USA

Neir Eshel
Undergraduate Student (Class of 2007), Princeton University, Bethesda, MD, USA

Alan J. Fischman, MD
Associate Professor, Department of Radiology, Harvard University, Massachusetts General Hospital Nuclear Medicine, Boston, MA 02114, USA

Michael J. Fisher, MD
Assistant Professor, Department of Pediatrics, University of Pennsylvania, Division of Oncology, Children's Hospital of Philadelphia, Philadelphia, PA 19104, USA

Marianne Glanzman, MD
Clinical Associate Professor, Department of Pediatrics, University of Pennsylvania School of Medicine, Division of Child Development and Rehabilitation, Children's Seashore House of the Children's Hospital of Philadelphia, Philadelphia, PA 19104, USA

Maria Green, RTNM
Team Leader, Nuclear Medicine, Department of Diagnostic Imaging, The Hospital for Sick Children, Toronto M5G 1X8, Canada

Klaus Hahn, MD
Professor, Head of the Department of Nuclear Medicine, University of Munich, Ludwig-Maximilians-University of Munich, D-80336 Munich, Germany

Olga T. Hardy, MD
Fellow, Departments of Endocrinology and Diabetes; Children's Hospital of Philadelphia, Core Laboratory, Children's Hospital of Philadelphia, Philadelphia, PA 19104, USA

Miguel Hernandez-Pampaloni, PhD
Research Assistant Professor, Department of Nuclear Medicine, University of Pennsylvania, Children's Hospital of Philadelphia, Philadelphia, PA 19104, USA

Marc P. Hickeson, MD
Assistant Professor, Department of Radiology, Division of Nuclear Medicine, McGill University, Royal Victoria Hospital, Montreal H3A 1A1, Canada

Rodney J. Hicks, MB BS (Hons), MD, FRACP
Professor, Department of Medicine, St. Vincent's Medical School, The University of Melbourne, Director, Center for Molecular Imaging, The Peter MacCallum Cancer Center, East Melbourne, Victoria, Australia

Robert Howman-Giles, MB BS, MD, FRACP, DDU
Clinical Associate Professor, Departments of Nuclear Medicine and Pediatrics and Child Health, The Children's Hospital at Westmead, University of Sydney, Sydney, Australia

Francis Jaubert, MD, PhD
Laboratoire de Anatomopathologie, Hôpital Necker-Enfants Malades, 75015 Paris, France

Paul R. Jolles, MD
Associate Professor, Department of Radiology, Director, Nuclear Medicine Residency Program, Virginia Commonwealth University Health System and Medical College of Virginia Hospitals, Richmond, VA 23298, USA

Joel S. Karp, PhD
Professor, Department of Radiology, University of Pennsylvania, Philadelphia, PA 19104, USA

Sue C. Kaste, DO
Member, Departments of Radiological Sciences and Hematology-Oncology, St. Jude Faculty, St. Jude Children's Research Hospital, Memphis, TN 38105, USA

Robin Kaye, MD
Assistant Professor, Department of Radiology, University of Pennsylvania, Chief, Interventional Radiologist, Children's Hospital of Pennsylvania, Philadelphia, PA 19104, USA

Geoffrey Levine, PhD, RPh, BCNP (Ret.)
Associate Professor, Departments of Radiology and Pharmaceutical Sciences, University of Pittsburgh, Schools of Medicine and Pharmacy, Director of Nuclear Pharmacy, Presbyterian University Hospital of the University of Pittsburgh Medical Center, Clinical Director of the Monoclonal Antibody Imaging Center, Pittsburgh Cancer Institute, Pittsburgh, PA 15213, USA

M. Beth McCarville, MD
Assistant Member, Department of Radiological Sciences, St. Jude Faculty, St. Jude Children's Research Hospital, Division of Diagnostic Imaging, Memphis, TN 38105, USA

Geoffrey McCowage, MB BS, FRACP
Senior Staff Specialist, Department of Oncology, The Children's Hospital at Westmead, Sydney, Australia

James M. Mountz, MD, PhD
Associate Professor, Departments of Neurology and Radiology, University of Pittsburgh Medical Center, Children's Hospital of Pittsburgh, Pittsburgh, PA 15213, USA

Suzanne Munson, BA
Medical Student (Class of 2007), Virginia Commonwealth University School of Medicine, Medical College of Virginia, Richmond, VA, USA

Robert M. Nelson, MD, PhD
Associate Professor, Departments of Anesthesiology, Pediatrics and Critical Care Medicine, University of Pennsylvania, Children's Hospital of Philadelphia, Philadelphia, PA 19104, USA

Claire Nihoul-Fekete, MD, PhD
Départment de Chirurgie Infantile, Hôpital Necker-Enfants Malades, 75015 Paris, France

Lorcan A. O'Tuama, MD
Professor, Departments of Radiology, Neuroradiology, and Nuclear Medicine, Virginia Commonwealth University Health System and Medical College of Virginia Hospitals, Richmond, VA 23298, USA

Christopher J. Palestro, MD
Professor, Departments of Nuclear Medicine and Radiology, Albert Einstein College of Medicine Bronx, New York, Chief of Nuclear Medicine, Long Island Jewish Medical Center, New Hyde Park, NY 11040, USA

Thomas Pfluger, MD
Associate Professor, Department of Nuclear Medicine, Ludwig-Maximilians-University of Munich, D-80336 Munich, Germany

Peter C. Phillips, MD
Professor, Departments of Neurology and Oncology, University of Pennsylvania, Director of Neuro-Oncology Programs, Children's Hospital of Philadelphia, Philadelphia, PA 19104, USA

Fabio Ponzo, MD
Assistant Professor, Department of Radiology, New York University School of Medicine, Nuclear Medicine, New York University Medical Centers, New York, NY 10016, USA

Josephine N. Rini, MD
Assistant Professor, Departments of Nuclear Medicine and Radiology, Albert Einstein College of Medicine, Bronx, New York, Attending Physician Nuclear Medicine, Long Island Jewish Medical Center, New Hyde Park, NY 11040, USA

Maria-João Santiago-Ribeiro, MD, PhD
Service Hospitalier Frédéric Joliot, Département de Recherche Médicale Direction des Sciences du Vivant, Commissariat à l'Energie Atomique, 91400 Orsay, France

Barry L. Shulkin, MD, MBA
Chief, Division of Nuclear Medicine, Department of Radiological Sciences, St. Jude Children's Research Hospital, Memphis, TN 38105, USA

Charles A. Stanley, MD
Professor, Division of Endocrinology, Department of Pediatrics, University of Pennsylvania, Chief, Children's Hospital of Philadelphia, Philadelphia, PA 19104, USA

Suleman Surti, PhD
Assistant Professor, Department of Radiology, Hospital of the University of Pennsylvania, Philadelphia, PA 19104, USA

Maria B. Tomas, MD
Assistant Professor, Departments of Nuclear Medicine and Radiology, Albert Einstein College of Medicine, Bronx, New York, Attending Physician Nuclear Medicine, Long Island Jewish Medical Center, New Hyde Park, NY 11040, USA

Stefaan Vandenberghe, PhD
Clinical Site Researcher, Philips Research, USA, Department of Radiology (PET Instrumentation Group), University of Pennsylvania, Philadelphia, PA 19104, USA

Jian Qin Yu, MD
Nuclear Medicine Fellow, Department of Radiology, Hospital of University of Pennsylvania, Children's Hospital of Philadelphia, Philadelphia, PA 19107, USA

Xiaowei Zhu, MS, DABMP
Director, Departments of Radiology Physics and Engineering, Children's Hospital of Pennsylvania, Philadelphia, PA 19104, USA

Hongming Zhuang, MD, PhD
Assistant Professor, Department of Radiology, Attending Physician, Nuclear Medicine Service, Hospital of the University of Pennsylvania, Philadelphia, PA 19104, USA

Section 1

Basic Science and Practical Issues

The Nuclear Imaging Technologist and the Pediatric Patient

Maria Green

For the nuclear imaging technologist, success in obtaining a high-quality imaging study in children is both challenging and rewarding. Imaging children for general nuclear medicine (NM) procedures requires versatile strategies that can be applied successfully to positron emission tomography (PET) imaging. This chapter discusses from the technologist's perspective the strategies for general NM imaging, the special considerations and requirements for PET imaging, and the appropriate use of sedation in the pediatric patient.

The role of the technologist is multifaceted when the focus is on imaging a pediatric patient. It is important to recognize that the technologist is working not only with a child who is anxious, frightened, or stressed, but also with parents or other family members who are anxious, frightened, or stressed. With careful planning, good communication, and some ingenuity, however, the technologist can create the right environment for a successful encounter. The goal should be to provide a quiet and friendly atmosphere with caring staff members who are calm and have a sympathetic approach and confidence in working with children. To achieve this end, it must be recognized that dealing with a child takes twice as long as dealing with an adult, and that patience is the key factor.

Technologists working in a pediatric center have the advantage of working in a culture that understands the unique needs of children and their families. Established techniques used on a regular basis ensure that high-quality images are obtained and that both the patients and parents leave satisfied (1).

The following should be kept in mind when dealing with the pediatric patient: the importance of communication appropriate for the child's stage of development; the need for flexible scheduling; the appropriate injection techniques; and the imaging environment, including the use of immobilization devices or safety restraints, distraction techniques, and the possibility of sedation when absolutely necessary.

Communication and Stages of Development

Imaging children of various ages is labor intensive and quite challenging, given the unpredictable nature of a child's behavior. A good pediatric imaging technologist should know what to expect from children at different ages, yet keep in mind that some children may be at different stages of maturity, psychosocial development, and cognitive capacity. There are many guides available that outline the various stages of child development (2). After assessing the patient by speaking with the parent and child, the technologist can effectively adjust techniques as required for the situation. Open and honest communication with parents is essential to gain cooperation and establish a good technologist–parent relationship. This can only benefit the child, who is greatly influenced by the parents' positive or negative attitude.

If at all possible, give the parents information beforehand about the procedure. Information sheets sent prior to the appointment or a phone call with preparation instructions will inform parents about what to expect. At the time of the appointment, the technologist should explain all the steps of the procedure in simple terms without using technical jargon. If the child is under the age of 8 years, the explanation should be given to the parents first. During the explanation, the technologist's full attention should be directed to the parents and he or she should not be multitasking at the same time. Tasks such as changing linen on the imaging table or manipulating a syringe can distract the parents' attention from the explanation. Explanations should include a reassurance about the safety of the procedure and radiation exposure, the need for the injection, timing of the images, how the imaging is done, the need for immobilization, the use of safety restraints, and other considerations necessary for the procedure such as bladder catheterization or sedation. It is also good practice to inquire about and record any medication that the child is currently taking and any known allergies. Because parents know their children best, ask them about previous experience with injections, intravenous (IV) placements, or catheterizations. Knowing how the child reacted previously or knowledge about unsuccessful IV sites can help the technologist decide on the best course of action.

It is important to repeat information to parents to ensure comprehension and to allow ample opportunity for questions. Parents overwhelmed by the hospital environment and their own personal circumstances may miss key points of the explanation. The technologist must be cognizant of the fact that parents have varying levels of understanding and some have a limited history of hospital experience. Technologists must also recognize that parents can be under a great deal of stress. Not only are they coping with an ill child, worrying about the procedure and the implications of the results, but also they may have had to take time off from work, arrange for the care of other children, and deal with transportation to and from the hospital or medical center.

Although infants and babies cannot understand verbal commands, they can and do react negatively to loud voices and rough handling. A soothing tone of voice and gentle treatment with warm hands help keep a baby from undue distress. Explanations in simple terms can be given to children starting at about the age of 3 years. Smiling to the child and using friendly facial expressions can make the child feel more at ease, as can having the child sit on a parent's lap to feel more secure in strange surroundings. The technologist should speak directly to the child and, if at all possible, should bend or crouch to the same level so as not to be towering above him or her. Because the child may not fully understand what is being said or may not be paying attention, the technologist can emphasize the explanation by either nodding or shaking his or her head. Younger children have short attention spans, so explanations should be brief and at the child's level of understanding. The technologist's approach should be nonthreatening to minimize fear and apprehension (2).

Children are more aware of what is going on than is generally acknowledged or appreciated, so try to be sensitive to their perception of what is happening around them. If the child appears to be frightened, ask what is frightening. It can be something totally different from what is assumed. For example, a child might be crying from a hidden discomfort or from misunderstanding a word used in the explanation. Reassure the child that you do not want to frighten him or her. Be truthful to gain a child's trust; however, be selective about the timing of the truth. Informing a child too far in advance of an injection can result in a buildup of anxiety that can be difficult to overcome when the time for the injection finally arrives. Try to explain how the child will feel or what to expect during the injection or the procedure, but do not dwell on the unpleasant aspects. Instead, try to have the child focus on getting the injection or the procedure done quickly, emphasizing that with his or her help the task can be completed sooner.

The technologist must be confident enough in dealing with a child to be in charge of all facets of the procedure. However, when the opportunity arises, the technologist may permit the child control of certain aspects by allowing the child to make some choices. The technologist can say that an injection, which is not a choice, is necessary for the test; however, if the child has several equally good injection sites, allow the child to choose one. Other examples of choices that a child can make include selecting whether to sit on a chair or on a parent's lap, or whether to image the knees or the back first on a bone scan if the order of the spot views is not important. After an injection, ask the child if he or she would like a bandage, as a technologist cannot assume that a child will want or accept having a bandage put on. Sometimes the appearance of a bandage will signify that it is "all done," and the child will be relieved that the injection is over; however, the child might be upset at having a bandage put on because it can be painful to remove.

Crying is a very important means of communication for children. Therefore, a technologist who is working with a child must be prepared to encounter this reaction and must take control of the situation. For babies, crying is the only means of communicating that something is wrong and will usually stop after the cause has been remedied. A baby can be comforted after an injection, fed when hungry, or covered with a blanket when cold. Children with limited verbal skills or life experiences will cry not only from pain but also from fear and anxiety. They must not be made to feel that they are behaving badly because of their crying. This is a normal reaction to a stressful situation and should not be confused with bad behavior. Parents sometimes feel the need to control this reaction and may want to discipline the child, which only adds more stress to the already-distraught child. A prepared technologist can circumvent this situation beforehand by explaining that certain aspects of the procedure, such as an injection or a catheterization, will be unpleasant or uncomfortable. The technologist can continue to say that crying is an expected and normal reaction from the child and that it can be tolerated.

Communication with school-age children is easier than with younger children, and the technologist can expect to have more of a dialogue with these children. As children get older, they are increasingly proud of their independence. Quite often, they are compliant with the technologist's requests as long as they understand what is going on and they feel that the technologist has been honest with them. Children aged 12 to 15 appreciate being treated as an adult. However, with this age group in particular, the technologist may be dealing with opposite extremes of emotional maturity.

Regardless of the patient's age, the technologist should keep in mind that instructions and information may be misunderstood or missed with the first explanation. Taking the time to repeat key points and giving the opportunity for the parents or patient to ask questions can be very beneficial to everyone involved.

Flexible Scheduling

Time is critical when dealing with the pediatric patient. Scheduling of procedures must allow for extra time and flexibility at every step in the process. As previously discussed, explanations to the parents and then to the child can be very time-consuming. Taking the time to find the optimum injection site is also very important, as a failed injection can make subsequent attempts much more difficult. The technologist must be prepared to accept that a patient injection can be as fast as 5 minutes or take as long as 30 minutes. And, finally, ample time must be allowed for the imaging procedure itself. Imaging young children for general NM procedures can often be done successfully and without sedation as long as the technologist has both the time and the patience to devote to the procedure. However, the technologist must image a child as quickly as possible to take advantage of a child's cooperation. If too much time is taken in setting up or positioning, a window of opportunity may be lost if the child becomes restless or bored. Keeping all of these factors in mind, one can easily appreciate that it takes about twice as long to complete a procedure on a pediatric patient as on an adult.

Injection Techniques

A successful injection is paramount when performing a procedure on the pediatric patient. A failed attempt can reduce the choices of viable injection sites and further distress the child. A partially delivered dose not only causes local discomfort but also reduces the count rate for imaging, increases the imaging time, and compromises image quality. "Hot" injection sites quite often end up in the field of view, as these are difficult to move out of the way when imaging small children or babies.

To ensure a successful injection, having an IV line established on the inpatient's hospital ward prior to the procedure is the most efficient step. The technologist will only need to reassure the child there will be no pain with the radiopharmaceutical administration into the IV site. However, this is not an option for the ambulatory outpatient, and the technologist will be required to perform a butterfly needle injection or to establish an IV line. A butterfly needle affords better maneuverability and flexibility than a straight needle because the tabs or "wings" can help direct the needle into a small superficial vein more easily. Some NM procedures, such as a Meckel's scan, diuretic washout study, or PET scan, require that an IV line is established; others require only injection by a butterfly needle.

The best method of injection with a butterfly needle is to have it attached to one port of a three-way stopcock with a 10-cc syringe of saline attached to the second port, the radiopharmaceutical dose attached to the third port, and everything secured to a small injection tray to hold it all firmly in place (Fig. 1.1). Once the butterfly needle is flushed through with saline, the needle can be inserted into the vein and patency verified by saline injection into the vein. After venous patency has been established, the radiopharmaceutical dose is delivered through the butterfly needle by opening the port to the dose syringe and depressing the plunger. Once the dose has been delivered, the stopcock is turned to open the port of the saline syringe, and saline is flushed through the butterfly needle again. The technologist can continue to flush out the dose syringe with saline to ensure that the patient has received the entire amount of radiopharmaceutical. Throughout the injection, the technologist must hold the patient securely near the injection site with one hand while using the other hand to quickly and efficiently deliver the radiopharmaceutical with the butterfly-stopcock system. An assistant, such as another technologist or other health care professional, is often required to help immobilize the hand, arm, or foot that is being injected and to ensure that other limbs will not interfere. Although parents may wish to help restrain the child for the injection, this is not an optimum choice as they may either hold too hard or not securely enough to be effective. Everyone involved must be prepared for the child's abrupt reaction to the injection, especially from a "calm" child who may not fully realize what is about to happen. *Never underestimate the strength of a baby or small child when a sudden surge of adrenaline occurs during the stress of an injection.* Table 1.1 lists key points for successfully injecting the pediatric patient.

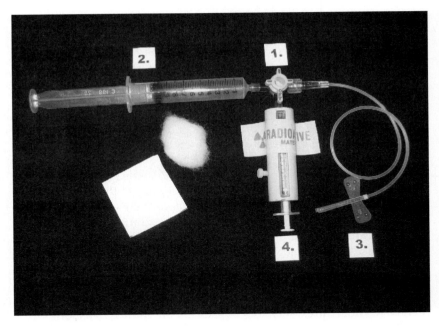

Figure 1.1. Injection tray is equipped with (1) a three-way stopcock, (2) a 10-cc syringe of normal saline, (3) a butterfly needle, and (4) a shielded radio-pharmaceutical dose syringe.

Table 1.1. Pediatric injection techniques: key points

1. For babies and small children good injection sites to consider are the back of the hand or the foot because these areas are easy to immobilize and the veins are more superficial (Figs. 1.2 and 1.3).

2. Use of a topical anesthetic may be of benefit to the child. However, if a young child has had a previously traumatic injection or IV experience, the child is already conditioned to expect another traumatic event and will react accordingly even though he or she may not be experiencing pain.

3. A paralyzed limb has impaired circulation, which may cause stasis of blood.

4. Dehydration may cause difficult venous access.

5. Keep in mind that for babies and small children, the tourniquet should be tight enough to restrict blood flow but not to interfere with arterial flow. While the technologist is assessing an area for veins, the tourniquet may need to be removed for a few seconds to allow the return of blood flow and then reapplied.

6. To help dilate blood vessels in a cold limb, apply a warm cloth.

7. Tap or rub the area to assist in detection of veins.

8. If an IV line is to be established, avoid using the hand of the baby's sucking thumb. The baby may want to suck a thumb to calm down after the IV insertion, and if it is not available he or she will take longer to settle.

9. If an IV line is to be established on a baby who has equally good sites in the hands and feet, consider using the feet to allow unrestricted movement of the hand and fingers.

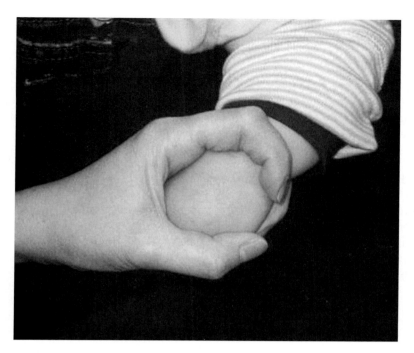

Figure 1.2. The fingers and wrist are held securely in a flexed position. This technique also extends and immobilizes the vein.

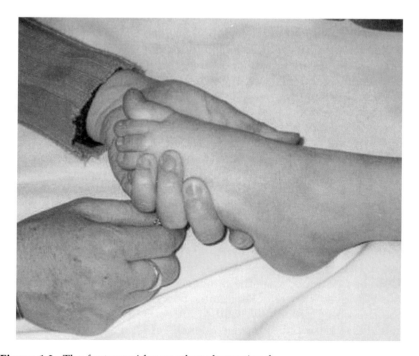

Figure 1.3. The foot provides another alternative for venous access.

Some patients have an indwelling central venous access line or port, and injection into this device may be allowed depending on the procedure ordered. Using sterile technique, the injection should be performed only by qualified personnel, and special attention must be paid to flushing the device well with saline. Failure to do so can result in radiopharmaceutical retention, resulting in a "hot spot" artifact in the chest. If the patient has symptoms or pathology in the chest, a peripheral site for injection should be used instead.

The Imaging Environment

Producing the optimum environment for imaging a child requires a combination of several elements. Creating a comfortable child-friendly atmosphere, allowing a fussy baby or child to settle down, and using various methods of distraction will help the technologist to obtain high-quality images.

A child-friendly room decorated with pictures on the walls (and on the ceiling above the gamma camera, if possible) helps to make the young child feel a bit more at ease and can also serve as a distraction from boredom. Removal of nonessential "scary"-looking equipment from the imaging room also reduces a child's fear in strange surroundings. Approaching the child in a gentle, nonthreatening manner without wearing a white lab coat can help to reduce fear in a child who associates unpleasant memories with strangers in white coats.

Although having toys available for a baby or young child to play with may seem like a child-friendly gesture, it is not recommended unless appropriate means are available for thorough cleaning of the toys for infection control; children of this age range readily put toys into their mouths. Instead the technologist can allow children to bring their own favorite toy or a blanket along for the scan. These items lend familiarity and comfort to strange surroundings. Placing the child's toy on the imaging table and showing the child what the scan involves may help to reduce fear and apprehension before the child gets on the table. Allowing the child to touch the camera face can also demonstrate that the camera will not hurt him or her.

For general imaging of babies and young children, selection of a single-head gamma camera, if available, is best. By positioning the camera head face up, underneath and touching the imaging table, the child can lie supine for posterior images. Not only does this allow the technologist better access to the child for immobilization and supervision, but also it eliminates the fear that a child will naturally have with the camera above him or her. This also allows the child better access to distractions such as watching a videotape. Anterior imaging can also be performed with the camera beneath the table and the child prone. However, the technologist must be meticulous with positioning, as the child might naturally want to lift his or her shoulders or keep turning his or her head. If this technique is used, the technologist must be prepared to hold any moving body parts for the duration of the acquisition.

When acquiring anterior images with the child supine and the camera above the child, care must be taken to prevent the child from bumping his or her head on the camera. The camera should be brought down as slowly and as closely as possible without touching the child because this action will certainly terrify a young child. A single-head camera also provides more flexibility by allowing the technologist to rotate or angle the camera head for the desired view if the child is uncooperative or cannot comply with the position.

It is important to continue with good communication throughout the imaging phase of the procedure. If the child is old enough to understand, it is best for the technologist either to explain in simple terms or show what is going to happen. The technologist can let the child know what is expected from him or her, such as "Lie down on your tummy" or "Keep still like a statue." Warn the child about any noises and bed or camera motion that might occur so as not to startle him or her. Let the child know when you need to touch or hold him or her. If clothing must be removed or a diaper is to be changed, the child will feel more at ease with a parent performing that function. During a diaper change, care should be taken to wash the area thoroughly to remove any evidence of urine contamination.

Allowing a parent to hold the child in the required position for an image might be comforting for the child; however, an untrained parent may not do an adequate job, and the view may need to be repeated. Repeating images only prolongs the procedure and increases the risk of losing the child's cooperation. *Speed is of the essence when dealing with the pediatric patient.* Because children do not like to be restricted, it is prudent for the technologist to release the restraint as soon as the imaging is complete (3). The technologist should try to position the child as quickly and as accurately as possible, because the child's behavior can be very unpredictable when restlessness or boredom sets in. When performing spot views for a whole-body scan, the technologist can allow the younger child to move in between the views to ward off restlessness. Saving the more difficult views (such as the anterior images with camera above the child) for the end can be a good strategy. By this time the child may have either become accepting of the procedure and surroundings or have fallen asleep.

A dual-head gamma camera for whole-body imaging of children 6 years and older can be quite successful. Some exceptional 3- to 5-year-olds can also tolerate whole-body imaging or simultaneous anterior and posterior spot views. Using a videotape or DVD player with age-appropriate movies for a distraction is a definite asset to promote compliance. For single photon emission computed tomography (SPECT) procedures, children under the age of 5 years usually need to be sedated due to the length of the acquisition and their inability to remain motionless. However, having good motion correction software available for SPECT reconstruction can help the technologist salvage an acquisition with a slight amount of motion.

Trying to induce natural sleep when imaging a baby or young child will yield much better results than having to restrain a wiggly child. Instructing the parents to wake their child a bit earlier on the morning of the procedure or having the child miss a usual nap time might work to the technologist's advantage. For the baby who does not have to be fasting, being fed before the scan can also help to induce sleep. By dimming the lights in the imaging room and providing a quiet environment, the child might relax enough to fall asleep. However, this strategy can backfire if the child becomes overtired.

Child safety is of paramount concern on the imaging table, and the use of safety straps is strongly recommended (Fig. 1.4). The technologist must always explain to the parent and child the need for the safety strap before putting it on. A child should never be left unattended while lying on an imaging table, and a busy technologist can enlist the help of a parent to stay beside the child when the technologist must leave the room. At the completion of the scan, it is prudent for the technologist to keep the child on the imaging table until the study has been checked. It is sometimes very difficult to have children return to the imaging table for more images once they have been allowed off (3).

Another challenge for the technologist is to ask a toilet-trained child to void. Children may see this as a choice that they can make, and uncooperative children can seize the opportunity to control the circumstances by refusing to void. Instead of asking, the technologist should *tell* the child that he or she must void before the test can begin, using words that are suitable to the child's level of understanding. The parents can advise the technologist which phrases or words are used at home for the younger, newly toilet-trained child, such as "go potty" or "pee." If the child does not feel the urge to void, encourage him or her to try anyway. It is best not to pressure the child, as this can soon become a power struggle among the child, parent, and technologist. Depending on the procedure, if the child cannot or will not void, the technologist must decide whether to continue with the scan and try to eliminate the bladder activity with lead shielding or with software

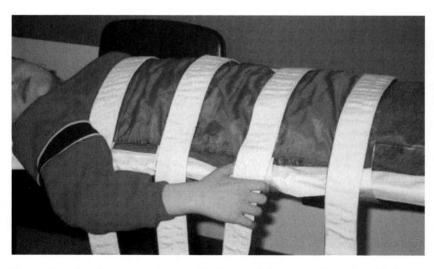

Figure 1.4. A safety strap, along with direct adult supervision, should always be used when a child is lying on the imaging table.

removal or wait until the child can comply by voiding. As a last resort, and with the referring clinician's consent, catheterize the bladder.

Because telling a baby or non–toilet-trained child to void is not an option, the technologist must be prepared to wait for the infant to void spontaneously; or, if the procedure requires it, catheterize the bladder. Having the child listen to the sound of running water from a tap or pouring warm water over the child's perineum may have limited success in stimulating bladder emptying. If these alternatives are not possible, techniques such as software removal of bladder activity or imaging with a lead shield overlying the bladder can be helpful.

To help build a good technologist–patient relationship, words of encouragement and praise can be given. If the child's efforts to hold still for the images or cooperate for the injection are recognized, the child will feel more involved and have greater self-esteem. Tokens of appreciation such as stickers given to the child at the end of the procedure are usually well received and sometime distract the child from any unhappy memories. Giving candies is strongly discouraged. However, if this type of reward is considered, the technologist must discreetly check with a parent first.

PET Imaging and the Pediatric Patient

Improvements in PET and PET/computed tomography (CT) technology that have resulted in increased image quality and decreased acquisition time have made PET imaging possible for routine pediatric applications. By utilizing the strategies and techniques used for general NM procedures, as previously discussed, PET imaging can be successfully tolerated by children.

This section focuses primarily on PET and PET/CT imaging using fluorine-18 fluorodeoxyglucose (FDG) for whole-body oncology studies. Special attention is given to patient preparation, including fasting and glucose levels, FDG administration, FDG uptake phase, and other technical considerations specific to PET and PET/CT imaging.

Patient Preparation

Communication continues to be one of the most essential steps for patient preparation. As discussed earlier, information about the procedure should be given to the parents beforehand, either by information sheets sent prior to the appointment or by a phone call with preparation instructions. Parents can be confused by the very complex nature of FDG-PET or PET/CT imaging, and ample time must be allotted to explain the study and to allow the parents an opportunity to ask questions.

For children undergoing a PET or PET/CT scan, this may not be their first experience in a nuclear medicine or CT department. They may have been examined previously as part of the initial diagnostic workup. If this is the case, a good technologist–patient/parent relationship may already have been established.

If no anesthetic will be used and there is sufficient time, the technologist should show the child the scanning room to describe how the scan will be performed. Key points to cover include the steps involved in the procedure, the need for an IV line and possible bladder catheterization, estimated time for each sequence, and the expectation of keeping the child inactive during the FDG uptake phase. To ensure that the fasting instructions have been followed, the technologist should take careful note about when the child last had something by mouth, including candies, gum, or any glucose-containing liquids or medications such as cough syrup; also take note of what the child ingested. All of the above should be discussed prior to the FDG injection in order to reduce the technologist's exposure to the high-energy photons of ^{18}F.

Because FDG is excreted by the kidneys, urine retention in the bladder can cause many difficulties with reconstruction and image interpretation. To eliminate these problems, bladder catheterization may be necessary. However, the timing of the bladder catheterization can be problematic. Ideally, the catheter should be inserted after an IV line has been established. Not only will this allow the child time to calm down prior to FDG administration, it also will further reduce the technologist's radiation exposure and avoid the possibility of urine contamination on the patient. If sedation is required for the scan, the child should be catheterized beforehand, because sedation does not eliminate the pain response and the child could become agitated (4,5). If general anesthesia is to be used, the child will not feel any pain and may be catheterized just prior to imaging after the induction of anesthetic. However, when catheterizing the child, one must work carefully and efficiently to avoid urine contamination and to keep radiation exposure of the catheterizing personnel to a minimum.

To reduce urinary retention in the upper tracts, administration of a diuretic may be considered if clinically appropriate (6).

Fasting and Glucose Levels

The same mechanism that makes FDG a desirable radiopharmaceutical to image glucose metabolism in tumors creates many challenges for the technologist and parents with respect to fasting and activity restrictions. Fasting is crucial prior to FDG injection so as to reduce glucose utilization and lower circulating insulin, thereby optimizing the target to background ratio (7). Whenever a baby or young child is kept fasting, predictably stress levels increase for parents, because a hungry child is also an unhappy child. The length of time fasting can vary from 4 hours for infants (8) to 6 to 8 hours for the older child (6). Most oral medications, if glucose-free, can be taken with water during the fasting period. Thirty minutes after injection, infants can be fed or a thirsty child can have some water (8); however, if sedation or general anesthesia is to be used, the child must remain fasting. If oral contrast is required, it can be given in a glucose-free liquid at the appropriate time prior to the CT (7). Administration of oral contrast prior to PET acquisition does not significantly complicate image interpretation (4).

Following fasting, some imaging centers assume stabilized blood glucose levels, whereas other centers take an actual measurement using a glucometer or obtain a serum glucose level from the laboratory to ensure the level is ≤150 mg/dL prior to FDG injection. For the diabetic child, management of blood glucose levels may require consultation with a diabetic-control specialist (6,7).

If the child is receiving intravenous fluids containing dextrose or total parenteral nutrition (TPN), the dextrose in the solutions will compete with the FDG uptake. So as not to compromise the PET study, administration of these fluids should be suspended for 6 hours prior to FDG injection (7).

Fluorodeoxyglucose Administration

The recommendation for pediatric use is 5 to 10 MBq/kg or 0.15 to 0.30 mCi/kg with a minimum dose of 37 MBq or 1 mCi (5). There appears to be no contraindication for FDG administration (9).

Although a successful injection is paramount in performing a general NM imaging procedure, it is more so for PET imaging. A "hot" injection site in the field of view can cause an artifact on reconstruction, and dose extravasation can result in lymph node uptake. Both situations may hinder the interpretation of the scan. A failed injection also increases the cost of performing the study, because the price of FDG is very expensive and the child may need to be rescheduled to another day. Rescheduling the child's PET scan not only delays provision of diagnostic results to the referring clinician but also increases parental stress and anxiety because the child will have to undergo the preparation and injection all over again. It has been reported that FDG injection into indwelling central venous lines/ports followed by thorough flushing with saline is acceptable (4,6). However, unless there is absolutely no other alternative, it is highly recommended to establish an IV line in a peripheral site instead. This action prevents possible radiopharmaceutical retention in the central line/port and interference on the scan. Furthermore, if the child requires intravenous contrast for a CT, a peripheral IV line may be necessary, as many centers do not use a power injector into a central line/port.

To ensure a successful injection, having an IV line established on the inpatient's hospital ward prior to the procedure is the most efficient step. The technologist will need only to check for venous patency and can reassure the child that there will be no pain with the radiopharmaceutical administration into the IV site. However, for the ambulatory outpatient, the technologist will need to establish an IV line and allow time for the child to calm down. Having the patient in a calm and relaxed state will minimize muscle uptake caused by excessive movement or muscle tension, both of which are likely to occur when a child has a needle injection. A butterfly needle is not recommended for FDG injections, as using a secure IV line will allow quick and successful delivery of the FDG, which will also reduce the technologist's radiation exposure.

Fluorodeoxyglucose Uptake Phase

Another challenging aspect of performing PET imaging in a child is the restriction of physical activity to minimize the uptake of FDG by the muscles. Physical activities such as muscle stress, tension, movement, or even talking increase muscle uptake, and trying to restrict these activities for a child can be difficult. To facilitate this goal, a quiet, dim room should be used for the child to rest, either in a lounge chair or on a comfortable stretcher, for at least 20 to 30 minutes, with imaging commencing about 60 minutes after injection (6). The room should be equipped with appropriate support equipment including a sink, oxygen, suction, and a restroom facility close by (7). The parents must understand the importance of inactivity during this phase and help to ensure minimal stimulation. The child can rest comfortably watching a quiet videotape or DVD movie, listening to soft music, or having a parent read to him or her. To reduce the radiation exposure to the parents, it is recommended that only one (nonpregnant) parent remain with the child for the duration of the uptake phase. Using a monitoring camera in the uptake room is a practical way for the technologist to supervise the child's status remotely. This serves two purposes, as the technologist will not have to disturb the quiet environment to check on the child and he or she will avoid additional radiation exposure.

Other means of reducing muscle uptake of FDG in certain situations include the use of muscle relaxants (6), which can also help calm an anxious or claustrophobic child, and sedation or general anesthesia. However, the length of time that a child would need sedation or general anesthesia for both the uptake and scan phases would be considerable. If resources are limited, the logistics for this course of action can be difficult, as monitoring by qualified personnel is required for both phases.

During the uptake phase, the child should be kept warm in order reduce the uptake of FDG in brown fat that can interfere with image interpretation (7). This can be accomplished by keeping the ambient temperature of the uptake room warm or by wrapping the child in heated blankets.

PET and PET/Computed Tomography Imaging

When the FDG uptake phase is over, the child must void just before entering the scanning room. This will eliminate the bladder activity from the images and ensure the child's bladder comfort for the duration of the lengthy scan. If the child has been catheterized, the technologist must position the drainage tube to keep the bladder continuously drained and to avoid overlapping the tube with the body.

Once in the room, the technologist can reassure the child that there will be no loud noises during the scan and continue with reassurances that although the scanner will never touch the child, for safety purposes a safety strap or restraint will be used. To reduce the risk of motion due to discomfort, the technologist can be creative and use various cushions, straps, and tape to keep the child in position for the study (8). To help ward off boredom, the child can listen to a music or storybook audiotape. If the head is not being imaged, watching a videotape or DVD can also be an option.

For whole-body imaging, the child is positioned with arms down, using the safety strap wrapped around the arms and torso to secure them in place. The technologist must pay special attention to having the child lying flat and not rotated so that the body will appear symmetrical in the reconstructed images. For patient safety and comfort, the technologist must make sure that any intravenous or catheter lines, oxygen tubing, straps, sheets, and monitoring equipment are safely arranged to allow free motion into and out of the scanner. Situating the child with his or her head out of the scanner as much as possible helps to reduce fear or claustrophobia. For the noncatheterized child, the pelvis should be imaged first to minimize the effects of the bladder filling; therefore, the imaging sequence can start with the pelvis and legs and move to the torso and head (5,6).

Attenuation correction for PET images is essential and can be obtained either by transmission imaging in a conventional PET scanner or by utilizing CT in a PET/CT scanner. For conventional PET, transmission images are obtained using a rotating rod source. The transmission scan (3 minutes per bed position) is acquired before the emission scan (4 to 7 minutes per bed position) (4,10). Therefore, a 60-cm, two-level (bed position) emission-transmission scan can be obtained in approximately 20 minutes. The number of bed positions and total acquisition time required for the study vary according to the size of the child, and the imaging procedure may take up to an hour.

With PET/CT technology, attenuation correction is obtained using spiral CT, which can be acquired in less than a minute. The patient is imaged from top to bottom. At completion, the child is ready to start the emission scan at the level of the pelvis in order to avoid the bladder activity. With an emission scan imaging typically lasting 5 minutes per bed position, a 60-cm, two-level study can be acquired in about 11 minutes (4).

Throughout the entire PET/CT procedure, the technologist, along with other personnel (such as a radiologist, nurse, or anesthesiologist if required), stay in the adjacent control room where the patient can be viewed through leaded glass; with an additional camera monitoring system, a closer view of the child can be obtained. This system is especially useful when a child is monitored while under sedation or anesthesia. Words of encouragement and support can be given to the child through a microphone during the scan. As the scan nears completion, informing the child that only a few minutes are left can help to maintain cooperation.

Following the PET scan, a diagnostic CT may also be ordered. The child may need to move his or her arms to an upright position if a CT is performed with the PET/CT scanner. However, for some complex CT protocols, the study may need to be done using a devoted CT scanner with CT technologists (4).

At the end of the emission-transmission or CT-transmission scans, the technologist reviews the acquired images to check for patient motion and completeness of the study. If all is in order, the child can leave the scanning room. If sedation or a general anesthesia has been used, the child will go to a recovery room until he or she can return to the hospital ward if an inpatient, or be discharged to go home if an outpatient. If sedation has not been given, the technologist or a nurse can take the child to a treatment room to remove the IV line and catheter (if used). Taking the child to another room for the removals serves many purposes. After leaving the scanning room, the child will finally feel that the procedure is done, and once the scanning room is vacant, preparation for the next patient can begin. Removal of an IV line or catheter can be time-consuming, and there is no need to occupy the scanning room for that purpose. Also, removing the catheter in another location other than the scanning room precludes the possibility of urine contamination on the imaging table. As previously mentioned, the technologist should ask the child first if he or she would like a bandage after the IV line is removed.

Again, words of encouragement and praise given for recognition of the child's cooperation will elevate his or her self-esteem and help to develop a good technologist–patient relationship. Stickers given as tokens of appreciation at the end of the procedure are usually well received and can divert the child from unpleasant memories. Because oncology patients return frequently for PET studies as part of their treatment, the technologist must realize that actions taken today may influence how the child and parents will react on the next appointment. In this sense technologists should consider themselves "goodwill ambassadors" and try to make the child's experience as positive as possible.

Sedation: The Technologist's Perspective

Sedation in the pediatric patient should never be used routinely but should be considered on an individual basis only. Most general nuclear medicine procedures can be performed without sedation and yield excellent results using the previously mentioned strategies. Many situations can be managed successfully by the technologist without sedation, as shown in Table 1.2. However, children of ages 8 months to 4 years require total immobilization by sedation for procedures such as bone scans, SPECT, and PET (11). Once it has been decided that sedation will be used, the technologist must involve other professionals in the administration, continuous monitoring, and recovery following the procedure. Guidelines and methods vary according to different departments and institutions, and the technologist must confirm that the required sedation preparation instructions have been followed before the child is injected for the scan. If a contraindication for sedation or discrepancy with preparation has been discovered, the sedation and scan should be postponed to another day. The technologist must communicate concisely with all involved individuals throughout the procedure to minimize any confusion and ensure a successful study.

Table 1.2. Alternatives to sedation

Situation	Alternative
Child crying from having an injection	• This is a normal and expected reaction from a child. A topical anesthetic can be applied; however, this will not eliminate a conditioned response to fear. • Once the injection or IV line has been established, reassure the child that all the "hurting" is finished. • Quickly distract the child's attention to more pleasant thoughts, such as going home, talking about a pet, or watching a videotape or DVD.
Child's restlessness during a lengthy scan	• Use distractions mentioned above. • If possible, allow the child to move or stretch between different images. • Have the child count down to the end of the acquisition, e.g., five, four, three, two, one—all done! • Try to induce natural sleep. If the child has been sleep deprived and cried a lot during the injection, he or she will be tired. Make the child comfortable, keep the area as quiet as possible, and dim the lights. • If fasting is not required, feeding the child prior to imaging can also induce natural sleep.
A parent's fear of the procedure	• Provide excellent communication about what the procedure involves and the expected reaction from the child. • Reassure the parent that a successful scan is possible without using sedation.
A parent's preconceived notion that the child is not capable of cooperating	• Often a child will react differently to a stranger's request and comply with the scan. • In some extreme situations, the technologist might ask the parent to leave the room. Once the parent is out of sight, the child may comply with the technologist because the child is no longer trying to control the parent.

Conclusion

Many unique and challenging issues must be considered when a nuclear imaging technologist is involved with a pediatric patient. Working with children requires patience, an active imagination, honesty, and flexibility. By adopting the techniques and strategies discussed in this chapter, the technologist can be confident that a high-quality study has been obtained and satisfied that the child and parent have had a successful and smooth encounter in the nuclear medicine department.

References

1. Gordon I. Issues surrounding preparation, information and handling of the child and parent in nuclear medicine. J Nucl Med 1998;39:490–494.
2. Veitch T. Pediatric nuclear medicine, part I: developmental cues. J Nucl Med Technol 2000;28:3–7.
3. Veitch T. Pediatric nuclear medicine, part II: common procedures and considerations. J Nucl Med Technol 2000;28:69–75.
4. Roberts E, Shulkin B. Technical issues in performing PET studies in pediatric patients. J Nucl Med Tecnol 2004;32:5–9.
5. Hossein J, Connolly L, Shulkin B. PET imaging in pediatric disorders. In: Valk P, Bailey D, Townsend D, et al., eds. Positron Emission Tomography: Basic Science and Clinical Practice. London: Springer-Verlag, 2003:756.
6. Hamblen S, Lowe V. Clinical ^{18}F-FDG oncology patient preparation techniques. J Nucl Med Technol 2003;31:3–10.
7. Kaste S. Issues specific to implementing PET-CT for pediatric oncology: what we have learned along the way. Pediatr Radiol 2004;34:205–213.
8. Borgwardt L, Jung Larsen H, Pedersen K, et al. Practical use and implementation of PET in children in a hospital PET centre. Eur J Nucl Med Mol Imaging 2003;30:1389–1397.
9. Kapoor V, McCook B, Torok F. An introduction to PET-CT imaging. Radiographics 2004;24:523–543.
10. Czernin J, Schelbert H. PET/CT imaging: facts, opinions, hopes and questions. J Nucl Med 2004;45:1S–3S.
11. Pintelon H, Jonckheer MH, Piepz A. Paediatric nuclear medicine procedures: routine sedation or management of anxiety? Nucl Med Commun 1994;15:664–666.

2

Sedation of the Pediatric Patient

Robin Kaye

Imaging pediatric patients provides many interesting challenges, not the least of which is keeping them motionless for the studies. Almost any imaging study is degraded, to a greater or lesser degree, by patient motion, and this can be particularly true for nuclear medicine studies where spatial resolution is an issue. Unfortunately, even the most cooperative child often cannot hold still for an imaging study of any length. This means that adequate sedation is one of the most important factors in performing high-quality imaging studies in children. This chapter discusses some of the basic concepts in pediatric sedation and suggests an approach to providing safe and effective sedation of children who are referred for PET scanning.

Background

In 1992 the American Academy of Pediatrics (AAP) revised its *Guidelines for Monitoring and Management of Pediatric Patients During and After Sedation for Diagnostic and Therapeutic Procedures* (1) and defined the goals of safe pediatric sedation. Other organizations, such as the American Society of Anesthesia (ASA) and the American College of Radiology (ACR), have also written such standards. In 2002 the ASA revised its practice guidelines for sedation and anesthesia by nonanesthesiologists (2), and in 2005 the ACR revised its guidelines for sedation of pediatric patients (3). The Joint Commission on Accreditation of Healthcare Organizations has adopted the concepts provided by the AAP guidelines, which has become a template for institutional policies and procedures for pediatric sedation in hospitals throughout the United States (4). The primary goal for sedation in the pediatric patient, as defined in these guidelines, is to guard the patient's safety and wellness in order to avoid sedation accidents.

In addition to patient safety, successful sedation of pediatric patients also has the goals of minimizing physical discomfort or pain, controlling behavior, minimizing negative psychological responses, and returning the patient to a state in which safe discharge is possible. All clinicians and support staff involved in the sedation of pediatric patients should understand and follow these guidelines. Further, it is highly advisable that, in order to ensure safe sedation of the pediatric patient undergoing imaging, a unified approach should be used in the radiology department and indeed throughout the entire institution (2,5–9) to help avoid errors that could potentially lead to sedation accidents.

To ensure that each of these goals is accomplished, several steps must be taken. First, the patient's present and past medical and surgical history must be thoroughly evaluated to find any possible problems that could affect sedation (Table 2.1).

Second, the patient should be fasting from solids (including formula or milk), breast milk, and clear liquids for an adequate period of time. Neonates and infants under 6 months of age should be NPO (nothing by mouth) for 2 hours for clear liquids, for 3 hours for breast milk, and for 4 hours for solids. Patients from 6 to 36 months of age should be NPO for 2 hours for clear liquids, for 3 hours for breast milk, and for 6 hours for solids. Patients over 36 months of age should be NPO for 2 hours for clear liquids and for 6 to 8 hours (at the physician's discretion) for solids. This regimen is recommended to decrease the risk of aspiration during sedation (Table 2.2). The only exception to these guidelines should be for those patients who require an oral medication, such as an antiseizure drug. These drugs are given prior to the procedure with small sips of water or other clear liquid at least 2 hours prior to the procedure.

Third, the sedation should be planned ahead of time, ideally based on a sedation protocol that includes a drug formulary that is comprehensive and appropriate for children of all ages and conditions. The appropriate sedative agents should be selected and doses calculated on a milligram per kilogram (mg/kg) basis, with a full understanding of

Table 2.1. Risk factors for sedation

Respiratory	Pneumonia, chronic lung disease, asthma tracheo- or bronchomalacia, sleep apnea, mediastinal mass
Cardiovascular	Cyanotic heart disease, congestive heart failure (CHF), hypotension, cardiomyopathy
Neurologic	Seizures, central respiratory depression
Gastrointestinal	Gastroesophageal reflux disease (GERD), hepatic dysfunction/failure
Genitourinary	Renal dysfunction/failure, dehydration, electrolyte disturbances
Systemic/other	Sepsis, allergies, medications, low hemoglobin
Syndromic	Macroglossia, micrognathia, chest wall deformity, craniofacial deformity scoliosis

Table 2.2. Risk factors for pulmonary aspiration of gastric contents

History of recent oral intake

Extreme obesity

Pregnancy

Patients with abnormal airway anatomy

Neurologic disorder
  Neurologic dysfunction
  Head trauma
  Deceased level of consciousness

Gastrointestinal disorders
  Bowel motility dysfunction
  Esophageal dysfunction
  Gastroesophageal reflux
  Gastrointestinal obstruction
  Prior esophageal surgery

Previous administration of pharmacologic agents
  Drugs that decrease gastric motility
  Drugs that produce loss of consciousness or depressed level of
    consciousness
  Drugs that produce loss of or reduce protective airway reflexes

their pharmacokinetics and pharmacodynamics. The selected agents should be titrated to effect, and sufficient time should be allowed to elapse between doses to achieve peak drug effect before administration of additional drugs. The doses of any pertinent reversal drugs should also be calculated ahead of time, although it is not necessary to have them drawn up for the procedure.

Fourth, if sedations are going to be performed, it is imperative to have high-quality monitoring equipment appropriate for all ages and sizes of children and an adequately trained group of sedation nurses with the knowledge and skills to properly monitor the patient during drug administration and during the procedure. Patients should also be monitored postprocedure to ensure that they are fully recovered from the effects of sedation before being released from medical supervision.

Fifth, there must be readily available resuscitation carts with medications and a full range of functioning age- and size-appropriate equipment, such as laryngoscopes, endotracheal tubes, oral airways, bags, and masks, to manage emergencies. One further precaution is the need for staff members to recognize their own limitations in experience and expertise; in those instances when the experience and expertise of the available staff are not sufficient, it is prudent to reschedule the examination for sedation by an anesthesiologist or other sedation specialist (Table 2.3).

Table 2.3. Circumstances that may require the assistance of an anesthesiologist or other specialist in sedation

Patient factors
  ASA class III or higher
  History of severe emotional or psychiatric illness
  History of major allergy or anaphylactic reaction
  Morbid obesity
  Sleep apnea
  Pregnancy
  Chemotherapy-induced cardiomyopathy
  Anatomic airway abnormalities
  Life-threatening underlying medical/surgical conditions
  History of difficult sedations
  Patients with a full stomach
  Patients with significant cardiac, pulmonary, renal, or central nervous system (CNS) dysfunction
Procedural factors
  Prolonged sedation
  Complex procedure
  New procedure
  Emergency procedure
  Procedure and patient suitable for regional block
  Procedure carried out in unusual position or geographic location
Miscellaneous factors
  Skilled personnel not available
  Inadequate facility or equipment

Levels of Sedation

Sedation is on a continuum from consciousness to unconsciousness and is a dynamic process. In children, in particular, progression along this continuum can be imperceptible and rapid, and may not depend so much on actual drugs and dosages but rather on individual responses. Because the level of sedation prescribes the intensity of monitoring, the team performing the sedation must be prepared to assess the true level of sedation and be prepared to increase the level of monitoring accordingly. There are three commonly described levels of sedation: conscious sedation, deep sedation, and general anesthesia. The differences between each of these levels should be well understood (Table 2.4).

Conscious sedation is defined as a medically controlled state of depressed consciousness in which protective reflexes are maintained, including the ability to maintain a patent airway and the ability of the patient to respond appropriately to verbal or physical stimuli. A true state of conscious sedation can be very difficult to attain in children. In our experience, most children require a deep level of sedation during procedures. Observation and monitoring of the pediatric patient who is medicated for conscious sedation includes continuous pulse oximetry, heart rate, intermittent respiratory rate, and blood pressure monitoring by a trained observer who frequently evaluates the patient but who may also participate in the procedure.

As compared to conscious sedation, deep sedation is a medically controlled state of depressed consciousness or unconsciousness in which the patient is not easily aroused and does not respond purposefully to verbal or physical stimuli and in which the patient may or may not maintain protective reflexes, including keeping a patent airway. In general, sedation protocols commonly used in radiology departments only very infrequently result in airway compromise. Monitoring for patients under deep sedation is significantly more intense than for those who are under only conscious sedation, as would be expected. The patient must have a working intravenous (IV) line; pulse oximetry and heart rate are continuously monitored; and vital signs (blood pressure, heart rate, and respiratory rate) are recorded every 5 minutes by an independent practitioner whose sole responsibility is to observe the patient's vital signs, airway patency, and adequacy of ventilation. Resuscitation equipment and medications must be readily available.

General anesthesia is a medically controlled state of unconsciousness in which protective reflexes are lost, the airway cannot be independently maintained, and the patient cannot respond to verbal or physical stimuli. Only specially trained physicians, or nurse anesthetists under their direct supervision, can provide general anesthesia.

The choice of whether to use sedation or general anesthesia is influenced by many factors: the physician's experience and expertise with sedation techniques and drugs, the ASA status of the patient, the availability of nurses trained in sedation techniques and patient monitoring, the institutional policy regarding sedation, and the length, complexity, and risk of the procedure to be performed. The risk of sedation-related complications increases directly or even exponentially with increasing ASA status (10). In general, patients with ASA I or II status are well suited for IV sedation by a radiology sedation team. Children with ASA class III status should be carefully evaluated and their condition and attendant risk factors carefully understood by the radiology sedation team before attempting IV sedation. ASA class IV status patients are most suitably cared for by an anesthesiologist or intensivist.

Table 2.4. Levels of sedation

Conscious sedation	Deep sedation	General anesthesia
Deep consciousness	Deep consciousness/ unconsciousness	Unconsciousness
Protective reflexes maintained	Protective reflexes may or may not be maintained	Loss of protective reflexes
Patent airway maintained independently	+/– Ability to maintain patent airway independently	Inability to independently maintain patent airway
Appropriate responses to verbal or physical stimuli	Inability to respond to verbal or physical stimuli appropriately	Inability to respond at all to verbal or physical stimuli

In addition, when there is a history of failed sedation, or when extreme patient cooperation is required, general anesthesia should be used.

Approach to Sedation

In our opinion any radiology department doing five or more cases per day that require medication to facilitate quality imaging should consider developing a sedation program. Performing that volume of cases using general anesthesia would be extremely challenging because, in our experience, most cases take at least 1.5 hours to complete.

Sedation by a radiology sedation team is preferred whenever possible because it allows easier, faster, and more flexible case planning and preparation and is less costly than general anesthesia. When sedation is chosen, formal protocols for preprocedural, intraprocedural, and postprocedural monitoring of the patient are imperative.

Although it is beyond the scope of this chapter to review all of the possible drugs that may be used, alone and in combination, to sedate children, I would like to describe the approach to sedation used by my department. We have used this method successfully and safely for many years, and although it is not the only approach that can be used, it is a time-tested one that can easily be adapted to use in a variety of settings. We use three main classes of agents for pediatric sedation: anxiolytics, barbiturate sedatives, and opioid analgesics. It is not important to know about all of the drugs available in each category. What is important is to choose a few of the drugs from each category and be familiar with their dosing, pharmacokinetics, and pharmacodynamics (e.g., time to peak effect, duration of action, and route of elimination), side effects, interactions with other sedative agents, and reversal agents (if any are available). Having a small, stable formulary that is familiar and predictable enhances the safety and effectiveness of the sedation program.

To successfully sedate children for the purposes of imaging or interventional procedures, the sedation team must carefully create a safe environment. In our opinion, safe and effective sedation facilitated by a team approach requires the presence of experienced pediatric radiology nurses, and in our practice we work very closely with these nurses. The radiology nurse is not only involved in obtaining pertinent information about medical history and physical examination, confirming preprocedure laboratory results, and acting as a liaison with the physicians and nurses caring for the patient in the hospital, clinic, or outside facility, but also dispenses sedation medications and monitors and records the patient's condition during and after sedation. It is these nurses who provide the backbone and consistency for an excellent sedation program. It is our preference to select nurses who have experience in an intensive care unit, pediatric transport, emergency room, or other area that cares for acutely ill children. However, nurses without this experience may also work well on a sedation team if they are trained and mentored to recognize and assess children who are at risk for problems and complications and take action when necessary.

Our approach to sedation is similar for diagnostic imaging or interventional procedures. As a rule we use single drugs, or two or more drugs in combination, that have the fastest time to action, the fewest untoward effects, and the shortest half-life, so that the return to baseline is as fast as possible. This approach enables us to discharge the patient to home or to the inpatient unit in the shortest time. Also, if untoward effects occur, they are as brief as possible.

We divide patients into two groups based on age: patients 1 year of age or less and patients who are older than 1 year. In children who are 1 year of age or less, the primary sedative is chloral hydrate. This drug may be given either by mouth or per rectum as a suppository. We rarely use the drug per rectum because of its variable absorption and less reliable onset of action.

In children 3 months of age or younger we usually begin with a dose of 50 mg/kg and in those older than 3 months of age we start with a dose of 75 mg/kg (or 1 g maximum single dose). In either group, the maximum total dose is 100 mg/kg or 1 g. The most common adverse effects of chloral hydrate are respiratory depression and occasionally hypotension. Chloral hydrate has no reversal agent and has a relatively long and somewhat unpredictable time to action, approximately 20 to 30 minutes, which is an obvious drawback. If the patient is not asleep in 20 to 30 minutes after the initial dose, one may want to consider giving a second dose of chloral hydrate or giving a second drug. Usually the determining factor in clinical practice is whether the patient has a functioning IV in place. Those children without IVs often receive a second dose of chloral hydrate, usually 25 to 50 mg/kg (again with a maximum total dose of 100 mg/kg or 1 g). Those patients who have a working IV may benefit from the addition of either Versed (0.05–0.1 mg/kg) or fentanyl citrate (1 μg/kg) to augment the sedation. In some cases in this age group, especially for short studies, a combination of Versed and fentanyl alone, given intravenously in the doses mentioned above, can also be used very successfully.

Children older than 1 year are most commonly sedated with a combination of intravenous drugs. Because anxiety is very frequently a part of the child's response to being in the hospital and to imaging studies, we almost always start with a dose of Versed, a benzodiazepine used frequently for anxiolysis, in doses of 0.1 mg/kg (or 3 mg maximum single dose). This drug has the added benefits of creating antegrade amnesia in most patients and of producing mild sedative effects.

We have found that when the patient's anxiety level is reduced by the use of Versed, the sedation is smoother and the total dose of sedation medication is often less, thereby reducing recovery time, and the overall experience for the patient (and the parents) is much less traumatic.

We administer the Versed 1 to 5 minutes before giving our primary sedative agent. The most common adverse effects of Versed are dose-related respiratory depression and occasionally paradoxical agitation.

Versed can be reversed by flumazenil in doses of 0.01 mg/kg to a maximum of 0.2 mg, but the patient needs to be carefully observed for re-sedation.

Our primary sedative agent is pentobarbital sodium (Nembutal). We use 3 mg/kg (or 100 mg maximum single dose) with a fast IV push as our initial dose. Although pentobarbital is an excellent and safe sedative, it has the undesirable property of creating hyperesthesia, and it has a long half-life leading to a relatively long time to return to presedation baseline. The most common adverse effects of pentobarbital are respiratory depression and occasionally emergence delirium. Pentobarbital has no reversal agent. To reduce the hyperesthesia effect and potentially reduce the total dose of pentobarbital needed, fentanyl citrate, a short-acting narcotic, can be added in doses of 1 μg/kg (or 50 μg maximum single dose) within minutes of giving pentobarbital. The most common adverse effects of fentanyl are respiratory depression and transient hypotension. Fentanyl can be reversed by naloxone in 0.01 mg/kg for children and 0.4 to 2 mg for adults, repeated as necessary, but the patient needs to be carefully observed for re-sedation. With this combination of three drugs, the vast majority of children will be sedated adequately to perform the diagnostic imaging study that is planned. If, after these drugs are initially administered the child is still moving, more drug or the addition of another drug is needed. The drug selected depends on the clinical state of the child. If the child is awake (eyes open, talking) a repeat dose of pentobarbital at 2 to 3 mg/kg is given.

If the patient is responding to noise, touch, or other stimuli without awakening, an additional dose of 0.1 mg/kg of Versed and/or 1 μg/kg of fentanyl citrate is given. Depending on the patient's status and the clinical situation, if the patient has been given two full rounds of drugs and is not adequately sedated, then there should be careful consideration given as to whether to administer a third round of drugs or to abandon the procedure and call a failed sedation. The maximum total doses that we use in most diagnostic settings are 7 mg/kg (or 300 mg) for pentobarbital, 3 μg/kg (or 150 μg) for fentanyl, and 0.3 mg/kg (or 5 mg) for Versed.

It should be remembered that the respiratory depressant effects of all three of the drugs used in this regimen are potentiated by one another and are additive. This requires rigorous monitoring of the patient and immediate treatment of any evidence of respiratory depression as soon as it is recognized. It is also important to remember that to maximize safety, fentanyl should always be diluted and injected slowly or added to the fluid in the drip chamber of the IV infusion set and dripped in slowly, over about 1 minute, to avoid severe respiratory depression, apnea, or the feared complication of "wooden chest syndrome." This syndrome of chest wall rigidity is a phenomenon during which the patient's chest wall muscles become spastic, making ventilation extremely difficult. Although the exact mechanism of these muscle contractions has yet to be identified, many authors have described success in reversing chest wall rigidity with either naloxone (Narcan) or muscle relaxants such as succinylcholine, with rapid resolution.

References

1. American Academy of Pediatrics. Committee on drugs: guidelines for monitoring and management of pediatric patients during and after sedation for diagnostic and therapeutic procedures. Pediatrics 1992;89: 1110–1115.
2. American Society of Anesthesiologists Task Force on Sedation and Analgesia by Non-anesthesiologists. Practice guidelines for sedation and analgesia by non-anesthesiologists. Anesthesiology 2002;96:1004–1017.
3. Towbin RB, Cardella JF, Barr JD, et al. ACR Practice Guideline for Pediatric Sedation/Analgesia. ACR Guidelines and Standards Committee of the Interventional and Cardiovascular Radiology Commission, Practice Guidelines and Technical Standards, Reston, VA. 2005:427–433.
4. Policy and Procedure for Intravenous Conscious Sedation. JCAHO Manual 1996:84–135.
5. Hoffman GM, Nowakowski R, Troshynski TJ, et al. Risk reduction in pediatric procedural sedation by application of an American Academy of Pediatrics/American Society of Anesthesiologists process model. Pediatrics 2002;109:236–243.
6. Holzman RS, Cullen DJ, Eichhorn JH, Philip JH: Guidelines for sedation by nonanesthesiologists during diagnostic and therapeutic procedures. The Risk Management Committee of the Department of Anaesthesia of Harvard Medical School. J Clin Anesthesiol 1994;6:265–276.
7. Guidelines for the elective use of pharmacologic conscious sedation and deep sedation in pediatric dental patients. Pediatr Dent 1993;15:297–301.
8. American Academy of Pediatrics. Committee on drugs: guidelines for monitoring and management of pediatric patients during and after sedation for diagnostic and therapeutic procedures: addendum. Pediatrics 2002;110:836–838.
9. Coté CJ: Sedation protocols—why so many variations? Pediatrics 1994; 94:281–283.
10. Fowkes FG, Lunn JN, Farrow SC, et al. Epidemiology in anaesthesia. III: mortality risk in patients with coexisting physical disease. Br J Anaesth 198;54:819–825.

3

The Biologic Effects of Low-Level Radiation

Martin Charron

Few topics engender more vigorous debate than the biologic effects of low-level radiation and selection of a mathematical model to predict the incidence of cancer. A recent review on radiation risk stated (1):

The A-bomb survivors represent the best source of data for risk estimates of radiation-induced cancer.

It is clear that children are ten times more sensitive than adults to the induction of cancer.

There are no assumptions, and no extrapolation indicated.

This chapter provides data that suggest that exactly the opposite of the above three statements applies; that is, I present a large amount of data indicating the linear no-threshold theory is erroneous. To that effect, this chapter discusses a review article (2) that scrutinized numerous scientific studies that arrived at drastically different conclusions. I present the information in four sections: the available experimental data, studies looking at the biologic effects of background radiation, the experimental evidence obtained from medical exposure to radiation, and in vitro studies.

First, let's look at the experimental data available on radiation risk. The only study that suggested a higher risk of cancer with low levels of radiation is the retrospective study by Ron and Modan (3) of 11,000 children treated for tinea capitis. The incidence of thyroid cancer was higher, especially in children less than 5 years old. Because the study was retrospective, the dose range was *estimated* to be 4.5 to 50 rem. But there are limitations of retrospective studies, as well as significant inaccuracies encountered in estimating radiation exposure. Also, a large proportion of the children received a dose (calculated to be) greater than 10 Rem. Therefore, it seems very inappropriate to draw any conclusion from this study, which was of dubious quality at best.

All the other studies, of much higher quality, done on the same topic have led to the opposite conclusions. A study of 14,624 infants less than

16 months of age treated for hemangioma did not reveal a higher incidence of cancer (4). Similarly, a Finland study of 1 million children, after the Chernobyl accident, did not reveal a higher incidence of cancer (5). Hjalmars et al. (6) reported no change in cancer incidence in a study of 1.6 million children in Sweden. The study by Rallison et al. (7), looking at the radiation fallout in Utah, reported similar results. Finally, a study of 35,074 patients who received diagnostic doses of iodine radioisotope ^{131}I did not find a higher incidence of cancer (8). Based on those studies of millions of children, it seems appropriate to conclude that low-level radiation does not increase the incidence of cancer, even in children.

We now review the conclusions stemming from studies about the biologic effects of background radiation. A Chinese study of 73,000 persons, comparing radiation doses of 96 mrem/yr versus 231 mrem/yr, found no difference in the incidence of cancer. Similarly, the study by Amsel et al. (9) comparing the incidence of cancer in a population of 825,000 patients living at an altitude of 1000 feet to the incidence in a population of 350,000 persons living at 3000 feet did not find a difference in the incidence of cancer between the two populations. One study comparing four groups living at different altitudes actually disclosed a negative dose-risk correlation (10). In the United States, a study looking at the radiation exposure of 1730 counties also found a negative dose-risk correlation (11). One more study of indoor radon exposure did not find any positive correlation (12).

As for the experimental evidence from medical exposure to radiation, a study by Saenger et al. (13) evaluated 33,888 Graves' disease patients treated with either surgery or with ^{131}I. The data revealed fewer complications in patient treated with ^{131}I. A study in 10,552 patients (8) and another study of 46,000 diagnostic doses of ^{131}I (14) did not disclose any higher incidence of cancer.

Looking at occupational exposure, data collected in approximately 200,000 persons (15–17) did not reveal an increase in cancer, notwithstanding that in one of those studies the mortality rate from cancer was lower in patients who were radiated! Also, the International Association for Research on Cancer study of 95,673 monitored radiation workers in the United States, the United Kingdom, and Canada found 3830 deaths for all cancers except leukemia but no deaths exceeding what was expected (18). No support for the linear no-threshold theory can be found here either. Finally, several studies have reported that workers who inhaled plutonium have lower lung cancer mortality rates than those not thus exposed (19–21). Contrary to impressions generated by the media, no record exists of cancer deaths resulting from human exposure to plutonium. Probably the most significant data on low-level radiation exposure in humans is still in the research stage, but preliminary results are interesting (22). In Taipei and other areas of Taiwan, 1700 apartment units were built using steel contaminated with cobalt 60, exposing 10,000 occupants for 16 years to an average, according to preliminary estimates, of 4.8 rem in the first year and 33 rem in total (23). From national

Taiwan statistics, 173 cancers and 4.5 leukemias would be expected from natural sources, and according to the linear no-threshold theory, there should have been 30 additional leukemias. However, a total of only five cancers and one leukemia have occurred among this group (23).

There are no statistically sound, well-designed studies that have validated the applicability of the linear no-threshold model at low doses (2). On the contrary, there is a suggestion that low-level exposure may be beneficial. This has been dubbed *hormesis,* and there are myriad of studies that suggest the beneficial effects of radiation. A study in human lymphocytes showed a protective effect of exposure from low-dose ^3H to subsequent exposure to 150 rem of x-rays (24). Shadley and Dai (25) found that preexposure of human lymphocytes to 5 rem reduces the number of DNA aberrations induced by 400 rem. Sanderson and Morely (26) found a decrease in mutagenesis. Kelsey et al. (27) found fewer mutations from 300 rem if human lymphocytes are preexposed to 1 rem of radiation. Shadley and Wolff (28) found a decrease in the number of DNA breaks if cells are irradiated with less than 20 rem. Fritz-Niggli and Schaeppi-Buechi (29) found lower embryonic mortality when *Drosophila melanogaster* eggs are exposed to 200 rem. Finally, ingenious experimental techniques have been developed for observing the effects of a single alpha particle hitting a single cell. Miller et al. (30) found that the probability for transformation to malignancy from N particle hits on a cell is much greater than N times the probability for transformation to malignancy from a single hit. This is a direct violation of the linear no-threshold theory, indicating that the estimated effects based on extrapolating the risk from high exposure, represented by N hits, greatly exaggerate the risk from low-level exposure as represented by a single hit.

The aforementioned data indicate that the linear nonthreshold model is unable to predict the biologic effects of low-level radiation, and consequently grossly overestimates the incidence of those effects. We shall demonstrate that this viewpoint that has exaggerated the risk from low-level exposure unduly poses a burden that is detrimental to the general welfare.

After a review of studies on natural, occupational, and medical exposure to radiation, health risk from low-level dose could not be detected above the "noise" of adverse events of everyday life (2). No available data confirm the hypothesis that children are more radiosensitive than adults (2). The evidence is consistent with the statement from the Health Physics Society that the health risk from the exposure to up to 10 rem is "either too small to be observed or nonexistent" (31). A sentiment has recently developed in the community of radiation health scientists to regard the risk estimates in the low-dose region that are based on the linear no-threshold theory as being grossly exaggerated or completely negligible (22). The data regarding leukemia among atomic bomb survivors (32) strongly suggest a threshold greater than 20 centisievert (cSv) (22). The evidence presented in that review leads to the conclusion that the linear nonthreshold theory fails badly in the low-dose region because it grossly overestimates the risk from low-level radiation (22).

A controversial analysis and interpretation by Pierce et al. (32) of some of the A bomb survivor data from Japan suggested that a linear model is valid at exposures as low as 50 millisievert (mSv) and that this is the lowest dose linked to a statistically significant radiogenic risk. In other independent analyses of the same data, a curvilinear dose-response also provided a satisfactory fit to the Japanese data (33). Heindenreich et al. (34), using the same data and applying different analytical methods, did not find any evidence for increased tumor rates below 200 mSv. Finally, if error bars are ignored (22), the points suggest a linear relationship with the intercept at a near-zero dose. The data themselves give no statistically significant indication of increased incidence of cancer for doses of less than 25 cSv. In fact, considering only the three lowest dose points, the slope of the dose-response curve has a 20% probability of being negative (risk decreases with increasing dose) (22).

The data largely comes from observation at relatively high doses and dose rate and do not suffice to define the shape of the dose-response curve in the millisievert dose range; however, it is noteworthy that "the dose-response curve for the overall frequency of solid cancers in the atomic-bomb survivors is not inconsistent with a linear function" (35). It is important to note that the rate of cancer in most populations exposed to low-level radiation has not been found to be detectably increased, and that in most cases the rate has appeared to decrease (35). The same report asserts that low-dose epidemiologic studies are of limited value in assessing dose-response relationship and have produced results with sufficiently wide confidence limits to be consistent with an increased effect, a decreased effect, or no effect. For some types of tumors there is actually a decrease in cancer frequency with exposure to radiation (35).

Finally, let us consider a legal interpretation in this country of the current scientific data. Recently, a U.S. federal court dismissed all 2100 lawsuits against GPU Nuclear Corporation that claimed radiation injury from the 1979 Three Mile Island accident because of lack of evidence that anyone had received doses greater than 100 mGy (36). The court determined that there is consensus within the scientific community that "at doses below 10 rems [100 mGy], the casual link between radiation exposure and cancer induction is entirely speculative." The Health Physics Society recommends against quantitative risk assessment of radiogenic health effects below an individual dose of 50 mGy in 1 year (36).

The former vice chancellor of Oxford University (37) stated that risk perception is intricate, as it involves fear and dread. However, an oversimplified algorithm is likely to prevent useful empirical application of radiation for the health benefit of children. In addition to the large number of studies we have reviewed, numerous scientific groups believe the linear no threshold model grossly overestimates the incidence of biologic effects, if any, of low-level radiation (38–49).

References

1. Hall EJ. Lessons we have learned from our children: cancer risks from diagnostic radiology. Pediatr Radiol 2002;32:700–706.
2. Ernst M, Freed ME, Zametkin AJ. Health hazards of radiation exposure in the context of brain imaging research: special consideration for children. J Nucl Med 1998;39(4):689–698.
3. Ron E, Modan B. Benign and malignant thyroid neoplasms after childhood irradiation for tinea capitis. J Natl Cancer Inst 1980;65:7–11.
4. Lundell M, Holm L. Mortality from leukaemia after irradiation in infancy for skin haemangioma. Radiat Res 1996;145:595–601.
5. Auvinen A, Hakama M, Arvela H, et al. Fallout from Chernobyl and incidence of childhood leukaemia in Finland. Br Med J 1994;309:151–154.
6. Hjalmars U, Kuldorf M, Gustaffson G, on behalf of the Swedish Child Leukaemia Group. Risk of acute childhood leukaemia in Sweden after the Chernobyl reactor accident. Br Med J 1994;309:154–157.
7. Rallison M, Dobyns B, Keating R, et al. Thyroid nodularity in children. JAMA 1975;233:1069–1072.
8. Holm L, Wilklund K, Lundell G, et al. Thyroid cancer after diagnostic doses of ^{131}I: a retrospective cohort study. J Natl Cancer Inst 1988;80:1132–1138.
9. Amsel J, Waterbor J, Oler J, Rosenwaike I, Marshall K. Relationship of site-specific cancer mortality rates to altitude. Carcinogenesis 1982;3:461–465.
10. Frigerio NA, Stowe RS. Carcinogenic and genetic hazard from background radiation. In: Biological and Environmental Effects of Low-Level Radiation. Vienna: International Atomic Energy Agency, 1976.
11. Cohen B, Colditz G. Tests of the linear no-threshold theory for lung cancer induced by exposure to radon. Environ Res 1994;64:65–69.
12. Blot W, Xu Z, Boice J, et al. Indoor radon and lung cancer in China. J Natl Cancer Inst 1990;82:1025–1030.
13. Saenger E, Thoma G, Tompkins E. Incidence of leukaemia following treatment of hyperthyroidism. JAMA 1968;205:855–862.
14. Hall P, Boice J, Berg G, et al. Leukaemia incidence after 131I exposure. J Natl Cancer Inst 1992;340:1–4
15. Kendall G, Muirhead C, MacGibbon B, et al. First analysis of the national registry for radiation workers: occupation exposure to ionizing radiation and mortality. Br Med J 1992;304:220–225.
16. Doody M, Mandel J, Boice JJ. Employment practices and breast cancer among radiologic technologists. J Occup Environ Med 1995;37:321–327.
17. Gilbert ES, Fry SA, Wiggs LD, Voelz GL, Cragle DL, Petersen GS. Analyses of combined mortality data on workers at the Hanford Site, Oak Ridge National Laboratory, and Rocky Flats Nuclear Weapons Plant. Radiat Res 1989;120:19–35.
18. Cardis E, Gilbert ES, Carpenter L, et al. Effects of low doses and low dose rates of external ionizing radiation: cancer mortality among nuclear industry workers in three countries. Radiat Res 1995;142:117–132.
19. Tokarskaya ZB, Okladlnikova ND, Belyaeva ZD, Drozhko EG. Multifactorial analysis of lung cancer dose-response relationships for workers at the Mayak Nuclear Enterprise. Health Phys 1997;73:899–905.
20. Voelz GL, Wilkinson CS, Acquavelle JF. An update of epidemiologic studies of plutonium workers. Health Phys 1983;44(suppl 1):493–503.
21. Gilbert ES, Petersen GR, Buchanan JA. Mortality of workers at the Hanford site: 1945–1981. Health Phys 1989;56:11–25.
22. Cohen BL. Review cancer risk from low-level radiation. AJR 2002;179:1137–1143.

23. Luan Y. The effects of low and very low doses of radiation on human health. Trans Am Nucl Soc 1999;18–23.
24. Olivieri G, Bodycote J, Wolff S. Adaptive response of human lymphocytes to low concentrations of radioactive thymidine. Science 1984;223:594–597.
25. Shadley J, Dai G. Cytogenic and survival adaptive responses in G-1 phase human lymphocytes. Mutat Res 1992;265:273–281.
26. Sanderson B, Morely A. Exposure of human lymphocytes to ionizing radiation reduces mutagenesis by subsequent ionizing radiation. Mutat Res 1986;164:347–351.
27. Kelsey K, Memisoglu A, Frenkel D, Liber H. Human lymphocytes exposed to low doses of x-rays are less susceptible to radiation-induces mutagenesis. Mutat Res 1991;263:197–201.
28. Shadley J, Wolff S. Very low doses of x-rays can cause human lymphocytes to become less susceptible to ionizing radiation. Mutagenesis 1987;2:95–96.
29. Fritz-Niggli H, Schaeppi-Buechi C. Adaptive response to dominant lethality of mature (class A) and immature (class B) oocytes of D. melanogaster to low doses of ionizing radiation: effects in repair-proficient (yw) and repair-deficient strains (mei 41D5 and mus 320DI). Int J Radiat Biol 1991;59:175–184.
30. Miller RC, Randers-Pehrson G, Geard CR, Hall EJ, Brenner DJ. The oncogenic transforming potential of the passage of single alpha particles thought mammalian cell nuclei. Proc Natl Acad Sci USA 1999;96:19–22.
31. Health Physics Society. Radiation risk in perspective: position statement of the Health Physics Society (adopted January 1996). In: Health Physics Society Directory and Handbook. 1998–1999. McLean, VA: Health Physics Society, 1998:238.
32. Pierce DA, Shimizu Y, Preston DL, Vaeth M, Mabuchi K. Studies of the mortality of atomic bomb survivors, report 12.1 Cancer: 1950–1990. Radiat Res 1996;146:1–27.
33. Little MP, Muirhead CR. Evidence for curvilinearity in the cancer incidence dose-response in the Japanese atomic bomb survivors. Int J Radiat Biol 1996;70(1):83–94.
34. Heindenreich WF, Jacob P, Paretzke HG. Exact solutions of the clonal expansion model and their application to the incidence of solid tumors of atomic bomb survivors. Radiat Environ Biophys 1997;36(1):45–58.
35. NCR Report No. 136. Evaluation of the linear-nonthreshold dose-response model for iodizing radiation. Recommendation of the National Counsel on Radiation Protection and Measurements. Society of Nuclear Medicine, June 4, 2001, pp. 279–286.
36. Mossman KL. The linear no-threshold debate: where do we go from here? Med Phys 1998;25(3):279–284.
37. Southwood TRE. Crookshank Lecture, risk from radiation—perception and reality. Clin Radiol 1994;49:1–6.
38. Stewart A. A-bomb data: detection of bias in the Life Span Study cohort. Environ Health Perspect 1997;105(6):1519–1521.
39. Kellerer AM, Nekolla E. Neutron versus gamma-ray risk estimates. Inferences from the cancer incidence and mortality data in Hiroshima. Radiat Environ Biophys 1997;36(2):73–83.
40. Heidenreich WF, Luebeck EG, Hazelton WD, Paretzke HG, Moolgavkar SH. Multistage models and the incidence of cancer in the cohort of atomic bomb survivors. Radiat Res 2002;158(5):607–614.
41. Pierce DA, Mendelsohn ML. A model for radiation-related cancer suggested by atomic bomb survivor data. Radiat Res 1999;152(6):642–654.

42. Kellerer AM. The effects of neutrons in Hiroshima. Implications for the risk estimates. C R Acad Sci III 1999;322(2–3):229–237.
43. Little MP, Muirhead CR. Curvature in the cancer mortality dose response in Japanese atomic bomb survivors: absence of evidence of threshold. Int J Radiat Biol 1998;74(4):471–480.
44. Hoel DG, Li P. Threshold models in radiation carcinogenesis. Health Phys 1998;75(3):241–250.
45. Sinclair WK. The linear no-threshold response: why not linearity? Med Phys 1998;25(3):285–290.
46. Stewart A. A-bomb data: detection of bias in the Life Span Study cohort. Environ Health Perspect 1997;105(suppl 6):1519–1521.
47. Kellerer AM. Radiation risk-historical perspective and current issues. J Radiol Prot 2002;22(3A):A1–10.
48. Ron E. Ionizing radiation and cancer risk: evidence from epidemiology. Radiat Res 1998;150(5 suppl):S30–41.
49. Heidenreich WF, Paretzke HG, Jacob P. No evidence for increased tumor rates below 200 mSv in the atomic bomb survivors data. Radiat Environ Biophys 1997;36(3):205–207.

4

Dosage of Radiopharmaceuticals and Internal Dosimetry

Xiaowei Zhu

Dosage of Radiopharmaceuticals

Radiopharmaceuticals are widely used for diagnostic imaging and radiation therapy. Although radiation therapy uses damage to living tissue to the advantage of the patient, this damage, however, is a limitation for the diagnostic application. Radiation dosages for specific indications are optimized based on thorough studies performed on animals and through clinical trials on human subjects prior to approval for clinical applications. Proper dosages are derived through careful study of pharmacokinetics, the physical characteristics of the radionuclide, metabolism of the subject, and the pharmacodynamics of the radiopharmaceutical in animal and human subjects. The chemical- and radiotoxicities and adverse reactions are well understood before an optimal and safe dosage is recommended. Doses are typically scaled by weight, or total body surface area, and reduced for children. The recommended dosage for a specific indication and route of administration are stated by the drug manufacturers in the package insert, and are readily available online.

Internal Radiation Dosimetry

To assess the effects of radiation on a living organ, it is important to understand and quantify radiation energy deposited and absorbed by that organ. This deposition/absorption of energy is called *radiation absorbed dose*. Internal radiation dosimetry involves the studying of energy absorbed by the organs from an internally deposited radionuclide. It includes the study of physical characteristics of radionuclides, pharmacokinetics and biokinetics of the radiopharmaceutical, as well as establishing assumptions and models for calculating absorbed radiation energy.

Radiation Absorbed Dose

Radiation absorbed dose is defined as the quantity of radiation energy absorbed by a unit mass of absorber material (e.g., bone marrow, body tissue, etc.). The SI unit for radiation absorbed dose is the *gray (Gy)*.

1 Gy = 1 joule energy absorbed/kg of absorber medium

However, the traditional unit *rad*, is used more commonly in the United States.

1 rad = 100 erg energy absorbed/g of absorber medium

1 rad = 0.01 Gy

Radiation absorbed dose is proportional to several key estimated components. These components include (1) the amount of radioactivity in the source organ, (2) the residence time of radioactivity in the source organ, (3) the type and amount of radiation energy emitted by the radioactivity in the source organ, and (4) the fraction of the emitting energy from the source that is absorbed by the target organ. The fraction is dependent on the geometric and anatomic relationship of the source to target organs.

To calculate the radiation absorbed dose, we need to quantify each component discussed above. Quantifying each component that contributes to the radiation absorbed dose can be difficult due to the complex nature of metabolic systems and to differences in patient anatomy. Therefore, the calculation of radiation absorbed dose is really an estimate of quantity based on standard anatomic and kinetic models and reasonable assumptions.

Absorbed Dose

Cumulated Radioactivity Ã
The radiation dose delivered from a source organ to a target organ is dependent on the amount of radioactivity in the source organ and the length of time the radioactivity resides in the source organ. Due to the continuous uptake and elimination of the radiopharmaceutical administered to the living system, and physical decay of the radionuclide, the radioactivity in each organ is a function of time. Mathematically, the *cumulated radioactivity*, $\tilde{A}$, can be expressed as

$$\tilde{A} = \int_0^\infty A(t)dt \tag{1}$$

where $A(t)$ is the radioactivity in source organ at the time of t (Fig. 4.1). $\tilde{A}$ accounts for the radioactivity in the organ, and how long it resided in source organ (component 1 and 2 discussed above). The units for $\tilde{A}$ are µCi-hr.

$A(t)$ is different from organ to organ, and varies in individual living systems. However, it can be estimated from studying the pharmacokinetics of the radiopharmaceutical of the source organ. A time-radioactivity curve can be established for each source organ by following the uptake and excretion of the radionuclide in the organ. $A(t)$ is a function of the physical and biologic decay of the radiophar-

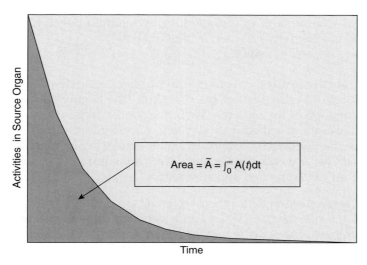

Figure 4.1. Time-activity curve. The area under is the curve is $\tilde{A}$, the accumulated radioactivity in the source organ.

maceutical. A simplified mathematical model of instantaneous and exponential elimination of the radiopharmaceutical in the source organ can be described as

$$A(t) = A_0 e^{-\lambda_e t} \tag{2}$$

and

$$\lambda_e = \lambda_p + \lambda_b \tag{3}$$

where λ_e is the effective decay constant, and λ_p and λ_b are the physical and biologic decay constants, respectively.

If the half-life is known, the decay constant can be calculated as

$$\lambda = \frac{0.693}{T_{1/2}}. \tag{4}$$

Therefore, equation 1 becomes

$$\tilde{A} = \frac{A_0}{\lambda_e} = 1.44 T_e A_0 \tag{5}$$

where T_e is the effective half-life.

Equilibrium Absorbed Dose Constant, Δ

The amount of radiation energy emitted per unit of accumulated radioactivity in the source organ can be calculated if the type, energy, and frequency of each emission of the radionuclide are known. If we designate E_i as the energy of the ith emission, n_i is the frequency of that emission. The amount of radiation energy emitted per unit of accumulated radioactivity can then be described as

$$\Delta_i = 2.13 n_i E_i \qquad (6)$$

where E_i is in MeV and Δ_i is in (g-rad/μCi-hr). Δ_i is defined as *equilibrium absorbed dose constant* of the ith emitter. The energy emitted from the ith emission of the radionuclide in the source organ is a product of the equilibrium absorbed dose constant, Δ_i, and accumulated radioactivity, $\tilde{A}$. If a radionuclide deposited in the source organ has more than one emission, the equilibrium absorbed dose constant should be calculated for each emission and summated.

Total Energy Absorbed by Target Organ, D

Due to the distance and attenuation between the source organ and target oranges, only a fraction of the energy emitted by the source organ is absorbed by the target organ. This fraction factor needs to be quantified so that the total absorbed dose by the target organ can be estimated.

Absorbed Fraction φ

The absorbed fraction depends on the geometric relationship of the source and target organ, the emission energy of the radionuclide, and the composition of the source organs, the target organ, and those organs in between. Mathematically, the absorbed fraction of the ith emission of the radionuclide can be expressed as $\phi_i(t_k \leftarrow s_j)$. The energy absorbed by the target organ, t_k, from the ith emission of the radionuclide in source organ, s_j, is equal to $\tilde{A}_j \phi_i(t_k \leftarrow s_j) \Delta_i$. So the total energy absorbed by target organ, t_k, from all emissions in the source organ, s_j, is

$$\text{Energy Absorbed (g-rad)} = \tilde{A}_j \sum_i \phi_i(t_k \leftarrow s_j) \Delta_i. \qquad (7)$$

Because the absorbed dose is defined as energy absorbed in unit mass, the dose delivered from the source organ, s_j, to the target organ, t_k, is

$$D(t_k \leftarrow s_j)(rad) = \left(\frac{\tilde{A}_j}{m_k}\right) \sum_i \phi_i(t_k \leftarrow s_j) \Delta_i \qquad (8)$$

where $\tilde{A}_j$ is the cumulated activity in source organ, s_j, and m_k is the mass of the target organ, t_k. The total dose to the target organ can be obtained by summing the doses from all the source organ of the body:

$$D(t_k)(rad) = \sum_j D(t_k \leftarrow s_j).$$

The calculation of absorbed fraction, ϕ, for each penetrating emission, for example, photons, is very complicated, as it is highly dependent on the energy of the radiation emission, the geometry between the target and source organs, and the characteristics of the tissue and organ. The range of ϕ is between 0 and 1 from the source organ to target organ (target organ can be the source organ itself) for photons with emitting energy >10 keV. When the target organ is the same as the source organ, and electron or photon energy is <10 keV, $\phi = 1$. If the target organ is a different organ, then $\phi = 0$. This assumes that the source organ will attenuate and absorb within itself the entire radiation energy when the radiation emission is a low-energy photon or a non-penetrating particle, such as an electron.

Specific Absorbed Dose Fraction, Φ

A rearrangement of equation 8, gives us

$$D(t_k \leftarrow s_j)(rad) = \tilde{A}_j \sum_i \frac{\phi_i(t_k \leftarrow s_j)}{m_k}\Delta_i. \qquad (9)$$

The term $\dfrac{\phi_i(t_k \leftarrow s_j)}{m_k}$, is defined as the specific absorbed fraction, $\Phi_i(t_k \leftarrow s_j)$. This is the fraction of the ith radiation emitter that is given off by the radionuclide in the source organ, s_j, and absorbed, per unit mass, by target organ t_k. Equation 9 can then be written as

$$D(t_k \leftarrow s_j)(rad) = \tilde{A}_j \sum_i \Phi_i(t_k \leftarrow s_j)\Delta_i. \qquad (10)$$

The specific absorbed fraction has been calculated using mathematical phantom models based on different age groups with complex mathematical simulations for source-target pairs. The results are a set of comprehensive tables of specific absorbed fractions for each reference age group. Table 4.1 is an example that was formulated by Oak Ridge National Lab (1). This example involves a 500 keV photon, the specific absorbed fraction from the kidney (source organ) to what could be considered the average liver of a 10-year-old (2.35E-2/kg or 2.35E-5/g).

A simplified quantity, *dose per cumulated activity*, or S value, has been calculated for the source-target organs for many radionuclides of interest. The S value of the source-target organs, pair j and k, is defined as $S(t_k \leftarrow s_j) = \sum_i \Phi_i(t_k \leftarrow s_j)\Delta_i$. This is calculated in the conventional units of rad/μCi-hr. Medical Internal Radiation Dose (MIRD) committee pamphlet No. 11 tabulated many of the most commonly used radionuclides for the standard adult phantom (2). Now Equation 10 can be rewritten as

$$D(t_k \leftarrow s_j)(rad) = \tilde{A}_j S(t_k \leftarrow s_j). \qquad (11)$$

The total dose $D(t_k)$ to target organ k is then described as

$$D(t_k) = \sum_j \tilde{A}_j S(t_k \leftarrow s_j). \qquad (12)$$

If the accumulated radioactivity in each source organ is known, one can calculate the total dose to the target organ by using the S-value table and summing up the dose delivered to the target organ from each

Table 4.1. Specific absorbed fraction of photon energy in kg-1: recommended values for a 10-year-old

Source = Kidneys

Target	Energy (MeV)											
	0.010	0.015	0.020	0.030	0.050	0.100	0.200	0.500	1.000	1.500	2.000	4.000
Adrenals	4.84E−03	5.22E−02	1.29E−01	1.57E−01	1.06E−01	7.46E−02	6.89E−02	6.69E−02	6.74E−02	6.21E−02	5.67E−02	4.40E−02
UB Wall	0.0	0.0	5.85E−07	2.95E−04	2.08E−03	2.49E−03	2.91E−03	3.29E−03	3.33E−03	3.23E−03	3.09E−03	2.64E−03
Bone Sur	1.39E−04	3.49E−03	1.40E−02	3.67E−02	3.90E−02	1.90E−02	1.06E−02	8.00E−03	7.26E−03	6.82E−03	6.45E−03	5.42E−03
Brain	0.0	0.0	0.0	5.72E−08	9.29E−06	5.32E−05	7.84E−05	1.31E−04	1.91E−04	2.33E−04	2.68E−04	3.65E−04
Breasts	0.0	0.0	3.85E−07	7.36E−04	2.82E−03	2.59E−03	3.19E−03	3.63E−03	3.53E−03	3.36E−03	3.21E−03	2.82E−03
St Wall	0.0	2.18E−05	1.78E−03	1.94E−02	2.80E−02	2.27E−02	2.08E−02	2.06E−02	1.92E−02	1.70E−02	1.53E−02	1.25E−02
SI Wall	5.55E−10	1.06E−04	3.50E−03	1.77E−02	2.70E−02	2.20E−02	2.06E−02	1.90E−02	1.73E−02	1.62E−02	1.52E−02	1.25E−02
ULI Wall	0.0	1.70E−05	1.61E−03	1.43E−02	2.70E−02	2.13E−02	1.76E−02	1.79E−02	1.64E−02	1.54E−02	1.45E−02	1.17E−02
LLI Wall	0.0	4.04E−07	1.18E−04	2.68E−03	5.43E−03	6.63E−03	6.04E−03	5.70E−03	5.63E−03	5.34E−03	5.05E−03	4.27E−03
Kidneys	5.37E+00	4.43E+00	3.21E+00	1.54E+00	5.95E−01	3.46E−01	3.56E−01	3.74E−01	3.54E−01	3.29E−01	3.06E−01	2.39E−01
Liver	8.35E−05	3.55E−03	1.58E−02	3.85E−02	3.75E−02	2.74E−02	2.49E−02	2.35E−02	2.19E−02	2.04E−02	1.91E−02	1.62E−02
Lng Tiss	0.0	5.05E−06	5.96E−04	5.35E−03	9.10E−03	7.87E−03	7.35E−03	6.81E−03	7.09E−03	6.34E−03	5.74E−03	5.15E−03
Muscle	3.13E−03	8.91E−03	1.43E−02	1.59E−02	1.16E−02	8.53E−03	8.27E−03	8.39E−03	8.04E−03	7.58E−03	7.14E−03	5.88E−03
Ovaries	0.0	1.55E−08	4.97E−05	2.30E−03	7.47E−03	8.85E−03	8.20E−03	8.49E−03	7.53E−03	6.96E−03	6.66E−03	6.24E−03
Pancreas	5.22E−10	3.99E−04	1.26E−02	6.20E−02	6.58E−02	4.69E−02	3.98E−02	4.04E−02	3.44E−02	3.02E−02	2.77E−02	2.36E−02
R Marrow	6.38E−05	1.33E−03	4.91E−03	1.23E−02	1.51E−02	1.38E−02	1.37E−02	1.35E−02	1.23E−02	1.14E−02	1.08E−02	8.81E−03
Skin	1.14E−04	7.68E−04	2.97E−03	5.28E−03	4.27E−03	3.41E−03	3.68E−03	4.08E−03	3.89E−03	3.94E−03	3.93E−03	3.31E−03
Spleen	2.92E−03	3.80E−02	1.13E−01	1.51E−01	9.95E−02	6.31E−02	5.57E−02	5.76E−02	5.31E−02	4.89E−02	4.55E−02	3.69E−02
Testes	0.0	0.0	1.53E−09	1.76E−05	3.60E−04	6.40E−04	8.50E−04	1.05E−03	1.16E−03	1.18E−03	1.20E−03	1.12E−03
Thymus	0.0	0.0	7.94E−08	1.13E−04	7.80E−04	1.89E−03	2.30E−03	2.50E−03	2.60E−03	2.64E−03	2.57E−03	2.21E−03
Thyroid	0.0	0.0	1.36E−10	5.08E−06	2.18E−04	6.20E−04	7.04E−04	7.71E−04	8.36E−04	9.48E−04	1.01E−03	9.37E−04
GB Wall	0.0	3.31E−05	3.69E−03	2.55E−02	5.26E−02	3.56E−02	2.48E−02	2.40E−02	2.00E−02	1.86E−02	1.80E−02	1.66E−02
Ht Wall	0.0	2.51E−08	4.81E−05	2.89E−03	7.30E−03	8.58E−03	7.65E−03	7.51E−03	7.66E−03	6.95E−03	6.32E−03	5.20E−03
Uterus	0.0	1.26E−09	1.72E−05	1.78E−03	6.39E−03	8.05E−03	6.87E−03	6.99E−03	7.56E−03	7.10E−03	6.57E−03	5.48E−03

Cristy M, Eckerman KF, Specific absorbed fraction of energy at various ages from internal photon source. IV. Ten-year-old. Oak Ridge National Laboratory Report ORNL/TM-8381:Vol. 4, 1987

Bone Sur: Bone Surface; GB Wall: Gall Bladder Wall; Ht Wall: Heart Wall; LLI Wall: Lower Large Intestine Wall; Long Tiss: Lung Tissue; R Marrow: Red Marrow; SI Wall: Small Intestine Wall; St. Wall: Stomach Wall; UB wall: Urinary Bladder Wall; ULI Wall: Upper Large Intestine Wall.

source organ. In absence of the S-value tables for other age groups, the S value can be calculated using tabulated Φ and Δ values, as discussed earlier.

Pediatric Dose Estimate

For pediatric patients, radiopharmaceutical dosages are based on a pediatric dosing schedule. There are many different dosing schedules. The most common ones are those using body weight or body surface areas as guides to scale the dose. Pediatric dose schedules consider many factors to scale down the dosage from that of adult to child, including organ doses, effective dose, and image quality.

However, absorbed radiation dose and effective dose to pediatric patients are not as simple as the dosing schedule. They are not just simple linear scaled-down doses of those for adult patients. As we discussed before, radiation doses to patients depend on geometric and anatomic relationships of source to target organs. Differences in pediatric organ size, density, and composition significantly change the geometric and anatomic relationships that were established for adult patient (or phantom). Differences of biokinetics, due to age-related differences in uptakes (e.g., thyroid uptake of iodine), and excretion (e.g., bladder voiding interval), must be considered when estimate radiation doses for pediatric patients.

Mathematical phantoms for age groups considering the geometric and anatomic variables have been well developed. They are typically for infants, and 1-, 5-, 10-, and 15-year-olds. Specific absorbed fraction has been calculated and tabulated (e.g., Table 4.1) for each age-specific phantom group. Combined with dose schedule, age-adjusted uptake and excretion parameters, pediatric radiation doses can then be estimated according to Equation 10.

Practical Approach to Internal Dose Estimate

The estimation of internal dose from a radionuclide in a human is rather a complicated process. Studies of biokinetic models of a particular radiopharmaceutical normally begin through investigations of the model in animals. Modeling data are collected starting with the initial amount of the radiopharmaceutical of interest that is injected into the animal. The percentage of the radionuclide that is taken up by the source organ is determined through imaging. Other pertinent data are collected through assays of blood and urine. These data points are then carefully plotted or fitted to an established mathematical model that describes the biokinetics of the radionuclides in each source organ. Complex regulatory requirements regarding human research subjects dictate that dose estimates in human subjects should conducted after successful animal studies. Many radiopharmaceuticals are not directly studied for pediatric applications because of complicated social and ethical issues related to conducting radiation research in children.

A wealth of information concerning internal dosimetry for the most commonly used radionuclides in nuclear medicine has been established and published, including dosimetry data for radionuclides used in positron emission tomography (PET) scanning (3–6). Pediatric dose estimates have also been calculated for different age groups based on adult biokinetics of radiopharmaceuticals and anatomic phantom models. Researchers have observed the differences between pediatric biokinetic models and those of an adult, especially in regard to infants, and so improvements in dosimetry data for pediatric patients continue. The Annals of International Commission on Radiological Protection (ICRP) Publication 53 provides biokinetic models and lists radiation doses to patients from the most commonly used radiopharmaceuticals in nuclear medicine (7). ICRP Publication 80 recalculated 19 of the most frequently used radiopharmaceuticals from ICRP 53 and added 10 more new radiopharmaceuticals (8). Tables 4.2 to 4.4 are absorbed-dose tables of several radiopharmaceuticals used for PET imaging, adapted from ICRP 80.

Table 4.2. Absorbed dose of ^{18}F-FDG (2-fluoro-2-deoxy-D-glucose)

^{18}F 109.77 min Organ	Absorbed dose per unit activity administered (mGy/MBq)				
	Adult	15 years	10 years	5 years	1 year
Adrenals	1.2E − 02	1.5E − 02	2.4E − 02	3.8E − 02	7.2E − 02
Bladder	1.6E − 01	2.1E − 01	2.8E − 01	3.2E − 01	5.9E − 01
Bone surfaces	1.1E − 02	1.4E − 02	2.2E − 02	3.5E − 02	6.6E − 02
Brain	2.8E − 02	2.8E − 02	3.0E − 02	3.4E − 02	4.8E − 02
Breast	8.6E − 03	1.1E − 02	1.8E − 02	2.9E − 02	5.6E − 02
Gall bladder	1.2E − 02	1.5E − 02	2.3E − 02	3.5E − 02	6.6E − 02
GI-tract					
Stomach	1.1E − 02	1.4E − 02	2.2E − 02	3.6E − 02	6.8E − 02
SI	1.3E − 02	1.7E − 02	2.7E − 02	4.1E − 02	7.7E − 02
Colon	1.3E − 02	1.7E − 02	2.7E − 02	4.0E − 02	7.4E − 02
(ULI	1.2E − 02	1.6E − 02	2.5E − 02	3.9E − 02	7.2E − 02)
(LLI	1.5E − 02	1.9E − 02	2.9E − 02	4.2E − 02	7.6E − 02)
Heart	6.2E − 02	8.1E − 02	1.2E − 01	2.0E − 01	3.5E − 01
Kidneys	2.1E − 02	2.5E − 02	3.6E − 02	5.4E − 02	9.6E − 02
Liver	1.1E − 02	1.4E − 02	2.2E − 02	3.7E − 02	7.0E − 02
Lungs	1.0E − 02	1.4E − 02	2.1E − 02	3.4E − 02	6.5E − 02
Muscles	1.1E − 02	1.4E − 02	2.1E − 02	3.4E − 02	6.5E − 02
Oesophagus	1.1E − 02	1.5E − 02	2.2E − 02	3.5E − 02	6.8E − 02
Ovaries	1.5E − 02	2.0E − 02	3.0E − 02	4.4E − 02	8.2E − 02
Pancreas	1.2E − 02	1.6E − 02	2.5E − 02	4.0E − 02	7.6E − 02
Red marrow	1.1E − 02	1.4E − 02	2.2E − 02	3.2E − 02	6.1E − 02
Skin	8.0E − 03	1.0E − 02	1.6E − 02	2.7E − 02	5.2E − 02
Spleen	1.1E − 02	1.4E − 02	2.2E − 02	3.6E − 02	6.9E − 02
Testes	1.2E − 02	1.6E − 02	2.6E − 02	3.8E − 02	7.3E − 02
Thymus	1.1E − 02	1.5E − 02	2.2E − 02	3.5E − 02	6.8E − 02
Thyroid	1.0E − 02	1.3E − 02	2.1E − 02	3.5E − 02	6.8E − 02
Uterus	2.1E − 02	2.6E − 02	3.9E − 02	5.5E − 02	1.0E − 01
Remaining organs	1.1E − 02	1.4E − 02	2.2E − 02	3.4E − 02	6.3E − 02
Effective dose (mSv/MBq)	1.9E − 02	2.5E − 02	3.6E − 02	5.0E − 02	9.5E − 02

Source: ICRP Publication 80 Radiation Dose to Patients from Radiopharmaceutical. Annals of ICRP 1998;28(3):10–49, with permission from the ICRP.

Table 4.3. Absorbed dose [methyl-^{11}C]thymidine

^{11}C 20.38 min Organ	Absorbed dose per unit activity administered (mGy/MBq)				
	Adult	15 years	10 years	5 years	1 year
Adrenals	2.9E − 03	3.7E − 03	5.8E − 03	9.3E − 03	1.7E − 02
Bladder	2.3E − 03	2.7E − 03	4.3E − 03	7.1E − 03	1.3E − 02
Bone surfaces	2.4E − 03	3.0E − 03	4.7E − 03	7.6E − 03	1.5E − 02
Brain	1.9E − 03	2.4E − 03	4.0E − 03	6.7E − 03	1.3E − 02
Breast	1.8E − 03	2.3E − 03	3.6E − 03	5.9E − 03	1.1E − 02
Gall bladder	2.8E − 03	3.4E − 03	5.2E − 03	7.9E − 03	1.5E − 02
GI-tract					
Stomach	2.4E − 03	2.9E − 03	4.6E − 03	7.3E − 03	1.4E − 02
SI	2.4E − 03	3.1E − 03	4.9E − 03	7.8E − 03	1.5E − 02
Colon	2.4E − 03	2.9E − 03	4.7E − 03	7.4E − 03	1.4E − 02
(ULI	2.4E − 03	3.0E − 03	4.8E − 03	7.7E − 03	1.4E − 02)
(LLI	2.3E − 03	2.7E − 03	4.5E − 03	7.1E − 03	1.3E − 02)
Heart	3.4E − 03	4.3E − 03	6.8E − 03	1.1E − 02	2.0E − 02
Kidneys	1.1E − 02	1.3E − 02	1.9E − 02	2.8E − 02	5.1E − 02
Liver	5.2E − 03	6.8E − 03	1.0E − 02	1.6E − 02	2.9E − 02
Lungs	3.0E − 03	3.9E − 03	6.2E − 03	9.9E − 02	1.9E − 02
Muscles	2.1E − 03	2.6E − 03	4.1E − 03	6.6E − 03	1.3E − 02
Oesophagus	2.2E − 03	2.8E − 03	4.3E − 03	6.9E − 03	1.3E − 02
Ovaries	2.4E − 03	3.0E − 03	4.8E − 03	7.6E − 03	1.4E − 02
Pancreas	2.7E − 03	3.4E − 03	5.3E − 03	8.3E − 03	1.6E − 02
Red marrow	2.5E − 03	3.1E − 03	4.8E − 03	7.6E − 03	1.4E − 02
Skin	1.7E − 03	2.1E − 03	3.4E − 03	5.6E − 03	1.1E − 02
Spleen	3.0E − 03	3.7E − 03	5.9E − 03	9.6E − 03	1.8E − 02
Testes	2.0E − 03	2.5E − 03	3.9E − 03	6.2E − 03	1.2E − 02
Thymus	2.2E − 03	2.8E − 03	4.3E − 03	6.9E − 03	1.3E − 02
Thyroid	2.3E − 03	2.9E − 03	4.7E − 03	7.8E − 03	1.5E − 02
Uterus	2.4E − 03	3.0E − 03	4.8E − 03	7.6E − 03	1.4E − 02
Remaining organs	2.1E − 03	2.6E − 03	4.2E − 03	6.8E − 03	1.3E − 02
Effective dose (mSv/MBq)	2.7E − 03	3.4E − 03	5.3E − 03	8.4E − 03	1.6E − 02

Source: ICRP Publication 80 Radiation Dose to Patients from Radiopharmaceutical. Annals of ICRP 1998;28(3):10–49, with permission from the ICRP.

Table 4.4. Absorbed dose ^{15}O-abeled water

^{15}O 2.04 min Organ	Absorbed dose per unit activity administered (mGy/MBq)				
	Adult	15 years	10 years	5 years	1 year
Adrenals	1.4E − 03	2.2E − 03	3.1E − 03	4.3E − 03	6.6E − 03
Bladder	2.6E − 04	3.1E − 04	5.0E − 04	8.4E − 04	1.5E − 03
Bone surfaces	6.2E − 04	8.0E − 04	1.3E − 03	2.3E − 03	5.5E − 03
Brain	1.3E − 03	1.3E − 03	1.4E − 03	1.6E − 03	2.2E − 03
Breast	2.8E − 04	3.5E − 04	6.0E − 04	9.9E − 04	2.0E − 03
Gall bladder	4.5E − 04	5.5E − 04	8.6E − 04	1.4E − 03	2.7E − 03
GI-tract					
Stomach	7.8E − 04	2.2E − 03	3.1E − 03	5.3E − 03	1.2E − 02
SI	1.3E − 03	1.7E − 03	3.0E − 03	5.0E − 03	9.9E − 03
Colon	1.0E − 03	2.1E − 03	3.7E − 03	6.2E − 03	1.2E − 02
(ULI	1.0E − 03	2.1E − 03	3.7E − 03	6.2E − 03	1.2E − 02)
(LLI	1.1E − 03	2.1E − 03	3.7E − 03	6.2E − 03	1.2E − 02)
Heart	1.9E − 03	2.4E − 03	3.8E − 03	6.0E − 03	1.1E − 02
Kidneys	1.7E − 03	2.1E − 03	3.0E − 03	4.5E − 03	8.1E − 03

Table 4.4. Absorbed dose ^{15}O-abeled water (*Continued*)

^{15}O 2.04 min Organ	Absorbed dose per unit activity administered (mGy/MBq)				
	Adult	15 years	10 years	5 years	1 year
Liver	1.6E − 03	2.1E − 03	3.2E − 03	4.8E − 03	9.3E − 03
Lungs	1.6E − 03	2.4E − 03	3.4E − 03	5.2E − 03	1.0E − 02
Muscles	2.9E − 04	3.7E − 04	6.1E − 04	1.0E − 03	2.0E − 03
Oesophagus	3.3E − 04	4.2E − 04	6.7E − 04	1.1E − 03	2.1E − 03
Ovaries	8.5E − 04	1.1E − 03	1.8E − 03	2.8E − 03	5.8E − 03
Pancreas	1.4E − 03	2.0E − 03	4.2E − 03	5.4E − 03	1.2E − 02
Red marrow	8.5E − 04	9.7E − 04	1.6E − 03	3.0E − 03	6.1E − 03
Skin	2.5E − 04	3.1E − 04	5.2E − 04	8.8E − 04	1.8E − 03
Spleen	1.6E − 03	2.3E − 03	3.7E − 03	5.8E − 03	1.1E − 02
Testes	7.4E − 04	9.3E − 04	1.5E − 03	2.6E − 03	5.1E − 03
Thymus	3.3E − 04	4.2E − 04	6.7E − 04	1.1E − 03	2.1E − 03
Thyroid	1.5E − 03	2.5E − 03	3.8E − 03	8.5E − 03	1.6E − 02
Uterus	3.5E − 04	4.4E − 04	7.2E − 04	1.2E − 03	2.3E − 03
Remaining organs	4.0E − 04	5.6E − 04	9.4E − 04	1.7E − 03	2.9E − 03
Effective dose (mSv/MBq)	9.3E − 04	1.4E − 03	2.3E − 03	3.8E − 03	7.7E − 03

Source: ICRP Publication 80 Radiation Dose to Patients from Radiopharmaceutical. Annals of ICRP 1998;28(3):10–49, with permission from the ICRP.

References

1. Cristy M, Eckerman KF. Specific absorbed fraction of energy at various ages from internal photon source. IV. Ten-year-old. Oak Ridge National Laboratory Report ORNL/TM-8381, vol. 4, 1987.
2. Snyder WS, Ford MR, Warner GG, et al. "S" absorbed dose per unit cumulated activity. Nm/MIRD Pamphlet No. 11. New York: Society of Nuclear Medicine, 1975.
3. Ruotsalainen U, Suhonen-Polvi H, Eronen E, et al. Estimated radiation dose to the newborn in FDG-PET studies. J Nucl Med 1996;37:387–393.
4. Hays MT, Watson EE, Stabin M, et al. MIRD dose estimate report No. 19: radiation absorbed dose estimates from 18F-FDG. J Nucl Med 2002;43:210–214.
5. Sorenson JA, Phelps ME. Physics in Nuclear Medicine. New York: Harcourt Brace Jovanovich, 1987.
6. Stabin MG, Stabbs JB, Toohey RE, et al. Radiation Dose for Radiopharmaceuticals, NEREG/CR. Radiation Internal Dose Center, Oak Ridge Institute of Science and Education, 1996.
7. ICRP Publication 53, Radiation Dose to Patient from Radiopharmaceutucal, Annals of ICRP, vol. 18, pp. 1–4. New York: Elsevier, 1988.
8. ICRP Publication 80, Radiation Dose to Patients from Radiopharmaceutical, Annals of ICRP, vol. 28, p. 3. New York: Elsevier, 1998.

5

Pediatric PET Research Regulations

Geoffrey Levine

Good intentions are necessary, but not sufficient, to conduct pediatric positron emission tomography (PET) research. This chapter provides direction to guide the process of conducting PET research in children.

Code of Federal Regulations (CFR)

When the executive rule-making voice of the government speaks, it does so officially through the Code of Federal Regulations (1). These are not the laws, per se, but rather the nitty gritty rules necessary to carry out the laws that are made by Congress. For example, Congress may pass a law to provide for a safe drug supply; the executive branch (e.g., the Food and Drug Administration, FDA) carries out the intent of the law and writes the rules (e.g., "Intravenous products shall be sterile and pyrogen-free").

Reading 21 CFR (Title 21 of the CFR, where the FDA rules are located) is about as exciting as reading the telephone book or the Internal Revenue Service regulations for preparing tax returns (until you come to that one paragraph that appears to justify your objective), but it is necessary. The judicial system interprets the regulations and may enforce compliance. Each agency of the executive branch of the government or each specific purpose for a set of regulations has a particular location. Title 10, for example, is where one finds radiation safety and safe use of radiopharmaceutical use in humans. Table 5.1 provides an example of several other locations within the CFR that may be of interest to the reader (3). In addition to the CFR, the various agencies issue letters, guidelines, interpretations, descriptions of courses, comments, request for comments, etc., in an effort to communicate with the public and research investigators, among others. And, like cement, the rules become more solidified with time. Occasionally, the book is opened for a rewrite, providing a glimpse into the "mind" of the government. One such opportunity appeared on November 16, 2004, in an open meeting at the FDA headquarters in which an update of the Radioactive Drug Research Committee (RDRC) regulations was being

Table 5.1. Some additional examples of codified federal policy

07 CFR Part 1C	Department of Agriculture
10 CFR Part 35	Human Use of Radiopharmaceuticals
10 CFR Part 745	Department of Energy
15 CFR Part 27	Department of Commerce
16 CFR Part 1028	Consumer Product Safety Commission
21 CFR Part 361.1	Radiopharmaceutical Use in Humans
40 CFR Part 26	Environmental Protection Agency
45 CFR Part 46	Public Welfare, Protection of Human Subjects
45 CFR Part 690	National Science Foundation

Note: There are source documents, regulations, amendments to regulations, Web sites, parts, subparts, preliminary documents for review, rewrites, updates, clarifications, and numerous other forms of communication.
Source: Data from ref. 2.

considered (4). The regulations will be examined shortly, particularly as they relate to PET research in children. Table 5.2 provides a resource list to facilitate communication (4,5,14).

Pathways Allowed by the Federal Regulatory System

There are three major routes to conduct research that are allowed by the federal regulatory system: (1) an investigational new drug (IND) application, (2) a physician-sponsored IND, and (3) the RDRC mechanism (6–8,15–21).

The full IND approach is the one taken by drug manufacturers who intend to obtain FDA approval to market a pharmaceutical to the general public, usually for commercial purposes. The manufacturer conducts physical, chemical, and biologic studies in vitro and then in animals prior to studies in humans (clinical trials, phases I, II, III described below), followed by postmarketing studies (phase IV), post–new drug approval. The pharmaceutical house has sufficient talent, expertise, and staff in its regulatory and medical departments to know how to proceed on its own.

A second pathway is the physician-sponsored IND, which usually involves studies with more than 30 subjects, can be conducted at one or multiple sites, and can involve agents that are new entities, new routes of administration, new dosage forms for existing or new drugs, new populations (including children) or disease states, new indications, etc. The physician or other qualified investigator (with a physician as co-investigator) is usually medical center or hospital based and will be required to fill out FDA forms 1571, 1572, and 1573 among possibly others. This process of how to compile, assemble, complete and submit the physician-sponsored IND has been reviewed broadly and in detail elsewhere (15).

A third pathway is the RDRC approach. Using this mechanism, the FDA delegates authority to a local committee to approve research studies (usually up to 30 patients, although the number can be higher under certain circumstances, for example, if FDA form 2915 is completed). The composition of the membership of that committee has FDA prior approval. Authority is given by this committee to investigators to conduct only phase I and phase II clinical trials, meeting very strict and specific criteria (see below). Under no circumstances are the results from such studies to be used to make clinical decisions for any of the participants in the study until the study is completed and the data are analyzed. In theory, the findings are investigational and remain unproven at this point. It is possible that approved clinical methods used to validate the research finding may be clinically helpful or of benefit to a study participant. For example, the findings from a computed tomography (CT) scan used to study the metabolism and distribution of a new diagnostic radiopharmaceutical such as a radio-labeled monoclonal antibody that was designed to locate a tumor, may find their way to the patient's or subject's medical record, but not information provided by the radiolabeled monoclonal antibody. This RDRC

Table 5.2. Selected reference sites and sources relative to pediatric PET research

Food and Drug Administration (December, 2004)	
Main telephone number	1-888-INFO-FDA
E-mail	http://www.FDA.gov
Drug information telephone number	1-301-827-4570
Pediatric Drug Development (PDD)	1-301-594-PEDS (7337)
E-mail	Pdit@cder.FDA.gov
Division of Drug Imaging and Radiopharmaceutical Drug Products (DMIRPD)	DMIRPD, RDRC Drug Program
E-mail	http://www.FDA.gov/cder/ regulatory/RDRC/default.htm.
Radioactive Drug Research Program	
Address	Food and Drug Administration Center for Drug Evaluation and Research Division of Medical Imaging and Radiopharmaceutical Drug Products HFD-160 Parklawn Building, Room 18R-45 5600 Fishers Lane Rockville, MD 20852 Attention: RDRC Team
Director	George Mills, MD
Senior manager	Capt. Richard Fejka, USPHS, RPh, BCNP
Clinical trials	
Government	http://www.Clinicaltrials.gov
United Healthcare Foundation	http://www.Unitedhealth-carefoundation.org/emb.html
Books	
Kowalsky RJ, Falen SW. *Radiopharmaceuticals in Nuclear Pharmacy,* 2nd ed. Available from the American Pharmaceutical and Nuclear Medicine Association, Washington, D.C. http://www.pharmacist.com/store/cfm	
Clinical evidence by the evidence-based update on more than 1000 medical conditions including clinical trials. British Medical Journal. Free of charge to healthcare professionals. http://www.unitedhealthcarefoundation.org/Emb.html	
Legislative Information Gateway to the Congressional Record and Congressional Committee Information. http://thomas.loc.gov	

Source: Data from refs. 4–13.

approach to conduct PET research in children is the one on which we concentrate in this chapter (6–8,16–18,21).

The Clinical Trial Process

The clinical trial is a biomedical or behavioral research study of human subjects that is designed to answer specific questions about biomedical or behavioral interventions (drugs, treatments, devices, or new ways of using known drugs, treatments, or devices). Clinical trials are used to determine whether new biomedical or behavioral interventions are safe, efficacious, and effective (17,18). Trials of an experimental drug, device, treatment, or intervention may proceed through four distinct phases. Sometimes more than one phase can be conducted at the same time. The actual number of subjects studied in each phase may depend in part on the incidence or prevalence of the disease state or condition being investigated.

Phase I

This phase entails testing in a small group of people (e.g., 20 to 80 subjects) to determine efficacy and evaluate safety (e.g., determine a safe dosage range) and identify side effects. A typical phase I trial of a new drug agent frequently involves relatively high risk to a small number of participants. The investigator and occasionally others have the only relevant knowledge regarding the treatment because these are the first human uses. The study investigator may be required to perform continuous monitoring on participant safety with frequent reporting to institute and center staff with oversight responsibility.

Phase II

This phase entails a study of a larger group of people (several hundred) to determine the efficacy and further evaluate safety. A typical phase II study follows phase I studies, and there is more information regarding risks, benefits, and monitoring procedures. However, more participants are involved, and the disease process confounds the toxicity and outcomes. An institute or center may require monitoring similar to that of a phase I trial or may supplement that level of monitoring with individuals with expertise relevant to the study who might assist in interpreting the data to ensure patient safety (17,18).

Phase III

This phase entails a study to determine the efficacy in large groups of people (from several hundred to several thousand) by comparing the intervention to other standard or experimental interventions, to monitor adverse effects, and to collect information to allow safe use. The definition includes pharmacologic, nonpharmacologic, and behavioral interventions given for disease prevention, prophylaxis, diagnosis, or therapy. Community-based trials and other population-based trials are also included. A phase III trial frequently compares a new treatment to a standard treatment or to no treatment, and treatment allocation may be randomly assigned and the data masked. These studies frequently involve a large number of participants followed for longer periods of treatment exposure. Although short-term risk is usually slight, one must consider the long-term effects of a study agent or achievement of significant safety or efficacy differences between the control and the study groups for the masked study. An institute or center may require a data safety monitoring board (DSMB) to perform monitoring functions. This DSMB would be composed of experts relevant to the study and would regularly assess the trial and offer recommendations to the institute or center concerning its continuation.

Phase IV

This phase entails studies done after the intervention has been marketed. These studies are designed to monitor the effectiveness of the approved intervention in the general population and to collect information about any adverse effects associated with widespread use. The controversy that appeared in the lay media in December 2004 as well as in medical publications (22) concerning adverse events associated with Vioxx and Celebrex is an example of a postmarketing discovery following new drug approval.

Radioactive Drug Research Committee Update Meeting and Transition

After more than a quarter of a century, it became obvious that technologic progress and events had surpassed the intent of the original 1975 FDA, RDRC regulations (6–8,16). During the current transition period (June 2005) and until the updated RDRC regulations are finalized, the 1997 FDA Modernization Act (FDAMA) provides a mechanism for the uninterrupted production of PET radiopharmaceutical by specifying that they should meet United States Pharmacopoeia (USP) monograph standards (23,24). An example of a PET radiopharmaceutical coming through that process was ^{18}F-fluorodeoxyglucose (FDG) injection, which received a new drug approval in less than 6 months after submission on August 5, 2004 (25).

RDRC Update Issues

Six issues or areas of concern, proposed by the FDA/RDRC, were placed on the agenda for discussion (4,5):

1. Pharmacologic issues
2. Radiation dose limits for adult subjects
3. Assurance of safety for pediatric subjects
4. Quality and purity
5. Exclusion of pregnant women
6. RDRC membership

As this chapter is being written, participants at the open meeting and other interested parties and organizations are submitting written comments for the record and for consideration regarding the updated regulations. Who could have predicted in 1975 how to best conduct research or manufacture pharmaceuticals (including radiopharmaceuticals), given the advent of monoclonal antibodies, cloning, stem cells, gene therapy, biologic response modifiers, and the growth of PET and other imaging modalities?

Vulnerable Populations

There are four populations addressed specifically in Title 45 part 46 of the Code of Federal Regulations, which deals with public welfare protection of human subjects (2,19–21):

Subpart A: Human subjects, research subjects, and volunteers as controls or normals

Subpart B: Additional protections for pregnant women, human fetuses, and neonates

Subpart C: Additional protections pertaining to biomedical and behavioral research in prisoners

Subpart D: Additional protections for children as subjects in research (21).

Assurance of Safety for Pediatric Subjects

Currently 21 CFR 361.1 (that FDA section of the code that deals with radiopharmaceutical research in humans) allows the study of radioactive drugs in subjects less than 18 years of age without an IND application, if the following conditions are met:

1. The study presents a unique opportunity to gain information not currently available, requires the use of research subjects less than 18 years of age, is without significant risk, and is supported with review by qualified consultants to the RDRC.
2. The radiation dose does not exceed 10% of the adult radiation dose as specified in 21 CFR 361.1 (b)(i) and, as with adult subjects, the following additional requirements are met:
3. The study is approved by an institutional review board (IRB) that conforms to the requirements of 21 CFR part 56.
4. Informed consent of the subject's legal representative is obtained in accordance with 21 CFR part 50.
5. The study is approved by the RDRC, which assures all other requirements of 21 CFR 361.1 are met (5,16).

Alternatively, when a study is conducted under an IND (as compared to a RDRC) in accordance with part 312 (21 CFR part 312), the sponsor must submit to the FDA the study protocol, protocol changes and information amendments, pharmacology/toxicology and chemistry information, and information regarding prior human experience with the same or similar drugs (see 21 CFR 312.22, 312.33, 312.30 and 312.31). Additionally, 21 CFR 32 requires that sponsors (of the IND) promptly review all information relevant to the safety of the drug obtained or otherwise received by the sponsor by any source, foreign or domestic. This includes information derived from any clinical or epidemiologic experience, reports in the scientific literature and unpublished scientific papers, as well as reports from foreign regulatory authorities. 21 CFR part 32 also requires that sponsors submit IND safety reports to the FDA (4,5).

Pediatric Concerns Considered for Update

Does 21 CFR 361.1 provide adequate safeguards for pediatric subjects during the course of a research project intended to obtain basic information about a radioactive drug, or should these studies be conducted only under an IND?

If we assume that 21 CFR 361.1 provides adequate safeguards for pediatric studies during such studies, given our present knowledge about radiation and its effects, can we conclude that the current dose limits would be appropriate to ensure no significant risk for pediatric participants? Should there be different dose limits for different pediatric groups (5)? At present, it is estimated that only about half of the RDRCs in conjunction with their IRBs consider approval of radioactive drug research in children. The operative phrase appears to be minimal risk.

Protections for Children Involved as Subjects of PET Research

There are three basic areas of concern in using children as PET research subjects: (1) conformity with IRB requirements, (2) radiation dosimetry of not more than 10% of the adult dose and in conformity with ALARA (as low as reasonably achievable) considerations, and (3) special considerations relevant to vulnerable populations (2,5,16,21). Under certain circumstances, the secretary of the Department of Health and Human Services (HHS) may waive some or all of the requirements of these regulations for research of this type (2,21).

Some Additional Protections Addressed in 45 CFR Part 46, Subpart D

To whom do the requirements to carry out the regulations apply?

To whom do the requirements apply as subjects, and who may give assent and grant permission for the children?

What are the IRB responsibilities related to children?

What protections are appropriate for research not involving greater than minimal risk?

What protections are appropriate for research involving greater than minimal risk but presenting the prospect of direct benefit to the individual subjects?

What protections should be required for research involving greater than minimal risk and no prospect of direct benefit to individual subjects but likely to yield generalizable knowledge about the disorder or condition?

What protections should be required for research not otherwise approvable that presents an opportunity to understand, prevent, or alleviate a serious problem affecting the health or welfare of children?

What is the requirement for permission by parents or guardians and for assent by children?

What protections should be required and who grants permission for children who are wards of the State? (21).

RDRC Specific Responsibilities Abstracted from the CFR

This section is taken directly from the minutes of the University of Pittsburgh Medical Center (UPMC) RDRC and Human Use Subcommittee (HUSC), Radiation Safety Committee, Dennis Swanson, M.S., Chairman (26).

In taking this action, the RDRC considered and assured that each of the following criteria were met:

1. The research study is intended to obtain basic information regarding the metabolism (including kinetics, distribution, and localization) of a radioactively labeled drug or regarding human physiology, pathophysiology or biochemistry. The research study is not intended for immediate therapeutic, diagnostic, or similar purposes or to determine the safety and effectiveness of the drug in humans for such purposes.

2. The research study involves the use of a radioactive drug(s), which will be prepared in accordance with a RDRC-approved drug master file or HUSC/RDRC Form 1002. The drug master file of HUSC/RDRC Form 1002 documents:

   a. that the amount of active ingredient or combination of active ingredient shall not cause any clinically detectable pharmacologic effect in humans as known based on pharmacologic dose calculations derived from data available published or other valid human studies;

   b. absorbed dose calculations based on the MIRD formalism and biologic distribution data available from the published literature or from other valid studies;

   c. that an acceptable method will be used to radioassay the drug prior to its use;

   d. that adequate and appropriate instrumentation will be utilized for the detection and measurement of the specific radionuclide;

   e. that the radioactive drug meets appropriate chemical, pharmaceutical, and radionuclidic standards of identity, strength, quality, and purity as determined by suitable testing procedures;

   f. that, for parenteral use, the radioactive drug is prepared in a sterile and pyrogen free form; and

   g. that the package and labeling of the radioactive drug is in compliance with the requirements of 21 CFR 361.1 and NRC (if applicable) and Commonwealth of Pennsylvania regulations regarding radioactive drugs.

3. For this specific research protocol:

   a. Scientific knowledge and benefit is likely to result from this study;
      — The proposed research is based on sound rationale derived from the published literature or other valid studies.
      — The proposed research is of sound design.

b. The radiation dose is sufficient and no greater than necessary to obtain valid data.
  — In consideration of available radioactive drugs, the radioactive drug used in the study has the combination of half-life, type of radiation, radiation energy, metabolism, and chemical properties that results in the lowest radiation dosimetry as needed to obtain the necessary information.
  — For adult subjects: the projected radiation dose to the whole body effective dose equivalent (EDE), active blood-forming organs, lens of eye, and gonads does not exceed 3 rem (single study) or 5 rem (annual and total dose), and the projected radiation dose to any other organ does not exceed 5 rem (single study) or 15 rem (annual and total dose).
  — For subjects under the age of 18 (if applicable), the projected radiation dose does not exceed 10% of the adult limits.
  — The projected radiation dose commitments address expected radionuclidic contaminants and x-ray and other radiation-emitting procedures performed as part of the research study.
c. The projected number of subjects is sufficient and no greater than necessary for the purpose of the study as supported by a statistical or other valid justification;
d. The proposed population is appropriate to the purpose of the study; and
  — The involvement of subjects less than 18 years of age, if applicable, is justified as (1) presenting a unique opportunity to gain information not currently available; and (2) necessitating the use of such subjects. The scientific review of research involving subjects less than 18 years of age is supported by qualified pediatric consultants to the RDRC.
  — Pregnancy testing, to confirm absence of pregnancy prior to administration of the radioactive drug(s), is performed on female subjects of childbearing potential.
e. The investigators are qualified by training and experience to conduct the proposed research study.
  — The research study involves, as a listed co-investigator, a physician "authorized user" recognized by the Radiation Safety Committee, University of Pittsburgh, as qualified to oversee the preparation, handling and use of the radioactive drug (26).

Illustrative Examples that Have Come to the UPMC-RDRC Requiring Directed Change, Correction, or Reconsideration

1. Not including the gallium-68 rod transmission scan to calibrate the PET scanner as part of the radiation dosimetry.
2. Submitting a phase III clinical trial to the RDRC.

3. Submitting an appropriate research protocol and informed consent for a study using ^{18}F-FDG to the IRB, but not the RDRC.

4. Inappropriate expression of radiation dose and risk to the patient in the informed consent. The UPMC has adopted a uniform radiation risk statement model which it recommends be used in both the consent and protocol, although other statements are also acceptable, for example, "Participation in this research study involves exposure to radiation from the two PET transmission scans, the one 12 mCi (a unit of radioactivity dosage) injection of [15-O] water, one 15-mCi dose of [11-C]WAY, and one 10-mCi injection of [11-C]raclopride. The amount of radiation exposure you will receive from these procedures is equivalent to a whole-body radiation dose of 0.47 rem (a unit of radiation exposure). This is less than 10% of the annual whole-body radiation exposure (5 rem) permitted to radiation workers by federal regulations. There is no minimum level of radiation exposure that is recognized as being totally free of the risk of causing genetic defects (cell abnormalities) or cancer. However, the risk associated with the amount of radiation exposure that you will receive from this study is considered to be low and similar to other everyday risks" (26).

5. While using magnetic resonance imaging (MRI) for co-registration with PET, performing the PET scan before MRI. A certain number of MRI subjects will be eliminated or withdrawn due to claustrophobia. If this is the case, then they have been exposed to the radiation dose unnecessarily.

6. A patient has a pregnancy test at a screening session 1 month prior to a research PET scan. The pregnancy test is due to the research nature of the PET scan. The pregnancy test should be conducted as close as possible to the time that the PET scan is scheduled; within 48 hours of PET.

7. A patient has a pacemaker and is going to have an MRI prior to a PET study. If there is a question of metal or metal fragment being attracted by the magnets, then an x-ray may be required. The x-ray is required as part of the research and thus should be included as part of the dosimetry table and consent.

8. A new drug that has been tested in thousands of mice to treat memory loss is to be trace radiolabeled and administered to humans as part of a multicenter trial of 50 patients at each site. Because the drug has never been given to a human (lack of a pharmacologic effect cannot be substantiated), and is a multicenter study with over 30 patients, it is best conducted under an IND. Even for a radiopharmaceutical, the mass of the administered radiolabeled compound currently must be quantified.

9. A physician wants to test a brachytherapy unit on his patients who have a tumor different from the one for which the FDA gave initial approval. There are 10 patients and he is comparing two types of seeds in two different cell types. This should not be submitted to the RDRC, but should be reviewed by the Human Use Subcommittee. The holder of the IND is a manufacturer of a radiation device.

10. A study comes before the RDRC that is so complicated that the members of the committee don't believe it can be carried out without losing data. The project is sent back for reconsideration because if the

data cannot be analyzed in a meaningful way, then subjects will have been exposed unnecessarily.

References

1. Fostering a culture of compliance. National Institutes of Health education and outreach seminar. Pittsburgh, July 15, 2004.
2. Administering and overseeing clinical research. Title 45 Public welfare. Part 46 Protection of human subjects. Revised November 13, 2001. Effective December 13, 2001. Subpart A—Federal policy for the protection of human subjects. Basic DHHS policy for the protection of human research subjects. In: Fostering a Culture of Compliance. National Institutes of Health education and outreach seminar. Pittsburgh, PA, July 15, 2004. http://ohrp.osophs.dhhs.gov/humansubjects/guidance/45cfr46. htm.
3. Fostering a culture of compliance. National Institutes of Health education and outreach seminar. Code of Federal Regulations. The common rule (Federal Regulations). Pittsburgh, PA, July 15, 2004. http://ohrp.osophs. dhhs.gov/ human subjects/guidance/45cfr46.htm.
4. Notice of public meeting—radioactive drugs for certain research uses. Radioactive Drug Research Committee (RDRC) program. Rockville, MD, November 16,2004. http://www.fda.gov/cder/regulatory/RDRC/ default.htm.
5. Agenda of public meeting—radioactive drugs for certain research uses. Radioactive Drug Research Committee (RDRC) program minutes. Rockville, MD, November 16, 2004. http://www.fda.gov/cder/meeting/ clinicalresearch/default.htm.
6. Positron emission tomography (PET) related documents. http://www. fda.gov/cder/regulatory/PET/default.htm.
7. What information does the RDRC review? Radioactive Drug Research Committee (RDRC) program. http://www.fda.gov/cder/regulatory/RDRC/ review.htm.
8. What are the responsibilities of the RDRC? Radioactive drug research committee (RDRC) program. http://www.fda.gov/cder/regulatory/RDRC/ Responsibilities.htm.
9. http://grants.nih.gov/grants/guide/notice-files/not98–084.html.
10. Having trouble keeping up with clinical trials? APhA-AAPM news you can use 4(2), October 28, 2004. http://www.pharmacist.com. Info-center@ apha.org.
11. Kowalsky RJ, Falen SW. Radiopharmaceuticals in Nuclear Pharmacy and Nuclear Medicine, 2nd ed. Washington, DC: APhA, 2004. http://www. Pharmacist.com/store.cfm.
12. Clinical evidence to help support the clinician's skillful use of scientifically valid and evidence based information. http://Unitedhealth carefoundation.org.ebm.html.
13. How do I find and track bills? Health Physics News 2005;33(1):3. http:// www.hps.org.
14. FDA meeting to focus on radioactive drugs for basic research. APhA-AAPM electronic newsletter. http://www.apha.net.org.
15. Levine G, Abel N. Considerations in the assembly and submission of the physician sponsored investigational new drug application. In: Hladik WB, Saha GB, Study KT, eds. Essentials of Nuclear Medicine Science. Baltimore: Williams & Wilkins, 1987:357–386.

16. Pediatric drug development. http://www.fda.gov/cder/pediatrics/index. htm.

17. NIH grants-general information glossary (NIH-grants policy statement, revised 12/01/03. In: Fostering a Culture of Compliance. National Institutes of Health education and outreach seminar. Pittsburgh, PA, July 15, 2004:6–15. http://www.grants.nih.gov/grants/terms_.htm.

18. NIH guide: NIH policy for data and safety monitoring, release date June 10, 1998. In: Fostering a Culture of Compliance. National Institutes of Health education and outreach seminar. Pittsburgh, PA, July 15, 2004. http://grants.nih.gov/grants/guide/notice-files/not98–084.html.

19. Administering and overseeing clinical research. Title 45 Public welfare. Part 46 Protection of human subjects. Revised November 13,2001. Effective December 13, 2001. Subpart B—additional protections for pregnant women, human fetuses and neonates involved in research. In: Fostering a Culture of Compliance. National Institutes of Health education and outreach seminar. Pittsburgh, PA, July 15, 2004. http://ohrp.osophs.dhhs. gov./humansubjects/guidance/45cfr46.htm.

20. Administering and overseeing clinical research. Title 45 Public welfare. Part 46 Protection of human subjects. Revised November 13, 2001. Effective December 13, 2001. Subpart C—additional protections pertaining to biomedical and behavioral research involving prisoners as subjects in research. In: Fostering a Culture of Compliance. National Institutes of Health education and outreach seminar. Pittsburgh, PA. July 15, 2004. http://ohrp.osophs.dhhs.gov/humansubjects/guidance/45cfr46.htm.

21. Administering and overseeing clinical research. Title 45 Public welfare. Part 46 Protection of human subjects. Revised November 13, 2001. Effective December 13, 2001. Subpart D—additional DHHS protections for children involved as subjects in research. In: Fostering a Culture of Compliance. National Institutes of Health education and outreach seminar. Pittsburgh, PA, July 15, 2004. http://ohrp.sosphs.dhhs.gov/humansubjects/ guidance/45cfr46.htm.

22. COX-2 inhibitors under scrutiny in wake of Rofecoxib withdrawal. APhA Drug Info Line 2004;1–2.

23. Food and Drug Administration Modernization Act of 1997. Title 21. Section 121. Positron emission tomography. http://www.fda.gov/cder/ regulatory/Pet/petlaw.html.

24. Radiopharmaceuticals for positron emission tomography-compounding. Chapter 823. US Pharmacopeia 20/National Formulary 25, 2002.

25. Update—new fludeoxyglucose F-18 injection PET drug approved in less than 6 months. http://fda.gov/cder/regulatory/pet/Fludeoxyglucose. htm.

26. Swanson DP. Radioactive drug research committee/human use subcommittee meeting minutes. University of Pittsburgh. Pittsburgh, PA, November 17, 2004.

6

Issues in the Institutional Review Board Review of PET Scan Protocols

Robert M. Nelson

The lack of reliable information on the use of medications for children has been addressed in the United States through two legislative initiatives: the Best Pharmaceuticals for Children Act (BPCA) of 2002 (1) and the Pediatric Research Equity Act (PREA) of 2003 (2). These two initiatives have stimulated pediatric pharmaceutical research, resulting in valuable information to guide the appropriate use of many medications (3). In addition, the National Institutes of Health now requires (as of 1998) that children be included in research unless there are scientific and ethical reasons not to include them (4). The resulting increase in pediatric research has led to concerns that the regulations governing pediatric research provide insufficient protection. This chapter refers to only the Food and Drug Administration (FDA) regulations governing research with children (21 CFR 50 and 56), as the use of radiopharmaceuticals in PET scanning is regulated by the FDA. Comparable regulations are found in 45 CFR 46, subparts A and D.

The FDA did not adopt additional safeguards for children in research (referred to as subpart D) until April 2001 (5). In passing the BPCA, the U.S. Congress also commissioned the Institute of Medicine (IOM) to review the adequacy of subpart D; their report was issued in March 2004. The IOM found that there are problems in the application of subpart D due to insufficient guidance and thus variable interpretation of key concepts (6).

The additional safeguards for children in research found in subpart D can be viewed as a further specification of the general requirement that the "risks to subjects are reasonable in relation to anticipated benefits, if any, to subjects, and the importance of the knowledge that may be expected to result" (21 CFR 56.111.a.2). Absent the prospect of direct benefit, the research risks to which children may be exposed must be restricted to either minimal risk (21 CFR 50.51) or a minor increase over minimal risk (21 CFR 50.53), depending on whether the children have the disorder or condition under investigation (5). If there is a prospect of direct benefit from the research intervention, the research risk must be justified by the anticipated benefit to the enrolled children (rather than by any knowledge that may result) (21 CFR 50.52) (5,7). Thus, to determine whether a research protocol involving children may proceed, an institutional review board (IRB) must assess (1) the level of risk, and (2) the prospect of direct benefit to the child presented by each research intervention or procedure (7).

This chapter examines the use of positron emission tomography (PET) scanning in research involving children from the perspective of the additional safeguards found in subpart D. The risks of the two major components of PET scanning (i.e., administration of the radiopharmaceutical tracer and procedural sedation) are discussed within this regulatory framework governing pediatric research. In the course of the analysis, key concepts from the pediatric research regulations that will be discussed include the component analysis of risk, minimal risk, minor increase over minimal risk, and disorder or condition (6). Finally, the relationship between subpart D(5) and other FDA regulations concerning the investigational use of radiopharmaceuticals (21 CFR 312 and 21 CFR 361.1) is discussed.

Component Analysis of Risk

The risks (i.e., potential harms) and benefits of each intervention or procedure included in a research protocol must be assessed independently. The potential benefits from one procedure should not be used to offset or justify the risks of another (IOM recommendation 4.6) (6). The application of this principle is fairly straightforward when the performance of one procedure does not depend on or require the performance of the other procedure. However, when the two procedures are dependent on each other, the analysis is more complex. In the case of a PET scan, the key procedural components for the purpose of risk analysis are the administration of the radioactive tracer and the necessary procedural sedation. Other risks such as the physical environment (e.g., an enclosed space and the possibility of claustrophobia) are less than those associated with computed tomography (CT) or magnetic resonance imaging (MRI) scans, as the child can be accompanied (and reassured) by a parent during the entire procedure. All of the other necessary procedures (e.g., venipuncture, placement of a peripheral intravenous catheter) are appropriately considered minimal risk given the limited duration (i.e., less than 2 hours) of a PET scan. Thus, the following discussion is limited to the risks of the radiotracer administration and procedural sedation.

Procedural sedation is usually required for the successful completion of the PET scan, given the need to reduce motion artifact. Thus, for the purpose of IRB analysis, the administration of the radiotracer, and the risk or benefit of radiation exposure, is the key component of the PET scan. If the PET scan, and thus the radiotracer administration, offers the prospect of direct benefit to the child undergoing the procedure, the radiation risks to which the child may be exposed can be greater than minimal risk assuming that the balance of potential harms and anticipated benefits is justified and comparable to any available alternatives (21 CFR 50.52) (5). As such, the risks of any procedural sedation necessary to complete the PET scan become part of this balancing of risks and benefits. However, if the PET scan does not offer the prospect of direct benefit to the child undergoing the procedure, the risks of the radiation exposure and any necessary procedural sedation must be no more than a minor increase over minimal risk for children with a disorder or condition (21 CFR 50.53) or no more than minimal risk for children without a disorder or condition (21 CFR 50.51) (5). In effect, the level of appropriate (and allowable) risk exposure associated with the procedural sedation depends on whether or not the results of the PET scan offer the child a prospect of direct benefit. A common mistake is to determine that the risk of a procedure that does not offer any prospect of direct benefit is no more than a minor increase over minimal risk but to fail to appreciate that the risks of any associated procedures must also be similarly restricted.

Administration of Radioactive Tracers

The risks of administering a radiopharmaceutical tracer can be divided into two aspects: (1) the risk from the compound to which the radioactive tracer is attached, and (2) the risk from the level of radiation exposure associated with the tracer. The risk from the compound itself is independent of the radiation risk and are discussed below (see Research Under an Investigational New Drug Application). The discussion here focuses on the general risks of radiation, and not on how one would determine the actual effective dose (ED) of radiation exposure to any given organ from individual radiopharmaceuticals. The scientific determination of the level of radiation exposure for any given radiopharmaceutical depends on such factors as the targeted receptor, blood flow to the area of interest, isotope and carrier compound half-life, mechanisms of metabolism and excretion, and so forth (8–10).

The Risks of Radiation Exposure

The data derived from atomic bomb survivors in Japan are the best available on the effects of ionizing radiation on a large human population (11). These data support the view that "the risk of solid cancers appears to be a linear function of dose" (12), perhaps down to a dose of about 5 rad (i.e., 5 rem) (12,13). Some argue that there is direct evidence of risk at low-level radiation exposure in the range of 600 mrem to 10 rem (13,14). Others place the lower limit of the range at which low-level ionizing radiation increases the risk of some cancers at 1 rem for acute exposure and 5 rem for protracted exposure (15). However, the risk of cancer is probably overestimated using these data, as "cancer rates may vary . . . due to other risk factors correlated with the exposure under investigation" (13).

The predominant model for describing the risks of low-level radiation (i.e., less than 10 rem) is the linear no-threshold (LNT) model. This theoretical model is based on two assumptions: "(a) any radiation dose can produce adverse effects such as cancer or genetic damage; [and] (b) the severity of adverse effects is directly proportional to the radiation dose received" (16). In support of this model, the dose-response relationship between low-level radiation and "the biological alterations that are precursors to cancer, such as mutations and chromosome aberrations," appears to be linear (17). Although the LNT model is the customary approach, "existing data do not exclude the possibility that there may be thresholds for such effects in the low-dose domain" (17).

The dose-response relationship between low-level radiation exposure and the risk of developing cancer cannot be precisely defined by extrapolating from observations at moderate-to-high doses (15,17). As a result, there is considerable debate about whether low-level radiation (i.e., less than 10 rem) increases the risk of developing cancer, with the data concerning the risk of low-level radiation exposure subject to wide interpretation (19,20). In addition, some data support the view that low-level radiation exposure may be protective (12,16,18–20). This possibility of "adaptive responses" (i.e., hormesis) further complicates the "assessment of the dose-response relationships for the genetic and carcinogenic effects of low-level irradiation" (17).

Critics argue that the LNT theory "grossly overestimates the risk from low-level radiation". In addition, no "statistically sound well-designed studies" (20) support the use of the LNT model at low-level radiation doses (16,20). The confidence limits from epidemiologic studies of the dose-response relationship of low-level radiation exposure are sufficiently wide "to be consistent with an increased effect, a decreased effect, or no effect" (20). Overall, "the health risk from low-level doses could not be detected above the 'noise' of adverse events of everyday life" (16). Proponents of the LNT theory, however, point out that the failure to find an increase in cancer, and the observation of a reduction in some instances, among populations exposed to low-level radiation does not contradict the LNT theory given the small increase that would be expected and the methodologic limitations of the studies. These limits are such that "it may never be possible to prove or disprove the validity of the LNT hypothesis" (17). However, there are no data that "suggest a threshold dose below which radiation exposure does not cause cancer" (21) nor "reliable data proving that radiation doses as used in diagnostic x-rays do induce cancer" (11).

In summary, there are three general views of the risk of low-level radiation exposure: (1) the relationship between potential harm and effective radiation dose is linear, with no level of radiation exposure being nonharmful (i.e., LNT model); (2) there is a threshold level of radiation below which there is no harm, with a linear relationship between potential harm and effective radiation dose above this threshold (i.e., threshold model); and (3) there is a threshold level of radiation below which there is benefit from enhanced cellular repair (i.e., hormesis model), with a linear relationship above this threshold. Below 1 rem effective radiation dose, there are no data that will discriminate among these three models. Between 1 and 5 rem effective radiation dose, the data are controversial, with the LNT model being the more favored approach. Above 5 to 10 rem, the linear relationship between potential harms and ED is generally accepted (with some difference of opinion on the lower limit of the range of this linear relationship).

Characterizing the Risks of Radiation

What level of radiation exposure should be considered "minimal risk" in light of the above data? Minimal risk is defined as follows: "The probability and magnitude of harm or discomfort anticipated in the research are not greater in and of themselves than those ordinarily encountered in daily life or during the performance of routine physical or psychological examinations or tests" (21 CFR 56.102i). Given the variability in the interpretation of minimal risk (22), the IOM recommended that minimal risk be interpreted "in relation to the normal experiences of average, healthy, normal children" (recommendation 4.1) (6). Children may be exposed to ionizing radiation during diagnostic radiologic studies; however, no such studies are performed as part of routine physical examinations of healthy children. Absent a disorder or condition, such as an injury, the interpretive standard of a healthy child appears to exclude diagnostic radiation exposure. However, children are exposed to background radiation from natural sources that ranges from 300 to 450 mrem per year depending on the altitude at which they live (19). Children are also exposed to additional radiation during such normal activities as air travel. Given the absence of data suggesting an increase in cancer at altitude, a one-time exposure to ionizing radiation that falls in the range of yearly environmental exposure would appear to qualify as minimal risk.

The IOM also recommended that the risks of research could be considered minimal if they were equivalent to the risks "that average, healthy, normal children may encounter in their daily lives or experience in routine physical or psychological examinations or tests" (recommendation 4.1) (6). Studies of radiation exposure from "background radiation, radon in homes, medical procedures, and occupational radiation in large population samples" have not demonstrated any additional health risks "above the 'noise' of adverse events of everyday life" (16). This conclusion is supported by the observation that "exposure to 1 rem [only] adds about 100 more genetic mutations" to the "average of 240,000 genetic mutations [that] occur spontaneously every day in the human body" (16). Although younger children are thought to be more susceptible to radiation-induced cancer (23), two reviews concluded that there are no data demonstrating higher risk to children of exposure to low-level radiation (14,16). What is the threshold level of radiation exposure which, if one remains below, could be considered minimal risk?

Proponents of the LNT interpretation of low-level radiation risk express concern that adopting the view of a radiation threshold below which the risk is zero may undermine efforts to minimize radiation exposure (12,19). Others argue that the LNT model imposes an undue regulatory burden that "is detrimental to the welfare of our society" (20). The minimal-risk standard does not require that the risks of the research be zero but rather that the risks be no different from those that are experienced by healthy children in the course of everyday life. One possible choice for the level of radiation exposure that presents no more than minimal risk can be taken from the 1996 Health Physics Society statement that the health risks from exposure up to 10 rem is "either too small to be observed or nonexistent" (24). A more conservative approach, taking into account more recently published data (12), would reduce the radiation level at which there is unobservable, and thus minimal, risk to 1 rem exposure (25). This approach is consistent with published research studies involving the exposure of healthy children to ionizing radiation that have been approved by an IRB (16).

Allowable Research Risk for Children with Conditions

Subpart D allows researchers to expose children with a disorder or condition to more than minimal risk, provided (among other conditions) that "the risk represents a minor increase over minimal risk" and "the intervention or procedure is likely to yield generalizable knowledge . . . that is of vital importance for the understanding or amelioration of the subjects' disorder or condition" (5). The IOM report recommends that a "minor increase over minimal risk" be interpreted "to mean a *slight increase* in the potential for harms or discomfort beyond minimal risk" (recommendation 4.2, emphasis added) (6). Based on the above discussion of the risks of radiation exposure, one could consider low-level radiation exposure falling between 1 and 5 rem as presenting only a minor increase over minimal risk. Even so, exposure to this level of radiation during research that does not offer the prospect of direct benefit is only justified if (a) the child has a disorder or condition, and (b) the research is likely to yield knowledge that is of "vital importance" for understanding or ameliorating the child's disorder or condition.

There are no guidelines on how to interpret the phrase "vital importance." At a minimum, the enrollment of children should be necessary (i.e., vital) to answer the research question (26). In addition, the requirement of having a disorder or condition should not be interpreted so broadly as to encompass all children. The IOM report recommends that "the term condition should be interpreted as referring to a specific (or a set of specific) physical, psychological, neurodevelopmental, or social characteristic(s) that an *established body of scientific evidence* or clinical knowledge has shown to *negatively affect children's health and well-being* or to increase their risk of developing a health problem in the future" (recommendation 4.3, emphasis added) (6). A normal stage of child development could be considered a condition provided that evidence exists that our lack of understanding of this condition may negatively affect children's health and well-being, perhaps through the use of an inappropriate medication dose. However, the inclusion of healthy children as a control group (i.e., those lacking the disorder or condition being studied) would not meet this standard. The exposure of children with a disorder or condition to greater research risk than other children has been the subject of criticism (27). The ethical justification of such exposure is not that children with a disorder or condition are otherwise exposed to greater risk. Rather, the exposure to greater risk (although limited to a slight increase over minimal risk) is justified by the necessity of such exposure to achieve vitally important scientific knowledge (26). Although exposing children without a disorder or condition to a minor increase over minimal risk in research would require review by a federal panel (7), the scientific necessity of such exposure is one of the "sound ethical principles" required for approval (21 CFR 50.54) (5).

Prospect of Direct Benefit

Children enrolled in research may be exposed to more than a minor increase over minimal risk provided that the intervention or procedure offers the prospect of direct benefit, "the risk is justified by the anticipated benefit" to the enrolled children, and "the relation of the anticipated benefit to the risk is at least as favorable to the subjects as that presented by available alternative approaches" (21 CFR 50.52) (5). For example, PET scanning may be a useful diagnostic test for localization of lesions such as tumors or collections of abnormal pancreatic islet cells when structural studies alone (i.e., CT or MRI scans) may not be sufficient (28). The risks of radiation from radiotracer administration would then be balanced by the benefits of a more appropriate clinical or surgical intervention and be comparable to the alternatives such as selective angiography or transhepatic portal venous sampling (in the case of insulin-secreting pancreatic islet cell tumors) (29). Absent direct benefit, or a justified balance of potential harms and benefits, the risks of the radiation exposure would need to be limited to no more than a minor increase over minimal risk. Although a restriction of radiation exposure to less than 5 rem likely would not prove limiting to research using PET scanning (30), the approach to procedural sedation would vary depending on the category of IRB approval (as discussed below).

Adequate Provisions for Parental Permission

Subpart D also requires that "adequate provisions are made for soliciting the assent of children and the permission of their parents or guardians." The child's assent can be waived only if the child is not capable of assent (e.g., too young or cognitively delayed) or the research offers a prospect of direct benefit that is not available outside of the research (21 CFR 50.55) (5). Setting aside the question of child assent, communicating the risks of low-level radiation exposure to parents is particularly challenging given the controversy over the interpretation of the data. At EDs below 1 rem (and some would argue below 5 rem), a consent document could state the following: "There is no evidence that radiation doses in the range that you will experience in this research cause any harm above that caused by the background radiation you experience every day." For higher doses where the assumption of the linearity of risk has greater merit, risks can be communicated in either numerical terms or in days of life lost. For example, in numerical terms: "Participation in this research study will increase your chances of getting cancer (dying) by 2/1000" (for a 5-rem ED exposure). Alternatively, this same risk can be expressed as 11 days of life lost over the next 15 years. The variation in background radiation over the course of 70 years is 7 rem (i.e., ±100 mrem per year), suggesting that this estimated difference of 11 days may be undetectable when compared to the effects of natural background radiation over the course of a lifetime (31). Thus, at the doses that may be considered to present minimal risk (<1 rem) or a minor increase over minimal risk (<5 rem), the consent document should reflect that the evidence to date shows no increase in the risks of radiation exposure when compared to natural background radiation.

Procedural Sedation for PET Scans

A child must remain still for the duration of a PET scan, which can range from 15 to 30 minutes or more. Thus children (especially young children) will need to receive some sedation to ensure that motion artifact does not undercut the quality of the PET scan. Depending on the type of scan and radiopharmaceutical used, the tracer may need to be administered prior to the sedation. The risks of procedural sedation thus need to be considered when evaluating the appropriateness of the PET scan.

The level of appropriate risk exposure during procedural sedation depends on whether the PET scan offers the prospect of direct benefit. If the PET scan offers the prospect of direct benefit, the procedural sedation may present more than minimal risk and should be performed in such a way that the PET scan is completed successfully. The risks of the procedural sedation should be minimized while a sufficient level of sedation is achieved to ensure a successful scan. If the PET scan does not offer the prospect of direct benefit, the risks of the procedural sedation must be restricted to only a minor increase over minimal risk. Children who are at increased risk from sedation (such as those with a difficult airway) should be excluded. The drugs used should have a wide therapeutic window between the dose necessary to achieve the needed level of sedation (i.e., without the loss of protective airway reflexes) and the risk of upper airway compromise and respiratory depression. Absent direct benefit, the end point of procedural sedation is to restrict risk even if the scan must be canceled due to an inadequate level of sedation. Finally, the provision of procedural sedation does not meet the criteria of minimal risk, thus restricting the performance of a nonbeneficial PET scan in children lacking a disorder or condition to those capable of remaining still without sedation for the necessary scanning time.

Investigational Use of Radiopharmaceuticals

The investigational use of a radiopharmaceutical may proceed under one of three FDA regulations: (1) the limited use of a radiopharmaceutical for basic research under the local jurisdiction of an authorized Radioactive Drug Review Research Committee (RDRC) (21 CFR 361.1), (2) the investigational use of a radiopharmaceutical that is exempt from the requirements for an investigational new drug (IND) application (21 CFR 312.2), or (3) the investigational use of a radiopharmaceutical under an IND application (21 CFR 312). In all three cases, the research use of the radiopharmaceutical must be reviewed by an IRB. In the first case under 21 CFR 361.1, the FDA has authorized the local RDRC to approve the "research only" use of a radioactive drug under specified conditions that classify the drug as "generally recognized as safe and effective." Otherwise the radioactive drug is considered to be an investigational new drug.

Local RDRC Review and Approval

A local RDRC may approve the use of a radioactive drug in a basic research protocol if (1) the administered compound (absent the radioactive material) is "safe and effective," and (2) the radiation dose is below specified levels. The drug may be "generally recognized as safe and effective" only when the "amount of . . . active ingredients to be administered shall be known not to cause any clinically detectable pharmacological effect in human beings . . . based on data available from published literature or from other valid human studies." Alternatively, "the total amount of active ingredients including the radionuclide shall be known not to exceed the dose limitations" under an IND application or the approved drug labeling (21 CFR 361.1). In effect, an RDRC cannot approve the use of a radioactive drug (even in trace amounts) without the knowledge gained from previous testing in humans under an IND application. The second condition is that the radiation dose fall below specified limits. For adults, the radiation dose must remain below 3 rem for a single dose or 5 rem for an annual and total dose to the "whole body, active blood-forming organs, lens of the eye, and gonads," and 5 rem for a single dose and 15 rem for an annual and total dose to "other organs." For research involving children less than 18 years of age, the radiation dose should not exceed 10% of these levels, e.g., 300 mrem and 500 mrem for a single dose to the "whole body, active blood-forming organs, lens of the eye, and gonads" and "other organs," respectively (21 CFR 361.1). The RDRC is not authorized to approve the use of radiation doses above these levels, but must refer the protocol to the FDA.

The radiation limits for local RDRC approval bear no relationship to the levels of radiation exposure that an IRB may approve under subpart D as either minimal risk or a minor increase over minimal risk. An IRB may approve, for example, a PET scan with an effective dose of 560 mrem in a 5-year-old child (30) under 21 CFR 50.53 (i.e., a minor increase over minimal risk given the procedural sedation necessary for preventing motion artifact), even though an RDRC would refer the research protocol to the FDA. Some investigators have argued for an increase in the upper limit on radiation exposure to be an effective dose of 2 rem for a single dose and 5 rem for an annual and total research-related dose for children with cancer and other chronic life-threatening diseases (32). However, these levels of radiation exposure may be approved by an IRB under 21 CFR 50.52 (absent direct benefit) or 21 CFR 50.53 (with direct benefit), provided that the radiopharmaceutical is considered under the IND regulations. Thus the regulatory hurdle per se is not the radiation limits of RDRC approval, but the requirement for an IND application (or exemption) under 21 CFR 312.

There are some additional criteria for RDRC approval under 21 CFR 361.1, including the following: (1) the amount and type of radioactive material that is administered should be the smallest amount necessary to perform the study; (2) the radiation exposure should be justified by the quality and importance of the resulting information; and (3) the study meets other requirements regarding qualifications of the investigator, proper licensure for handling radioactive materials, selection and consent of research subjects, quality and purity of radioactive drugs used, research protocol design, reporting of adverse reactions, and approval by an appropriate IRB. All of these additional requirements are consistent with the general criteria for IRB approval of research found in 21 CFR 56.111. In addition, for a research protocol involving children to be approved by an RDRC, the study must present "a unique opportunity to gain information not currently available," involve no "significant risk," and require the use of children to answer the scientific question. These additional RDRC protections for research involving children are also consistent with the safeguards of subpart D, provided that "no significant risk" is interpreted to mean no more than a minor increase over minimal risk. Finally, the RDRC is required to submit an annual report of all locally approved protocols to the FDA. When a protocol involves children (i.e., subjects less than 18 years of age), this report needs to be submitted immediately upon approval (21 CFR 361.1).

Research Under an Investigational New Drug Application

The investigational use of a radioactive drug falls under the IND regulations (21 CFR 312) if it does not meet the criteria for local RDRC approval as "generally recognized as safe and effective." A clinical investigation involving a drug product that is "lawfully marketed in the United States" is exempt from the requirement for an IND application if (among other requirements) (1) the study is not intended to support a new indication, any other significant change in drug labeling, or product advertising; and (2) the study "does not involve a route of administration or dosage level or use in a patient population or other factor that significantly increases the risks (or decreases the acceptability of the risks) associated with the use of the drug product" (21 CFR 312.2). As of January 2005, the only PET tracer that has been approved by the FDA is fluorine-18 fluorodeoxyglucose (^{18}F-FDG) injection (33). The only approved pediatric indication is for localization of seizure foci in epilepsy. The recommended dose of 2.6 mCi would result in an estimated absorbed radiation dose to the urinary bladder (as the organ with the highest exposure across all age groups) of 11.2 rem in a newborn (3.4 kg), 4.4 rem in a 1-year-old (9.8 kg), 2.4 rem in a 5-year-old (19 kg), 1.6 rem in a 10-year-old (32 kg), and 1.0 rem in a 15-year-old (57 kg) (33). It is conceivable that an IRB could determine that the investigational use of ^{18}F-FDG within these dosage guidelines would not require an IND application (assuming all of the conditions of 21 CFR 312.2 are met), even for other pediatric indications. However, an IND would be required for all other PET drugs.

The requirement for an IND application as part of pediatric PET drug development creates both a regulatory and financial burden. It is unlikely that 21 CFR 312 and 21 CFR 361.1 will be revised to alter the limits on local RDRC approval or the requirements for an IND for PET drug development. However, there may be some flexibility available to the FDA in determining the necessary preclinical database for allowing the initial human testing of PET drugs. For example, the European Agency for the Evaluation of Medicinal Products (EMEA) issued in 2003 a position paper on the nonclinical safety studies necessary to support clinical trials with a single microdose of a PET drug (34). A "microdose" is defined as less than 1% of the dose of the test substance that is expected to yield a pharmacologic effect up to a maximum dose of 100 µg. The EMEA proposal would simplify the preclinical safety studies necessary to justify the first human use to an extended single-dose toxicity study in one nonhuman species and genotoxicity studies (34). As yet the FDA has not issued guidance that would establish an exploratory IND process for PET radiopharmaceuticals under 21 CFR 312.

Conclusion

The empirical data on the effects of low-level radiation exposure support the view that an ED of less than 1 rem is minimal risk and an ED of between 1 and 5 rem is a minor increase over minimal risk. If the PET scan is being performed for research purposes only and offers no direct benefit to the child subject, the radiation ED should be limited to below 1 rem (for healthy children) and to below 5 rem (for children with the disorder or condition under study). If the PET scan offers the prospect of direct benefit, the level (and risks) of radiation exposure that may be justified is balanced against the benefits of the information for the child subject (as would be the case for any radiation exposure during the provision of clinical care).

An IRB must consider the risks of different approaches to procedural sedation and of the stable isotope compound carrying the radioactive tracer, before making a decision about the overall acceptability of the research under subpart D. Absent the prospect of direct benefit from the PET scan, the risks of procedural sedation and the stable isotope compound need to be limited to a minor increase over minimal risk for children with a disorder or condition for the research to be approvable under 21 CFR 50.53 (5). The need for any procedural sedation disqualifies the research from being considered minimal risk (21 CFR 50.51) (5). Some stable isotope compounds would present no more than minimal risk, such as naturally existing metabolic compounds and compounds administered with microdosing techniques (34). If the PET scan offers the prospect of direct benefit, the risks of procedural sedation and the stable isotope carrier compound need to be considered in the overall balancing of the risks and potential benefits of the research (21 CFR 50.52) (5).

References

1. Best Pharmaceuticals for Children Act. Public Law 107-109. In: 115 Stat. 107th Congress. 2002:1408–1424.
2. Pediatric Research Equity Act of 2003. Public Law 108-155. In: 117 Stat. 108th Congress. 2003:1936–1943.
3. Roberts R, Rodriguez W, Murphy D, Crescenzi T. Pediatric drug labeling: improving the safety and efficacy of pediatric therapies. JAMA 2003;290(7): 905–911.
4. National Institutes of Health. NIH Policy and Guidelines on the Inclusion of Children as Participants in Research Involving Human Subjects. March 6, 1998. http://grants.nih.gov/grants/guide/notice-files/not98-024.html.
5. Food and Drug Administration. 21 CFR Parts 50 and 56: Additional Safeguards for Children in Clinical Investigations of FDA Regulated Products. Federal Register 2001;66(79):20589–20600.
6. Field MJ, Behrman RE, eds. Ethical Conduct of Clinical Research Involving Children. Washington, DC: National Academies Press, 2004.
7. Nelson RM. Analysis of Research Protocols Involving Children: Combining Subparts A and D. 2004. http://www.fda.gov/ohrms/dockets/ac/04/briefing/2004-4066b1_25_Nelson.ppt.
8. Lu JQ, Ichise M, Liow JS, Ghose S, Vines D, Innis RB. Biodistribution and radiation dosimetry of the serotonin transporter ligand 11C-DASB determined from human whole-body PET. J Nucl Med 2004;45(9):1555–1559.
9. Newberg AB, Plossl K, Mozley PD, et al. Biodistribution and imaging with (123)I-ADAM: a serotonin transporter imaging agent. J Nucl Med 2004; 45(5):834–841.
10. Seltzer MA, Jahan SA, Sparks R, et al. Radiation dose estimates in humans for (11)C-acetate whole-body PET. J Nucl Med 2004;45(7):1233–1236.
11. Herzog P, Rieger CT. Risk of cancer from diagnostic x-rays. Lancet 2004;363(9406):340–341.
12. Hall EJ. Lessons we have learned from our children: cancer risks from diagnostic radiology. Pediatr Radiol 2002;32(10):700–706.
13. Pierce DA, Preston DL. Radiation-related cancer risks at low doses among atomic bomb survivors. Radiat Res 2000;154(2):178–186.
14. Brenner DJ. Estimating cancer risks from pediatric CT: going from the qualitative to the quantitative. Pediatr Radiol 2002;32(4):228–223; discussion 42–44.
15. Brenner DJ, Doll R, Goodhead DT, et al. Cancer risks attributable to low doses of ionizing radiation: assessing what we really know. Proc Natl Acad Sci USA 2003;100(24):13761–13766.

16. Ernst M, Freed ME, Zametkin AJ. Health hazards of radiation exposure in the context of brain imaging research: special consideration for children. J Nucl Med 1998;39(4):689–698.

17. Upton AC. The state of the art in the 1990'S: NCRP report No. 136 on the scientific bases for linearity in the dose-response relationship for ionizing radiation. Health Phys 2003;85(1):15–22.

18. Cohen BL. Cancer risk from low-level radiation. AJR 2002;179(5):1137–1143.

19. Frush DP, Donnelly LF, Rosen NS. Computed tomography and radiation risks: what pediatric health care providers should know. Pediatrics 2003; 112(4):951–957.

20. Charron M, Lentle BC. Is it really this simple? Pediatr Radiol 2003; 33(11):811–814; author reply 5–7.

21. de Gonzalez AB, Darby S. Risk of cancer from diagnostic x-rays: estimates for the UK and 14 other countries. Lancet 2004;363(9406):345–351.

22. Shah S, Whittle A, Wilfond B, Gensler G, Wendler D. How do institutional review boards apply the federal risk and benefit standards for pediatric research? JAMA 2004;291(4):476–482.

23. Preston DL, Shimizu Y, Pierce DA, Suyama A, Mabuchi K. Studies of mortality of atomic bomb survivors. Report 13: solid cancer and noncancer disease mortality: 1950–1997. Radiat Res 2003;160(4):381–407.

24. Health Physics Society. Radiation risk in perspective: position statement of the Health Physics Society (adopted January 1996). In: Health Physics Society Directory and Handbook 1998–1999. McLean, VA: Health Physics Society, 1998:238.

25. Hall EJ. Reply. Pediatr Radiol 2003;33:815–817.

26. Nelson RM. Including children in research: participation or exploitation? In: Santoro M, Gorrie T, eds. Ethics and the Pharmaceutical Industry. Cambridge: Cambridge University Press, 2005.

27. Ross LF. Do healthy children deserve greater protection in medical research? [see comment]. J Pediatr 2003;142(2):108–112.

28. Fekete CN, de Lonlay P, Jaubert F, Rahier J, Brunelle F, Saudubray JM. The surgical management of congenital hyperinsulinemic hypoglycemia in infancy. J Pediatr Surg 2004;39(3):267–269.

29. Adzick NS, Thornton PS, Stanley CA, Kaye RD, Ruchelli E. A multidisciplinary approach to the focal form of congenital hyperinsulinism leads to successful treatment by partial pancreatectomy. J Pediatr Surg 2004;39(3): 270–275.

30. Stabin MG, Gelfand MJ. Dosimetry of pediatric nuclear medicine procedures. Q J Nucl Med 1998;42(2):93–112.

31. Royal HD. Radiation Dose Limits for Adult Subjects. 2004. http://www. fda.gov/cder/meeting/clinicalResearch/royal1.ppt.

32. Gelfand MJ. Pediatric Nuclear Medicine and the RDRC Regulations. 2004. http://www.fda.gov/cder/meeting/clinicalResearch/gelfand.ppt.

33. Anonymous. Update—New Fludeoxyglucose F 18 Injection PET Drug Approved in Less than 6 Months. Food and Drug Administration, 2004. http://www.fda.gov/cder/regulatory/pet/Fludeoxyglucose.htm.

34. Committee for Proprietary Medicinal Products, the European Agency for the Evaluation of Medicinal Products. Position Paper on Non-Clinical Safety Studies to Support Clinical Trials with a Single Microdose. 2003. http://www.emea.eu.int/pdfs/human/swp/259902en.pdf.

7

Ethics of PET Research in Children*

Suzanne Munson, Neir Eshel, and Monique Ernst

Positron emission tomography (PET) technology offers clinical researchers the opportunity to gain unprecedented understanding of the neurobiologic correlates of pediatric illness. In contrast to other forms of functional neuroimaging, PET provides direct information on neurochemical activity, such as neurotransmitter function in the human brain (1). Such data may prove invaluable to the understanding of brain maturation and the development of novel pharmacologic treatments for children. However, because PET is a radionuclear medicine technique and children are classified as a vulnerable population requiring special safeguards, PET utilization in pediatric research is controversial. The involvement of healthy children in PET research is an especially contentious issue, and to date fewer than a dozen such studies have been conducted in the United States.

This chapter examines the ethics of pediatric PET imaging in the context of a hypothetical research study, as it is formulated and submitted to the institutional review board (IRB) for approval. First, issues that must be considered by the principal investigator (e.g., scientific significance and risk/benefit ratio) are addressed. Guidelines for minimizing risk to pediatric participants are reviewed. Next, the role of the IRB in determining the study's risk level and in protecting the children involved in medical research is outlined. Also discussed are the implications of recent case law concerning nontherapeutic research that poses greater than minimal risk, as well as IRB member liability.

The Role of the Principal Investigator

In our hypothetical study, we wish to investigate the neurobiology of attention-deficit/hyperactivity disorder (ADHD), a prevalent pediatric psychiatric disorder, with poorly understood neurobiochemical

*The views stated herein do not necessarily represent the official views of the National Institute of Mental Health, the National Institutes of Health, the Department of Health and Human Services, or any other agency of the United States Government.

etiology (2,3). We propose a methodology that involves PET with intravenous administration of raclopride, a radioligand used to measure the concentration of dopamine (D2) receptors in the brain. Proposed subjects for the first stage of the study are boys of ages 9 to 17 years (see discussion of inclusion criteria that follows). Two groups will be studied: individuals with ADHD and individuals with no psychiatric history. Before submitting the study to the IRB for review, it is essential (1) to establish scientific significance and evaluate scientific yield of the proposed methodology, and (2) to delineate the risk/benefit ratio to the participants involved. Potential ethical concerns should be addressed in the context of these two facets of the proposal.

Scientific Significance, Scientific Yield, and Ethical Considerations

Why is the proposed study scientifically significant? First, ADHD is a disorder that primarily affects children; it is the most prevalent psychiatric condition in the pediatric population (4). Recent statistics estimate a 3% to 10% prevalence rate of pediatric ADHD in the United States, and as many as 30% of children with the disorder either do not respond to or cannot tolerate the side effects of conventional (stimulant) treatment (5). Second, although ADHD has been found to be associated with altered dopamine function (6–8), the neurobiochemical mechanisms underlying such alternations are unclear. Therefore, this study is necessary to answer key questions regarding the postsynaptic functional integrity of the dopamine system in children with ADHD. Data obtained may aid in the design of more effective pharmacologic treatments for children suffering from the disorder.

Ethical concerns must be weighed against the scientific relevance and salience of the proposed study (9). Furthermore, the principal investigator should demonstrate that the study has been designed to maximize scientific yield and minimize risk to participants involved. Thus, it should be established that (1) PET is the only methodology that can be used to answer the scientific question, (2) the scientific question can be answered only in children, and (3) healthy controls are necessary for the interpretation of the findings.

Why PET?

When reviewing the study, IRB members may question why PET is proposed when less invasive functional neuroimaging tools are available. Functional neuroimaging methods, for example, PET, single photon emission computed tomography (SPECT), functional magnetic resonance imaging (fMRI), magnetic resonance spectroscopy (MRS), and magnetoencephalography (MEG), differ in the nature of the recorded signal (e.g., radioactive counts for PET and SPECT, electromagnetic energy for fMRI and MEG), physiologic variables (e.g., cerebral blood flow for PET, SPECT, and fMRI; glucose metabolism and receptor density for PET and SPECT), temporal and spatial resolution, cost, and associated risks (10). Positron emission tomography is the only technique that allows direct assessment of neurotransmitter function and thus can help to answer proposed scientific questions. It enables investigators to assess regional dopamine function and to parse out its different elements (e.g., presynaptic vs. postsynaptic). However, PET is associated with unique medical risks (delineated below) that raise ethical issues for its use in pediatric populations, especially when healthy children are involved.

Why Children?

Why must the proposed study involve children? A seemingly simple way to avoid ethical conflict would be to study adults with ADHD. However, findings from prior neuroimaging studies suggest that the developing brain is structurally and functionally distinct from the adult brain. In a review of 25 magnetic resonance imaging (MRI) studies of the developing brain, Durston et al. (11) cite age-associated volumetric changes in several brain structures. Although the basal ganglia decrease in volume with age, the amygdala and hippocampus increase in volume. Giedd et al. (12) found that these developmental changes in brain morphometry also vary according to gender. Amygdala volume increases significantly in males, and hippocampal volume in females. In addition, PET studies have revealed functional differences between the developing and mature brain. Chugani (13) reported that pediatric rates of cerebral glucose metabolism differ from those of adults, and that metabolism rates vary significantly throughout childhood. After birth, glucose metabolism rates rise steadily until age 4, when they are twice that of adults. Between the ages of 4 and 10, metabolism rates remain high, and then gradually decline to reach adult values by age 16 to 18. Additionally, Chugani found that metabolic rates in the developing brain differ by brain region. In newborns, glucose metabolism rates are highest in sensorimotor cortex, thalamus, brainstem, and cerebellar vermis, but as the infant grows, metabolic rates increase in occipital lobe, temporal lobe, and eventually frontal cortex.

Considering these structural and functional differences, the neuropathology associated with neurologic and psychiatric illnesses may also differ in the developing and mature brain. For example, studies of children and adults with ADHD reveal neurobiochemical differences between the two groups. Blood or cerebrospinal concentrations of the dopaminergic metabolite homovanillic acid (HVA) have been found to be abnormal in children with ADHD (14,15) but not in adults with ADHD (16,17). Cerebral glucose metabolism levels have been found to be abnormally low in adults with ADHD (18) but unaltered in adolescents with ADHD (19,20). Most significant are PET-based findings that children with ADHD exhibit different abnormalities in dopaminergic function than adults with ADHD (6,7). Such age-associated neurobiochemical changes may explain why certain psychiatric medications are effective in adults but not in children (e.g., tricyclic antidepressants for major depressive disorder) (21). Furthermore, they suggest that the proposed scientific question cannot be answered based on inferences from adult data.

Another consideration is the age of the children. The younger the children who are subjects in a study, the more stringent are the safeguards. This is particularly important with regard to the capacity of children to assent to participate in a study. In our study, 9 years of age was selected as the inferior age limit because, by age 9, healthy children are believed to possess the cognitive maturity necessary to understand the research process and evaluate the risks involved in participation (22). However, there is much debate on this topic, with some arguing that the age of assent should be as high as 14 (23).

Why Healthy Controls?

Although there is some debate over whether it is better to enroll healthy or affected children in nonbeneficial research (24), PET studies of children with ADHD are generally more likely to receive IRB approval than studies of healthy children, who are less likely to benefit from participation (1). In previous pediatric PET studies, researchers have utilized several methods to mitigate ethical objections to the inclusion of healthy controls (25). The first is to scan healthy siblings of children affected by the condition under investigation. Siblings may indirectly benefit from increased knowledge of ADHD, a disorder with probable genetic etiology that may be inherited by their own children (26). However, the use of siblings as healthy controls can reduce the scientific yield if the siblings carry a common genetic vulnerability that influences brain function, even if behavioral symptomatology is not expressed. A second method, applied by Chugani et al. (27), is to study unaffected brain regions of children with transient neurologic disorders, such as epilepsy. This method is also suboptimal, because neurologic disorders may induce changes in cerebral function that increase variability and lead to results difficult to interpret. A third method, utilized by both Bentourkia et al. (28) and Chugani et al. (29), is to retrospectively select control children who had been scanned as part of a diagnostic evaluation, but whose results had been negative, indicating an absence of neurologic abnormalities. This method is also problematic because the medical or behavioral problems that prompted a diagnostic PET scan undermine these subjects' status as truly "healthy" controls. A fourth method is to study only children with ADHD and correlate PET results with symptom severity (30). However, this method reduces the investigators' ability to elucidate the neural mechanisms of the disorder because no comparisons can be made to the healthy brain. Thus, although these alternative methods may be more ethically feasible, the use of nonrelated, nonsymptomatic children as healthy controls remains the gold standard for optimizing scientific yield.

Once scientific significance is established, and issues related to scientific yield are addressed, the principal investigator must demonstrate that the study has a favorable risk/benefit ratio (i.e., the risks to the subjects involved are lower than or at least proportionate to the benefits to the subject and society) (9,31). In addition, the investigator should demonstrate that the study design minimizes risks and maximizes benefits to participants involved.

Optimizing the Risk/Benefit Ratio

Risks

Risks for participants in pediatric PET protocols include (1) physical side effects associated with the venous line; (2) stress related to the procedure (e.g., possible claustrophobic reaction, difficulty lying still, anxiety provoked by medical environment); and (3) radiation exposure.

Risks related to the insertion of the venous line include transient redness, swelling, or bruising. A topical anesthetic such as eutectic mixture of local anesthetics (EMLA) cream can be used to numb the site of needle puncture, which tends to reduce discomfort and anxiety. Adequate preparation can significantly reduce stress related to the procedure. Before the scan, children should visit the room where the procedure will take place and ideally spend time in a PET simulator. Simulation can help to desensitize the subject to the medical environment. Furthermore, it can allow the research team to determine if the subject will have a claustrophobic reaction once inside the scanner. Optimal simulation should replicate any environmental elements (e.g., background noise, lights) that may be anxiety provoking for children during the actual scan. Children, especially those with ADHD, often have difficulty remaining still during a PET scan. Placing the child's head on an inflatable pillow and allowing him to watch a video can alleviate this problem.

The most ethically concerning of these risks is exposure to radiation because of its association with genetic mutation and carcinogenesis. Three common misconceptions regarding this association may bias the evaluation of pediatric PET studies: (1) any radiation dose can produce cancer or genetic damage, (2) the severity of adverse effects is directly proportional to the radiation dose received, and (3) children are more radiosensitive than adults (32). Ernst et al. (32) conducted a comprehensive review of studies of low-level radiation exposure from various sources (background, occupational, and medical) to assess the health hazards of radiation exposure in the context of brain imaging research. Findings indicated that the incidence of cancer in individuals exposed to low-level radiation, defined as 10 to 20 rem (roentgen equivalents in man, the conventional unit for dose equivalent), cannot be detected above the incidence rate of cancer in the general population. Although the majority of the studies available for review did not include children, there were no definitive findings of higher risks associated with younger age (younger than 5 years old) following exposure to low-level radiation.

One possible exception is data from an Israeli longitudinal study conducted by Ron et al. (33), who tracked the incidence of thyroid tumors following childhood exposure to radiation. A total of 11,000 subjects who had been treated with scalp irradiation for tinea capitis as children and 16,000 controls were followed between 1950 and 1972. Age at treatment ranged from 1 to 15 years, with a mean of 7.1 years. The authors concluded that an estimated thyroid dose of 9 cGy (9 rem) was linked to a fourfold [95% confidence interval (CI) = 2.3–7.9] increase of malignant thyroid tumors and a twofold (95% CI = 1.3–3.0) increase of benign thyroid tumors. In addition, younger age at exposure was found to be associated with higher risk, particularly in children younger than 5 years. In a more recent study, Juven and Sadetzki (34) examined the medical records of 4900 of Ron et al.'s subjects and also noted a possible association between childhood exposure to ionizing radiation and benign pituitary adenoma. An important limitation of both studies is the lack of a true measure of radiation exposure; radiation doses administered during treatment were estimated based on post-hoc measurements of representative exposures assumed to be analogous to the original exposures. In addition, although the mean radiation dosage was estimated to be 9.3 rem, dosage ranged from 4.5 to 50.0 rem. Thus, a proportion of the subjects were exposed to radiation dosages that significantly exceeded the low-level threshold. Therefore, it is problematic to draw generalized conclusions regarding exposure to low-level radiation based on the findings of these two studies.

Billen (35) examined the relationship between exposure to radiation and spontaneous DNA damage, and found that the biologic impact of low-level radiation at the cellular level is proportionally low in comparison to the frequency of daily spontaneous genetic mutations. Each day, an average of 240,000 genetic mutations spontaneously occur in the human body. Radiation exposure of a single rem adds approximately 100 mutations to this number.

In addition, research has provided evidence in support of hormesis, a theory that exposure to low-dose radiation may be beneficial. Studies conducted by Sanderson and Morley (36) and Kelsey et al. (37) demonstrated that previous low-level radiation can have a protective effect during subsequent high-dose radiation exposure by stimulating chromosomal repair mechanisms.

Despite these findings, many scientific questions remain to be answered before definitive conclusions can be made regarding the effects of low-dose radiation exposure during a PET scan. As relevant research evolves, the Food and Drug Administration (FDA) has developed vigilant guidelines to protect children, who may be more vulnerable to radiation exposure on account of smaller size and ongoing tissue growth. Currently, the FDA restricts the use of radioactive drugs in research involving minors to 0.3 rem in a single dose (or 0.5 rem cumulative annual dose) to the whole body, active blood-forming organs, lens of the eye, and gonads (32,38,39). This dose is one tenth of that mandated for adults. Furthermore, 0.5 rem is at least 20 times lower than the low-level exposure in the studies reviewed by Ernst et al. (32) (i.e., 10–20 rem). As of 1998, the highest research radiation dose used in imaging studies of healthy children 12 and older was 0.06 rem to the whole body (32,38,39).

As an additional safeguard, when large medical institutions conduct human research studies that involve exposure to non–medically indicated ionizing radiation, a local radiation safety committee (RSC) or radioactive drug research committee (RDRC) reviews the study prior to or concurrently with the IRB review. Members of these committees provide the principal investigator and IRB with an estimated percentage risk (in terms of increased likelihood for the development of fatal cancer) associated with participation in studies such as the one proposed here. If the maximum permitted pediatric radiation dosage is administered (0.3 rem in a single dose, or 0.5 rem cumulative annual dose), this increase in percentage risk is approximately 0.000025.

When designing pediatric PET protocols, the principal investigator should take all possible steps to minimize radiation exposure to the subjects involved. In a PET study of adolescent girls with ADHD, Ernst et al. (19) implemented several methodologic adjustments to reduce the amount of tracer injected: they lengthened the scan acquisition time, thus recovering image resolution lost due to the lower injected dose; and they allowed subjects to void during the study, thus removing the tracer from the bladder, which is the organ with the highest level of exposure during [18F] fluorodeoxyglucose PET scans. When possible, researchers should also utilize new developments in PET technology, such as the emergence of highly sensitive three-dimensional (3D) cameras that permit the use of lower doses of radioactive tracer.

Another important consideration for the investigator is to use a design that minimizes the number of subjects exposed to risks. In the proposed study, only male subjects are included in the first phase of the trial. This decision was made in light of evidence of neurobiologic differences between males and females (12) and the fact that ADHD is predominately a male disorder (40). Enrolling only males effectively reduces the number of subjects exposed to radiation, while maintaining scientific validity.

Benefits

What are the potential benefits for participants in the proposed study? King (41) defines three possible types of research benefits: (1) direct (benefit arising from receiving the intervention being studied), (2) collateral or indirect (arising from being a subject), and (3) aspirational (benefit to society or future patients arising from the results of the study). According to these definitions, only collateral and aspirational benefits are available to subjects in the proposed study because it is nontherapeutic. For children with ADHD, collateral benefits may include a free psychiatric evaluation, physical exam, and an opportunity to learn more about their disorder. Healthy controls may also benefit from free evaluations and examinations, as well as a sense of altruism gained from volunteering to help other children (38). Furthermore, participation in a research protocol can be a valuable learning experience. Not only will subjects gain exposure to a hospital setting, but they can also learn about how scientific research is conducted. Research teams may augment this learning experience by engaging the child in the research process (e.g., explaining to a curious child how neuroimaging "works" or providing the child with an image of his or her brain and a certificate of appreciation).

The proposed study also has potential scientific benefits at large, as ADHD affects thousands of children in the United States and is associated with academic impairments, social dysfunction, poor self-esteem, and increased likelihood for substance abuse (5). Studies such as the one proposed are essential for elucidating the neurobiologic correlates of the disorder. Findings will likely assist in the development of safe and effective treatment. Furthermore, because the proposed study includes healthy controls, PET data collected can provide critical insight into dopaminergic function during normal development. Such information is critical to the understanding of plasticity of the maturing brain and may help to identify critical periods of neural vulnerability as well as potential compensation and opportunity for treatment.

After delineating these potential benefits and contrasting them to potential risks, the principal investigator concludes that the risk/benefit ratio for the study is favorable and submits the protocol to the IRB for approval.

The Role of the Institutional Review Board

The IRB is charged with two main functions, which are often conflicting. Although its primary goal is to protect individual participants in medical research, it is also expected to facilitate research that is critical to the evolution of medical care. The board's members are guided by Title 45, Part 46 of the Code of Federal Regulations (CFR) (42), which outlines ethical and legal obligations of persons and institutions conducting or supporting research involving humans. The CFR mandates that each institution conducting federally funded research adhere to the principles for the protection of human subjects set forth in the Belmont Report (43). These principles include (1) beneficence, which requires that researchers maximize benefits and minimize harm; this principle also entails that all approved protocols have a favorable risk/benefit ratio; (2) respect for persons, which recognizes the autonomy of individuals, while requiring protection for people with diminished autonomy (such as children); this principle is implemented via informed consent and assent; and (3) justice, which requires equitable selection and recruitment, as well as fair treatment of research subjects.

Beneficence and Risk Classification

The first objective of the IRB is to classify the risk level of the proposed study (e.g., minimal risk, minor increase over minimal risk, or more than a minor increase over minimal risk). Subpart D of the CFR ("Additional DHHS Protections for Children Involved as Subjects of Research") prohibits IRBs from approving pediatric research that poses more than a minor increase over minimal risk and does not offer the prospect of direct benefit to participants. The level of risk, as well as whether there is prospect of direct benefit to participants, determines the provisions necessary for the study to be approved and conducted, as outlined in Figure 7.1. In subsection 46.102 (i), the CFR suggests the following definition for minimal risk:

Minimal risk means that the probability and magnitude of harm or discomfort anticipated in the research are not greater in and of themselves than those ordinarily encountered in daily life or during the performance of routine physical or psychological examinations or tests.

Given that the study's risk classification determines its approval, this definition is a paramount guideline for IRB deliberations. However, the definition contains several ambiguities.

First, risks "ordinarily encountered in daily life" can vary significantly among children, depending on their age, socioeconomic class, and physical environment. In terms of the proposed study, it can be argued that children who routinely fly on airplanes or frequently receive medical x-rays "ordinarily" encounter risks of radiation exposure. In fact, a cross-country flight and a chest x-ray each contribute approximately 0.003 rem (44). Does this mean that these children should be permitted to participate in the PET study, whereas children who do not "ordinarily" encounter risks of radiation exposure should be excluded? Furthermore, "examinations or tests" that are routine for a child with a medical disorder such as ADHD may not be routine for a healthy child. This disparity raises the question of whether the study's risk classification should differ for patients and healthy controls. A child with ADHD who is accustomed to a clinical setting may tolerate certain procedures (e.g., psychiatric interviews) better than a healthy child. On the other hand, ADHD could render a child more vulnerable to research-associated risks (e.g., psychological stress from an inability to lie still in the scanner). Although there is some agreement that the minimal risk standard should be based on risks in the lives of the general population, the lack of a more specific definition produces unnecessary complications. Furthermore, IRB deliberations may be hindered by the fact that the CFR does not provide definitions for the terms *minor increase over minimal risk* and *direct benefit*.

Considering the ambiguous nature of CFR guidelines, it is not surprising that risk categorization varies greatly among IRBs. Shah et al. (45) presented a series of hypothetical research vignettes to 188 randomly selected chairpersons of IRBs in the United States and asked them to categorize the risks and benefits involved for a healthy 11-year-old participant. Data collected demonstrated marked variability in the risk determinations. For example, when asked to designate the risk category of MRI (without sedation), 48% of IRB chairpersons surveyed selected minimal risk, 35% selected minor increase over minimal risk, and 9% selected more than a minor increase over minimal risk. Disparities were also noted in the categorization of direct benefits of participation. Only 60% of the chairpersons surveyed considered added psychological counseling to be a direct benefit of participation in a study. Furthermore, 10% considered participant payment to be a direct benefit, even though the IRB guidebook explicitly states that it should not be (46). McWilliams et al. (47) and Rogers et al. (48) demonstrate how variations in the categorization of risks and benefits can

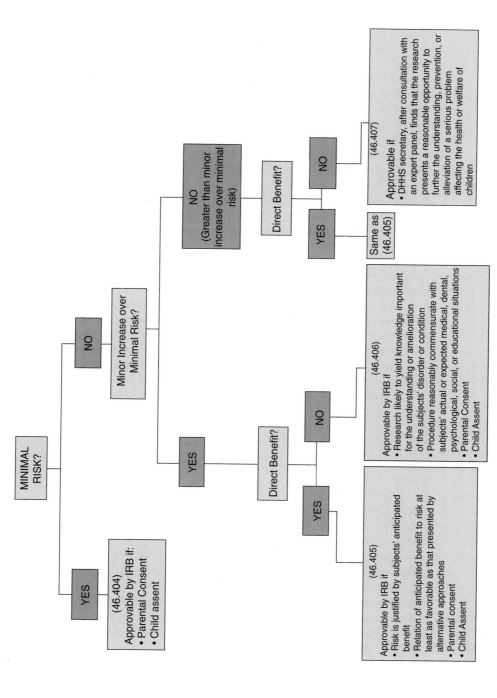

Figure 7.1. Institutional review board risk assessment flowchart. Based on CFR 46, Protection of Human Subjects, subpart D, Additional DHHS Protections for Children Involved as Subjects in Research.

complicate the review of multicenter protocols, which must be approved by the IRBs of each institution involved.

Variability in IRB review standards can be detrimental in two ways: either children may be subjected to undue risk, or potentially beneficial research may not be approved on account of inappropriate risk categorization. To prevent such consequences, more specific definitions for the terms *minimal risk, minor increase over minimal risk*, and *direct benefit* should be provided within the CFR. For example, Nicholson (49) provides a list of ordinary daily risks to which research risks can be compared to determine minimal risk (39). Furthermore, considering the fact that some IRB members lack clinical experience, neutral medical experts should be called upon to educate the committee when unfamiliar procedures (such as PET scanning) are proposed to ensure that risk categorization is not biased by misconception.

According to CFR 46.404, if the IRB categorizes the proposed study as minimal risk, it may be conducted as long as proper consent and assent is obtained. However, based on IRB classifications of comparable studies (45), our proposed study will likely be deemed greater than minimal risk, with no prospect of direct benefit to healthy subjects involved. If the study is categorized as a minor increase over minimal risk, CFR 46.606 (the subject condition requirement) should be considered by the IRB. This section permits research that is "likely to yield generalizable knowledge about the subject's disorder or condition." Thus, this section clearly sanctions the approval of the proposed study if children with ADHD are the only subjects included. How can this section be interpreted for the study of healthy controls? One could argue that the terms *disorder* and *condition* are ambiguous. For example, the IRB at the Children's Hospital in Los Angeles approved a computed tomography study of bone development in which 50 healthy girls were briefly exposed to 0.10 rem of radiation (50). Findings yielded increased knowledge on differences in bone density in developing African-American and Caucasian females. Can race be considered a "condition" in accordance with CFR guidelines? If so, what about childhood or adolescence? If the term is interpreted broadly, one could argue that in addition to elucidating the neuropathology of ADHD, including healthy control children will likely yield generalizable knowledge about the neurobiology of development, or the "condition" of immaturity itself.

Alternatively, if the proposed study is categorized as greater than minor increase over minimal risk, CFR 46.407 may be applicable. According to this section, the IRB may submit an unapprovable research study for higher review if it is believed to "present an opportunity to understand, prevent, or alleviate a serious problem affecting the health or welfare of children." Approval may be granted by the secretary of the Department of Health and Human Services (DHHS) after public review and consultation with an expert panel. In the 18 years following the 1983 adoption of 45 CFR 46, only two unapproved pediatric research studies were considered under section 46.407. However, in 2001 alone, the secretary of DHHS received 26 requests for higher review (51). Research proposals previously reviewed under CFR 46.407

are listed on the Web site of the Office for Human Research Protection (OHRP) (http://www.hhs.gov/ohrp/children/index.html# researchproposals). One protocol on this list, "HIV Replication and Thymopoiesis in Adolescents," is comparable to the proposed PET study because it involves healthy adolescents (ages 13 to 24) and radiation exposure (during a computed tomography scan and intravenous infusion of deuterium-labeled glucose solution). The OHRP recommended that the DHHS approve this study but stipulated that the risks involved must be clearly defined in the consent documentation (i.e., by including the specific amount of radiation to which each subject will be exposed and a statement that a CT scan is associated with more radiation exposure than a chest x-ray). The marked increase in pediatric protocols submitted under CFR 46.407 is likely a reflection of recent legal and ethical scrutiny of clinical research studies.

Issues Related to Informed Consent and Assent

After issues related to beneficence have been addressed, the IRB should ensure that the proposed study upholds the second principle set forth in the Belmont Report (43): respect for persons. Thus, the IRB must critically evaluate the proposed consent and assent process. According to federal guidelines, children under 18 must assent to participation in clinical research. In addition, their parents (or legal guardians) must sign consent forms for their child to participate (52). For the consent/assent process to be valid, participants must possess competence, knowledge, and a desire to participate in the study not influenced by undue coercion (38).

Competence implies that the participant has the cognitive ability to arrive at a rational decision to participate in the study. In a review of literature assessing assent by minors, Leikin (22) concludes that by age 9, healthy children have sufficient cognitive capacity to make a valid decision as to whether to participate in a research study. In accordance with these findings, the minimum age for subjects in the proposed study is 9 years. However, there is ongoing debate on this topic, with some investigators proposing a more stringent age cutoff for assent (23), and IRBs varying widely in their requirements (53). Until the federal regulations explicitly include a minimum age, it is likely that this debate will continue. Regardless, it is critical that the investigator use age-appropriate language when providing an explanation of the purpose of the study and the procedures involved. Psychiatric disorders, often associated with characteristics such as paranoia, apathy, and impaired insight, may hinder a child's cognitive processing and ability to provide informed assent. Considering comorbidity of pediatric ADHD and psychiatric disorders such as anxiety, depression, and oppositional defiant disorder (54), subjects should receive a complete psychiatric interview before the PET scan. Furthermore, if the presence of a psychiatric disorder (other than ADHD) is suspected during the consent process, the principal investigator should carefully question the child to ensure that his or her motivation to participate in the study is psychologically sound.

Knowledge entails that the participant has been fully informed of the protocol methodology as well as all possible risks and benefits involved in participation. In its 2001 report on improving informed consent for research radiation studies, the NIH Radiation Safety Committee provided model language to clearly inform subjects of potential radiation-related risks (55). The template includes disclosure of the effective radiation dose to be administered before the PET scan and a comparative estimation of typical radiation exposure from natural background sources. Furthermore, it recommends disclosure of the estimated amount of risk associated with the research-related radiation exposure in terms of increased possibility of fatal cancer. The NIH Radiation Safety Committee provided the following sample clause as a guideline for informing research participants of the risks of low-dose radiation exposure comparable to that which would occur during a PET scan:

One possible effect that could occur at these [radiation] doses is a slight increase in the risk of cancer. Please be aware that the natural chance of a person getting a fatal cancer during his/her lifetime is about 25 percent. The increase in your chance of getting a fatal cancer, as a result of the radiation exposure received from this study, is [insert percent increase calculated by Radiation Safety Committee]. Therefore, your total risk of fatal cancer may increase from 25 percent to (25 + calculated increased risk). This change in risk is small and cannot be measured directly. Compared with other everyday risks, such as flying in an airplane or driving a car, this increase is considered slight.

The IRB should ensure that consent documents for the proposed study adhere to these recommended guidelines to guarantee that participants are fully informed with regard to potential risks.

It is the responsibility of the investigator to ensure that the child's decision to participate in the study is completely voluntarily and not unduly influenced by financial need, parental pressure, or psychological coercion. The compensation of minor participants in medical research studies is a controversial topic frequently debated by IRBs. Major ethical questions include whether to compensate the parent or the child, whether to consider the economic status of the family when determining compensation, and whether the compensation should be correlated with risk involved (38). If compensation is provided for the child, its perceived value may differ based on the child's age, cognitive abilities, and socioeconomic status. Regardless, financial motivation should never preclude the child from carefully considering the risks involved in participating in a PET study. If there is any concern that compensation may be an undue influence, a neutral observer should monitor the consent/assent process to counterbalance investigator bias. Also, after parental consent is obtained, investigators should meet with the child alone to discuss his or her motivation for participation and ensure that there is no undue parental coercion before assent is elicited. There is some debate over whether researchers should meet with the child before the parent rather than after, but both processes are reasonable and should be left up to the individual investigator to decide.

Furthermore, it is critical that the child understands that he or she can withdraw from the study at any time without providing a reason and without loss of any previously attained benefits or financial compensation. Throughout the course of the study, the research team should strive to facilitate feelings of autonomy in the child participant. This can be accomplished by asking children how they feel about the prospect of a PET scan, having them fill out feedback forms, and having them make simple procedural decisions (e.g., which seat they want to sit in, which snack they would like to eat after completing the scan). Such simple steps increase the likelihood that the child will share concerns and questions with the research team, thus remaining a willing participant in the PET study.

Justice

The third ethical principle set forth in the Belmont Report is justice, which compels the IRB to monitor the selection of research subjects at two levels: the individual and the social (43). To uphold individual justice, the IRB should ensure that subjects for the proposed study are not preferentially selected or excluded on the basis of race, ethnicity, or socioeconomic class. For example, the proposed study includes only boys, which may be considered unjust if the principal investigator had not provided a scientific rationale, or stated intentions to include girls in subsequent phases of the study. According to the Belmont report, social justice "requires that a distinction be drawn between classes of subjects (e.g., adults and children) that ought, and ought not, to participate in any particular kind of research, based on the ability of members of that class to bear burdens." In the past, children have been excluded from research studies because they are considered less able to bear the burden of potential risks involved than adult subjects. However, excluding children from medical research precludes them from its benefits and could potentially cause them harm. For example, if research studies are not conducted to elucidate the neurobiochemical etiology of ADHD in children, it will be difficult to develop novel treatments for the disorder. Furthermore, attempts to extrapolate data from adult studies may lead to the development of treatments that are unsafe or ineffective for the pediatric population (9). Such consequences seem to be in conflict with the concept of "fairness in distribution" of the benefits of research, an ideal also included in the Belmont Report's definition of justice.

In 1998, two policy initiatives were introduced to ensure that children are not unnecessarily excluded from the benefits of research (56). First, the NIH mandated that children be included in all human research conducted or supported by their institution unless there are sound scientific and ethical reasons to exclude them (57). Second, in response to the fact that 70% of all medications do not include sufficient data for use in children (45,58), the FDA developed the Best Pharmaceuticals for Children Act, which provided patent extension incentives to drug companies that tested their products in children (52). Although such initiatives promote the approval of the proposed study, they should not preclude a careful consideration of the risks involved.

Recent Case Law and Implications

There is currently no known case law involving PET imaging in children. However, in the past 5 years, three highly publicized legal cases have raised controversial questions regarding human research studies involving greater than minimal risks and whether individual IRB members can be held legally liable for approving such studies if injury occurs. Challenges to the integrity of clinical research made during these three cases are especially likely to influence IRB review of ethically controversial pediatric research studies, such as the one proposed here.

The first case involved a lead abatement research study conducted by the Kennedy-Krieger Institute (KKI) (59). Between 1993 and 1995, researchers monitored dust lead levels in three groups of homes in a low-income Baltimore neighborhood, each treated with a different lead abatement method. Blood lead levels of children living in the homes were periodically sampled, and parents were reimbursed $15. In 2000, two families involved in the study filed suit against KKI, claiming that they had not been fully informed of the risks involved in the study and were not advised when their children's blood lead levels rose (60). In response, the Maryland Court of Appeals issued the following opinion:

> It is not in the best interest of any healthy child to be intentionally put in a non-therapeutic situation where his or her health may be impaired, in order to test methods that may ultimately benefit all children (61).

Thus, the court ruled that a parent or guardian cannot consent to a child's participation in nontherapeutic research in which there is any risk of injury or damage to the child's health (i.e., minor increase over minimal risk) (60). In addition, the court criticized the "IRB's attempt to manufacture a therapeutic value" for the KKI study (61). Two months later, the court clarified its ruling, seeming to conform again to federal regulations (62). And in 2002 the Maryland legislature essentially nullified the court's objections, allowing all research that is consistent with the federal regulations, which includes studies involving a minor increase over minimal risk (63). Nevertheless, the case instigated public and legal challenges to the integrity of pediatric research and the role of the IRB.

In 2001 *Robertson v. McGee* (64) set legal precedent by including 12 members of the University of Oklahoma IRB as defendants. The case involved a cancer vaccine trial that was suspended after an audit cited inadequate protections for human subjects. The OHRP was called to investigate, and concluded that the IRB had failed to "ensure that additional safeguards were included in the study" to protect subjects, many of whom were terminally ill. Based on these allegations, negligence counts were filed against the IRB members in the legal suit that followed (65).

In the aftermath of these cases, IRB members are likely to be increasingly cautious when reviewing studies such as the one proposed. Positron emission tomography imaging may be classified in a higher risk category, and the inclusion of healthy controls is unlikely to be approved. Furthermore, the IRB may be more likely to submit the study (under CFR 46.407) to the DHHS for higher review to avoid legal liability issues. And although there are no known examples of successful lawsuits against bioethicists or IRB members, the possibility of such a lawsuit may make individuals hesitant to provide advisory services to IRBs or serve on the committee. These circumstances threaten both the future of clinical studies and the welfare of research participants.

Conclusion

Pediatric PET research presents novel opportunity for scientific discovery, as well as unprecedented ethical issues warranting careful evaluation. Several conclusions can be drawn from the hypothetical PET study presented in this review: First, we have established the unique utility of PET to study neurobiochemical function, such as the mechanisms of dopamine modulation in children with ADHD. Second, because developmental differences mitigate any extrapolation from adult data, PET studies such as the one proposed here must be conducted in children. Third, including healthy children is the only way to maximize scientific yield and learn about normal neurobiologic development. Fourth, pediatric PET studies are associated with considerable potential risks, as well as significant collateral and aspirational benefits to participants. The principal investigator should take all possible procedural steps, including those outlined in this review, to optimize this risk/benefit ratio. It is hoped that these four conclusions may serve as a guideline in the design of future PET studies.

This chapter also yields several suggestions regarding the IRB evaluation of pediatric PET research. First, it is essential that board members be accurately informed of the risks associated with pediatric PET, especially in terms of radiation exposure. Second, the definition of *minimal risk* should be clarified and definitions should be provided for the terms *minor increase over minimal risk* and *direct benefit* within the CFR so that IRB deliberations are not clouded by ambiguity or misconception. Third, the IRB should ensure that risks associated with PET are fully disclosed in the consent documentation, as outlined by the NIH Radiation Safety Committee. Fourth, in accordance with the principle of justice, children are entitled to benefit from advances in scientific research, such as those that may be gained by conducting the proposed study. Therefore, it is critical that recent case law not bias the IRB's evaluation of the risks and benefits of pediatric PET studies. The IRBs are charged with the vital responsibility of protecting individual children while allowing research needed to improve overall pediatric medical care. It is hoped that the recommendations outlined in this chapter will aid in the ethical considerations needed to fulfill this responsibility.

References

1. Ernst M. PET in child psychiatry: the risks and benefits of studying normal healthy children. Prog Neuropsychopharmacol Biol Psychiatry 1999;23(4): 561–570.
2. Biederman J, Faraone SV. Current concepts on the neurobiology of attention-deficit/hyperactivity disorder. J Atten Disord 2002;6(suppl 1): S7–16.
3. Castellanos FX, Tannock R. Neuroscience of attention-deficit/hyperactivity disorder: the search for endophenotypes. Nat Rev Neurosci 2002;3(8): 617–628.
4. Leung AK, Lemay JF. Attention deficit hyperactivity disorder: an update. Adv Ther 2003;20(6):305–318.
5. Daley KC. Update on attention-deficit/hyperactivity disorder. Curr Opin Pediatr 2004;16(2):217–226.
6. Ernst M, Zametkin AJ, Matochik JA et al. High midbrain (18F)DOPA accumulation in children with attention deficit hyperactivity disorder. Am J Psychiatry 1999;156(8):1209–1215.
7. Ernst M, Zametkin AJ, Matochik JA et al. DOPA decarboxylase activity in attention deficit hyperactivity disorder adults. A (fluorine-18)fluorodopa positron emission tomographic study. J Neurosci 1998;18(15):5901–5907.
8. Krause KH, Dresel SH, Krause J, et al. The dopamine transporter and neuroimaging in attention deficit hyperactivity disorder. Neurosci Biobehav Rev 2003;27(7):605–613.
9. Vitiello B, Jensen PS, Hoagwood K. Integrating science and ethics in child and adolescent psychiatry research. Biol Psychiatry 1999;46(8):1044–1049.
10. Ernst M, Rumsey J. Functional Neuroimaging in Child Psychiatry. Cambridge: Cambridge University Press, 2000.
11. Durston S, Hulshoff Pol HE, Casey BJ, et al. Anatomical MRI of the developing human brain: what have we learned? J Am Acad Child Adolesc Psychiatry 2001;40(9):1012–1020.
12. Giedd JN, Castellanos FX, Rajapakse JC, et al. Sexual dimorphism of the developing human brain. Prog Neuropsychopharmacol Biol Psychiatry 1997;21(8):1185–1201.
13. Chugani HT. A critical period of brain development: studies of cerebral glucose utilization with PET. Prev Med 1998;27(2):184–188.
14. Castellanos FX, Elia J, Kruesi MJ, et al. Cerebrospinal fluid monoamine metabolites in boys with attention-deficit hyperactivity disorder. Psychiatry Res 1994;52(3):305–316.
15. Shaywitz BA, Cohen DJ, Bowers MB Jr. CSF monoamine metabolites in children with minimal brain dysfunction: evidence for alteration of brain dopamine. A preliminary report. J Pediatr 1977;90(1):67–71.
16. Ernst M, Liebenauer LL, Tebeka D, et al. Selegiline in ADHD adults: plasma monoamines and monoamine metabolites. Neuropsychopharmacology 1997;16(4):276–284.
17. Reimherr FW, Wender PH, Ebert MH, et al. Cerebrospinal fluid homovanillic acid and 5–hydroxy-indoleacetic acid in adults with attention deficit disorder, residual type. Psychiatry Res 1984;11(1):71–78.
18. Zametkin AJ, Nordahl TE, Gross M, et al. Cerebral glucose metabolism in adults with hyperactivity of childhood onset. N Engl J Med 1990;323(20): 1361–1366.
19. Ernst M, Cohen RM, Liebenauer LL, et al. Cerebral glucose metabolism in adolescent girls with attention-deficit/hyperactivity disorder. J Am Acad Child Adolesc Psychiatry 1997;36(10):1399–1406.

20. Zametkin AJ, Liebenauer LL, Fitzgerald GA, et al. Brain metabolism in teenagers with attention-deficit hyperactivity disorder. Arch Gen Psychiatry 1993;50(5):333–340.

21. Ambrosini PJ. A review of pharmacotherapy of major depression in children and adolescents. Psychiatr Serv 2000;51(5):627–633.

22. Leikin S. Minors' assent, consent, or dissent to medical research. IRB 1993;15(2):1–7.

23. Wendler D, Shah S. Should children decide whether they are enrolled in nonbeneficial research? Am J Bioeth 2003;3(4):1–7.

24. Wendler D, Shah S, Whittle A, et al. Nonbeneficial research with individuals who cannot consent: is it ethically better to enroll healthy or affected individuals? IRB 2003;25(4):1–4.

25. Hinton VJ. Ethics of neuroimaging in pediatric development. Brain Cogn 2002;50(3):455–468.

26. Shastry BS. Molecular genetics of attention-deficit hyperactivity disorder (ADHD): an update. Neurochem Int 2004;44(7):469–474.

27. Chugani HT, Phelps ME, Mazziotta JC. Positron emission tomography study of human brain functional development. Ann Neurol 1987;22(4):487–497.

28. Bentourkia M, Michel C, Ferriere G, et al. Evolution of brain glucose metabolism with age in epileptic infants, children and adolescents. Brain Dev 1998;20(7):524–529.

29. Chugani HT, Phelps ME. Imaging human brain development with positron emission tomography. J Nucl Med 1991;32(1):23–26.

30. Rosa Neto P, Lou H, Cumming P, et al. Methylphenidate-evoked potentiation of extracellular dopamine in the brain of adolescents with premature birth: correlation with attentional deficit. Ann N Y Acad Sci 2002;965:434–439.

31. Emanuel EJ, Wendler D, Grady C. What makes clinical research ethical? JAMA 2000;283(20):2701–2711.

32. Ernst M, Freed ME, Zametkin AJ. Health hazards of radiation exposure in the context of brain imaging research: special consideration for children. J Nucl Med 1998;39(4):689–698.

33. Ron E, Modan B, Preston D, et al. Thyroid neoplasia following low-dose radiation in childhood. Radiat Res 1989;120(3):516–531.

34. Juven Y, Sadetzki S. A possible association between ionizing radiation and pituitary adenoma: a descriptive study. Cancer 2002;95(2):397–403.

35. Billen D. Spontaneous DNA damage and its significance for the "negligible dose" controversy in radiation protection. Radiat Res 1990;124(2):242–245.

36. Sanderson BJ, Morley AA. Exposure of human lymphocytes to ionizing radiation reduces mutagenesis by subsequent ionizing radiation. Mutat Res 1986;164(6):347–351.

37. Kelsey KT, Memisoglu A, Frenkel D, et al. Human lymphocytes exposed to low doses of X-rays are less susceptible to radiation-induced mutagenesis. Mutat Res 1991;263(4):197–201.

38. Arnold LE, Zametkin AJ, Caravella L, Korbly N. Ethical Issues in Neuroimaging Research with Children. In: Ernst M, Rumsey JM, eds. Functional Neuroimaging in Child Psychiatry. Cambridge: Cambridge University Press, 2000:99–109.

39. Arnold LE, Stoff DM, Cook E Jr, et al. Ethical issues in biological psychiatric research with children and adolescents. J Am Acad Child Adolesc Psychiatry 1995;34(7):929–939.

40. Biederman J, Mick E, Faraone SV, et al. Influence of gender on attention deficit hyperactivity disorder in children referred to a psychiatric clinic. Am J Psychiatry 2002;159(1):36–42.
41. King NM. Defining and describing benefit appropriately in clinical trials. J Law Med Ethics 2000;28(4):332–343.
42. U.S. Department of Health and Human Services. Protection of Human Subjects. 45 CFR §46. 2001.
43. National Commission for the Protection of Human Subjects of Biomedical and Behavioral Research. The Belmont Report: Ethical Principles and Guidelines for the Protection of Human Subjects of Research. Washington, DC: U.S. Government Printing Office, 1979.
44. Austin Radiological Association. Radiation Safety and Medical Imaging. 2004. http://www.ausrad.com/rse_le_p_radsafe.shtml
45. Shah S, Whittle A, Wilfond B, et al. How do institutional review boards apply the federal risk and benefit standards for pediatric research? JAMA 2004;291(4):476–482.
46. Office for the Protection from Research Risks. Protecting Human Research Subjects: Institutional Review Board Guidebook. Washington DC: U.S. Government Printing Office, 1993.
47. McWilliams R, Hoover-Fong J, Hamosh A, et al. Problematic variation in local institutional review of a multicenter genetic epidemiology study. JAMA 2003;290(3):360–366.
48. Rogers AS, Schwartz DF, Weissman G, et al. A case study in adolescent participation in clinical research: eleven clinical sites, one common protocol, and eleven IRBs. IRB 1999;21(1):6–10.
49. Nicholson R. Medical Research with Children: Ethics, Law, and Practice. Oxford: Oxford University Press, 1986.
50. Gilsanz V, Roe TF, Mora S, et al. Changes in vertebral bone density in black girls and white girls during childhood and puberty. N Engl J Med 1991;325(23):1597–1600.
51. Meeting of the National Human Research Protections Advisory Committee. The meeting was held in Washington, DC, 2002.
52. Alexander D. Regulation of research with children: the evolution from exclusion to inclusion. J Health Care Law Policy 2002;6(1):1–13.
53. Whittle A, Shah S, Wilfond B, et al. Institutional review board practices regarding assent in pediatric research. Pediatrics 2004;113(6):1747–1752.
54. Jensen PS, Hinshaw SP, Kraemer HC, et al. ADHD comorbidity findings from the MTA study: comparing comorbid subgroups. J Am Acad Child Adolesc Psychiatry 2001;40(2):147–158.
55. Radiation Safety Committee NIH. Improving Informed Consent for Research Radiation Studies. 2001. http://www.nih.gov/od/ors/ds/rsb/rsc/forms/informed_consent.pdf
56. Baylis F. Mandating research with children. IRB 1999;21(1):10–11.
57. National Institutes of Health. NIH Policy and Guidelines on the Inclusion of Children as Participants in Research Involving Human Subjects. 1998. http://grans2.nih.gov/grants/guide/notice-files/not98-024.html
58. Center for Drug Evaluation and Research and US Food and Drug Administration. Offices of Drug Evaluation Statistical Report 89-233530. Rockville, MD: U.S. Department of Health and Human Services, 1989.
59. *Ericka Grimes v. Kennedy Krieger Institute, Inc.* August 16, 2001. Maryland Court of Appeals.
60. Nelson RM. Nontherapeutic research, minimal risk, and the Kennedy Krieger lead abatement study. IRB 2001;23(6):7–11.
61. Sharav VH. Children in clinical research: a conflict of moral values. Am J Bioeth 2003;3(1):W-IF.

62. Mastroianni AC, Kahn JP. Risk and responsibility: ethics, Grimes v Kennedy Krieger, and public health research involving children. Am J Public Health 2002;92(7):1073–1076.

63. Wendler D, Forster H. Why we need legal standards for pediatric research. J Pediatr 2004;144(2):150–153.

64. *Dawanna Robertson, et al. v. J. Michael McGee, MD, et al.* January 29, 2001. U.S. District Court in Tulsa, Okla.

65. Anderlik MR, Elster N. Lawsuits against IRBs: accountability or incongruity? J Law Med Ethics 2001;29(2):220–228.

8

Physics and Instrumentation in PET

Roberto Accorsi, Suleman Surti, and Joel S. Karp

The radioactive decay of many radioisotopes generates penetrating photons capable of escaping outside the matter in which the isotopes are located. From this radiation it is possible to image the spatial distribution of such isotopes inside an object. However, by itself the detection of a single photon outside the body of a patient carries minimal information on the location of its origin, unless some device capable of connecting the detection with the emission location is used. These devices are the optics of the imaging instrument and they identify, in combination with a position sensitive radiation detector, a line in space (the line of response, LOR) along which the photon must have originated (Fig. 8.1A,B). The LOR data are manipulated in reconstruction software to produce three-dimensional (3D) images of the activity distribution. When imaging humans, it is necessary to use photons capable of escaping undeflected from a few centimeters of tissue. The energy of these photons is such that their path cannot be bent by reflection (mirrors), refraction (lenses), or diffraction as in visible light optics. Nuclear scintigraphy and single photon emission computed tomography (SPECT) instrumentation resort to absorptive collimation, in which photons are selectively passed or absorbed depending on their emission location and angle of incidence on the optics. The drawback of this approach is that the wide majority of photons are lost before image reconstruction. For example, typical parallel-hole collimators [low energy—technetium-99m (^{99m}Tc; 140 keV); general purpose] pass on the order of 1 in 10,000 (10^{-4}) photons, but sensitivity is even lower for high-resolution and high-energy collimators, which need lower acceptance angles and thicker septa, respectively. Although sensitivity can be recouped by trading off resolution (as with high-sensitivity collimators) or field-of-view (as with converging collimators), it is the concept of absorptive collimation itself that implies an inefficient use of emitted photons.

For isotopes decaying by positron emission, an alternative approach is possible. Because two back-to-back photons are emitted, if both photons are detected, the LOR is immediately identified with no need of discarding any photons incident on the detector (Fig. 8.1C). Greatly

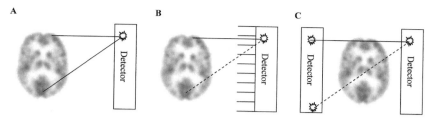

Figure 8.1. Pictorial representation of the identification of lines of response in nuclear imaging. A: Single photon imaging. With no collimation optics present it is impossible to establish the path of incoming photons. B: Single photon imaging. The presence of a collimator gives information on the path of incoming photons. In this case the detected photon must have come from the anterior part, rather than the posterior part, of the brain. Photons not parallel to the bores of the collimator are absorbed and thus lost. C: Positron emission tomography. When radioactive decay results in the emission of two colinear photons, it is possible to determine the path of the photons without a collimator. In principle, no incoming photons are lost.

increased sensitivity to incoming photons is one advantage of positron emission tomography (PET) over SPECT. Another is that most biologically significant elements (e.g., C, N, and O) have positron but no single photon emitting isotopes with practical half-lives. Radioisotope marking of biologically significant molecules is therefore usually more natural with PET rather than SPECT isotopes.

When compared to other techniques such as ultrasound, magnetic resonance imaging (MRI), and computed tomography (CT), PET is characterized, as is SPECT, by relatively poor spatial resolution but excellent sensitivity because the signal is generated by a number of atoms on the order of picomoles. Because the biodistribution of the radiotracer, rather than anatomic structures, is imaged in nuclear imaging, PET is most appropriate when functional information is sought.

Dedicated PET scanners have evolved in a number of different configurations over the years. Today, the most common design presents several rings of small scintillator crystals coupled to photomultiplier tubes (PMTs). In whole-body scanners, the ring diameter is about 80 to 90 cm. Together, all rings form a cylinder with a height limited by cost considerations to about 15 to 25 cm. These dimensions may be sensibly different in scanners designed for other, often specialized, purposes, such as brain, breast, and small animal imaging. Brain and animal scanners need a small transverse field of view and can be designed with a smaller radius to improve solid angle coverage, and thus increase sensitivity. If coincident events connecting many different rings are accepted, the scanner is said to operate in 3D mode. If only events originating in the plane of each ring (and, typically, a few adjacent rings) are collected, the scanner is said to operate in two-dimensional (2D) mode instead. In many 2D systems, septa are used to separate the rings and are retractable to allow both modes of operation on the same scanner.

The literature is rich with thorough presentations of PET (1,2). This chapter presents an essential summary of PET physics, instrumentation, and operation principles, with observations on the relevance of the concepts presented in pediatric applications. First, the physics at the basis of PET is discussed. Aspects influencing the performance of detection instrumentation are emphasized. The discussion of PET instrumentation starts from the parameters and the trade-offs involved in the choice of the scintillating material. Next, the different schemes that can be used to arrange the scintillating material in the scanner are presented. These schemes mainly concern how the light into which high-energy photons are converted in the scintillator is conveyed to the electronics. The data correction procedures necessary to achieve quantitatively accurate images are described next. Finally, the parameters used in the assessment of scanner performance and a brief overview of the choices available for image reconstruction are presented. Some considerations specific to the pediatric applications of PET close this chapter.

Radioactive Decay and Positron Emission

Radioactive decay of unstable isotopes usually occurs through three modalities: α, β, and γ. In its turn, β decay is subdivided in three different types: β^+, β^-, and electron capture (EC). β^+ decay follows the scheme

$$_Z^A X \rightarrow _{Z-1}^A Y + e^+ + \nu \qquad (1)$$

where X and Y indicate the chemical species of the mother and daughter nuclei, respectively, Z is the atomic number (number of protons, which also identifies the chemical species) of the nucleus X, A its mass number (number of protons plus neutrons, which identifies the isotope within the species), e^+ is a positron, and ν a neutrino. The decay is governed by quantum mechanical laws (3) that select at random the kinetic energy E of the positron emerging from the decaying nucleus in the range from almost zero to a maximum possible value E_{max}, which depends on the isotope $^A X$. Table 8.1 shows values of E_{max} for sample PET isotopes.

As the radiotracer decays, the rate at which positrons are emitted declines over time. The activity A of the sample is defined as the average number of decays per unit over a short time interval. It varies with time according to the relationship

$$A(t) = A(t = 0)e^{-\lambda t} \qquad (2)$$

where t is time and λ is the decay constant governing the rate of decay. It is the probability of decay of the isotope per unit time and is a physical constant for every isotope. λ is also connected to the half-life of the isotope, $\tau_{1/2}$, which is defined as the time it takes for the activity to halve, through the relationship

Table 8.1. Decay data for some positron emitters

Isotope	Half-life	Branching ratio of β^+ decay	E_{max} (MeV)	Production
^{11}C	20.4 min	>0.99	0.960	Cyclotron
^{13}N	9.97 min	>0.99	1.198	Cyclotron
^{15}O	122.2 s	>0.999	1.732	Cyclotron
^{18}F	110 min	0.97	0.633	Cyclotron
^{22}Na	2.6 y	0.90	0.545	Reactor
^{64}Cu	12.7 h	0.17	1.673	Cyclotron
^{68}Ga	67.6 m	0.89	2.921	Daughter of ^{68}Ge
^{82}Rb	1.27 m	0.95	3.379	Daughter of ^{82}Sr
^{124}I	4.17 d	0.23	1.535	Cyclotron

Source: Data from Chang J. Table of Nuclides, KAERI (Korea Atomic Energy Research Institute). Available at http://atom.kaeri.re.kr/ton/.

$$\tau_{1/2} = \frac{\ln 2}{\lambda} \tag{3}$$

as it can be worked out from Equation 2. The half-lives of isotopes of interest in nuclear medicine range from seconds to years. In SPECT, the most widely used isotope, ^{99m}Tc, has a half-life of about 6 hours. For PET, the half-life of fluorine 18 (^{18}F) is approximately 2 hours. This is about ideal because this is enough time to allow for isotope production, radiopharmaceutical synthesis, dose delivery, and imaging time while minimizing the dose burden to the patient, which also depends on $\tau_{1/2}$. The decay constant λ is related to the number N of nuclei present in the sample and the activity by the relationship

$$A = \lambda N. \tag{4}$$

It should be noted that Equation 2 governs the rate of decay of nuclei, which is not always the same as the rate of emission of positrons. In fact, different modes of decay may be available to a nucleus. For example, iodine 124 (^{124}I) undergoes β^+ decay only in 23% of the cases; in the remaining 77% the decay mode is EC, which does not produce any positrons. In such cases, it is important to account for this branching ratio when estimating the rate of positron emission from the decay rate of the nuclei. If the problem is to predict the decay over time of a certain type of activity measured at some other point in time, Equation 2 can be applied without worrying about the branching ratio, which is already accounted for in the measurement.

Interaction with Matter

Positron Annihilation

After decay, the positron leaves the site of emission and slows down in the surrounding material. As the positron is a relatively light, charged particle, it undergoes large-angle scattering interactions with other charged particles, which result in a tortuous path. The distance

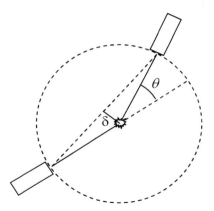

Figure 8.2. The small (~0.5-degree) deviation from 180 degrees in the emission of annihilation photons due to the residual momentum of the $e^- - e^+$ pair causes the corresponding line of response to be slightly misplaced (by the distance δ) from the annihilation site. This error is small, but it does limit the ultimate resolution of PET scanners. Compton scattering results in misplacement of events for the same basic reason, that is, because an angular deviation θ is introduced. In this case, misplacement is much more severe because θ is usually much greater than 0.5 degrees.

traveled from the nucleus, that is, the range of the particle, depends on the energy E with which the photon is emitted, the density of the surrounding material, as well as on the trajectory followed. The range is longer for positrons emitted with higher E. Maximum and average values of the range are found in the literature. For ^{18}F, carbon 11 (^{11}C), nitrogen 13 (^{13}N), and oxygen 15 (^{15}O) the average range is 0.6, 1.1, 1.5, and 2.5 mm, respectively.

During slowdown or once it has come to rest, the positron may combine with a surrounding electron and annihilate, that is, undergo a reaction in which positron and electron disappear and their total energy is converted into two or more photons. Fortunately, the great majority of annihilations results in the simultaneous emission of two (almost) back-to-back photons, each with an energy of 511 keV (4). The distance that each of the two annihilation photons must cover to reach the scanner depends on where the annihilation took place, so that the two photons can reach the scanner at slightly different times. However, this relative delay cannot be larger than a few nanoseconds (billionths of a second). The basic idea of PET is to attribute an event to an LOR every time that two photons are detected in approximate time coincidence.

Because the positron travels some distance from the nucleus before annihilation, annihilation photons are not generated at the site of the emitting nucleus, as happens for single photon emitters. Consequently, the nucleus can be located only approximately, the approximation worsening for increasing positron range. A second physical factor that intrinsically limits the spatial resolution of PET scanners is that annihilation photons are not emitted exactly along the same line (i.e., at a relative 180 degrees) in the laboratory frame of reference (5). This means that the annihilation site in general does not lie exactly on the line connecting the detection locations of the two photons (Fig. 8.2).

The ensuing positioning uncertainty δ is proportional to the diameter of the scanner (6) and reaches about 2 mm for a diameter of 90 cm. With current technology, this is one of the main factors limiting the resolution of whole-body PET scanners.

Gamma Attenuation, Scattering, and Random Coincidences

Annihilation photons may undergo interaction with surrounding materials before detection. Photons in the energy range relevant to PET interact with matter through two principal mechanisms: photoelectric absorption and Compton scattering. In photoelectric absorption, a photon is absorbed in an interaction with an atom in the surrounding material.

Effectively, the final result of a photoelectric event is that the photon disappears. Because in PET both annihilation photons need to be detected to form a valid event, photoelectric absorption of either photon outside the detector is sufficient to lose the annihilation event for image formation. Depending on the location and direction of the annihilation, the likelihood of attenuation changes, with higher losses for emission points lying deep within the patient. Therefore, attenuation must be compensated to obtain realistic images and quantitative data. Attenuation correction strategies for PET are described below and are based on the observation that, unlike in SPECT, in a collected event the total photon path crosses the object from side to side (Fig. 8.3). If a point source located anywhere along this line emits N_0 photons per unit time along the line, the rate at which events are recorded is

$$C = N_0\, e^{-\mu\rho D} \qquad (5)$$

where μ is the mass attenuation coefficient of the material, which is known from its atomic composition and the energy of the photons, and ρ is its density. The key point is that the factor $e^{-\mu\rho D}$ can be obtained by direct measurement. In fact, if an external source of known activity A_0 is placed at one end of a given LOR, the count rate A measured at the other end of the LOR is given by

$$A = A_0\, e^{-\mu\rho D}. \qquad (6)$$

Therefore, the factor $e^{-\mu\rho D}$ can be obtained experimentally from the ratio A/A_0 and then used to divide the coincident count rate C to recover the activity N_0. Note that this applies for sources anywhere along the LOR, that is, at any depth in the object.

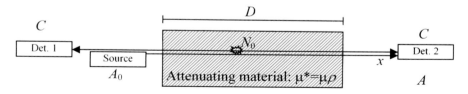

Figure 8.3. Attenuation correction in PET. The count rate recorded at detector 2 is C when exposed to annihilation photons in coincidence with detector 1 and A when exposed to the source of intensity A_0. The line connecting detector 2 to the source is separate from that connecting it to detector 1 only for illustration purposes.

For 511-keV photons in biologic materials, Compton scattering is much more likely to occur than photoelectric absorption. In Compton scattering, the photon loses some energy and its path is deviated by an angle θ (Fig. 8.2). The scattering angle is again selected in a random process governed by quantum mechanical laws (e.g., ref. 7). The energy of the scattered photon is related to θ by the Compton equation:

$$E'_\gamma = \frac{E_\gamma}{1 + \dfrac{E_\gamma}{m_e c^2}(1 - \cos\theta)}$$

(7)

where E_γ is the energy of the incident photon, m_e is the rest mass of the electron, and c is the speed of light. The product $m_e c^2$ is a physical constant and its value is 511 keV. The Compton equation shows that photons emerge from scattering with an energy that depends on the scattering angle. For example, for $\theta = 0$, or forward scattering, which is the limiting case in which the photon is not scattered at all, $E'_\gamma = 511$ keV; for $\theta = \pi$, which is the case of backscattering, that is, when the photon turns back, $E'_\gamma = 170$ keV. Unlike attenuation, scattering does not necessarily remove events from image reconstruction. Rather, it usually causes the incorrect association of a significant fraction of events to LORs, through the same basic mechanism of Figure 8.2, but in a much more dramatic way because of the much larger angular deviation involved. It is not at all uncommon that scatter events are assigned to LORs not even passing through the object, which does not happen for true events (i.e., unscattered events coming from the same annihilation) except for the much smaller effect of non-colinearity. Scatter events, in principle, could be rejected by measuring the energy of incoming photons and then accepting only those arriving with the correct energy, that is, 511 keV. As discussed below, existing equipment allows only an approximate measurement of the energy of photons, so that it is necessary to accept events with a measured energy of less than 511 keV to avoid discarding too many true events. Therefore, in practice, only photons whose measured energy is above a certain threshold (set at less than 511 keV) are accepted. This threshold is selected by setting the low-level discriminator (LLD) of the scanner. Because the Compton equation shows that E'_γ decreases as θ increases, increasing the LLD means confining θ closer to zero. From Figure 8.2, it is possible to see that this minimizes the error introduced. Whereas a high LLD setting does minimize the impact of scattering events, it has also other implications, as we shall see, and it cannot, alone, completely solve the problem of scatter contamination of the data; other methods, described below, are needed for full scatter compensation. The scattered photon can undergo further scattering, still governed by the same equations. Such events, as well as those in which both annihilation photons are scattered once, are referred to as multiple scattering.

Another type of spurious event, besides scattering events, can also enter the image. If more than one nucleus decays at approximately the same time, and for both events one of the two photons is lost, it is still possible that the two survivors are detected in coincidence. In this case a LOR is mistakenly associated to the unrelated photons (Fig. 8.4). This

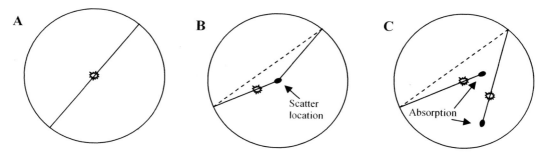

Figure 8.4. Pictorial representation of (A) a true coincidence, (B) a scatter event, and (C) a random coincidence. In B and C, the dashed line represents the line of response to which the event is assigned. It coincides with the path of the photons (solid line) only in case A.

type of event is called a random coincidence. The likelihood of random coincidences depends on the level and spatial distribution of activity and the temporal width of the coincidence window, as well as the geometry of the object. To appreciate this, it is helpful to consider that after the detection of a first photon above the LLD, the scanner waits up to a time τ for the photon emitted simultaneously to arrive. The time interval 2τ is called the time coincidence window. If the rate at which the first event is recoded is N events per unit time, then the rate at which random coincidences occur in the scanner is τN^2. Time coincidence windows are usually set between 6 and 12 ns (billionths of a second, i.e., 10^{-9} s), depending on the scintillator.

PET Instrumentation

It is desirable to detect photons with high spatial, energy, and time resolution, with high sensitivity and count rate capabilities, all at reasonable cost. Different classes of detectors of high-energy photons have long been under development; no single class, however, offers the best performance in all respects. For example, solid-state detectors offer the best energy resolution, but their sensitivity is usually low, especially when their cost and availability over a large area are considered.

Commercial clinical PET cameras are based on scintillation detectors. In these systems, the photon interacts with a scintillating material, which converts the photon energy into visible or near-visible light. These low-energy photons are then conveyed to PMTs for conversion into an electrical signal. The front end of the PMT is the photocathode, which is a thin element of material capable of absorbing light photons and emitting electrons (called photoelectrons, because they are released by incident light) in proportion to the number of absorbed photons. Electrons are then multiplied by a cascade of electrodes (dynodes) to generate a measurable current and voltage, which is the output of the PMT. In summary, the role of the PMT is to convert the light emitted in the scintillator into an electric signal that is directly proportional to the intensity of the light signal. A much more compact alternative to PMTs are photodiodes. These are semiconductor devices capable of playing the same role. To date, their use has been hampered by their cost and instability with respect to fluctuations of temperature and applied voltage, and, often, the consequent need for cooling.

The electric signal generated by the PMT is then sent through pulse processing electronics that collect and process signals from the entire scanner. The part of this processing most typical of PET is the identification of events in time coincidence and their location on the detector for assignment to a LOR. Scanner designs differ mainly in the choice of the scintillator and the way light is conveyed (coupled) to PMTs.

Scintillating Material

Scintillators commonly considered for PET are listed in Table 8.2 along with some properties that characterize their performance. An ideal scintillator would have high sensitivity, that is, it would detect all incoming photons and record their energy and location of interaction accurately. Moreover, the timing properties of scintillators are also important because with fast scintillators a narrow time coincidence window can be used, which reduces the rate at which random coincidences are acquired as well as dead time effects (see below).

High sensitivity can be obtained with large volumes of scintillators. However, it is also important to be able to stop photons in a small volume to obtain precise positioning and thus high-resolution images. The thickness of a material necessary to absorb photons is regulated by the product $\mu^* = \mu\rho$ (e.g., see Equation 5). Materials with a high value of μ^* can stop photons within a relatively small distance and are preferred.

As already mentioned, an accurate energy measurement is important to differentiate scattering from true coincidence events. Figure 8.5 is a pictorial representation of the response of a real detector. This figure shows the number of incoming photons as a function of their measured energy. The peaks centered on 511 keV are due to 511-keV photons; because not all of these photons are exactly at 511 keV, it is evident that a real detector does not always measure energy accurately. This is due to a number of factors. An accurate measurement requires that, first, all the energy of the photon be deposited in the detector; second, that all deposited energy be transformed into light and converted into current with minimal fluctuations and losses; and, third, that all the current be collected and analyzed by pulse processing electronics.

Table 8.2. Properties of some scintillators used in PET

	NaI(Tl)	BGO	LSO	GSO	BaF$_2$	LaBr$_3$
Attenuation coefficient μ^* (cm^{-1})	0.34	0.95	0.87	0.7	0.45	0.47
Effective Z	50.6	74.2	65.5	58.6	52.2	46.9
Light output (photons/keV)	38	8	25	13	10	60
Light decay constant (ns)	230	300	40	60	0.6	25

BaF$_2$: Barium Fluoride; BGO: Bismuth Germanate; GSO: Gadolinium Oxyorthosilicate; LaBr$_3$: Lanthanum Bromide; LSO: Lutetium Oxyorthosilicate; NaI(Tl): Sodium Iodide.

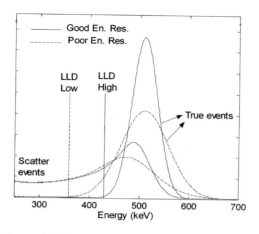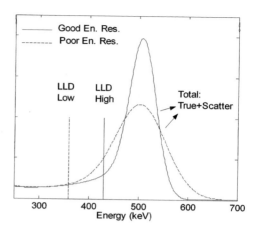

Figure 8.5. Energy spectrum for scintillators with good (solid line) and poor energy resolution (En. Res.) (dash). On the left true and scattering events are shown separated but in reality these events are indistinguishable to the detector; only the sum of the two curves is available (right). For a scintillator with good energy resolution it is possible to set the low-level discriminator (LLD) at a higher level to reject scatter with minimal loss of true events.

For the incoming photon to deposit all its energy, it is important that the photon-crystal interaction be a photoelectric rather than a Compton event. Because the likelihood of Compton scattering is proportional to the atomic number Z of the medium, whereas the likelihood of a photoelectric event is proportional to Z^5, scintillators with a high Z (or effective Z for compounds) are preferable to maximize the fraction of events with full energy deposition.

It is not possible to entirely avoid statistical fluctuations, which are also an inherent part of the detection mechanism. In fact, the number of light photons n produced by a high-energy (gamma) photon is determined in a random process. For this reason, photons having the same energy produce a varying n. Other statistical processes are involved in the conversion of photons to photoelectrons and in the multiplication of electrons inside the PMT. Because the energy of the event is measured by collecting over time (integrating) the PMT current, the final effect is an imperfect energy measurement, distributed approximately along a gaussian curve, which results in the peaks in Figure 8.5. A statistical analysis of the process shows that energy resolution, which gets worse as the gaussian becomes wider, depends mainly on the light yield of the scintillator. Table 8.2 shows the light output of different scintillators. A high light output minimizes relative fluctuations in the current and is associated with good energy resolution. Figure 8.5 also shows the case of two scintillators: one with good and one with poor energy resolution. From inspection of the peaks in the figure, good energy resolution allows a more precise measurement of the energy.

Photons that undergo Compton scattering in the patient (and thus have an energy of less than 511 keV) and deposit their full energy in the detector give the contribution shown to the left of the peaks in Figure 8.5. The measured energy of these photons is also blurred by the statistical fluctuations just described. From Figure 8.5 it is clear that scatter and true events cannot be completely separated on the basis of their measured energy. However, blurring is less pronounced when energy resolution is good, which allows a relatively better separation of true from scatter events. This observation determines the choice of the LLD of the scanner. From a scatter rejection point of view, the LLD should be as high as possible. However, when the LLD is increased, eventually true events are also discarded. Optimizing the LLD setting, then, involves optimizing a trade-off between maximum sensitivity to true events and minimum sensitivity to scatter events. The advantage of good energy resolution is that it is possible to operate with a higher LLD setting, and thus reject comparatively more scatter, before a significant number of true events is lost. For the same number of true events relatively fewer scatter events are collected, which means that image processing in scanners based on a scintillator with good energy resolution can start from better estimates of the true distribution of the radiotracer.

It is important to recognize that other factors also affect energy resolution, such as size of the scintillator, homogeneity of the light output, how the scintillators are coupled to the PMTs, and the successive pulse processing. For example, to maximize energy resolution, a long time should be allowed to collect all the PMT current (integration time). However, this is at odds with the necessity of being able to process separately the next incoming event as soon as possible, that is, to achieve high count rate capabilities, which demand that integration times be kept as short as possible. Because the integration time is mainly driven by the time interval over which light is emitted, the rate at which scintillators emit light is also an important performance parameter. Table 8.2 lists decay times for different scintillators. In this case, a small value indicates a fast scintillator and thus is a desirable property. Energy resolution, then, is related to light output, but it cannot be directly inferred from it.

The data in Table 8.2 summarize all the physical parameters important for the evaluation of different scintillators. For example, NaI(T1): sodium iodide [NaI(T1)] has higher light output (and better energy resolution) than bismuth germanate (BGO) and lutetium oxyorthosilicate (LSO), for which sensitivity is much better, with LSO being also significantly faster. BGO has a much higher attenuation coefficient than NaI(Tl), and thus higher sensitivity, but the reduced light output affects negatively its energy resolution. LSO has almost the same attenuation coefficient of BGO, and is much faster than both BGO and NaI. GSO is almost as fast as LSO and in the past has offered better energy resolution at the price of reduced sensitivity. Recent improvements in LSO crystal production have led to energy resolution similar to GSO. Slight variations to the composition of LSO have recently been tested [e.g., lutetium (yttrium) oxyorthosilicate [L(Y)SO], mixed lutetium silicates (MLSs), and lutetium pyrosilicates (LPSs)]. Most of these crystals have properties similar to LSO. It is possible that scanners based on such scintillators will be developed commercially in the near future. Commercial PET scanners based on NaI(Tl), BGO, LSO, and GSO have been deployed on the field. Scanners utilizing barium fluoride (BaF_2) and lanthanum bromide ($LaBr_3$) are of particular interest in PET instrumentation research because their fast decay times open the possibility of time-of-flight (ToF) PET. This technique is characterized by low image noise, which compensates for the disadvantage of the relatively low sensitivity of these materials. BaF_2 was among the first scintillators considered for ToF PET; more recently, interest has been focusing on $LaBr_3$ because its timing performance is competitive with BaF_2 (8) and its superior light output and energy resolution are expected to result in improved spatial resolution and rejection of scatter events.

Light Coupling and Spatial Assignment of Events

The discussion has so far focused on the efficiency of the detection of one of the two annihilation photons and on the accuracy of the measurement of its energy. Different techniques are used to identify the position at which incoming photons are detected. A possible approach is to consider them as different compromises between two extreme designs.

In the first design, a large, continuous crystal is used and the position of the event is read as in a conventional Anger (gamma) camera. In this design, the light following an interaction is shared by several PMTs facing the crystal (Fig. 8.6A) (9,10). The position of the event is calculated by a weighted average of the coordinates of the center of each PMT, where the weights are determined by the light intensity seen by

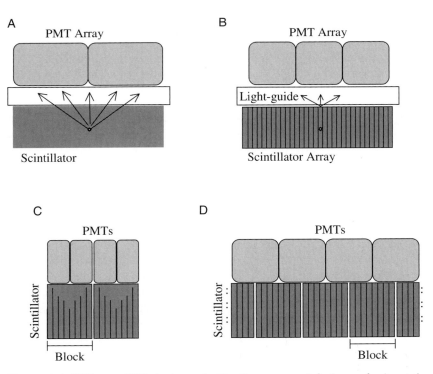

Figure 8.6. Different PET designs. A: Continuous crystal, Anger logic positioning. B: Pixelated crystal, Anger logic positioning. C: Block detectors (two shown). D: Block detectors (quadrant sharing). In designs C and D, light is allowed to spread within each block.

each PMT. This positioning strategy is often called Anger logic, after the name of its developer. For this scheme to work, light needs to spread to several PMTs to allow an accurate calculation of the position. The energy of the event is calculated from the sum of the signals from all PMTs. The same statistical fluctuations that limit energy resolution, then, affect the spatial localization of the event and thus spatial resolution. For this reason, Anger logic designs perform best with scintillators with a high light output. The typical intrinsic resolution of an Anger camera is about 3 mm in SPECT applications but is worse (~5 mm) for PET applications, due to the thicker crystals (25.4 mm NaI vs. 9.3 mm NaI) used to achieve reasonable sensitivity at the energy of the more penetrating 511-keV photons. The major disadvantage of this design is that, following each event, light invades a significant portion of the large crystal and its detection involves several PMTs. Consequently, a large area of the detector is not available for recording other events. This leads to high dead time and decreased maximum count rates.

In the second design, the scintillator is cut in an array of very small crystals (pixels), each of which is connected to a single light detector (one-to-one coupling). The advantage of a pixelated design is that the intrinsic spatial resolution of the detector is about half the size of the pixels, which can be cut to a cross section of a few millimeters. A second advantage is that, because pixels are entirely independent, count rate capabilities are much improved. Whereas the continuous crystal design has been implemented in a commercial clinical scanner, one-to-one coupling has been implemented only in small animal and brain research scanners. Its drawbacks are significantly increased cost and complexity because of the large number of small light detectors needed, as well as compromised energy resolution, especially as crystals are made smaller. Hence its application to systems that use fewer pixels and light detectors.

Most commercial clinical scanners follow neither of these designs but rather different degrees of compromise between the two extremes. A first architecture, conceptually relatively close to the continuous-crystal design, connects small, independent crystals to a light guide, which is then read out by PMTs in an Anger logic configuration (11) (Fig. 8.6B). The design of the crystals and the light guide carefully limits the number of PMTs involved in the detection of a photon; because scintillation light is not allowed to invade the whole crystal, fewer PMTs are involved and the count rate capability is improved. In the block detector architecture (12), groups of crystals (typically an 8×8 cluster) are connected to a 2×2 array of PMTs (Fig. 8.6C). The light generated in each crystal is allowed to spread in a controlled manner within the block (this is why crystals are formed by cutting slots of different depths in a block of scintillator) to only four PMTs, which, by use of Anger logic over this very limited area, can identify the crystal in which detection occurs. In yet another design, PMTs assigned to a block are replaced by larger PMTs straddling quadrants of adjacent blocks (quadrant sharing block geometry) (13).

An important parameter for comparison is the encoding ratio, which is the average number of crystals per PMT. For a given number of crystals of a given size (i.e., for comparable field of view and resolution), independently of the scintillator used, the encoding ratio is inversely proportional to the number of PMTs used. If large PMTs are used, fewer are needed to cover all crystals and the encoding ratio is large. This reduces cost; however, large PMTs also result in reduced count rate capability, because each PMT must serve a large area. Large PMTs are typically used with the continuous light guide and the continuous or pixelated crystal geometry discussed above, which have the advantage of uniform light collection over large areas. This uniformity benefits the energy resolution of the scanner. The best energy resolution is obtained in conjunction with scintillators with high light output. At the other end of the spectrum, scintillators with a low light output are best used with smaller PMTs in a block detector geometry. This has the advantage of more independent modules, which benefits the count rate, but energy resolution is sacrificed with cost and system complexity, which increase because of the larger number of PMTs needed.

Depth of Interaction

To locate accurately the annihilation photons, the scintillator in an ideal scanner would be infinitely dense and thin. To achieve workable sensitivity, real scanners must use scintillators with thickness on the order of 20 to 30 mm, which are not negligible values. Reconstruction algorithms, however, assume that photon detection takes place at the crystal surface. Figure 8.7 illustrates how this results in a degradation of spatial resolution far from the center of the scanner. The degradation increases with the thickness of the crystals as well as with the distance from the center of the scanner, where it vanishes. At 10 cm from the center, it is typically a few tenths of a millimeter. Depth of interaction, thus, is not likely to play a major role in general and especially in pediatric PET for younger patients, who are imaged only at the center of the scanner. Several schemes have been proposed to mitigate the

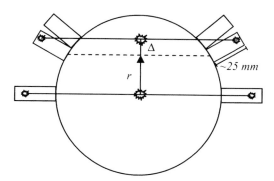

Figure 8.7. Pictorial representation of event misplacement due to depth of interaction. Due to penetration, photons can be detected well inside the crystals, but, because no information on the depth of interaction is available, reconstruction algorithms assume that detection takes place at the inside surface of the crystal. At the center of the scanner this has no consequences; however, depending on the radial position r and the length of the crystals, depth of interaction can result in the assignment of the event to an incorrect line of response (LOR) (i.e., to the dashed rather than the solid line).

problem [e.g. (14,15)], but to date none has yet been implemented in a commercial system.

Data Acquisition, Correction, and Image Reconstruction

When coincident photons are detected, the event is assigned to the LOR corresponding to the two detection locations and stored. The number of events detected in each LOR is the basic output of the scanner. These raw data are the starting point of image reconstruction. The scanner also acquires other data for the various corrections necessary, for example, for random events, scattering, and attenuation.

Detected events whose energy is above the energy threshold (the LLD) are often called single events. If a second single event is detected inside the time coincidence window, a prompt coincidence is obtained. This is not necessarily a true event because photons may have undergone scattering or may have originated from different nuclei ("random" event). Ideally, only true events should be used for reconstruction, but all three kinds are inevitably present in the acquired data, in varying proportions depending on the activity present in the field of view of the scanner, its distribution, and that of the scattering material, along with acquisition parameters such as the time coincidence window and the LLD setting, and the geometry of the scanner, which can be designed for 2D or fully 3D imaging.

The simplest PET scanner is composed of a single ring of detectors and thus is capable of acquiring data only in a single transverse plane, that of the ring. Extension to 3D imaging can follow different avenues. The most straightforward is to stack rings of detectors axially and, at the same time, to use tungsten septa to narrow the angle of acceptance of each ring to admit only events originating in the plane of that ring and of a few adjacent rings. In this design, rings operate independently (2D geometry). An alternative is to allow all rings to see the entire object, in which case a fully 3D geometry is realized.

Purely transverse data are sufficient for reconstruction of a 3D volume by stacking 2D transverse images, each generated independently from a 2D reconstruction of 2D data. The advantage of 3D geometry is its higher sensitivity. The elimination of the septa, however, increases the sensitivity to true as well as to random and scatter coincidences, for which the increase can be higher than for true events. Three-dimensional geometry affects scanners based on different scintillators to different degrees. In general, it places a premium on scintillators with good energy resolution (which can use a higher LLD and therefore are relatively less sensitive to scatter events) and fast timing (which are relatively less sensitive to random events and can better handle the increased count rate). It is mainly because of scatter that, in practice, in spite of the development of specific correction methods, 3D scanners based on crystals with relatively low energy resolution have not yet achieved performance consistently superior to 2D scanners, with effects measurable in terms of contrast recovery and detectability (16). This fact increases the emphasis on the scatter and random coincidence compensation methods described below.

As compared to SPECT, PET data lend themselves to correction for physical effects such as attenuation and scatter rather naturally, paving the way for quantitative imaging, that is, for the evaluation of the activity per unit volume present in the object. To reach this goal, considerable effort has been spent in the development of accurate correction methods.

Normalization

Reconstruction algorithms usually rely on the assumption of an ideal scanner, that is, one for which all parts of the detector ring are uniformly sensitive to incoming photons. In real scanners, a number of factors deviate from this assumption. Normalization is a procedure that corrects the raw data to restore the conditions of an ideal scanner with uniform sensitivity prior to reconstruction. Normalization techniques can be based on the acquisition of data on the scanner, on mathematical models, or on a combination of these two methods (17–21). Regardless of the technique used, normalization data do not need to be acquired for every study. However, because some factors, especially the calibration of the electronics, may drift over time, normalization should be part of quality control procedures and carried out periodically.

Attenuation Correction

As previously discussed, accurate attenuation correction can be achieved from knowledge of the attenuation exponentials $e^{-\mu\rho D}$ for every LOR (22–24). In the simplest methods, these are determined from the emission image by assuming that all regions containing activity have uniform attenuation. Attenuation exponentials are then determined automatically for each LOR by calculating the length of its intersection with these regions. These approaches work well for rather homogeneous parts of the body, such as in brain scans, and have the advantage of introducing no noise into image reconstruction. However, they rely on the assumption of uniform attenuation and so they are much less accurate for irregular distributions of the scatter medium, as in the chest, where the lungs present an attenuation coefficient significantly different from adjacent regions. In these situations, attenuation is better measured with a transmission scan, in which the patient is exposed to an external source of photons. In dedicated PET scanners, line sources of either germanium 68/gallium 68 (^{68}Ge/^{68}Ga) (511 keV) or cesium 137 (^{137}Cs) (662 keV) (25–27) have been used. In PET-CT scanners, it is possible to take advantage of the superior resolution and accuracy of CT data for attenuation correction. However, care must be taken in rescaling the attenuation data from the energy of the measurement (about 60 keV) to 511 keV and in considering the effects of contrast agents, if used. Another potential concern is the incorrect spatial alignment (registration) of the data, which are now effectively acquired on two different scanners, and the consistency of PET with CT data, in which the effects of the patient's breathing may be different due to the much shorter duration of the scan.

The effect of attenuation correction is usually obvious in PET images: corrected studies restore activity in the inner parts of the body to its correct, higher level. Because photons are attenuated more when more material is present, the magnitude of the correction is directly related to the size of the patient.

Random Events Subtraction

Different correction methods for random events are available. Some involve processing of the acquired data, but the most accurate approach requires that additional data with a delayed timing window also be acquired. A delayed timing window is one accepting events coming within a time τ after a time (the delay) much larger than τ has elapsed since the detection of the first event. These are the so-called delayed coincidences. In true and scatter events, the two photons identifying the LOR originate from the same nuclear decay and thus arrive at the scanner separated by a time shorter than τ. Therefore, these events are excluded from the delayed coincidences. On the other hand, random coincidences involve the decay of two different, unrelated nuclei, which happen to produce annihilation photons at the same time by chance. The method of the delayed coincidences assumes that this chance is the same as the chance of producing the photons with a time difference equal to the delay. In summary, delayed coincidences contain only random events that, although not the very same that are part of the image, are still an excellent estimate that can be subsequently subtracted from the data collected with no delay, that is, the actual scan. Whereas subtraction of noisy data from noisy data increases image noise, averaging techniques [also known as variance reduction techniques (28,29)] have been developed to minimize this problem.

The number of collected random events is proportional to the time coincidence window τ and the square of the singles count rate. Thus, their impact is less relevant in scanners based on a fast scintillator (for which τ can be set to a small value) and when low activity is present in the field of view. Because this is usually the case in pediatric PET, especially for younger patients, it is expected that the magnitude of the correction for random events will be smaller than for adults.

Scatter Correction

Accurate scattering correction is vital for accurate quantification, especially in fully 3D scanners, where the open geometry increases sensitivity to scatter events more than to true events.

In theory, because the energy of each incoming photon is available after its detection, scatter could be rejected by simply discarding all detected photons whose energy is not the 511 keV expected for an unscattered photon. In practice, because detectors do not have perfect energy resolution, scattered photons may appear as true events and vice versa. As previously discussed, a careful choice of the LLD minimizes the number of scatter events collected without unduly sacrificing sensitivity to true events. However, some scatter events are still accepted, and for a complete correction additional data processing is necessary.

Different approaches to the problem have been proposed and have evolved over the years (30–37). Most take advantage of the fact that the scatter distribution is very smooth, that is, even though it can be markedly asymmetric, it varies slowly across the field of view, and it is not very sensitive to sudden variations in the object. Recently, the steady increase in affordable computational capacity has made practical techniques that estimate the spatial distribution of scatter directly from physical principles. These are single scatter simulation (SSS) and Monte Carlo (MC) algorithms (38–40). The calculation starts from the estimate of the distribution of the activity provided by the uncorrected image and the estimate of the scattering medium provided by the attenuation scan. Application of physical laws such as Equation 7 generates an estimate of the scatter distribution, which is then subtracted from the uncorrected image to generate a more accurate estimate of the activity distribution. This estimate is still incorrect because it is still based on the uncorrected image. However, the procedure can be repeated to improve accuracy, until further repetitions do not produce significant corrections. Such techniques have the advantage of being patient-specific and equally applicable to uniform (e.g., brain) and nonuniform (e.g., chest) regions. Single scatter simulation explicitly estimates only single scatter and incorporates the effects of multiple scatter only indirectly; MC techniques can be applied to model accurately both single and multiple scatter (41–43), which can be as much as single scatter in large patients. However, at present, MC methods still need more computational resources than routinely available and in most cases do not seem to provide significant advantages over SSS. Therefore, most clinical systems use different implementations of SSS, which has proven to provide very good estimates, except perhaps for the very heaviest patients, and superior performance than previous correction techniques (40).

Because the effect of scatter is to add a rather smooth, featureless background, the effects of scatter on the image are not as evident as those of attenuation. Nevertheless, scatter correction can have a quite dramatic impact on the extraction of quantitative data, especially from cold regions, that scatter tends to "fill in." In this case scatter correction algorithms should restore the correct, lower intensity. As for attenuation, the relative impact of scatter on image quality is directly related to the size of the patient, large patients being more affected. For this reason, the magnitude of the scatter correction is less relevant for smaller and lighter patients. Furthermore, in this population the large majority of scatter is single scatter, for an accurate estimate of which relatively simple methods such SSS are already routinely available.

Dead Time and Decay Correction

Dead time is the amount of time during data acquisition in which the scanner is not available for processing new incoming events because it is busy processing previous ones. Data are usually acquired over a given length of time (real time); in the presence of dead time the scanner will be available only for a fraction of the real time (called the live time), and, accordingly, the recorded number of events is smaller than that which would be recorded in the absence of dead time. Correction for dead time involves multiplying the acquired data by a factor that will restore this number.

Dead time increases with the count rate in the scanner. In general, correction is necessary when data acquired at different count rates need to be compared in some way. This is the case in whole-body studies, where images are formed by juxtaposing images of adjacent sections of the body, each containing a different activity (and thus affected by different dead time); in dynamic studies, because decay and redistribution of the radiotracer cause the count rate to change; and in the evaluation of quantitative measures, such as standard uptake values (SUVs), in which the number of counts is important in an absolute, not only in a relative, sense.

At low count rates, events arrive sparsely in time and it is unlikely that an event will be lost because others have just been detected, so the dead time correction is small and may not be necessary. This is the case in many pediatric studies, in which the injected dose is typically low. However, dead time correction does not present any particular disadvantages and is usually always enabled.

It is often also necessary to correct the data for the radioactive decay of the isotope. This is obtained by keeping record of the time t elapsed between some reference time (e.g., injection) and each study, and then by multiplying the acquired data by the decay factor $e^{\lambda t}$. This multiplication restores the activity of each data set to that which would have been recorded at the reference time, thus making the data comparable to those acquired at a different time.

Figure 8.8 compares the same coronal slice of the clinical study in Figure 8.9B before and after correction for attenuation, scatter, and

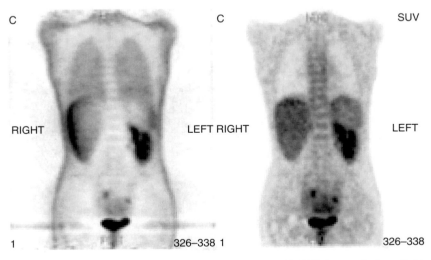

Figure 8.8. Reconstructed fluorodeoxyglucose (FDG)-PET image before (left) and after (right) correction for attenuation and scattering. Both include correction for random events, which is performed online during data acquisition.

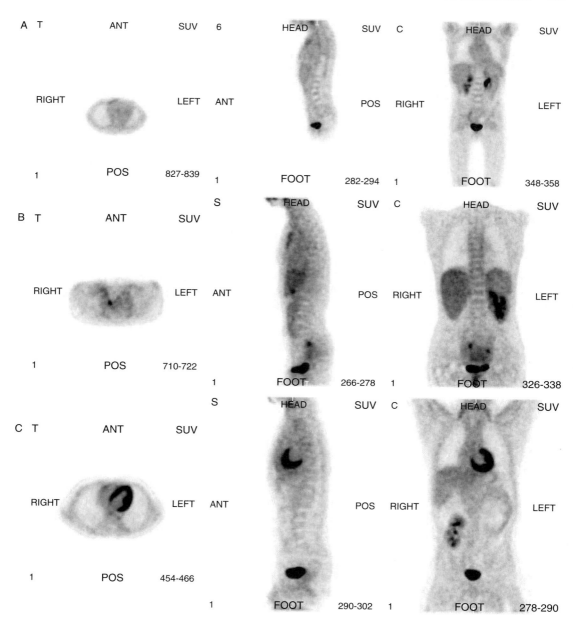

Figure 8.9. Sample whole body FDG clinical scans. A: 6-year-old girl (18 kg); B: 13-year-old girl (52.3 kg); and C: 19-year-old man (72.7 kg). Shown are representative transverse, sagittal and coronal slices.

random events. Other than the obvious artifact in slices containing the bladder, which is due to the attempt at reconstructing inconsistent data, relevant features are that before correction contrast in the lungs vs. surrounding tissue is inverted; that the sides of the body appear to have increased uptake; that the liver has not uniform uptake; and that the contrast at the site of the lesion (in the uterus) is also different from that in the corrected image.

Image Reconstruction Algorithms

A complete discussion of image reconstruction algorithms is clearly outside the scope of this overview. Only a brief summary of the most common methods used in PET imaging, with qualitative, general comments, is provided. For a more detailed overview, the interested reader is referred to the overviews offered elsewhere (44,45).

The problem of image reconstruction is to calculate the distribution of activity inside an object from the raw data. In PET, these are usually generated in the form of counts for each LOR. Most algorithms first rearrange the data in sinograms, which represent the projection of the object along a parallel, evenly spaced beam in all directions. In the 2D case, image reconstruction is similar to the reconstruction of SPECT data from a parallel-hole collimator. In every single view of the projection data, depth information has been lost, but mathematical analysis shows that if projections are taken from angles covering continuously at least 180 degrees, it is still possible to reconstruct exactly the object, slice by slice, by combining data from all directions. The image of a 3D volume is then obtained by stacking all the 2D slices. In 3D geometry, data from LORs connecting different scanner rings (i.e., for oblique tilt angles) are also acquired. The problem of fully 3D reconstruction is that these LORs cross several transverse slices; thus, it is not immediately possible to process them separately in the same way as each transverse slice.

Two different classes of algorithms are used in both 2D and 3D PET image reconstruction: analytic and iterative methods. An example of an analytic algorithm is filtered back projection (FBP), which in its 2D version is analogous to the algorithm used in other imaging modalities. Modifications of the algorithm (e.g., 3D reprojection) were introduced to handle 3D data. A common solution is the use, before reconstruction, of a rebinning algorithm to reorganize oblique into transverse data, which are then processed with 2D algorithms. The simplest approach is single-slice rebinning (SSRB) (46), which assumes that oblique data can be projected directly onto regular transverse slices, but more advanced techniques that rely on less drastic approximations, such as FOurier REbinning (FORE) (47), reduce the loss of axial resolution introduced by rebinning. The main advantage of analytic algorithms, in both 2D and 3D reconstruction, is their speed; their main drawback is that statistical noise in the data is not modeled.

Iterative algorithms handle explicitly data noise and also offer the opportunity to model more precisely the geometry of even complex scanners as well as other effects such as attenuation and scatter; however, more precise models imply much longer reconstruction times, which is the main limitation of the technique even in basic applications. Iterative algorithms start from a guess of the image and then use a computer model of the scanner and physics to predict the projection data that such guess would have generated. Comparison to the data actually acquired provides a correction factor, which is applied to the first guess to obtain a second. Iterations are continued until a satisfying image is reached. Further iteration is usually not worth the additional time and may be even harmful because excessive iteration eventually results in undesired effects such as divergence and noise amplification. Iterative algorithms differ in how updates are calculated. The most widely used method is the maximum likelihood expectation maximization (MLEM) algorithm (48,49), which estimates the object for which the probability of acquiring the data that were actually acquired is maximum. Execution can be accelerated by different variants of the algorithm, the most popular of which is ordered subset expectation maximization (OSEM) (50). Other algorithms, such as row action maximum likelihood algorithm (RAMLA) (51–53), achieve stable performance through the use of a well-chosen relaxation parameter that forces a gradual and consistent convergence toward a solution for the consistent portion of the data. Current clinical scanners implement both 2D and 3D versions of iterative algorithms. A popular solution is to use a 2D iterative algorithm, typically OSEM, in place of an analytic method after FORE. A more advanced solution is to incorporate in the iterative algorithm (e.g., RAMLA), a model of the 3D geometry. In this sense, this approach provides "fully 3D" reconstruction.

Overall, iterative algorithms are credited with better imaging performance than analytic algorithms. Their performance is particularly advantageous in whole-body studies and in low-count situations. However, especially in situations in which computational time is a limiting factor, analytic algorithms still provide a useful alternative.

Time-of-Flight Scanners

Lines of response are identified from the location of interaction of the two annihilation photons with the detector. Time-of-flight scanners are also capable of detecting the difference in the time of arrival of the two photons, from which it is possible to calculate the location of the annihilation along the LOR. In principle, this would completely locate the event in 3D, and thus altogether eliminate the need for reconstruction. Unfortunately, this is only a theoretical possibility. In fact, to locate the event along the LOR within, say, 5mm, it would be necessary to detect a time difference of about 30ps (30 millionths of a millionth of a second). In practice, with scintillators currently available, it is possible to identify time differences about an order of magnitude larger (i.e., about 300ps), which corresponds to several centimeters—hardly enough to eliminate the need for image reconstruction. However, time information is still helpful. In fact, reconstruction of conventional PET data starts from the sum of events originating on the whole LOR. Therefore, noise propagation is more pronounced when LORs intersect a wide object, as, for example, in large patients. In ToF PET, this sum can be divided in the contributions due to different sections of the LOR, which provides relative containment of the propagation of statistical noise. Accordingly, all other factors being equal, the main advantage of ToF PET is in reduced image noise and the advantage is more significant for large patients. With current technology, thus, it is doubtful that

ToF PET will offer advantages in pediatric PET due to the small size of the patients.

System Performance

This section discusses very briefly some parameters of interest in the evaluation of the performance of PET scanners.

Resolution

The resolution of PET scanners can be obtained by measuring the size of the reconstructed image of a point source much smaller than the resolution of the scanner. From this definition, it is evident that a small numerical value is desirable. Modern whole-body clinical scanners have a resolution of 4 to 6 mm in the center of the field of view (FoV). Much better values, down to about 1 mm resolution, have been achieved in research scanners specifically designed for small-animal imaging (54,55). However, in clinical studies, images are typically reconstructed to reduce noise, which worsens resolution to about 10 mm.

Count Rate

The count rate is the rate at which events are acquired. In PET scanners a distinction is made between the rate at which photons are detected individually (singles rate) and the rate at which coincident events are acquired. Clearly, the two are related. In a typical scanner, the singles rate is a factor of about one thousand higher than the coincident count rate. Whereas it is an important performance parameter, the count rate includes all types of event. Because only true events are useful for image reconstruction, some other figure of merit should be used in the determination of the optimal dose.

Noise Equivalent Count Rate

The performance of a PET scanner is usually characterized with a figure of merit that, unlike the count rate, can also account for the presence of scatter and random coincidences along with true events. This is the noise equivalent count rate (NECR) (56). If T is the rate of collection of true events and R and S are, respectively, the collection rates of random and scatter events, then

$$NECR \equiv \frac{T^2}{T+S+R} \tag{8}$$

which assumes random correction with smoothing. The NECR has been shown to be proportional to the square of the signal-to-noise ratio in which signal is given by the true events and noise is the combined statistical fluctuation due to noise from all types of event.

The NECR is often plotted vs. the activity in the field of view of the scanner or its concentration in a standard phantom. These are the

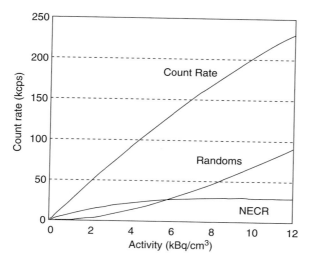

Figure 8.10. Sample noise equivalent count rate (NECR) curve of a whole-body clinical scanner (Allegro, Philips Medical Systems). The NECR is plotted vs. the activity concentration present in a 20×70 cm (diameter $\times$ height) phantom. Total (true + scatter + random) coincident count rate and random coincidences are also shown separately in this example. The typical dose at our institution is $5.18\,kBq/cm^3$ ($0.14\,\mu Ci/mL$).

NECR curves, an example of which is given in Figure 8.10. The NECR usually presents a maximum. The maximum is determined mainly by the rapid increase of the random count rate, also shown in Figure 8.10. Other factors being equal, desirable properties are high values of the NECR occurring at activity levels of interest in clinical practice. The activity corresponding to the maximum NECR provides an indication of the optimal operation point of the scanner. The optimal dose, however, is also determined by other factors not accounted for in the NECR curve, such as the accuracy of corrections for scatter and random events and radiation safety limits. In particular, note that once a significant fraction of the peak NECR is reached, further increase in the activity results only in progressively minor improvements in the NECR, so that the additional dose burden to the patient may not be entirely justified. For these reasons, injection doses are typically lower than the activity corresponding to the peak NECR.

These considerations show that NECR curves contain a simple, although not complete, summary of scanner performance. For this reason, NECR curves should be considered cautiously. For example, when the task is lesion detection, a better figure of merit is lesion detectability as assessed in human observer studies. Though it is possible to measure the sensitivity and specificity for the detection of lesions in PET images, these studies require data that are difficult and time-consuming to acquire, and the method of acquiring the data has not yet been standardized. For these reasons, they are not yet part of the standard protocols for the evaluation of the performance of clinical scanners.

Overview and Performance of Today's Clinical Scanners

Early PET scanners were designed as 2D systems. As solutions for the challenges of 3D imaging were developed (i.e., count rate as well as scatter and randoms correction), scanners with both 2D and 3D capability were introduced. Today, most scanners on the market operate only in 3D. This trend is also connected to the substitution of slow scintillators (mainly BGO and NaI) with significantly faster materials, such as GSO, LSO, and, more recently, LYSO, whose properties are very similar to LSO. Commercial scanners are still based on different light coupling designs, chiefly the block and the pixelated Anger detector configurations. Resolution is directly connected to the size of the crystals used, which is usually in the lower end of the range from 4 to 8 mm. Typical axial FOVs range from 15 to 18 cm. Most scanners currently sold today are sold as PET/CT units.

The fluorodeoxyglucose (FDG) scans in Figure 8.9 were acquired on one (Allegro, Philips Medical Systems Cleveland, Ohio) of the whole-body scanners currently installed at the PET center of the University of Pennsylvania. Figure 8.9A shows a 6-year-old girl (18 kg) with a history of neuroblastoma. The image shows no definite evidence of active neoplastic process. The FDG uptake is diffusely increased in the bone marrow due to the administration of colony-stimulating factors, with the exception of the midthoracic to the upper lumbar spine, where uptake is decreased, likely due to radiation therapy. Figure 8.9B shows a 13-year-old girl (52.3 kg) evaluated for possible lymphoma. The image shows two small foci of increased FDG activity in the superolateral aspect of the uterus bilaterally of uncertain etiology. Figure 8.9C shows a 19-year-old man (72.7 kg) with a history of Hodgkin's disease and a right kidney transplant. Increased uptake in the neck is likely a normal variant of muscle uptake due to contraction. Also, the transplanted kidney is visualized. The rest of the FDG distribution is normal. The absence of focal areas of abnormal FDG uptake suggests the absence of active neoplastic disease. Unattenuated 511-keV photon pairs from the center of the body vary from 20% of all events for the first patient to a little less than 10% in the heaviest. The fraction of scatter events increases with the weight of the patient from about 25% to about 35% for these three patients.

Physics Considerations in Small-Patient Imaging

The diseases to which PET has been applied for diagnosis and evaluation in adults are infrequent in pediatrics. Nevertheless, in certain applications, pediatric PET is taking up a more important role, specifically in brain imaging (epilepsy) as well as in whole-body imaging (bone tumors, lymphoma, neuroblastoma) (57). To date, no special scanners have been expressly designed for pediatric imaging; only adult scanners are used.

The pediatric population covers the range of patient sizes from newborns to young adults. Though the same considerations that apply to adults apply to children, imaging of small patients offers advantages and poses challenges for the optimal use of the instrumentation. The most obvious advantage is that in a small patient attenuation and scatter are relatively low. Also, the 3D mode should be particularly competitive for quantitative accuracy because the magnitude of the scatter compensation necessary is relatively lower. Sensitivity is particularly important to keep dose and scan time at a minimum, which may be particularly desirable in this population. On the other hand, energy resolution may be less of a concern because of the reduced need for scatter rejection. Finally, fast timing may not be necessary because of the low activity. Therefore, scanners based on high-sensitivity scintillators may be attractive in pediatrics in spite of their energy and timing resolution.

As for the overall geometry of the scanner, a smaller transverse field of view may be sufficient, especially for newborns and infants. Dedicated brain and small animal scanners were developed to take advantage of similar opportunities. It makes sense, then, to accommodate a patient sufficiently small in a brain scanner, which is designed to provide better resolution and higher sensitivity over a smaller and longer field of view than a whole-body scanner. This solution may be practical only for very few patients, likely not enough to justify the acquisition of a special purpose scanner at most institutions.

Conclusion

In pediatric PET imaging, the same scanners designed for adult imaging are used successfully. In general, PET image quality depends on the weight of the patient for a given scan time. In lighter patients, attenuation and scatter are minimized, which results in improved image quality. This is often the case in pediatric imaging, especially for younger patients. Alternatively, the improvement in image quality can be traded off for reduced scan time at constant image quality. The main challenge, in particular for the smallest patients, comes from the need for improved resolution and sensitivity, especially when lower tracer concentrations are used to minimize the dose burden to a young population. These needs can be answered with a scanner design with prolonged axial and reduced transverse field of view (and patient port). The result would then be a design similar to the adult brain scanners present at some research institutions. Operation in 3D mode seems particularly appealing again because of the low scatter and random fractions expected in pediatric studies. For the same reason, especially if low levels of activity are preferred for radiation exposure considerations, scintillators with high stopping power may be very competitive compared to less efficient or faster materials, even at the cost of relatively poor energy resolution and timing properties.

References

1. Valk PE, Bailey DL, Townsend DW, Maisey MN. Positron Emission Tomography: Basic Science and Clinical Practice. New York: Springer-Verlag, 2003.

2. Bendriem B, Townsend DW. The Theory and Practice of 3D PET. New York: Kluwer Academic Publishers, 1998.
3. Krane KS. Introductory Nuclear Physics. New York: Wiley, 1987.
4. Harpen MD. Positronium: review of symmetry, conserved quantities and decay for the radiological physicist. Med Phys 2004;31:57–61.
5. De Beneditti S, Cowan CE, Konneker WR, et al. On the angular distribution of two-photon annihilation radiation. Phys Rev 1950;77:205–212.
6. Levin CS, Hoffman EJ. Calculation of positron range and its effect on the fundamental limit of positron emission tomography system spatial resolution. Phys Med Biol 1999;44:781–799.
7. Evans RD. The Atomic Nucleus. New York: McGraw-Hill, 1955.
8. Surti S, Karp JS, Muehllehner G. Image quality assessment of LaBr3-based whole-body 3D PET scanners: a Monte Carlo evaluation. Phys Med Biol 2004;49:4593–4610.
9. Karp JS, Muehllehner G, Mankoff DA, et al. Continuous-slice PENN-PET: a positron tomograph with volume imaging capability. J Nucl Med 1990;31:617–627.
10. Adam LE, Karp JS, Daube-Witherspoon ME, Smith RJ. Performance of a whole-body PET scanner using curve-plate NaI(Tl) detectors. J Nucl Med 2001;42:1821–1830.
11. Surti S, Karp JS, Freifelder R, Liu F. Optimizing the performance of a PET detector using discrete GSO crystals on a continuous lightguide. IEEE Trans Nucl Sci 2000;47:1030–1036.
12. Nutt R, Casey M, Carroll LR, Dahlbom M, Hoffman EJ. A new multi-crystal two-dimensional detector block for PET. J Nucl Med 1985;26:P28.
13. Wong WH, Uribe J, Hicks K, Hu GJ. An analog decoding BGO block detector using circular photomultipliers. IEEE T Nucl Sci 1995;42:1095–1101.
14. Moses WW, Derenzo SE. Design studies for a PET detector module using a pin photodiode to measure depth of interaction. IEEE Trans Nucl Sci 1994;41:1441–1445.
15. Casey ME, Eriksson L, Schmand M, et al. Investigation of LSO crystals for high spatial resolution positron emission tomography. IEEE Trans Nucl Sci 1997;44:1109–1113.
16. El Fakhri G, Holdsworth C, Badawi RD, et al. Impact of acquisition geometry and patient habitus on lesion detectability in whole-body FDG-PET: a channelized Hotelling observer study. Presented at IEEE Nuclear Science Symposium and Medical Imaging Conference, Norfolk, VA, 2002.
17. Defrise M, Townsend DW, Bailey D, Geissbuhler A, Michel C, Jones T. A normalization technique for 3D PET data. Phys Med Biol 1991;36:939–952.
18. Bailey DL, Townsend DW, Kinahan PE, Grootoonk S, Jones T. An investigation of factors affecting detector and geometric correction in normalization of 3–D PET data. IEEE Trans Nucl Sci 1996;43:3300–3307.
19. Badawi RD, Lodge MA, Marsden PK. Algorithms for calculating detector efficiency normalization coefficients for true coincidences in 3D PET, Phys Med Biol 1998;43:189–205.
20. Badawi RD, Marsden PK. Developments in component-based normalization for 3D PET. Phys Med Biol 1999;44:571–594.
21. Badawi RD, Ferreira NC, Kohlmyer SG, Dahlbom M, Marsden PK, Lewellen TK. A comparison of normalization effects on three whole-body cylindrical 3D PET systems. Phys Med Biol 2000;45:3253–3266.
22. Carroll LR, Kertz P, Orcut G. The orbiting rod source: improving performance in PET transmission correction scans. In: Esser PD, ed. Emission Computed Tomography: Current Trends. Society of Nuclear Medicine, New York, 1983.

23. Huesman RH, Derenzo SE, Cahoon JL, et al. Orbiting transmission source for positron tomography. IEEE Trans Nucl Sci 1988;35:735–739.
24. Daube-Witherspoon M, Carson RE, Green MV. Postinjection transmission attenuation measurements for PET. IEEE Trans Nucl Sci 1988;NS-35:757–761.
25. deKemp RA, Nahmias C. Attenuation correction in PET using single photon transmission measurement. Med Phys 1994;21:771–778.
26. Karp JS, Muehllehner G, Qu H, Yan XH. Single transmission in volume-imaging PET with a Cs-137 source. Phys Med Biol 1995;40:929–944.
27. Smith RJ, Karp JS. Post-injection transmission scans in a PET camera operating without septa with simultaneous measurement of emission activity contamination. IEEE Trans Nucl Sci 1996;43:2207–2212.
28. Casey ME, Hoffman EJ. Quantitation in positron emission computed-tomography. 7. A technique to reduce noise in accidental coincidence measurements and coincidence efficiency calibration. J Comput Assist Tomogr 1986;10:845–850.
29. Badawi RD, Miller MP, Bailey DL, Marsden PK. Random variance reduction in 3D PET. Phys Med Biol 1999;44:941–954.
30. Karp JS, Muehllehner G, Mankoff DA, et al. Continuous-slice PENN-PET—a positron tomograph with volume imaging capability. J Nucl Med 1990; 31:617–627.
31. Cherry SR, Huang SC. Effects of scatter on model parameter estimates in 3D PET studies of the human brain. IEEE Trans Nucl Sci 1995;42:1174–1179.
32. Bergstrom M, Martin W, Pate B. A look at anatomical and physiological brain images. Dimensions Health Serv 1983;60:36.
33. Hoverath H, Kuebler WK, Ostertag HJ, et al. Scatter correction in the transaxial slices of a whole-body positron emission tomograph. Phys Med Biol 1993;38:717–728.
34. Bailey DL, Meikle SR. A convolution-subtraction scatter correction method for 3D PET. Phys Med Biol 1994;39:411–424.
35. Bendriem B, Trebossen R, Frouin V, Syrota A. A PET scatter correction using simultaneous acquisitions with low and high lower energy thresholds. Presented at 1993 IEEE Nuclear Science Symposium and Medical Imaging Conference, San Francisco, CA, 1993.
36. Grootoonk S, Spinks TJ, Sashin D, Spyrou NM, Jones T. Correction for scatter in 3D brain PET using a dual energy window method. Phys Med Biol 1996;41:2757–2774.
37. Adam LE, Karp JA, Freifelder R. Energy-based scatter correction for 3–D PET scanners using NaI(Tl) detectors. IEEE Trans Med Imaging 2000;19: 513–521.
38. Ollinger JM. Model-based scatter correction for fully 3D PET. Phys Med Biol 1996;41:153–176.
39. Watson CC, Newport D, Casey ME, deKemp RA, Beanlands RS, Schmand M. Evaluation of simulation-based scatter correction for 3-D PET cardiac imaging. IEEE Trans Nucl Sci 1997;44:90–97.
40. Accorsi R, Adam LE, Werner ME, Karp JS. Optimization of a fully 3D single scatter simulation algorithm for 3D PET. Phys Med Biol 2004;49: 2577–2598.
41. Levin CS, Dahlbom M, Hoffman EJ. A Monte-Carlo correction for the effect of Compton-scattering in 3-D PET brain imaging. IEEE Trans Nucl Sci 1995;42:1181–1185.
42. Holdsworth CH, Levin CS, Farquhar TH, Dahlbom M, Hoffman EJ. Investigation of accelerated Monte Carlo techniques for PET simulation and 3D PET scatter correction. IEEE Trans Nucl Sci 2001;48:74–81.

43. Holdsworth CH, Levin CS, Janecek M, Dahlbom M, Hoffman EJ. Performance analysis of an improved 3-D PET Monte Carlo simulation and scatter correction. IEEE Trans Nucl Sci 2002;49:83–89.

44. Lewitt RM, Matej S. Overview of methods for image reconstruction from projections in emission computed tomography. Proc IEEE 2003;91:1588–1611.

45. Defrise M, Kinahan PE, Michel C. Image reconstruction algorithms in PET. In: Valk PE, Bailey D, Townsend DW, Maisey MN, eds. Positron Emission Tomography: Basic Science and Clinical Practice. New York: Springer-Verlag, 2003:91–114.

46. Daube-Witherspoon ME, Muehllehner G. Treatment of axial data in three-dimensional PET. J Nucl Med 1987;28:1717–1724.

47. Defrise M, Kinahan PE, Townsend DW, Michel C, Sibomana M, Newport DF. Exact and approximate rebinning algorithms for 3D PET data. IEEE Trans Med Imaging 1997;11:145–158.

48. Shepp L, Vardi Y. Maximum likelihood reconstruction for emission tomography. IEEE Trans Med Imaging 1982;MI-1:113–122.

49. Lange K, Carson R. EM reconstruction algorithms for emission and transmission tomography. J Comput Assist Tomogr 1984;8:306–316.

50. Hudson HM, Larkin RS. Accelerated image reconstruction using ordered subsets of projection data. IEEE Trans Med Imaging 1994;13:601–609.

51. DePierro AR. On some nonlinear iterative relaxation methods in remote sensing. Matematica Aplicada Computacional 1989;8:153–166.

52. Browne JA, DePierro AR. A row-action alternative to the EM algorithm for maximizing likelihoods in emission tomography. IEEE Trans Med Imaging 1996;15:687–699.

53. Daube-Witherspoon ME, Matej S, Karp JS. Assessment of image quality with a fast fully 3D reconstruction algorithm. In: Siebert JA, ed. 2001 IEEE Nuclear Science Symposium and Medical Imaging Conference. Piscataway, NJ: Institute of Electrical and Electronics Engineers, 2002:M14–12.

54. Jeavons AP, Chandler RA, Dettmar CAR. A 3D HIDAC-PET camera with sub-millimetre resolution for imaging small animals. IEEE Trans Nucl Sci 1999;46:468–473.

55. Tai YC, Chatziioannou AF, Yang YF, et al. MicroPET II: design, development and initial performance of an improved microPET scanner for small-animal imaging. Phys Med Biol 2003;48:1519–1537.

56. Strother SC, Casey ME, Hoffman EJ. Measuring PET scanner sensitivity—relating count rates to image signal-to-noise ratios using noise equivalent counts. IEEE Trans Nucl Sci 1990;37:783–788.

57. Jadvar H, Connolly LP, Shulkin BL. PET imaging in pediatric disorders. In: Valk PE, Bailey D, Townsend DW, Maisey MN, eds. Positron Emission Tomography: Basic Science and Clinical Practice. New York: Springer-Verlag, 2003:755–774.

9

How to Image a Child by PET–Computed Tomography

Sue C. Kaste and M. Beth McCarville

Positron emission tomography (PET)–computed tomography (CT), which merges functional and anatomic imaging, is likely to herald a new generation of imaging modalities. Despite increasing interest and expertise in PET-CT, incorporation of such new technology into any department can be a challenge. Each department has its individual needs, personality, strengths, and weaknesses. The organization and integration of such imaging equipment must reflect these individual institutional and departmental characteristics, plus available supporting resources and the characteristics of patient cohorts.

The applicability of PET/PET-CT is well demonstrated in the adult population, particularly for oncologic and seizure imaging. It has only recently been applied in pediatrics, and therefore experience in the logistics and techniques for imaging children and adolescents are limited. Similarly, the diagnostic sensitivity and specificity of PET/PET-CT and its effect on patient management and outcomes are still largely uncharacterized.

This chapter addresses several issues raised by pediatric application of PET-CT. It is written primarily from the vantage point of a dedicated tertiary-care pediatric institution. However, it also addresses issues that can be expected to arise when children are scanned in a predominantly adult department. This chapter does not address all concerns, but rather lays a foundation for the implementation of this exciting new technique in the practice of pediatric imaging.

Pre-Scanning Considerations

Interaction with Patient and Family

Efficient and successful completion of the examination requires the cooperation of the patient and family, proper patient preparation, and relief of patient and family anxiety. An inviting, comfortable, child-friendly environment should greet the patient and family upon arrival to minimize their anxiety. At the time of scheduling, the patient and family should be advised of the pre-scan fasting requirements, adjustment of potential hypoglycemic medications, the need for quiet rest during the equilibrium phase, the expected length of the examination, and the sharing of results with the appropriate family members.

Pre-scan education should be directed at both the parents and the patient. The amount of information that children can understand and their ability to participate in procedures are typically underestimated (1–4). However, children are not small adults, and interactions with them should be age-appropriate (1–4). The family should be instructed in radiation safety, with emphasis on maintaining maximum distance from the patient during the uptake phase. We typically permit one family member to remain with a young child during the uptake phase. However, pregnant family members and siblings should not be present after fluorine-18 fluorodeoxyglucose (^{18}F-FDG) has been administered. If a single adult arrives with the young patient and siblings, care for the siblings may be a matter of urgency. Therefore, the family should be advised to arrange for child care before the appointment, or provisions for such care should be proactively arranged by the institution or department.

The same principles of radiation safety must be extended to ancillary personnel, who should also be monitored for radiation exposure. This precaution applies particularly to those in prolonged close proximity to the patient, such as sedation nurses and anesthesiologists. A rotation schedule like that used for nuclear medicine technologists may be needed in some departments. Such provisions depend on the number of PET-CT cases per day, staff availability, and departmental and institutional resources. In some cases, movable clear shields may be used to enhance the protection of personnel and family members from radiation.

Scheduling and Logistics

Coordination of Related Services

Numerous institutional departments and services must coordinate their efforts in order to successfully care for the pediatric patient and obtain the optimal PET-CT imaging. Figure 9.1 shows many of the resource components that must be organized. The key to successful completion of the study is communication and coordination of the many services involved. The role of each component is briefly addressed below.

The PET/PET-CT study begins with a request for the examination by the health care provider. The request should include the age of the patient, details about why the examination is needed, pertinent medical history (e.g., allergies, current medications, history of diabetes, surgery), need for sedation/general anesthesia, and whether an interpreter is needed.

Upon receipt of the request, the scheduler must identify potential scheduling conflicts (e.g., other imaging studies, clinic appointments, sedation requirements, laboratory tests). The range of services needed and their availability for the individual patient must be identified. Upon verification of the PET/PET-CT appointment, the patient or

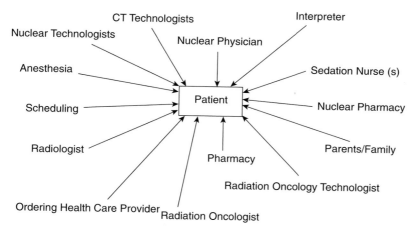

Figure 9.1. Diagram of the interaction of the multiple departments and personnel necessary for coordination of PET/PET-CT.

family is given the appointment time, preexamination preparation instructions, and contact information should the patient or family have questions.

Behind-the-scenes preparation includes the scheduling of a sedation team member or anesthetist, an interpreter if needed, reservation of the uptake room and PET/PET-CT scanner, identification of needed nuclear medicine or CT technologists, and scheduling of a recovery area in the event that sedation or anesthesia is used.

When the PET/PET-CT study is scheduled, order details entered into the scheduling system appear on the work schedules of the diagnostic imaging or nuclear medicine department, depending on the institution. This item on the schedule prompts the nuclear medicine technologist to interact with the nuclear pharmacy to ensure that the ^{18}F-FDG dose will be available at the appropriate time. The designated radiologist or nuclear medicine physician responsible for the study reviews the order details and prescribes the patient positioning, anatomic areas to be assessed, and possible use of contrast material.

If the information obtained from the PET/PET-CT study is to be used for radiation therapy treatment planning, direct interaction with the designated radiation oncologist and radiation therapy technologist is needed to facilitate PET/PET-CT data acquisition. This interaction is particularly important when PET/PET-CT images are to be electronically merged with information stored in computer programs used to design the radiation therapy treatment plan.

The primary health care provider and the institutional pharmacy should be notified of a PET/PET-CT study on an inpatient to allow adjustment of diabetic medications, intravenous fluids, and total parenteral nutrition.

In an institution such as ours that has central scheduling and electronic order entry, coordination of some of the resources can be built into the order set for the PET/PET-CT. Similarly, patient preparation instructions can be automatically printed at the time of scheduling and given to the patient or appropriate family member. These instructions can be linked to the electronic medical record for the reference of house staff and nursing personnel.

In the absence of electronic scheduling, the needed services are usually coordinated by the scheduler, who phones each department to request that the needed services be available at the agreed-upon appointment time. One central person should be responsible for relaying the appointment information to the patient or accompanying family member.

Additional scheduling considerations may be necessary when pediatric patients undergo PET/PET-CT imaging in a predominantly adult department. Scheduling adjustments might include specified days of the week for pediatric imaging, a special waiting area with child-appropriate activities, pediatric-oriented informational brochures, and child life personnel who interact with patients and family members. To further minimize patient and family anxiety, consideration should also be given to placement of the intravenous access by pediatric specialists before the patient reports to the imaging department.

Diagnostic CT Imaging Performed Simultaneously with PET/PET-CT
Contemporary PET-CT units merge state-of-the-art CT and PET elements, allowing routine diagnostic CT imaging and PET scans to be performed independently of each other. In our institution, PET-CTs take priority over routine diagnostic CTs on the PET-CT unit. However, any unscheduled table time on the PET-CT unit may be used for routine CTs, biopsies, radiation therapy planning, etc. Such prioritization varies among institutions and depends on the number of CT scanners, the number of PET-CT scanners, and the number and types of cases. Similarly, scheduling of imaging for clinical management, as opposed to studies driven by research protocols, reflects the caseload of the institution.

The level of demand for PET-CT studies shortly after installation of our equipment allowed the use of the PET-CT unit for both a PET-CT and a diagnostic CT on the same patient, when so ordered. The orders were designed so that the CT could be ordered within the PET-CT order; it was not necessary to schedule them separately. The two studies could be completed within a single 60-minute appointment time. This scheduling method made efficient use of the imaging table, shortened patient visits, minimized patient inconvenience, and averted any need for multiple administration of sedation or anesthesia. The imaging department member responsible for the PET-CT would prescribe the studies in such a way as to minimize radiation exposure to the patient and optimize the information obtained. Low-dose CT parameters are typically used for the attenuation-correction CT, and standard CT imaging parameters are used for the diagnostic study. However, a diagnostic-quality CT scan using a higher milliampere-second (mAs) setting than routinely used for the attenuation-correction CT can be used for used for PET-CT and eliminates the need to perform two separate CT scans. If needed, display field of view (DFOV) can retrospectively be changed. An additional 10 to 15 minutes of postprocessing time on the system console is needed to convert the image data into an acceptable diagnostic CT. This method would typically include the oral administration of contrast material before the attenuation-correction CT is performed. Intravenous contrast material would be administered during the attenuation-correction CT. Like others, we have found that the intravenous nonionic contrast and low-density oral contrast media used with diagnostic CT are compatible with PET-CT (4–10).

Patients and parents can be confused by the need to maintain glucose restriction when diagnostic CTs are coordinated with PET-CT. We find that both intravenous (IV) and oral contrast agents used for diagnostic CTs can be used in pediatric PET-CT without compromising the PET-CT study. In fact, as others have reported (4,5), IV and oral contrast can improve interpretation of the PET-CT, particularly in studies of small children with limited retroperitoneal fat and in differentiation of vessels from lymph nodes and tumors that lack ^{18}F-FDG avidity in the mediastinum and neck. However, oral contrast agents must be taken with sugar-free beverages. We provide a choice of flavored sugar-free mixes to our patients. In a department such as ours, where CT and PET-CT technologists are shared and the examinations are performed in adjacent suites, sugar-free beverage mixes for oral contrast agent could be offered to all patients undergoing CT, whether or not PET-CT is also scheduled. Such an approach might minimize patient confusion but places the burden of dispensing the beverages on the technologists and the department. The logistics of such a practice depend on the department and the institution.

Arm position also becomes an issue when the two types of studies are combined; this consideration is discussed below (see Patient Positioning).

With increasing demand for PET-CT studies, we will likely begin performing on the PET-CT unit only those diagnostic CT studies that require sedation or anesthesia. All others will be scheduled on the standard diagnostic CT unit. The diagnostic CT is most often performed as a completely separate study after completion of the PET/PET-CT. This method optimizes use of the PET/PET-CT scanner for its specialized purpose, allows the patient to rest between studies, and allows more flexibility in the administration of oral and intravenous contrast.

Patient Preparation

Forcing of sugar-free beverages or intravenous fluids before administration of ^{18}F-FDG can help to clear background avidity and improve image interpretation. Oral administration of fluids must be coordinated with the need for sedation or anesthesia (discussed below).

To minimize competition between physiologic glucose and ^{18}F-FDG, patients are typically instructed to fast overnight for early morning studies and for a minimum of 4 hours before studies performed later in the day. Departments may request an NPO (nothing by mouth) period of 4 to 8 hours before ^{18}F-FDG administration (4,11–16). The difference largely reflects patient age and the need for sedation or general anesthesia.

Adherence to an NPO instruction can be particularly challenging in pediatrics. Despite the best efforts of parents and health care providers, pediatric patients seem to have an endless hidden repository of sugar-laden treats. Although a single gummy worm may not adversely affect FDG uptake in an adolescent, a bag of jelly beans can potentially block FDG uptake in a 6-year-old, thus prompting cancellation of the study and the possible waste of the FDG dose.

When studies are performed on inpatients, similar coordination and education should be implemented with the nursing staff, pharmacy, sedation team, and primary care service. There is a real possibility that an inpatient may arrive in the nuclear medicine suite while receiving intravenous fluids, not uncommonly with added dextrose [e.g., dextrose 5% in water (D_5W) with 50g added dextrose, total parenteral nutrition, etc.]. For this reason, the need for fasting and avoidance of glucose-laden solutions must be communicated to the primary health care service, nursing staff, and pharmacy. Further, management of serum glucose levels in diabetics may be more complicated than adherence to NPO restrictions. Modification of patient diet or medication should be coordinated by the responsible service or individual in collaboration with nuclear medicine, the patient, technologists, and other ancillary personnel.

Medications and liquids that might not readily be appreciated as containing sugars include diphenhydramine (Benadryl) liquid and cough medicines flavored with sugar syrups. Direct questioning of the patient or accompanying adult about the use of such medications is thus necessary.

Serum glucose should be assayed before the radioisotope is injected. Typically, a serum glucose concentration below 200mg/dL is adequately low to allow FDG uptake into metabolically active tissues. Some departments prefer to maintain a glucometer in the nuclear medicine suite and incorporate a serum glucose check into the pre-scan preparation. In other institutions, serum glucose is determined in the main laboratory and expeditiously reported to nuclear medicine before FDG injection.

Uptake Phase

During the uptake phase (after ^{18}F-FDG injection and prior to imaging), the patient should rest quietly in a warm, nonthreatening environment designed to allay anxiety (Fig. 9.2). A nonpregnant parent, guardian, or health care provider may sit with young children but must adhere to radiation protection guidelines. If the patient is to undergo imaging of the axial and appendicular body, then quiet resting activity may be allowed. Such activity includes watching an age-appropriate video, listening to a story, or listening to music. It can be quite a challenge to keep a toddler or young child at quiet rest for up to an hour after injec-

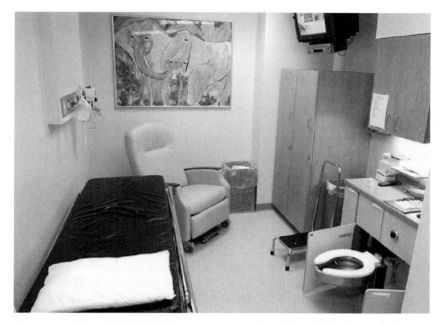

Figure 9.2. The PET/PET-CT uptake room should be fully furnished, comfortable, and nonthreatening for the patient and accompanying adult. Note the wall-mounted television. A ceiling-mounted video camera by which the patient is constantly monitored is located in the corner opposite the television.

tion; even such seemingly negligible activity as chewing gum, talking, or playing video games may complicate FDG interpretation.

If the patient is to undergo PET/PET-CT imaging of the brain, then any stimulation of the central nervous system should be kept to a bare minimum. The room should be darkened, quiet, and soothing. If possible, eye shields should be used to prevent visual stimulation, which can prompt occipital activity. Similarly, videos, music, and talking are avoided.

Uptake of ^{18}F-FDG by thermogenic "brown fat" can complicate image interpretation. The uptake of ^{18}F-FDG by brown fat has been attributed to the ambient outdoor temperature (17–19). It is seen more often in females than males and occurs more often in children and young adults than in older patients (17–19). Rats exposed to a cold room for several hours prior to imaging showed stimulation of ^{18}F-FDG uptake (19). The effect of brief exposure to cool or cold temperatures in humans has not been verified. However, this finding in rats suggests that a warm equilibrium room or possibly the use of an extra blanket or heavier clothing may minimize the ^{18}F-FDG avidity of brown fat. Such uptake can potentially complicate imaging interpretation, particularly when PET is performed without correlative CT imaging (11,12,17–21).

For patients who are extremely restless or anxious, quiet rest may be facilitated by the use of anxiolytic drugs during the equilibrium phase. We do not typically administer such agents. However, if a patient is noted to be particularly restless during the equilibrium phase or scan-ning at our institution, or if children have a prior history of anxiety during studies at other institutions, anxiolytics are considered for future studies.

Patient monitoring begins with the registration of the patient in the imaging department and continues from the time of injection until completion of post-scan recovery. At our institution, the patient is injected with ^{18}F-FDG in the uptake room. This room is constantly mon-itored by a video camera, which allows real-time viewing of the patient and the room from the PET/CT scanning console area directly across the hall.

Scanning of the Patient

Timing of Imaging

Positron emission tomography imaging should be timed in coordina-tion with the chemotherapy cycles to prevent their affecting the results of studies. Imaging done for staging purposes should be performed before induction chemotherapy or other therapeutic intervention.

The timing of follow-up imaging may be more variable. However, we have found that the optimal time to assess the response to therapy is probably just before the next course of therapy. This strategy mini-mizes any potential "flare" response from chemotherapy, granulocyte colony-stimulating factor, radiation therapy, or even radiofrequency ablation. A flare response typically occurs within 2 days of chemother-apy or radiation therapy. Similarly, postoperative changes are most apparent during the first several weeks after surgery. Therefore, we prefer to wait at least 2 to 3 weeks after surgery before performing follow-up imaging.

Standardization of technique is important to allow the comparison of studies, particularly when response is to be quantified by imaging. As many patients with cancer undergo serial imaging for assessment of treatment response, a log of prior imaging parameters or inclusion of these parameters in the dictated report is helpful to ensure consis-tent imaging. These include radiopharmaceutical dose, equilibration time, two- or three-dimensional image acquisition, patient height and weight, and patient positioning.

One potentially overlooked aspect of standardization is synchrony of the PET-CT clock with the clock used to determine dose assay times. The "hot lab" clock is typically used to calculate the dose of ^{18}F-FDG at the time of injection, and the clock in PET-CT is used to determine the time that scanning is initiated. Dose quantification for the study at the time of scanning will be inaccurate if these two clocks are not synchronized.

Immobilization of the Patient

Patient immobilization is paramount in obtaining well-registered PET/CT studies with minimal motion artifact. Difficulty in maintaining immobilization is dependent on several factors: child age, medical condition, pain level, physical positioning of the patient on the scanning table, and length of time to complete the study (which is partly dependent on patient size).

There are several standard immobilization techniques that may be used with PET/CT. Swaddling may be considered for very young or small infants and children, particularly for short studies. This technique may be particularly effective if the scanning time can be coordinated with the patient's usual nap time. Immobilization is optimized by ensuring that the patient is comfortable and warm and that any potential pain has been controlled.

More sophisticated immobilization techniques include special cushions similar to those used in radiation oncology: the child is placed on a cushion that is filled with tiny plastic balls and is fitted to the contour of the patient by vacuum extraction. For more cooperative children, patient positioning may be maintained by using sandbags, rolled towels, or pillows held in place by strategically placed strips of tape or Velcro straps.

Certainly immobilization is optimized when the patient is sedated under general anesthesia. In such cases, the anesthesiologist is in control of the patient and positioning must adhere to the needs of the anesthesiologist in the interest of patient safety.

Sedation and General Anesthesia

As with other lengthy pediatric procedures, sedation or general anesthesia may be necessary to complete the PET-CT examination. This is particularly true when imaging very young children who cannot cooperate, those who are mentally impaired, and for the few who demonstrate claustrophobia (11). For some patients, adequate pain control may be all that is needed to complete the study. Our practice is to employ sedation or anesthesia only for the imaging phase of the examination. Rarely, sedation may be needed during the equilibrium phase as well, but such a practice considerably extends the sedation/anesthesia time.

We calculated that 11.3% (16/142) of patients who underwent PET-CT at our institution during the months of September through November 2004 received sedation or anesthesia. We performed eight studies in children aged 0 to 4 years, 28 studies in 5- to 10-year-old children, 74 studies in 11- to 18-year-olds, and 32 studies in patients older than 18 years. Of these, 10 patients aged 22 months to 7 years received intravenous sedation. General anesthesia was administered to five patients aged 23 months to 20 years. One additional patient received intravenous medication for pain control.

The preferred method of sedation/anesthesia varies by institution, department, resources, and patient demographics; detailed discussion is beyond the scope of this chapter. However, it should always be administered according to the published guidelines of the American Academy of Pediatrics and the American Society of Anesthesiologists (22,23). At our institution, sedation/anesthesia falls under the auspices of the Department of Anesthesia. Under the direction of anesthesiologists or sedation physicians, nurse anesthetists and members of the nursing sedation team assess the patient prior to sedation and administer the sedation, or in the case of nurse anesthetists, general anesthesia. They monitor the patient throughout the examination until full recovery.

Other potential mechanisms for patient care and administration of sedation/anesthesia include management by a sedation pediatrician dedicated solely to this task or by the attending pediatrician, radiologist, intensivist, or emergency room physician. Regardless of the mechanism for managing the patient under sedation/anesthesia, qualified personnel whose only responsibility is the care and safety of the patient must be in attendance throughout the study.

The need for sedation/anesthesia affects study scheduling, the need for supportive staff and resources, and the use and timing of oral contrast administration. We have strict NPO requirements designed according to the practice guidelines of the American Academy of Pediatrics and the American Society of Anesthesiologists (22,23) that prohibit oral contrast ingestion less than 2 hours prior to sedation. These patients may require separate appointments for PET/PET-CT and a diagnostic CT for which opacification of the gastrointestinal tract is needed. We make every effort to minimize the number of potential sedations, contrast administrations, and appointments for the patient while optimizing the use of imaging and staffing resources. However, patient imaging must be managed on a case-by-case basis as discussed above.

Patient Positioning

The standard position for PET imaging is the position of comfort with the patient supine and arms at the sides or over the head if the patient can tolerate the position. If the primary site of interest is in the head or neck, then the arms should be placed alongside the torso. However, this position causes significant streak artifacts on the CT images, often limiting the utility of the images. This is particularly problematic when a diagnostic CT and PET-CT are combined in a single study. If the arms are positioned over the patient's head, then additional imaging stations are required to fully image the upper extremities in total body PET/PET-CT studies. This position is also difficult for patients to maintain during the prolonged PET imaging phase of the study. In such cases, positioning pads or cushions may be helpful. A possible alternative is to lay the patient's arms across the abdomen; however, this position is more difficult to accurately reproduce on subsequent studies. Arm positioning is a particular issue when the primary disease—or metastatic site—is in the upper extremity.

The positioning of the patient is also dictated by the need for sedation/anesthesia, which requires that the airway and the ability to monitor vital signs be given priority. As with any procedure, the physical condition of the patient plays a significant part in positioning. This can be particularly challenging in young or lightly sedated children.

The patience and creativity of the technologists or parents in working with the patient are often the key to successful imaging.

One aspect of positioning that might not be readily apparent is the alignment of the patient positioning for the PET/PET-CT study with the position used for radiation therapy. This positional coordination allows improved merging of image data with the treatment planning data. It may be necessary to scan patients in the prone position or on the positioning cushions as done for administration of therapeutic radiation. Therefore, the imaging team should interact with the radiation oncology team.

Scanning Sequence

Whether a whole-body study (vertex to toes) or a targeted study (e.g., head, torso, pelvis) is performed should be decided by the information needed to care for the patient. In many cases, a PET/PET-CT study is used for tumor staging. In such cases, detection of distant metastatic disease is important for selecting the appropriate treatment strategy. In other cases, determination of the response of a primary brain tumor or the presence of residual disease in a site of previous surgery or radiofrequency ablation may entail a study limited to the area of interest.

Tracer activity in a full bladder can cause significant reconstruction artifacts and may obscure important pathology. To prevent problems caused by the bladder filling between the time scanning is initiated and the time the pelvis is imaged, we image the pelvis first and then scan cephalad through the head in the first set of acquisitions. The rest of the body (pelvis through legs) is scanned in the second set of acquisitions. Between the two sets of acquisitions, the patient is able to void if necessary. Although this method of scanning reduces artifact caused by a distended, radioisotope-filled bladder, it adds 25 to 30 minutes to the appointment.

An alternative method is to use bladder catheterization with gravity drainage. The bladder catheter should be placed prior to imaging but after the child has been sedated/anesthetized to minimize trauma to the patient. If the catheter is placed at a later time during the procedure, the remaining sedation may be inadequate to maintain the child's comfort. A bladder catheter may be needed for children who are to receive sedation/anesthesia, as such medications predispose the patient to bladder activity (11). To avoid catheter artifact, a drainage catheter should be long enough to position the drainage bag outside of the imaging field.

Technologists' Roles

State mandates regulating the licensing and handling of radiopharmaceuticals vary to a certain degree and should be consulted during planning for PET and PET-CT. The roles of the CT technologist and the nuclear medicine technologist must be addressed by each institution. The interest and skills of the available technologists, staffing limitations, and physical location of the equipment, together with compliance with regulatory mandates, help to define technologists' roles. In some institutions, staffing and familiarity with the operation of a CT scanner may dictate that the CT technologist perform the actual scanning procedure after radiopharmaceutical injection by the nuclear medicine technologist. In other institutions, the nuclear medicine technologists learn CT scanning techniques and are responsible for completion of the entire study.

There are currently no formalized specialty registries for certification of PET-CT technologists. However, the American Society of Radiologic Technologists (ASRT) and the Society of Nuclear Medicine Technologist Section (SNMTS) are collaboratively designing a supplementary training curriculum that will address the needs of practicing technologists who wish to obtain competency in this new modality. The best source of information on local regulatory mandates and legislation is the Radiation Safety Office under which the PET/PET-CT facility operates and under which the technologists practice. Additional useful Web sites include those of the Nuclear Regulatory Commission (http://www.nrc.gov), the American Society of Radiologic Technologists (http://asrt.org), the Society of Nuclear Medicine (http://snm.org), the American Registry of Radiologic Technologists (http://www.arrt.org), and the Nuclear Medicine Technology Certification Board (http://www.nmtcb.org).

When we began PET-CT imaging, the nuclear medicine technologists accompanied the patient to the uptake room, injected the radiopharmaceutical, and transferred monitoring of the patient and completion of the study to the CT technologists. After the appropriate equilibrium time, the patient would be instructed to void and transported across the hall to the PET-CT scan room by the CT technologist, who would complete the patient scanning and image processing. If a diagnostic CT was also ordered, it would be completed during the same appointment time. After scanning was complete, the patient was dismissed by the CT technologists or observed by the sedation/anesthesia team until recovery.

Currently, our nuclear medicine technologists are responsible for all phases of the PET-CT examination. If a diagnostic CT has also been ordered, then one of the CT technologists performs that study separately. A diagnostic CT is currently ordered with PET/PET-CTs in approximately 80% of cases in our institution. This number varies by institution. Transfer of technologist responsibility and transfer of patients between scanners is facilitated in our department by design of the CT imaging suite. The dedicated CT scanner and the PET-CT scanner occupy adjacent rooms with a shared console area.

Conclusion

Positron emission tomography–computed tomography is an exciting imaging modality that merges functional and anatomic information and that is expected to refine assessment of disease and response to therapy. Though in its infancy, particularly for imaging children and adolescents, it shows great promise in the detection and monitoring of disease. Special logistical procedures should be implemented for the care, safety, and monitoring of pediatric patients. This chapter serves as a starting point for planning and implementing PET-CT imaging in pediatrics.

References

1. Tates K, Meeuwesen L. "Let mum have her say": Turntaking in a doctor-parent-child communication. Counseling 2000;40:151–162.
2. Rushforth H. Practitioner review: communicating with hospitalised children: review and application of research pertaining to children's understanding of health and illness. J Child Psychol Psychiatry 1999;40:683–691.
3. Jay SM, Elliott CH, Ozolons M, et al. Behaviourial management of children's distress during painful medical procedures. Behav Res Ther 1985;23:513–520.
4. Borgwardt L, Larsen HJ, Pedersen K, et al. Practical use and implementation of PET in children in a hospital PET centre. Eur J Nucl Med Molec Imag 2003;30(10):1389–1397.
5. Dizendorf EV, Treyer V, von Schulthess GK, et al. Application of oral contrast media in coregistered positron emission tomography-CT. AJR 2002;179:477–481.
6. Antoch G, Freudenberg LS, Strattus J, et al. Whole-body positron emission tomography-CT: optimized CT using oral and IV contrast materials. AJR 2002;179:1555–1560.
7. Nakamoto Y, Chin BB, Kraitchman DL, et al. Effects of nonionic intravenous contrast agents at PET/CT imaging: phantom and canine studies. Radiology 2003;227(3):817–824.
8. Cohade C, Osman M, Nakamoto Y, et al. Initial experience with oral contrast in PET/CT: phantom and clinical studies. J Nucl Med 2003;44(3):412–416.
9. Cohade C, Wahl RL. Applications of positron emission tomography/computed tomography image fusion in clinical positron emission tomography—clinical use, interpretation methods, diagnostic improvements. Semin Nucl Med 2003;33(3):228–237.
10. Roberts EG, Shulkin BL. Technical issues in performing PET studies in pediatric patients. J Nucl Med Technol 2004;32:5–9.
11. Shulkin BL. PET imaging in pediatric oncology. Pediatr Radiol 2004;34(3):199–204.
12. Kaste SC. Issues specific to implementing PET-CT for pediatric oncology: what we have learned along the way. Pediatr Radiol 2004;34(3):205–213.
13. Roberts EG, Shulkin BL. Technical issues in performing PET studies in pediatric patients. J Nucl Med Technol 2004;32(1):5–9.
14. Jadvar H, Connolly LP, Shulkin BL, et al. Positron-emission tomography in pediatrics. Nucl Med Annu 2000;53–83.
15. Wahl RL. Principles of cancer imaging with fluorodeoxyglucose. In: Wahl RL, Buchanan JW, eds. Principles and Practice of Positron Emission Tomography. Philadelphia: Lippincott Williams & Wilkins, 2002:100–110.
16. Bar-Shalom R, Yefremov N, Guralnik L, et al. Clinical performance of PET/CT in evaluation of cancer: additional value for diagnostic imaging and patient management. J Nucl Med 2003;44:1200–1209.

17. Yeung HWD, Grewal RK, Gonen M, et al. Patterns of 18F-FDG uptake in adipose tissue and muscle: a potential source of false-positives for PET. J Nucl Med 2003;44:1789–1796.

18. Cohade C, Mourtzikos KA, Wahl RL. "USA-Fat": prevalence is related to ambient outdoor temperature—evaluation with 18F-FDG PET/CT. J Nucl Med 2003;44:1267–1270.

19. Cohade C, Osman M, Pannu HK, et al. Uptake in supraclavicular area fat ("USA-Fat"): description on 18F-FDG PET/CT. J Nucl Med 2003;44(2): 170–176.

20. Tatsumi M, Engles JM, Ishimori T, et al. Intense (18)F-FDG uptake in brown fat can be reduced pharmacologically. J Nucl Med 2004;45(7):1189–1193.

21. Hudson MM, Krasin MJ, Kaste SC. PET imaging in pediatric Hodgkin's lymphoma. Pediatr Radiol 2004;34(3):190–198.

22. American Academy of Pediatrics: Committee on Drugs. Guidelines for monitoring and management of pediatric patients during and after sedation for diagnostic and therapeutic procedures. Pediatrics 1992;89:1110–1117.

23. American Society of Anesthesiologists: Task Force on sedation and analgesia by non-anesthesiologists. Practice guidelines for sedation and analgesia by non-anesthesiologists. Anesthesiology 2002;96:1004–1017.

10

Coincidence Imaging

Girish Bal, Stefaan Vandenberghe, and Martin Charron

The concept of using gamma cameras to detect the 511 keV γ rays, arising from the annihilation of a positron, was first implemented by H.O. Anger in the late 1950s (1–4). These cameras were capable of acquiring planar images of low-energy single photons as well as acquiring tomographic images of 511-keV photons in the coincidence mode. In the absence of a collimator, the resolution and sensitivity of the images obtained using the coincidence mode was far superior to that obtained using a collimated single photon emission computed tomography (SPECT) system. However, due to the limited count rate capability, slow computational speed, and lack of algorithms to process the acquired coincidence data, coincidence imaging was not widely used for clinical applications. Further, the limited availability of the fast decaying positron emitting tracers, coupled with limited reimbursement from the insurance companies, temporarily halted the development of gamma camera–based positron emission tomography (GCPET) systems (5,6).

In the mid-1990s, significant improvements were made to overcome the count rate limitations of the sodium iodide [NaI(Tl)]-based gamma cameras (7–11). These improvements coupled with the establishment of regional distribution centers for fluorine-18 fluorodeoxyglucose (FDG) resulted in renewed interest in GCPET as a cost-effective alternative to dedicated positron emission tomography (PET) systems. Furthermore, the relatively long half-life of FDG, compared to other positron tracers, enabled longer acquisition times so as to obtain statistically significant counts for a faithful reconstruction. The convenience of performing both single photon and positron imaging on the same scanner made GCPET an attractive option, in terms of cost-effectiveness, for many nuclear medicine departments around the world.

Single Photon Emission Computed Tomography Imaging of 511-keV Photons

Apart from the fact that GCPET can be used to image the biodistribution of positron tracers in coincidence mode, they can also be used to image the 511-keV photons as single photons using an ultra-high energy collimator. In this imaging protocol, the annihilation photons are detected as single photons that successfully pass through the collimator holes. To compromise between the ability to detect a sufficient number of 511-keV photons and at the same time achieve reasonable spatial resolution, collimators with thick lead septa and long bores were designed. For example, an ultra-high energy parallel-hole collimator consisting of hexagonal holes with a diameter of 5.08 mm (flat side to flat side), septal thickness of 3.43 mm, and bore length of 77 mm was designed for FDG-SPECT imaging using a three-head gamma camera (12) (Fig. 10.1). This system had a spatial resolution of about 11 to 15 mm full width half maximal (FWHM) for a point source placed at a distance of 10 cm from the collimator and a sensitivity of about two counts per second per microcurie (μCi) per detector.

In spite of the thick septa, some septal penetration is inevitable, resulting in a loss of resolution as well as an increase in the background activity in the projection data. This background tends to degrade the contrast of the reconstructed image, thereby degrading the detectability of lesions smaller than 2 to 3 cm (13,14). Hence, 511-keV SPECT is

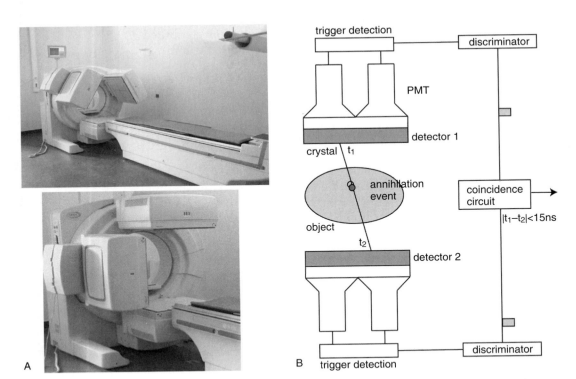

Figure 10.1. A: A three-head gamma camera–based positron emission tomography (GCPET) system (Philips Irix 3000). The three heads can be placed at different gantry angles with respect to each other and can be used for both routine SPECT as well as for coincidence imaging. B: A schematic representation of the coincidence circuit used in a GCPET system. For a coincidence event to be detected, the two photons must be detected within the 15-ns timing window and should lie within the specified energy range.

not widely used for the detection of tumors in patients. On the other hand, for cardiologic applications, several clinical studies have shown that FDG SPECT is capable of providing diagnostic information similar to that obtained using a dedicated PET system (13,15–24). The gantry with an ultra-high energy collimator (weighing about 150 kg each) is rotated around the patient so as to obtain complete tomographic information. For cardiac imaging, using a dual-head GCPET system, the two detectors can be placed either 90 degrees (18) or 180 degrees apart (19). For the 90-degree geometry, the detector is rotated from 45 degrees right anterior oblique to 45 degrees left posterior oblique, so as to measure projections closer to the heart walls. The projection data is saved in a 64 × 64 matrix with a pixel size of about 7 mm. The large pixel size, large hole diameter, and increased septal penetration result in reconstructed cardiac images with limited spatial resolution. To recover the lost resolution and contrast, an iterative reconstruction algorithm that models the depth-dependent geometric point spread function is used (25). Reconstructed images obtained using the resolution recovery algorithm were found to give improved qualitative and quantitative images for both phantom as well as patient studies. The resolution recovery algorithm plays a critical role, especially in dynamic FDG-SPECT studies (26) where the poor resolution of the reconstructed images can significantly affect the bias in the kinetic rate parameters.

Coincidence Detection Using GCPET

A SPECT camera requires wide range of hardware and software modifications to facilitate the detection of high-energy coincidence photons (Fig. 10.1). Some of these modifications and their effects on image acquisition and image quality are described in detail in the next few sections of this chapter. The most significant of these changes were increasing the crystal thickness and modifying the electronics so as to identify the coincidence photons from the large number of high-energy photons detected by the system.

Crystal Properties

Traditional gamma cameras used in SPECT, were built of NaI(Tl) crystals with a thickness of 9.5 mm. The thickness of these crystals was sufficient for low-energy photons as they had a photo-peak detection efficiency of 100% for 70-keV photons (201-Tl) and detection efficiency of 84% for 140-keV photons [technetium-99m (^{99m}Tc)]. However, for 511-keV photons, the photo-peak detection efficiency of a 9.5-mm NaI(Tl) crystal is reduced to just 13%. To make matters worse, in the coincidence-imaging mode both 511-keV photons need to be detected simultaneously. Thus the combined photo-peak detection efficiency of the 511-keV coincidence events is 13% × 13% = 1.69%. To overcome this problem of reduced detection efficiency, the use of thicker crystals was proposed (3,27), thereby increasing the probability of photon interactions in the crystal.

Table 10.1 shows the detection efficiency of NaI crystals of varying thicknesses. Increasing the thickness to 19.1 mm results in a corresponding increase in detection efficiency to 24% for 511-keV photons. Hence, in the coincidence mode the combined efficiency of the two 511-keV photons is 24% × 24% = 5.76%. This increase in efficiency in the coincidence mode corresponds to a total improvement of 3.3 times compared to a 9.5-mm crystal. Figure 10.2 shows the maximum true coincidence count rates, measured using an unattenuated point source, for various crystal thickness and dead times (28).

Recently, manufacturers have tried using NaI(Tl) crystals that are 2.5 cm thick. Increasing the crystal thickness tends to degrade the spatial resolution of the SPECT images. To overcome this problem, orthogonal grooves (1.3 cm deep) are cut into the crystal surface facing the photomultiplier tube (PMT), thereby reducing the light spread in the crystal (29). These grooves contain the light within each block, thereby providing improved resolution for SPECT as well as for coincidence imaging. Further, for SPECT imaging it was observed that the low-energy high-resolution (LEHR) collimator plays a dominating role in determining the overall resolution of the system. For a ^{99m}Tc point source placed at a distance of 10 cm from the LEHR collimator, the difference in resolution between a 9.5-mm and 19.1-mm-thick crystal was found to be just 0.2 mm (30).

In spite of the improved gain observed by increasing the crystal thickness, NaI(Tl) crystals have a very poor stopping power compared to crystals such as BGO, LSO, and GSO. On the other hand, the energy resolution and relative light output of the NaI crystals are far better than those of the other crystals, thereby enabling better scatter correction using multiple energy windows (Table 10.2) (31). To improve the detection efficiency of both low- and high-energy photons, new detectors consisting of different crystals sandwiched together were proposed. Such detectors are usually made up of a combination of NaI and LSO crystals (32) or by combining YSO and LSO crystals (33,34). In these detectors, NaI/YSO were used for the detection of low-energy single photons, whereas LSO was used to detect the high-energy annihilation radiation. The events originating from the two crystals are separated using a pulse shape discriminator, as the scintillation light decay time is different for the two crystals [14 nanoseconds (ns) for LSO and 17 ns for YSO].

Table 10.1. Photo-peak detection efficiency versus crystal thickness in gamma camera–based positron emission tomography (GCPET)

Crystal thickness (mm)	^{201}Tl 70 keV (%)	^{99m}Tc 140 keV (%)	^{67}Ga 300 keV (%)	^{18}F 511 keV (%)
9.5	100	84	33	13
12.7	100	91	41	17
15.9	100	95	48	21
19.1	100	98	54	24

Source: Data from Patton and Turkington (6), with permission of the Society of Nuclear Medicine.

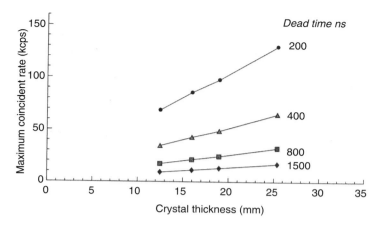

Figure 10.2. Plot of maximum true count rate for different crystal thickness and different dead times used. A maximum polar half acceptance angle of 20 degrees was used for these measurements. [*Source:* Hillel et al. (115), with permission of Institute of Physics and Engineering in Medicine.]

Acquisition Geometry

Two- and three-head gamma cameras are widely used for GCPET imaging. As these scanners are incapable of acquiring complete data from the 3D image space, using just one gantry position, they are rotated around the patient at an angular rate based on the tracer used and the tracer kinetics of the physiologic process under investigation. For example, some GCPET systems can acquire dynamic 360-degree data in just 5 seconds for the fast sampling of the three-dimensional (3D) distribution of FDG during a dynamic cardiac study (26). The limiting factor for the rotation speed is determined based on the number of coincidence photons detected per location of the gantry head, which in turn depends on the tracer used, attenuation, and system sensitivity. For the two-head configuration, the two detectors are placed 180 degrees apart and rotated around the patient for 180 degrees so as to obtain complete data (35,36). However, for the three-head GCPET systems, the three heads can be placed at a wide range of mutual angles (37). As will be explained later, the relative locations of the heads were

Table 10.2. Properties of different scintillation crystals

Crystal	Density (g/cm³)	Attenuation coefficient (cm⁻¹)	Relative light output (%)	Decay time (ns)	Energy resolution at 511 keV (%)
NaI (Tl)	3.7	0.34	100	230	8
BGO	7.1	0.95	15	300	12
LSO	7.4	0.87	50–80*	40	10
GSO	6.7	0.70	20–40*	60	9

*Light output is dependent on cerium concentration and read-out device (PMT or APD).
Source: Tarantola et al. (31).

found to affect the sensitivity of the system (38–40). The measured projection data are then corrected using *rotational weights* along with other compensations before reconstruction (41).

Coincidence Electronics

To measure the three-dimensional distribution of positron-emitting tracers in the body, the GCPET system is operated in the coincidence mode, either in the absence of a collimator or using a coarse scatter reducing collimator (5,42,43). Absence of the collimator tends to increase the acceptance angle of the incident photons, thereby significantly increasing the number of photons detected by the system. In PET, the location of the positron decay is determined by the coincidence circuitry. The two 511-keV photons arising from a positron annihilation are emitted 180-degrees (±0.5 degrees) apart. By detecting both events in coincidence, the line that passes through the annihilation location (also called line of response, LOR) can be easily determined. This approach is also called *electronic collimation*, as a photon interaction on one detector is not used in the reconstruction without a corresponding coincidence event detected on the second detector. For coincidence, the two photons should be detected within a timing window of 15 ns after the detection of the first event (Fig. 10.1B) (8).

The timing window is selected such that it is large enough to take into account (1) the time of flight of the two photons, (2) the scintillation time, and (3) the time taken by the electronics to register an event. For a detected coincidence event, the energy of the incident photons, the gantry angle, and the coordinate where the event was detected on each detector is recorded. Events that are detected within the specified timing window are called *true coincidences* (Fig. 10.2). The rate of true coincidences of a point source placed in air is given by, $R_t = A\varepsilon^2 d\Omega$, where A is the total activity in the source, ε is detection efficiency, and $d\Omega$ is the smallest solid angle subtended by the point source with each detector (5). The detection efficiency term ε is squared as the annihilation photons have to be detected by both detectors in order to be recorded as a true coincidence event.

Due to the finite width of the detectors, attenuation of the photon, scatter within the patient, and poor detection efficiency of the NaI(Tl) crystal, it is possible that one of the annihilation photons is detected whereas the other photon is not detected at all. Such single photon interactions are called *single events* and the count rate of single interaction is given by $R_s = 2A\varepsilon d\Omega$ (5). Single photons tend to decrease the sensitivity of the system due to the dead time associated with the detection of each event. For every coincidence photon that is detected, about 100 or more singles are detected by the GCPET system (6). If two of these single events from different decays are detected on both detectors well within the timing window, then they are considered as a coincidence event (Fig. 10.3). Such coincidence photons are called *random coincidences* as they provide erroneous positional information regarding the location of the annihilation event. The number of random coincidence events detected is proportional to the coincidence timing window and

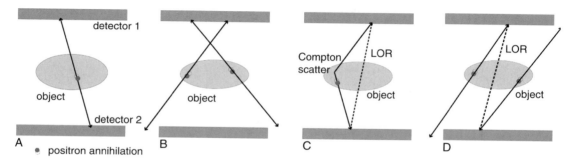

Figure 10.3. Schematic representation of *true, single, scattered,* and *random* coincidence events. A: A *true* coincidence event is detected when both photons from the same annihilation do not scatter in the object and are detected within the specified timing window and energy range. B: When only one of the annihilation photons is detected, then the detected even is called a *single*. C: *Scattered* photons are those where one of the annihilation photons undergoes Compton scatter in the patient and is still detected. These photons contribute to an erroneous line of response (shown by the dotted line). D: The GCPET system considers the simultaneous detection of two singles from different annihilations within the timing window as a true coincidence. Such events are called *randoms* and tend to reduce the contrast of the reconstructed image.

the number of singles detected by each head. Thus the random rate increases proportional to the square of the activity compared to true coincidences that are proportional to the activity. The ratio of detected random coincidence to true coincidence is given by $R_r/R_t = 8A\varepsilon d\Omega$ (5). Hence, to reduce randoms, it is desirable to keep the timing window as short as possible (31).

Another contamination that affects the contrast and resolution of the reconstructed image is scatter (Fig. 10.3). If one of the annihilation photons undergoes Compton scatter in the patient and is detected within the timing window, then an incorrect location is recorded for that particular annihilation event. The energy lost by the scattered photon is proportional to the scatter angle. For large scatter angles, the energy loss is significant; hence such coincidence events can easily be eliminated by increasing the lower threshold of the energy window. However, for small scatter angles, the energy lost is not significant and hence cannot be discriminated against (44). Combining the above-mentioned effects, the total coincidence count rate for a GCPET is given by $R_{total} = R_t + R_r + R_s$, where R_s is the contribution from the scattered photon.

Count Rate Capabilities

True coincidences account for just 1% of the total counts detected by a GCPET system. The relatively low coincidence fraction is caused by the attenuation in the patient, low detection efficiency of the crystals, limited solid angle of the accepted photons, and detection of scatter as well as random photons emitted from the patient (10). A tremendous improvement in the count rate capabilities was required to achieve significant improvements in the detection of the coincidence photons.

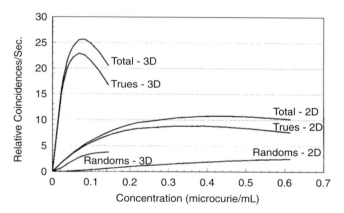

Figure 10.4. Coincidence count rate curves for a dual-head GCPET system. The plots shows the measured relative coincidences for a cylindrical phantom (22 cm diameter × 20 cm long with uniform activity) plotted for different activity concentration. [*Source:* Patton and Turkington (6), with permission of the Society of Nuclear Medicine.]

Patton and Turkington (6) plotted the relative coincidence count rate as a function of concentration for a cylindrical phantom that is 20 cm long and 22 cm in diameter (Fig. 10.4) (45). A delayed timing window was used for the correction of the random coincidence events. From this example, it was observed that the true coincidence peaked at 0.35 mCi/mL for 2D and at 0.07 mCi/mL for the 3D configurations. The decrease in trues after certain concentration was due to the corresponding increase in the singles that were being detected. This led to an increase in the dead time of the system as well as an increased detection of random events in the coincidence timing window. Thus, to detect lesions with good contrast, activity corresponding to about 7×10^5 counts per second in 2D mode (6) and about 20×10^5 counts per second in 3D mode (46) should be injected in the patient. In this scenario, the true coincidence will be about 7×10^3 counts per second in 2D mode and about 20×10^3 counts per second in the 3D mode (47). On the other hand, dedicated PET systems are capable of acquiring 3 to 6×10^5 true coincidences per second. Hence, to obtain reconstructed images with similar noise properties as a dedicated PET system, the acquisition time of the GCPET system will have to be increased correspondingly.

To detect the high count rates of about 20×10^5 events per second, some of the following hardware modifications were implemented in the traditional gamma camera. As will be explained in the next few sections, these modifications were (1) pulse clipping technique, (2) local centroid calculation, (3) use of graded absorbers, and (4) use of coarse slat collimators.

Pulse Clipping Technique
The decay time of light in a NaI(Tl) crystal for an absorbed 140-keV gamma ray is about 230 ns. A typical gamma camera integrates the light output for about 900 ns to get a good spatial as well as energy resolu-

tion of the absorbed low-energy photon. When a 511-keV photon is absorbed, it takes just 75 ns to emit the same amount of light as emitted by a 140-keV photon with an integration time of 900 ns. Due to this fast rise time for 511-keV photons, the integration time window of the GCPET system can be clipped to 200 ns (4). The remaining scintillation energy of the absorbed 511-keV photon is estimated by using a pulse-tail extrapolation technique (10). However, this extrapolation can cause a small degradation in the energy resolution of the GCPET system. Once an event is detected, an additional time interval of 80 ns is used to reset the system. Hence, the crystal is ready to detect the next event after a total dead time of 280 ns compared to 900 ns used by a dedicated SPECT system (10,36). As shown in Figure 10.2, decreasing the dead time was found to drastically improve the count rate capability of the system.

Local Centroid Calculation

In a dedicated PET system, the detector is made up of about 12,000 to 19,000 individual crystals (31). These crystals are grouped together into blocks of 6 × 6 or 8 × 8 and coupled to a set of four PMTs. The total light from the PMTs is used to determine the energy of the incident photon; the relative light in the tubes is used to determine the spatial location where the photon hits the crystal. On the other hand, in GCPET, a single crystal is used and the relative location of the incident photon is determined by using Anger position logic. At high count rates, multiple photons could be simultaneously incident on the crystal at different spatial locations. In this case, the PMTs with the highest signal are identified and the positions of the multiple events are determined separately by considering the six local PMTs that are in the immediate vicinity of the PMT with the maximum count (48,49). Thus, events that are spatially separate but incident on the crystal simultaneously can be detected. Further, to reduce the pulse pileup and to properly position the detected events, the scintillation crystal is electronically subdivided into multiple regions, such that each region is connected to a separate set of electronics (50). These modifications dramatically enhanced the count rate capability of the GCPET systems, enabling them to handle very high count rates with very limited loss in energy as well as spatial resolution.

Gantry Shielding and Graded Absorbers

The lead shielding surrounding the detector head of a gamma camera needs to be significantly increased so as to attenuate the stray 511-keV photons emitted from the volume outside the coincidence FOV. However, this increased lead shielding tends to increase the weight of the detector head significantly as the FWTM thickness of lead for 511-keV photons is about 13.5 mm while that of 140-keV photons is just 0.9 mm. Hence, this additional weight should be taken into consideration during the design of the rotating gantry for the GCPET system.

To reduce the detection of low-energy scattered photons, thin metal sheets were placed around the patient to act as a *graded absorber* (4,51). The sheets were made of thin layers of lead, tin, and copper (about 1 mm each) with the material of lowest atomic number placed toward the NaI crystal. The sheet made of a lower atomic number helps to absorb the characteristic x-rays produced from the Compton interactions of the 511 gamma rays in lead. If this setup is implemented correctly, then a significant reduction in the scatter component is observed in the measured data.

Apart from improving the count rate, another advantage of the setup explained above is that the Compton interactions in the crystal can now be used for image reconstruction, using the dual-energy window algorithm explained later. Further, the graded absorbers will be effective in imaging PET tracers such as rubidium 81 (^{81}Rb), bromine 76 (^{76}Br), iodine 124 (^{124}I), and indium 111 (^{111}In) that emit a wide range of gamma rays along with a positron (52). However, in a clinical environment, it is impractical to attach the graded absorbers permanently to the gantry, as the GCPET system is used for both SPECT imaging of low-energy single photons as well as for coincidence imaging of high-energy photons.

Slat Collimation

To improve the number of true coincidences while minimizing the detection of singles and scattered photons from the patient, parallel slat collimators were often used. The lead slats were oriented perpendicular to the axis of rotation so as to limit the detection of the photons originating outside the field of view FOV (53–55). These slats, when arranged perpendicular to the crystal, are analogous to the interslice septa often used in dedicated PET scanners. Such parallel slat collimators help to create a pseudo-2D geometry in which a larger number of annihilation events from the corresponding trans-axial plane are detected, compared to those detected from the neighboring planes. The effects of the height, septal thickness, and septal penetration of these slats on the image quality were studied in detail (53,56), and an approximate slat height of 64 mm, lead thickness of about 3 mm, and septal separation of about 13 mm were observed to be good for high count rate studies.

To overcome the 2D nature of the parallel slat collimators, new designs based on axially converging slat collimators have been evaluated (43,56,57). These collimators provide significant improvement in the true coincidence events detected from the center of the FOV and at the same time provide more effective shielding of the scattered photons originating outside the region of interest. Another approach to increase true events is to use a traditional LEHR collimator instead of a parallel slat collimator for coincidence imaging (58).

Spatial Resolution

Collimators play an important role in determining the spatial resolution of a SPECT system. However, in coincidence imaging, the absence of the collimator helps to drastically improve the spatial resolution of the system. In this case, the spatial resolution of the system is determined by (1) positron range corresponding to the path traveled by the positron before annihilation (up to 3 mm), (2) noncolinearity of emission angle (180 ± 0.5 degrees) caused due to the nonzero momentum of the positron and electron during annihilation, and (3) the intrinsic response function of the system (5,59). The intrinsic response function of the system in turn depends on a wide range of parameters. One of the main contributors to the intrinsic response function is crystal thickness. Increasing the thickness of the crystal tends to degrade the spatial resolution due to the light spread in the crystal. For a 2.5-cm-thick crystal, the intrinsic resolution is about 10mm FWHM for 140-keV photons and about 7.7mm FWHM for 511-keV photons (4). Thus the resolution of the coincidence photons in the image space between the two detectors A and B is given by $R_I = 0.5\sqrt{R_A + R_B}$ (about 5.4mm FWHM). Similarly, the spatial resolution in the image space for the 1-cm and 1.6-cm-thick crystals can be calculated using the values given in Table 10.3.

On the other hand, reducing the thickness of the crystal reduces the sensitivity of the system. As will be explained later, in such systems with poor sensitivity, coincidence events from the photo-peak–Compton window are also accepted as true coincidences. However, these coincidence events are contaminated with scattered photons from the patient. As shown in Figure 10.3, these coincidence events tend to assign a wrong line of response during reconstruction, thereby increasing the background activity and reducing the contrast as well as the resolution of the reconstructed image. For a 1.6-cm crystal, inclusion of the photons from the Compton window was found to degrade the resolution by an additional 0.5mm (30).

Another major factor that degrades resolution is incidence angle of the coincidence photons. Large incidence angles tend to degrade the spatial resolution due to the uncertainty in determining the entry point. The problem of incident angle is more pronounced in GCPET compared to dedicated PET systems due to the longer axial FOV. One approach to limit the incidence angle is the use of axial-slat collimators that tend to limit the acceptance angle of the incident photons in the axial direction. Another approach is to place the two detectors as far apart as possible. Though this approach reduces the incident angle, it could magnify the noncolinearity effect of the annihilation event (180 ± 0.5 degrees).

The spatial resolution of the GCPET system for a point source in air is about 8.5mm in 2D mode, with an acceptance angle of 2 degrees and about 10mm with an acceptance angle of 16 degrees. Further, due to

Table 10.3. Effect of using dual-window technique on spatial resolution and sensitivity

Crystal interaction	Spatial resolution (mm)	Relative sensitivity
Photo-peak–photo-peak	4.5	1
Photo-peak–photo-peak plus photo-peak–Compton	5.0	3
Photo-peak–photo-peak plus photo-peak–Compton plus Compton-Compton	5.2	4

Source: Patton and Turkington (6), with permission of the Society of Nuclear Medicine.

the flat surface of the crystal, less deterioration in the spatial resolution is observed as the point source is moved away from the axis of rotation in a given transaxial slice. For a physical phantom experiment using a dual-head clinical scanner with 1.6-cm-thick crystal, $54 \times 40\,cm$ surface area, 8-degree acceptance angle, and 73 cm separation, the smallest detectable spheres were 8, 12, and 16 mm for a sphere to background ratio of $10:1$, $5:1$, and $3:1$, respectively (60).

Apart from degrading the intrinsic resolution, oblique rays can cause serious degradations in the spatial resolution of the reconstructed image, depending on the rebinning algorithm used. As will be explained later, algorithms such as single-slice rebinning (SSRB) tend to place oblique coincidence photons, emitted from a point further away from the axis of rotation, in the wrong transaxial plane. Hence, to improve resolution, more accurate rebinning algorithms such as Fourier rebinning (FORE) (61) should be used for the oblique photons.

Some of the other factors that affect the intrinsic resolution of the system to a lesser extent are (1) local centroid approach, (2) pulse clipping, (3) geometric calibration of the system (62), and (4) relative position of the detector heads in a three-head system (40).

Dual-Energy Window Technique

Most SPECT systems were designed to image gamma rays below 400 keV. Hence, to image 511-keV photons, it was necessary to expand the energy range of the pulse height analyzers so as to effectively detect both low- and high-energy photons simultaneously. Similarly, uniformity and linearity corrections were also extended into the high-energy range to enable faithful detection of incident photons over a wide energy range.

As shown in Table 10.2, NaI(Tl) crystals have a lower attenuation coefficient for 511-keV photons compared to other crystals used in dedicated PET systems. This resulted in poor overall sensitivity of the GCPET system. To increase the sensitivity, a 30% energy window centered at 511 keV was used. It was found that, apart from increasing the sensitivity, the wide energy window also helped to reduce the nonuniformities arising from any drift in photo peak during an acquisition (28). However, only 23% of all detected coincidence events fall in the peak-to-peak energy window of both detectors. On the other hand, about 20% of the 511-keV photons incident on the crystal undergo one or two Compton interactions in the crystal. Schematic representation of this effect is shown in Figure 10.5, where some of the 511-keV photons, incident on the crystal, undergo either photoelectric/Compton interaction, depositing all the energy in the crystal, or only Compton interaction and escape from the crystal. These escaped photons deposit less energy compared to those that are completely absorbed by the crystal.

Unlike the photons that undergo Compton scatter in the patient body, the photons that undergo Compton interaction in the crystal still possess the correct spatial information for the location of the annihila-

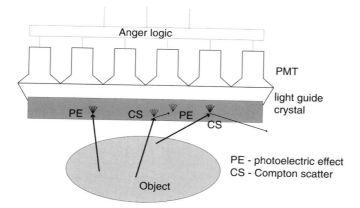

Figure 10.5. Schematic representation of the different photon interactions in the crystal for 511-keV photons. Some photons undergo both photoelectric as well as Compton interactions, depositing all the energy in the crystal, whereas others undergo only Compton interaction, depositing only part of their total energy in the crystal.

tion event. Hence, to increase the sensitivity of the system, a dual-energy window technique (4,10) was used. In this technique, coincidence events that are detected in the photo-peak energy window in the first detector and in the Compton energy window in the second detector are also accepted as a *true coincidence* (Fig. 10.6). This approach was found to increase the sensitivity of the system by three times at the cost of a small resolution loss of about 0.5 mm (6). The spatial resolution and relative sensitivity of a 22-cm-diameter and 20-cm-long phantom images using a 15.9-mm NaI (Tl) crystal is shown in Table 10.4. Note that the loss in resolution is relatively small compared to the large increase in sensitivity for the same acquisition time.

If we assume the low-energy scatter photons are successfully eliminated by the graded absorber and slat collimators explained above, then the Compton interactions of the 511-keV photons in the crystal will lie around 310 keV in the energy spectrum (28). Figure 10.6 shows the typical energy spectrum of a FDG scan on each detector. Depending on the total number of counts detected and the relative number of scattered photons present, the Compton scatter window can be selected anywhere from 100 to 350 keV. In a clinical environment, the dual-energy window was found to be favorable for GCPET systems with thin crystals used along with graded absorbers and slat collimators. However, for thick crystals (2.5 cm), the dual-energy window technique was found to decrease the contrast and resolution of the reconstructed image for certain clinical applications (63,64). This reduction in contrast is significant, especially if the coincidence photons detected in the Compton energy window of both detectors are used in the reconstruction. Hence, this technique should be tested for each specific application, though overall the technique was found to give improved images for most GCPET applications (65).

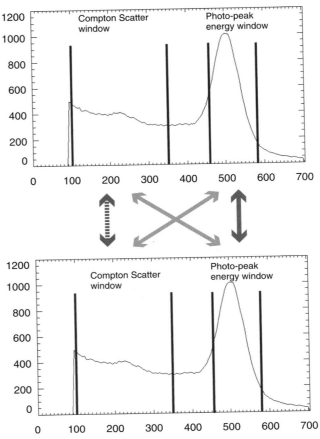

Figure 10.6. Typical energy spectrum of an FDG scan, from a patient. In the dual-energy window technique, counts from both the photo-peak energy window as well as the Compton scatter window (100–350 keV) were used in the reconstruction. The reduced counts in the lower energy range are due to the effective attenuation of the low-energy photons by the graded absorber and slat collimators. Photons below 100 keV were not detected for this study.

Geometric Sensitivity

The geometric sensitivity of a voxel in the image space is the detection probability of the isotropic photons emitted from that voxel in a complete study. Hence, the geometric sensitivity of a voxel includes effects such as total solid angle subtended by the voxel with a detector overall detector positions and detector efficiency of the crystal due to the incident angle of the accepted photon. Because the solid angle of incidence of the accepted photon varies with the relative location of the voxel in the image space, the overall sensitivity profile in the FOV is nonuniform and spatially varying. Some of the major parameters that affect the shape of the sensitivity profile are (1) number of heads used, (2) head configuration, (3) angular spacing in a 360-degree acquisition, (4) radius of rotation, (5) coincidence acceptance angle used, and (6) detector crystal dimensions (40,66–68).

Table 10.4. General features of various GCPET systems

Camera	ADAC	Marconi	SMV	GE	Siemens
Camera design feature					
Crystal thickness (inches)	5/8	3/4	1/2 or 5/8	5/8	5/8
Number of heads	2	2 or 3	2	2	2
Detector spacing (cm)	60–81	25–71	71	20–54	40–72
FOV axial (cm)	38	39	54	40	39
FOV transaxial (cm)	51	53	40	51	53
Features of head electronics					
High count rate mode	Yes	Yes	Yes	Yes	Yes
Pulse clipping	Yes	Yes	No	Yes	No
Cut off time for pulse clipping (ns)	320	225	N/A	225	N/A
Local centroiding	Yes	Yes	No	No	No
Coincidence window (ns)	15	10	15	<15	12
Collimation options					
Open frames	Yes	Yes	Yes	Yes	No
Axial collimation	No	Yes	Yes	Yes	Yes
Recommended	Open frames	Axial collimation	Axial collimation	Axial collimation	Axial collimation
Energy window options					
Photo-peak window (%)	30	30	45	20	20
Compton window recommended	Yes	No	No	Yes	Yes
Energy values of events stored	Yes	Yes	No	Yes	No
Energy window selection at processing	No	Yes	No	Yes	No
Reconstruction options					
Maximum polar half angle (degrees)	16	12	20	8	7.5
Rebinning	FORE/ SSRB	SSRB	FORE/ SSRB	SSRB	MSRB/ SSRB
2D reconstruction	OSEM/ FBP	OSEM/ FBP	OSEM/ FBP	OSEM/ FBP	OSEM/ FBP
Full 3D reconstruction	No	No	Yes	Yes	Yes
Attenuation correction	Yes	Yes	WIP	Yes	No
Scatter correction	Yes	No	WIP	WIP	Yes
Decay correction	Yes	Yes	Yes	Yes	Yes
Random correction	Yes	No	Yes	WIP	Yes
Sensitivity correction	Yes	Yes	Yes	Yes	Yes
Transmission source for attenuation correction	^{137}Cs moving point sources	^{133}Ba moving point sources	^{153}Gd multiple stationary point sources	X-ray CT scan	N/A

Source: Fleming and Hillel (28), with permission of the Institute of Physics and Engineers in Medicine.

The nonuniform sensitivity of the GCPET system can drastically affect lesion detectability in clinical studies and hence needs to be either measured accurately or modeled so that it can be compensated during reconstruction (66,69). Measuring the spatially varying geometric sensitivity for every clinical radius of rotation and for every head configuration (especially for three-head) is impractical, and hence an accurate simulated model of the geometric sensitivity is preferred. For a fixed gantry location, the sensitivity is calculated by integrating the detector efficiency over the solid angle formed by the voxel and the intersection of the first detector with the projection of the second detector on the plane of the first detector (Fig. 10.7) (67). The geometric sensitivity for that voxel is then calculated by adding the corresponding values obtained over all gantry angles. For a dual-head configuration placed 180 degrees apart, the projection of one detector plane onto the other is a rectangle, whereas for any other gantry angle the projection takes the shape of a trapezium as shown in Figure 10.7 (68,70,71).

The sensitivity profile of a two-head GCPET system placed 180 degrees apart is shown in Figure 10.8A. In this case, the acquisition model is 2D with the axially acceptance angle of the incident photons limited to just 9 degrees. Slat collimators were used to reduce the detection of scattered photons and events with larger incident angles. The gantry was rotated around the FOV to obtain a complete data set.

The sensitivity profile was observed to drop linearly as one moves away from the axis of rotation. To increase the acceptance solid angle per gantry location and thereby increase the geometric sensitivity, the use of additional detector heads was proposed (37,38). In such cases,

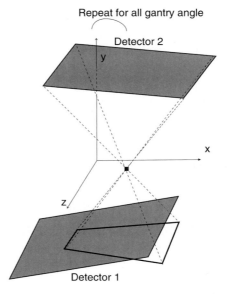

Figure 10.7. Geometry illustration of the solid angle subtended by a point in the image space with respect to the two detectors. The second detector is projected through the point on to the first detector to analytically measure the accepted solid angle for that point in the image space.

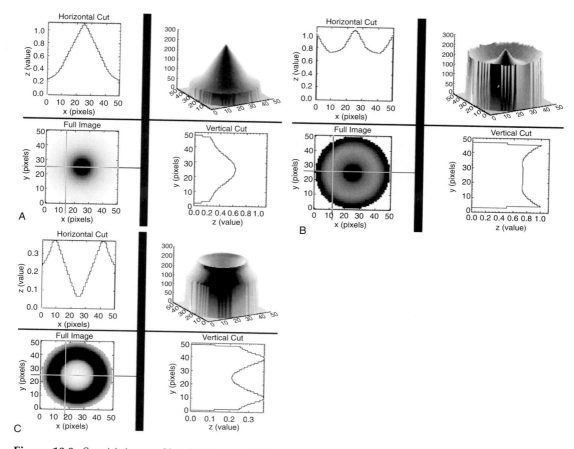

Figure 10.8. Sensitivity profile of different GCPET systems with a 50-cm square crystal and a radius of rotation of 40 cm. A: The sensitivity of a two-head configuration placed 1800 apart. B: Three-head triangular configuration where the heads are placed 1200 apart. C: Three-head U-shaped configuration where the second and third heads are placed at 900 and 1800 with respect to the first head.

the shape of the sensitivity profile was found to be relatively uniform and varied depending on the mutual angle among the three heads during the image acquisition (40,47,66). For example, Figure 10.8B shows the transaxial sensitivity profile for a U-shaped three-head configuration, where the detector heads were placed at 0, 90, and 180 degrees. In this case, the geometric sensitivity of the voxel for a particular gantry location is measured by adding the sensitivity obtained by considering any two heads at a time. The sensitivity at the center of FOV for the U-shaped and dual-head configurations was found to overlap perfectly (47). However, as one moves away from the axis of rotation, the profile through the U-shaped configuration was found to be more uniform compared to the dual-head case.

Another triple-head configuration that is often used for brain imaging is equilateral triangle configuration where the three heads were placed 120 degrees apart. The sensitivity profile of this configuration was found to show less variation for a small radius of rotation.

However, on increasing the radius of rotation, the sensitivity at the axis of rotation was found to decrease drastically and eventually reach zero (Fig. 10.8C).

Attenuation Correction

Attenuation compensation plays a very important role in GCPET imaging. The image degradation effects of attenuation are far more severe in GCPET compared to routine SPECT, as both photons should successfully pass through the patient in order to be detected. That means, in spite of the lower attenuation coefficient of the 511-keV photons (about $0.095\,cm^{-1}$ for soft tissue, 0.12 to $0.14\,cm^{-1}$ for bone, and 0.03 to $0.04\,cm^{-1}$ for lungs) compared to 140-keV photons (about $0.15\,cm^{-1}$ for soft tissue, $0.28\,cm^{-1}$ for bone, and $0.043\,cm^{-1}$ for lungs) the total length traveled by the single photon in the attenuating medium is less than that traveled by the 511-keV coincidence photons. Thus for GCPET, the effect of attenuation is independent of the relative depth at which the annihilation took place in the body and more dependent on the total attenuation in the LOR.

Noncompensation for attenuation in GCPET results in poor quantification, regional nonuniformities, distorted reconstruction of organs with high activity, and inability to detect lesions located near organs with high uptake (72). The nonuniformity in the image is caused as photons from low attenuated regions, such as from the lungs or the periphery of the patient, have a higher probability of being detected compared to photons from regions located deep within the body. For example, the reconstructed images in Figure 10.9 show a high uptake in the lungs and peripheral regions for the uncorrected case. Such artifacts were found to disappear with proper attenuation compensation giving a faithful representation of the tracer distribution (73).

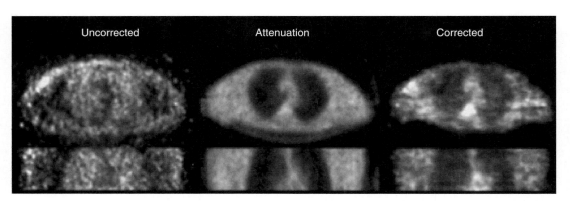

Figure 10.9. Transaxial (top row) and coronal (bottom row) slices through the uncorrected emission image, attenuation map, and attenuation-corrected emission image of a male patient (weight 73.9 kg, height 175.3 cm). The lungs and periphery of the patient look bright in the uncorrected emission images, and it is difficult to differentiate between the different organs. On the other hand, the attenuation corrected image is closer to the true representation of the tracer distribution in the patient. [*Source:* Laymon et al. (73), with permission of the Society of Nuclear Medicine.]

For attenuation correction, obtaining an accurate representation of the attenuation map is crucial. Initial attenuation correction algorithms used attenuation maps consisting of crude body contours and uniform attenuation coefficients during image reconstruction (74). These algorithms were fast to implement and gave reasonable images for brain imaging. However, for cardiac imaging, such algorithms were found to cause artifacts and distortions in the reconstructed image. To overcome this problem, transmission scans were obtained using a transmission source that emits single photons with a different energy from that sof the coincidence photons. Due to the excellent energy resolution of NaI(Tl) crystal, the transmission and emission scans can be performed either simultaneously or sequentially. Some of the widely used radioisotopes for transmission scans are cesium 137 (^{137}Cs) (662-keV photons and 30-year half-life) (72,75,76), gadolinium 153 (^{153}Gd) (photons varying from 41 to 103 keV, 242 days half-life) and barium 133 (^{133}Ba) (mostly 356-keV photons, 10 year half-life) (77,78). The transmission scans were obtained by either moving the point sources linearly with every gantry angle (79) or using multiple line sources (73,80) attached to any one of the detector heads. The gantry was then rotated around the patient to obtain complete data set.

A sufficient number of counts needs to be acquired so as to obtain good attenuation maps with very few statistical variations. To reduce down-scatter, some manufacturers recommended performing the attenuation scans after injecting the patient but before acquiring the emission image. This step gives time for tracer uptake and at the same time helps to reduce motion artifacts and patient misregistration during image reconstruction. In such imaging protocols, the transmission source is shielded in a tungsten case during the emission scan.

Another approach to obtain a high-quality attenuation map is to attach an extended x-ray computed tomography (CT) scanner to the GCPET system (30,81). The added advantage of the CT scanner is the availability of anatomic information that can be fused with the positron image for better region localization. Even though high-resolution images can be obtained using the CT scanner (~1 mm), the scans are reconstructed into 128×128 slices so as to match the array size of the attenuation map with that of the GCPET system. Depending on the size of the coincidence imaging detector, the transmission scan is obtained using a helical orbit by translating the patient bed through the FOV of the CT scanner. The x-ray tube is operated around 140 kVp and 2.5 mA to reduce the radiation dose to the patient from the photoelectric absorption of low-energy photons (30,72).

The transmission scans are acquired as either a fan-beam or a cone-beam projection and reconstructed to obtain the attenuation map. The values of the attenuation maps are then corrected so that they correspond to the attenuation coefficient of the 511-keV photons. A blank transmission scan is also acquired without the patient in the FOV. Finally the attenuation coefficients of the patient and blank scans are reprojected for the imaging geometry used in GCPET acquisition. Dividing the reprojected blank image with a reprojected transmission image gives the attenuation correction factors that are used in the scaling of the emission projections during reconstruction.

Image Reconstruction

The process of image reconstruction transforms the information from the projection space to the image space. The algorithms used to solve this inverse problem can be broadly divided into (1) analytical or (2) iterative reconstruction algorithms. In this section, we discuss the process of rebinning the coincidence events into planar projections along with a few analytic as well as iterative reconstruction algorithms that are widely used in GCPET imaging (82).

Data Rebinning

As in a dedicated PET system, the measured data in a GCPET system can be either rebinned directly into sinograms or saved in a *list-mode* format. If the projection data are acquired using axial slat collimators arranged perpendicular to the axis of rotation, then the acquired data are treated as 2D with limited interaction between transaxial planes. On the other hand, if the projection data are acquired without using a slat collimator, then the projection data is fully 3D with the LOR not being restricted to any particular transaxial plane. In this case the axial acceptance angle can be as large as 30 degrees and hence the reconstruction of this fully 3D data is computationally time-consuming and memory intensive.

Different rebinning algorithms have been developed to sort the 3D data into a stack of ordinary 2D data sets. In these rebinned data sets, the detected coincidence events are organized as a set of 2D sinograms. These rebinned data can then be considered equivalent to the data obtained by the scanner in the 2D mode. However, due to the increased counts measured in the 3D mode, the rebinned 2D data tend to be less noisy. To get faithfully reconstructed images, rebinning algorithm needs to be (1) fast, (2) accurate (i.e., based on an exact analytical inversion formula), and (3) stable with respect to noise (61). Three of the widely used rebinning algorithms for GCPET systems are single-slice rebinning (SSRB), multislice rebinning (MSRB), and Fourier rebinning (FORE).

Single Slice Rebinning

As shown in Figure 10.10A, SSRB is the simplest rebinning algorithm where the oblique LOR is rebinned to a slice lying axially midway between the two detectors in coincidence (83). In this algorithm, the angle made by the oblique LOR and the transaxial plane is totally ignored. Hence, this method is accurate for rebinning photons emitted from the axis of rotation. However, as one moves away from the axis of rotation, the rebinning algorithm places the coincidence events in the wrong transaxial slice, resulting in distortions in the reconstructed image. Figure 10.11A,B shows the reconstructed image of various point sources placed transaxially at various distance from the axis of rota-

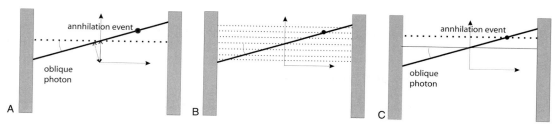

Figure 10.10. Schematic representation of (A) single-slice rebinning (SSRB), (B) multislice rebinning (MSRB), and (C) Fourier rebinning (FORE) algorithms.

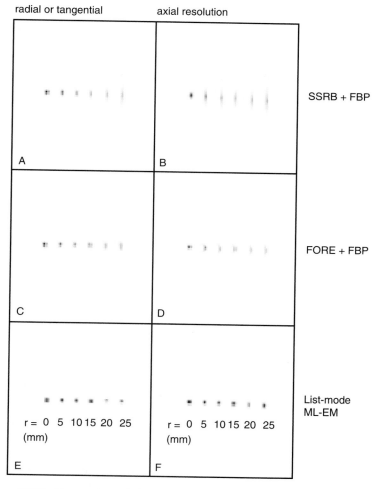

Figure 10.11. Reconstructed images of a phantom consisting of 12-point sources placed 5mm apart in the axial and transaxial direction. The reconstructed images were obtained using (A,B) SSRB combined with FBP, (C,D) FORE combined with FBP, and (E,F) list-mode reconstruction.

tion. For the reconstructed image obtained using SSRB and filtered backprojection (FBP), the resolution recovery for the point source located further from the axis of rotation is degraded drastically. To limit this degradation of resolution, the acceptance angle (angle between LOR and the transaxial plane) of the detected photons is limited depending on the clinical application. In dedicated PET systems, this acceptance angle is limited to ±10 degrees. However in GCPET, due to the wider axial size of the crystals (about 40 cm compared to 25 cm for dedicated PET) the acceptance angle can be as high as ±30 degrees (84). Increasing the acceptance angle results in a gain in sensitivity, whereas reducing the acceptance angle gives images with better resolution especially for voxels further away from the axis of rotation. This trade-off of sensitivity versus resolution dependence on acceptance angle was investigated in detail by D'Asseler et al. (40).

Multislice Rebinning
To overcome the limitations of SSRB, it was proposed that the oblique LOR contributes to the sinograms of all the transaxial slices it traverses equally (85) (Fig. 10.10B). This algorithm, like SSRB, is fast and can be performed online during data acquisition. Though this method is a better approximation than SSRB, it results in a 1D blurring in the axial direction. This axial blurring is rectified using a 1D filter but results in degraded noise properties compared to SSRB.

Fourier Rebinning
Another algorithm very often used in GCPET is Fourier rebinning (61). This algorithm is based on the frequency distance relationship and is much more accurate than SSRB and MSRB. Figure 10.11C,D shows the reconstructed image obtained using FORE and FBP (86). The resolution recovery of the FORE algorithm for point sources placed at a distance from the center is far better than those obtained using SSRB. Though FORE is a bit slow compared to SSRB, it is still an order of magnitude faster than 3D reprojection algorithm (3DRP) (87) and can faithfully reconstruct images with acceptance angles of up to 35 degrees (88).

Imaging Geometry

The objective of GCPET imaging is to visualize the 3D distribution of the radiopharmaceutical administered to the patient. As shown in Figure 10.12, $f(x, y, z)$ is the unknown 3D distribution of the radiopharmaceutical, whereas $p_{\theta,\phi}(u, v)$ is the 2D parallel ray projection measured along the polar angle θ and azimuthal angle ϕ. The coordinates u and v are in the image plane and are parallel to the unit vectors $\underline{\alpha}$ and $\underline{\beta}$. The vectors $\underline{\alpha}$, $\underline{\beta}$, and $\underline{\theta}$ are orthogonal to each other, and the vector $\underline{\alpha}$ lies in the x-y plane, whereas the projected image plane (on the crystal) is orthogonal to the vector $\underline{\theta}$. Hence, the vector $\underline{\theta}$ defines the direction of the parallel line integrals passing through the function $f(\underline{x})$, and detected at the crystal. The unit vector $\underline{\theta}$ makes a polar angle θ with the positive z-axis and an azimuthal angle ϕ with the positive

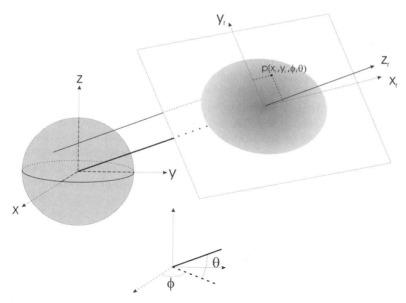

Figure 10.12. The unknown three-dimensional (3D) distribution is denoted as $f(\underline{x})$, whereas $p_{\theta,\phi}(u, v)$ is the two-dimensional (2D) projection measured at polar angle θ and azimuthal angle ϕ. The cartesian coordinate system $\underline{x} = (x, y, z)$ is used to represent the image space, whereas $\underline{t} = (t, u, v)$ is used to represent the projection space. The unit vector $\underline{\theta}$, $\underline{\alpha}$, and $\underline{\beta}$ are orthogonal to the (t, u, v) coordinates and the unit vector $\underline{\alpha}$ lies in the x-y plane. The projection plane is orthogonal to the unit vector $\underline{\theta}$. Hence, $\underline{\theta}$ denotes the direction of the line integrals that pass through the 3D image $f(\underline{x})$ and are measured to give the 2D projections $p_{\theta,\phi}(u, v)$.

x-axis. For convenience, let's denote the cartesian coordinate system in the image space as $\underline{x} = (x, y, z)$ and in the projection space as $\underline{t} = (t, u, v)$. From Figure 10.12 and by definition, $\underline{\theta} = (\sin\theta\cos\phi, \sin\theta\sin\phi, \cos\theta)$, $\underline{\alpha} = (-\sin\phi, \cos\theta, 0)$, and $\underline{\beta} = (-\cos\theta\cos\phi, -\cos\theta\sin\phi, \sin\theta)$. The coordinate conversions from the image space to the projection space and vice versa are obtained by $x = t\underline{\theta} + u\underline{\alpha} + v\underline{\beta}$ where $t = \underline{x}.\underline{\theta}$, $u = \underline{x}.\underline{\alpha}$, and $v = \underline{x}.\underline{\beta}$.

The unknown 3D tracer distribution $f(\underline{x})$ is assumed to be continuous and exists only within the boundary of the patient. In other words, the function $f(\underline{x}) = 0$ outside the patient. The detector on which the 2D projections are measured is assumed to be large enough that the projections from the 3D image $f(\underline{x})$ is not truncated in any of the views. The 2D projections measured at the polar angle θ and at the azimuthal angle ϕ are given by

$$P_{\theta,\phi}\left(u\big|_{u=\underline{x}.\underline{\alpha}}, v\big|_{v=\underline{x}.\underline{\beta}}\right) = \int_{-\infty}^{\infty} f(t\underline{\theta} + u\underline{\alpha} + v\underline{\beta})dt \tag{1}$$

The values of θ and ϕ can be varied such that we get a set of detector locations at which the 2D projections are measured. This set of projections is referred to as the *imaging geometry* of the system denoted by

Ω. An easy way to graphically represent the imaging geometry is to denote each projection $p_{\theta,\phi}(u, v)$ as a dot on a unit sphere, corresponding to the spherical angles θ and ϕ. This unit sphere is also called Orlov's sphere (89). Plotting the imaging geometry on the Orlov sphere helps to determine whether the necessary and sufficient conditions are satisfied, to faithfully reconstruct $f(\underline{x})$. The imaging geometry Ω can be considered to be complete, and a faithful reconstruction can be obtained by inverting Equation 1, provided the imaging geometry Ω intersects every great circle on the Orlov sphere.

Let us now illustrate some of the 3D imaging geometries used in PET, as well as in GCPET, on the Orlov sphere. The simplest 3D imaging geometry is the one obtained by using a parallel slat collimator and rotating the GCPET system around the longitudinal axis of the patient for 360 degrees. The data are acquired in the 2D mode, and the projection data is rebinned as a set of 2D parallel projections. If we assume the longitudinal axis of the patient as the z-axis on the Orlov sphere, then this geometry corresponds to an equatorial circle perpendicular to the z-axis on Orlov's sphere. The center of this equatorial circle coincides with the center on the sphere as shown in Figure 10.13A. This equatorial circle is also called a *great circle* and the geometry is mathematically denoted as $\Omega_{2\pi} = \{\underline{\theta}; \theta = \pi/2, \phi \in [0, 2\pi)\}$.

A popular PET geometry is the equatorial band on the Orlov sphere that can be obtained by either rotating an uncollimated 2D planar GCPET detector around the longitudinal axis of the patient or using a stationary truncated spherical/cylindrical PET detector. For the GCPET system the data are acquired in the fully 3D mode with the oblique rays considered as parallel ray projections. As shown in Figure 10.13B, the parallel projections are obtained for the polar angle θ ranging from $\pi/2 - \psi$ to $\pi/2 + \psi$ and for the azimuthal angle ϕ varying from 0 to 2π. Mathematically this geometry is represented as $\Omega_{B(\psi,0,2\pi)} = \{\underline{\theta}; \theta = [\pi/2 - \psi, \pi/2 + \psi), \phi \in [0, 2\pi)\}$.

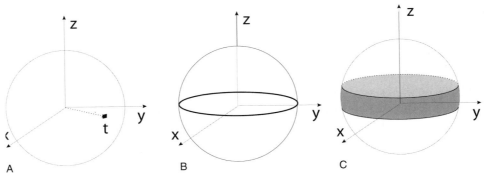

Figure 10.13. A: A 2D parallel projection on the Orlov sphere is represented as a dot corresponding to the vector direction of the measured projection. B: The imaging geometry obtained using a GCPET system in the 2D mode for a 360-degree rotation of the gantry around the patient. C: The imaging geometry on the Orlov sphere for a 3D acquisition using a GCPET system. In this case the imaging geometry takes the shape of an equatorial band.

The shape of the imaging geometry helps to graphically establish whether the unknown image $f(\underline{x})$ is sampled completely as well as to determine the shape of the point-spread function (PSF) $h(\underline{x})$ used in the backprojection filtering (BPF) algorithm. In the next section, we describe the BPF algorithm used for 3D image reconstruction.

Analytical Reconstruction Algorithm

Backprojection Filtering

The 3D backprojected image $b(\underline{x})$ is obtained by simply smearing back the values in the 2D projection data $p_{\theta,\phi}(u, v)$ along the vector direction $-\underline{\theta}$. The above step is repeated for all projections measured along the imaging geometry Ω to give the backprojected image

$$b(\underline{x}) = \iint_{\Omega} P_{\theta,\phi}\left(u|_{u=\underline{x}.\underline{\alpha}}, v|_{v=\underline{x}.\underline{\beta}}\right)\sin\theta\, d\theta\, d\phi,$$

where $\underline{x}$ is a point in the 3D image space. The dot products $\underline{x}.\underline{\alpha}$ and $\underline{x}.\underline{\beta}$ help to determine the u and v locations in the projection space, which contributes to the point $\underline{x}$. This step is repeated for all locations $\underline{x}$ in the image space to get the 3D backprojected image. However, the simple backprojection step results in a backprojected image $b(\underline{x})$ that is equal to the original image $f(\underline{x})$ convolved with a 3D PSF $h(\underline{x})$ given by

$$b(\underline{x}) = \int_{-\infty}^{\infty}\int_{-\infty}^{\infty}\int_{-\infty}^{\infty} f(\underline{x}-\underline{x}')h(\underline{x}')d\underline{x}'.$$

This PSF depends on the imaging geometry and can be expressed as

$$h(\underline{x}) = \frac{\chi_{\Omega}(\underline{x})}{\|\underline{x}\|^2} \quad \text{where} \quad \chi_{\Omega}(\underline{x}) = \begin{cases} 1 & if\left(\dfrac{\underline{x}}{\|\underline{x}\|} \in \Omega\right) \\ 0 & otherwise \end{cases}$$

Hence, to get the function $f(\underline{x})$ back, we need to deconvolve the PSF from the backprojected image, a step also known as BPF. The deconvolution is implemented as a division in the Fourier domain to give

$$f(\underline{x}) = F_{3D}^{-1}\{F(\underline{v})\} = F_{3D}^{-1}\{B(\underline{v})/H(\underline{v})\},$$

where $F(\underline{v}) = \int_{-\infty}^{\infty}\int_{-\infty}^{\infty}\int_{-\infty}^{\infty} f(\underline{x})\exp(-i\pi\underline{x}.\underline{v})d\underline{x}$ and likewise for $B(\underline{v})$ and $H(\underline{v})$. The capital letters are used to denote the functions in the Fourier domain, whereas in the cartesian coordinate system $\underline{v} = (v_x, v_y, v_z)$ is used. The 3D BPF filter function $G(\underline{v})$ can be denoted as

$$G(\underline{v}) = \begin{cases} 1/H(\underline{v}) & if\ H(\underline{v}) \neq 0 \\ 0 & otherwise \end{cases}.$$

The multiplication of the BPF $G(\underline{v})$ with the Fourier transform of the backprojected image $B(\underline{v})$ compensates for the variations in the sampling density due to the imaging geometry given by

$$f(\underline{x}) = F_{3D}^{-1}\{F(\underline{v})\} = F_{3D}^{-1}\{B(\underline{v})/H(\underline{v})\} = F_{3D}^{-1}\{B(\underline{v})\}G(\underline{v})\} \dots \text{ for all } H(\underline{v}) \neq 0 \quad (2)$$

In the above equation, if $H(\underline{v}) = 0$ for any $\underline{v}$, then the imaging geometry does not satisfy Orlov's condition. Such imaging geometries can lead to limited angle artifacts in the reconstructed image (90).

The 3D Fourier transform of the PSF gives us the 3D transfer function $H(\underline{v})$ in the Fourier domain. A 3D illustration of this transfer function tells us the sampling density of all frequencies in the Fourier domain. As mentioned by Schorr and Townsend (91), determining the 3D transfer function from the PSF is a complicated and lengthy process and is largely dependent on the imaging geometry used. Thus, for a given imaging geometry, finding the 3D closed-form solution for $H(\underline{v})$ is nontrivial and has been solved only for few imaging geometries. Some of the previous work done in determining $H(\underline{v})$ were (1) by Tanaka (92) for the 4π geometry; (2) by Pelc (93), Colsher (94), Ra et al. (95), and Defrise et al. (96) for the equatorial band; (3) by Schorr and Townsend (91) for the planar stationary PET detector; (4) by Pelc (97), Knutsson et al. (98), Harauz and vanHeel (99), Defrise et al. (100), and Wessell (101) for the ectomography case; and (5) by Bal et al. (102) for a circular arc on the Orlov's sphere. Once the 3D transfer function is determined, then finding its inverse to obtain the BPF $G(\underline{v})$ is trivial.

One of the advantages of the imaging geometry dependent closed-form expression for $H(\underline{v})$ and $G(\underline{v})$ is the elimination of tedious geometry-dependent numerical integration in equation (2). Thus, the implementation of the 3D BPF algorithm, used to determine the function $f(x)$, is simplified and accurate results can be obtained. Apart from BPF, another analytical reconstruction algorithm widely used to invert Equation A is filtered backprojection (FBP), which is preferred over BPF as (1) the filtering and the reconstruction process can be done simultaneously as the data are being acquired, (2) less computer memory is required to store the filter, and (3) the support of the BPF algorithm is not compact. In the next section, we explain some of the basic principles of FBP.

Filtered Backprojection (FBP)

The relationship shown in Equation 1 can also be written in the Fourier domain using the central section theorem (CST) (103) as

$$P_{\theta,\phi}(v_u, v_v) = F(v_u\underline{\alpha} + v_v\underline{\beta}).$$

This means the 2D Fourier transform of the projection $p_{\theta,\phi}(u, v)$ is the same as a planar slice through the 3D Fourier transform of the unknown function $f(x)$ (Fig. 10.14). This 2D plane is perpendicular to the unit vector $\underline{\theta}$ and passes through the origin of the 3D function $F(\underline{v})$. In other words, each projection $p_{\theta,\phi}(u, v)$ contains some information corresponding to certain frequencies of the 3D function (103,104). Hence, a set of projections that satisfies Orlov's condition is needed to sample all the 3D frequencies of the function $F(\underline{v})$.

In the above example, four variables are required to define the projection data $p_{\theta,\phi}(u, v)$ obtained from a 3D image, whereas only two vari-

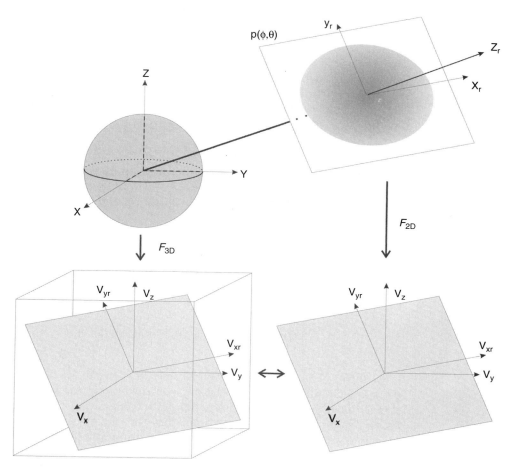

Figure 10.14. The central section theorem shows that the 2D Fourier transform of the projection data, in a certain direction, corresponds to a slice through the 3D Fourier transform of the 3D image.

ables are sufficient to define the measured projections from a 2D object. For the 3D case, if the imaging geometry does not satisfy Orlov's condition, then the reconstructed image will contain limited angle artifacts. On the other hand, if the imaging geometry oversamples certain frequencies and satisfies Orlov's condition, then an infinite number of valid filters can be determined. In this chapter, we determine the "optimal" factorizable filter that can be obtained, assuming all projections have the same noise level. This optimal 2D FBP filter is determined by taking central sections through the inverse of the transfer function $H(\underline{v})$.

In FBP, the 2D projection data $p_{\theta,\phi}(u, v)$ is first convolved with a 2D filter $g_{\theta,\phi}(u, v)$ and then backprojected onto a 3D matrix. The 2D filter for each projection depends on the direction of the measured projection $\underline{\theta}$ and the imaging geometry Ω of the system. Hence, a set of 2D FBP filters corresponding to the angle at which the projection data was measured is determined. The 2D filters are then convolved with the corresponding projections, to obtain the set of filtered projections. The convolution operation in the spatial domain can be replaced by a multiplication operation in the Fourier domain. In the Fourier domain, the 2D filter $Q_{\theta,\phi}(v_u, v_v)$ is obtained by taking the central section through the 3D filter $G(\underline{v})$ along a plane normal to $\underline{\theta}$ given by

$$Q_{\theta,\phi}(v_u, v_v) = G(v_u\underline{\alpha} + v_v\underline{\beta}).$$

The inverse Fourier transform of the function obtained by multiplying the 2D filter with the 2D Fourier transform of the projection image, gives us the filtered projection in that direction represented as

$$p_{\theta,\phi}^*(u, v) = F_{2D}^{-1}\{P_{\theta,\phi}(v_u, v_v) \times Q_{\theta,\phi}(v_u, v_v)\}.$$

Hence, in this method, the 2D filter "precorrects" the measured projections, for the blurring caused by the imaging geometry–dependent PSF. The filtered projections are then backprojected along the imaging geometry, to give the 3D reconstructed image

$$f(\underline{x}) = \iint_{\Omega} P_{\theta,\phi}^*\left(u\big|_{u=\underline{x}.\underline{\alpha}}, v\big|_{v=\underline{x}.\underline{\beta}}\right)\sin\theta d\theta d\phi.$$

A fully 3D reprojection algorithm (87) based on the above principle of filtered backprojection was developed for GCPET and widely used for image reconstruction (60). Some of the advantages of using analytical reconstruction algorithms are (1) increased accuracy, (2) ease of implementation, and (3) reduced computational effort resulting in the reconstruction of the 3D volume in a very short period of time.

Iterative Reconstruction Algorithm

The speed and simplicity of analytical reconstruction have made it the method of choice for clinical applications. However, using analytic methods it is difficult to model and compensate for the numerous image degradation factors such as scatter, spatially variant sensitivity, and asymmetric point-spread function. Iterative algorithms, on the other hand, can compensate for these degradation factors better than analytic algorithms. Yet iterative algorithms were not liberally used in the past due to limitations in computing power. Now with the increasing computing capabilities of modern-day computers, the development and use of iterative algorithms is becoming increasingly popular for image reconstruction.

Maximum Likelihood Expectation Maximization Algorithm

In GCPET, iterative reconstruction algorithms based on statistical properties such as maximum likelihood expectation maximization (MLEM) (105,106), OSEM (107,108), conjugate gradient (109), and COSEM (70) are widely used. Statistical methods try to statistically find the most probable value of the image vector F for the measured projection P. For example, the MLEM algorithm was designed to maximize the posterior probability of the reconstructed image for a given projection data with Poisson statistics, whereas the iterative expectation maximization (EM) procedure of the MLEM algorithm maximizes the log likelihood function with respect to F. Thus the log likelihood function increases with each iteration, and hence the EM algorithm always converges to a more likely solution. Mathematically, the MLEM algorithm is written as

$$f_i^{new} = \frac{f_i^{old}}{\sum\limits_{j=0}^{M} a_{ji}} \sum\limits_{l=0}^{M} a_{li} \frac{p_l}{\sum\limits_{k=0}^{N} a_{lk} f_k^{old}}$$

where f_i^{new} and f_i^{old} are vectors representing the current (updated) and previous estimates of the image. The summation over j and l is the backprojection of all the bins for all projection angles, whereas the summation over k is the projection of the previous image estimate. The element a_{ji} corresponds to the probability that a photon emitted by the ith pixel will be detected at the jth bin (i.e., a_{ji} is an element of the transfer or projection matrix A while its transpose A^T is a backprojection matrix). The algorithm converges, that is, $f_i^{new} = f_i^{old}$ when $p_l = \sum\limits_k a_{lk} f_k^{old}$. If the initial estimate and the transfer matrix are nonnegative, then the final image is nonnegative. Further, because it is easy to model the image degradation factors in the transfer matrix, the images obtained using MLEM can be potentially better than those obtained using analytical algorithms such as FBP.

Thus, the MLEM algorithm is capable of reconstructing images with a decent degree of quantitative accuracy and hence preferable for clinical applications. However, the MLEM algorithm is extremely slow and requires many iterations to reconstruct the original image. To solve this problem, a variation of MLEM called OSEM is routinely used for clinical applications. OSEM is very similar to MLEM, except that the projection data are ordered into subsets and the image is updated after going through every projection in a subset, given by

$$f_i^{new} = \frac{f_i^{old}}{\sum\limits_{j \in S_n} a_{ji}} \sum\limits_{l \in S_n} a_{li} \frac{p_l}{\sum\limits_{k \in S_n} a_{lk} f_k^{old}}$$

where S_n is the nth subset of the projection data. During reconstruction, the image is updated after using all the projection bins in a subset, that is, the image estimate is updated multiple times in an iteration depending on the number of subsets used. These multiple updates in turn accelerate the convergence speed of the OSEM algorithm by a factor proportional to the number of subsets used (107). A detailed study comparing OSEM and FBP reconstruction for dual-head coincidence imaging was performed by Gutman et al. (110). They observed that though the OSEM reconstructed images showed better visual quality, the overall detectability of lung nodules using the two methods was similar for a large set of patient studies.

Summarizing the above discussions, the five main steps of an iterative algorithm are (1) start with an initial estimate of the image to be reconstructed, (2) simulate a measurement using the image estimate mentioned in step 1, (3) compare the original measurement and the simulated measurement, (4) update the image estimate based on the above comparison in step 3, and (5) repeat steps 2, 3, and 4 until the image converges, or for some predetermined number of iterations or until some stopping criterion is reached.

List-Mode Reconstruction

The measured data obtained using GCPET system can be either rebinned or stored as list-mode data. In list-mode format each coincidence event is stored sequentially and each stored event contains the detection position on both detectors as well as the energy information of the two photons. In routine GCPET scans, the acquired number of coincidence events is typically about 20×10^3 counts per second. Because GCPET systems have a larger axial aperture compared to dedicated PET, rebinning the sparse data into large set of 2D projections over a large number of azimuthal and polar angles results in a huge number of mostly empty bins. In such cases, it is advantageous to save the data in a list-mode format (70,71,111). To reconstruct these data, by avoiding rebinning the data during reconstruction, a maximum likelihood expectation maximization (MLEM)–based list mode reconstruction approach has been developed (70,111–114). The MLEM list-mode algorithm is given by

$$f_l^{(t+1)} = \sum_{j=1}^{N} \frac{P(A_j/l)f_l^{(t)}}{T \sum_{i=1}^{M} P(A_j/i)s_i f_l^{(t)}}$$

where $f_i^{(t)}$ is the expected number of photons emitted from source voxel i per unit time and t is the iteration number. A total acquisition time is denoted by T, the total number of measured LORs is equal to N, and the number of voxels is equal to M; $p(A_j/l)$ is the probability that a detected event from voxel l leads to a measurement in LOR j, whereas the term $\sum_{i=1}^{M} P(A_j/i)s_i f_l^{(t)}$ is the forward projector that calculates the value that will be measured at LOR j with a distribution $f_l^{(t)}$ and sensitivity s_i. Various modifications of the above MLEM based list-mode algorithm have been proposed and used clinically (70,111,114).

As shown in Figure 10.15, small improvements in the resolution and contrast were observed for the list-mode reconstructed images compared to FBP and MLEM reconstructed images of single-slice rebinned data. The patient data was obtained using axial collimation with a maximum acceptance angle of 9 degrees (114).

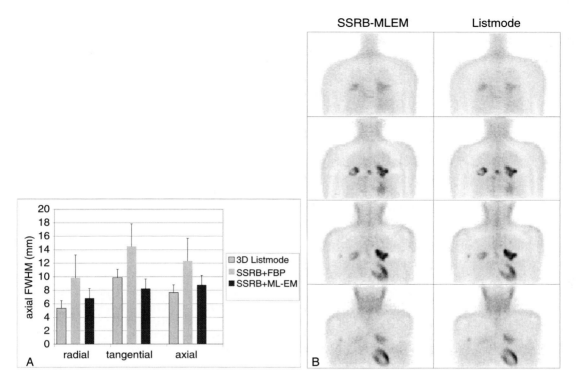

Figure 10.15. A: Resolution of the reconstructed image along the radial, transaxial, and axial direction, for 3D list-mode, SSRB + FBP and SSRB + MLEM reconstruction. B: Different coronal slices through a patient data after 20 iterations of SSRB + MLEM and 20 iteration of list-mode reconstruction.

Commercial GCPET Systems

Table 10.5 lists features provided by various GCPET manufacturers over the years (28). Though this list is not exhaustive and is constantly being updated by the manufacturers, it serves as a good starting point to understand the various hardware and software modifications that went into the design of GCPET systems.

Table 10.5. Photo-peak detection efficiency versus crystal thickness in GCPET

Crystal thickness (mm)	^{201}Tl 70 keV (%)	^{99m}Tc 140 keV (%)	^{67}Ga 300 keV (%)	^{18}F 511 keV (%)
9.5	100	84	33	13
12.7	100	91	41	17
15.9	100	95	48	21
19.1	100	98	54	24

Source: Data from Patton and Turkington (6), with permission of the Society of Nuclear Medicine.

References

1. Anger HO, Gottschalk A. Localization of brain tumors with the positron scintillation camera. J Nucl Med 1963;77:326–330.
2. Anger HO. Scintillation camera. Rev Sci Instrum 1958;29:27–33.
3. Muehllehner G. Positron camera with extended counting rate capability. J Nucl Med 1975;16(7):653–657.
4. Muehllehner G, Buchin MP, Dudek JH. Performance parameters of a positron imaging camera. IEEE Trans Nucl Sci 1976;23(1):528–537.
5. Jarritt PH, Acton PD. PET imaging using gamma camera systems: a review. Nucl Med Commun 1996;17(9):758–766.
6. Patton JA, Turkington TG. Coincidence imaging with a dual-head scintillation camera. J Nucl Med 1999;40(3):432–441.
7. Karp JS, Muehllehner G, Mankof FD, et al. Continuous-slice PENN-PET: a positron tomograph with volume imaging capability. J Nucl Med 1990;31(5):617–627.
8. Smith RJ, Karp JS, Muehllehner G. The count rate performance of the volume imaging PENN-PET scanner. IEEE Trans Med Imag 1994;13(4): 610–618.
9. Miyaoka RS, Lewellen TK, Kim JS, et al. Performance of a dual headed SPECT system modified for coincidence. Proc IEEE Nucl Sci Symp 1995;3:1348–1352.
10. Nellemann P, Hines H, Braymer W, Muehllehner G, Geagan M. Performance characteristics of a dual head SPECT scanner with PET. In: Proceedings of the IEEE Nuclear Science Symposium, San Francisco, 1995; 1751–1755.
11. Coleman RE. Camera-based PET: the best is yet to come. J Nucl Med 1997;38(11):1796–1797.
12. Leichner PK, Morgan HT, Holdeman KP, et al. SPECT imaging of fluorine-18. J Nucl Med 1995;36(8):1472–1475.
13. Martin WH, Delbeke D, Patton JA, et al. FDG-SPECT: correlation with FDG-PET. J Nucl Med 1995;36(6):988–995.
14. Burt R. Dual isotope F-18 FDG and Tc-99m RBC imaging for lung cancer. Clin Nucl Med 1998;23(12):807–809.
15. Chen EQ, MacIntyre WJ, Go RT, et al. Myocardial viability studies using fluorine-18–FDG SPECT: a comparison with fluorine-18–FDG PET. J Nucl Med 1997;38(4):582–586.
16. Bax JJ, Cornel JH, Visser FC, et al. Prediction of recovery of myocardial dysfunction after revascularization. Comparison of fluorine-18 fluorodeoxyglucose/thallium-201 SPECT, thallium-201 stress-reinjection SPECT and dobutamine echocardiography. J Am Coll Cardiol 1996;28(3): 558–564.
17. Bax JJ, Visser FC, Blanksma PK, et al. Comparison of myocardial uptake of fluorine-18–fluorodeoxyglucose imaged with PET and SPECT in dyssynergic myocardium. J Nucl Med 1996;37(10):1631–1636.
18. Matsunari I, Yoneyama T, Kanayama S, et al. Phantom studies for estimation of defect size on cardiac (18)F SPECT and PET: implications for myocardial viability assessment. J Nucl Med 2001;42(10):1579–1585.
19. Srinivasan G, Kitsiou AN, Bacharach SL, Bartlett ML, Miller-Davis C, Dilsizian V. [18F]fluorodeoxyglucose single photon emission computed tomography: can it replace PET and thallium SPECT for the assessment of myocardial viability? Circulation 1998;97(9):843–850.
20. Martin WH, Delbeke D, Patton JA, Sandler MP. Detection of malignancies with SPECT versus PET, with 2-[fluorine-18]fluoro-2-deoxy-D-glucose. Radiology 1996;198(1):225–231.

21. Martin WH, Jones RC, Delbeke D, Sandler MP. A simplified intravenous glucose loading protocol for fluorine-18 fluorodeoxyglucose cardiac single-photon emission tomography. Eur J Nucl Med 1997;24(10):1291–1297.

22. Delbeke D, Videlefsky S, Patton JA, et al. Rest myocardial perfusion/metabolism imaging using simultaneous dual-isotope acquisition SPECT with technetium-99m-MIBI/fluorine-18–FDG. J Nucl Med 1995;36(11):2110–2119.

23. Sandler MP, Videlefsky S, Delbeke D, et al. Evaluation of myocardial ischemia using a rest metabolism/stress perfusion protocol with fluorine-18 deoxyglucose/technetium-99m MIBI and dual-isotope simultaneous-acquisition single-photon emission computed tomography. J Am Coll Cardiol 1995;26(4):870–878.

24. Burt RW, Perkins OW, Oppenheim BE, et al. Direct comparison of fluorine-18–FDG SPECT, fluorine-18–FDG PET and rest thallium-201 SPECT for detection of myocardial viability. J Nucl Med 1995;36(2):176–1769.

25. Zeng GL, Gullberg GT, Bai C, et al. Iterative reconstruction of fluorine-18 SPECT using geometric point response correction. J Nucl Med 1998;39(1):124–130.

26. DiBella EVR, Gullberg GT, Ross SG, Christian PE. Compartmental modeling of ^{18}FDG in the heart using. In: Proceedings of IEEE Nuclear Science Symposium, Albuquerque, NM, 1997:1460–1463.

27. Muehllehner G. Effect of crystal thickness on scintillation camera performance. J Nucl Med 1979;20(9):992–993.

28. Fleming JS, Hillel P. Basics of Gamma Camera Positron Emission Tomography. New York: Institute of Physics and Engineering in Medicine, 2004.

29. Sossi V, Morin O, Celler A, Rempel TD, Belzberg A, Carhart C. PET and SPECT performance of the Siemens HD3 E.Cam/sup duet//spl reg/: a 1″ Na(I) hybrid camera. IEEE Trans Nucl Sci 2003;50(5):1504–1509.

30. Patton JA, Delbeke D, Sandler MP. Image fusion using an integrated, dual-head coincidence camera with x-ray tube-based attenuation maps. J Nucl Med 2000;41(8):1364–1368.

31. Tarantola G, Zito F, Gerundini P. PET instrumentation and reconstruction algorithms in whole-body applications. J Nucl Med 2003;44(5):756–769.

32. Schmand M, Dahlbom M, Eriksson L, et al. Performance of a LSO/NaI(Tl) phoswich detector for a combined PET/SPECT imaging system. J Nucl Med 1998;39(5):9P.

33. Dahlbom M, MacDonald LR, Eriksson L, et al. Performance of a YSO/LSO phoswich detector for use in a PET/SPECT. IEEE Trans Nucl Sci 1997;44(3):1114–1119.

34. Dahlbom M, MacDonald LR, Schmand M, Eriksson L, Andreaco M, Williams C. A YSO/LSO phoswich array detector for single and coincidence photon. IEEE Trans Nucl Sci 1998;45(3):1128–1132.

35. Swan WL. Exact rotational weights for coincidence imaging with a. IEEE Trans Nucl Sci 2000;47(4):1660–1664.

36. Lewellen TK, Miyaoka RS, Jansen F, Kaplan MS. A data acquisition system for coincidence imaging using a conventional dual head gamma camera. IEEE Trans Nucl Sci 1997;44(3):1214–1218.

37. Matthews CG. Triple-head coincidence imaging. In: Proceedings of IEEE Nuclear Science Symposium, Seattle, 2000:907–909.

38. Soares EJ, Germino KW, Glick SJ, Stodilka RZ. Determination of three-dimensional voxel sensitivity for two- and three-headed coincidence imaging. IEEE Trans Nucl Sci 2003;50(3):405–412.

39. D'Asseler Y, Vandenberghe S, Matthews CG, et al.—Three-dimensional geometric sensitivity calculation for. IEEE Trans Nucl Sci 2001;48(4):1451.

40. D'Asseler Y, Vandenberghe S, Matthews CG, et al. Three-dimensional geometric sensitivity calculation for three-headed coincidence imaging. IEEE Trans Nucl Sci 2001;48(4):1446–1451.

41. Swan WL. Exact rotational weights for coincidence imaging with a continuously rotating dual-headed gamma camera. IEEE Trans Nucl Sci 2000;47(4):1660–1664.

42. D'asseler Y, Vandenberghe S, Koole M, et al. A method for the calculation of the geometric sensitivity for stationary 3D PET using a triple-headed gamma camera. Eur J Nucl Med 2001;28(8):1007.

43. Kadrmas DJ, Rust TC. Converging slat collimators for PET imaging with large-area detectors detectors. IEEE Trans Nucl Sci 2003;50(1):17–23.

44. Hamilton DI, Riley PJ. Diagnostic Nuclear Medicine. New York: Springer, 2004.

45. Karp JS, Daube-Witherspoon ME, Hoffman EJ, et al. Performance standards in positron emission tomography. J Nucl Med 1991;32(12):2342–50.

46. Budinger TF. PET instrumentation: what are the limits? Semin Nucl Med 1998;28(3):247–267.

47. Vandenberghe S, D'Asseler Y, Koole M, Van de Walle R, Lemahieu I, Dierckx RA. Physical evaluation of 511 keV coincidence imaging with a gamma camera. IEEE Trans Nucl Sci 2001;48(1):98–105.

48. Mankoff DA, Muehllehner G, Karp JS. The high count rate performance of a two-dimensionally position-sensitive detector for positron emission tomography. Phys Med Biol 1989;34(4):437–456.

49. Mankoff Da, Muehllehner G, Karp JS. The effect of detector performance on high count-rate PET imaging with a tomograph based on position-sensitive detectors. IEEE Trans Nucl Sci 1988;35(1):592–597.

50. Mankoff DA, Muehllehner G, Miles GE. A local coincidence triggering system for PET tomographs composed. IEEE Trans Nucl Sci 1990;37(2):730–736.

51. Muehllehner G, Jaszczak RJ, Beck RN. The reduction of coincidence loss in radionuclide imaging cameras through the use of composite filters. Phys Med Biol 1974;19(4):504–510.

52. Sandstrom M, Tolmachev V, Kairemo K, Lundqvist H, Lubberink M. Performance of coincidence imaging with long-lived positron emitters as an alternative to dedicated PET and SPECT. Phys Med Biol 2004;49(24):5419–5432.

53. Joung J, Miyaoka RS, Kohlmyer SG, Harrison RL, Lewellen TK. Slat collimator design issues for dual-head coincidence Imaging systems. IEEE Trans Nucl Sci 2002;49(1):141–146.

54. Glick SJ, Groiselle CJ, Kolthammer J, Stodilka RZ. Optimization of septal spacing in hybrid PET using estimation task performance. IEEE T Nucl Sci 2002;49(5):2127–2132.

55. Groiselle CJ, Glick SJ. Using the bootstrap method to evaluate image noise for investigation of axial collimation in hybrid PET. In: Proceedings of IEEE Nuclear Science Symposium, 2002:782–785.

56. Groiselle CJ, D'Asseler Y, Kolthammer JA, Matthews CG, Glick SJ. A Monte Carlo simulation study to evaluate septal spacing using triple-head hybrid PET imaging. IEEE Trans Nucl Sci 2003;50(5):1339–1346.

57. Rust TC, Kadrmas DJ. Survey of parallel slat collimator designs for hybrid PET imaging. Phys Med Biol 2003;48(6):N97–104.

58. Di Bella EVR. Gamma camera PET with low energy collimators: characterization and correction of scatter. IEEE Trans Nucl Sci 2002;49(5):2067–2073.

59. Cherry SR, Sorenson JA, Phelps ME. Physics in Nuclear Medicine, 3rd ed. Philadelphia: Saunders, 2003.

60. Miyaoka RS, Kohlmyer SG, Lewellen TK. Hot sphere detection limits for a dual head coincidence imaging. IEEE Trans Nucl Sci 1999;46(6):2185–2191.

61. Defrise M, Kinahan PE, Townsend DW, Michel C, Sibomana M, Newport DF. Exact and approximate rebinning algorithms for 3–D PET data. IEEE Trans Med Imaging 1997;16(2):145–158.

62. Wang W, Matthews CG. Geometric calibration of a triple-head gamma-camera PET system. In: Proceedings of IEEE Nuclear Science Symposium, 2000:16/44–16/48.

63. Boren EL Jr, Delbeke D, Patton JA, Sandler MP. Comparison of FDG PET and positron coincidence detection imaging using a dual-head gamma camera with 5/8–inch NaI(Tl) crystals in patients with suspected body malignancies. Eur J Nucl Med 1999;26(4):379–387.

64. Visvikis D, Fryer T, Downey S. Optimisation of noise equivalent count rates for brain and body FDG imaging using gamma camera PET. IEEE Trans Nucl Sci 1999;46(3):624–630.

65. Thompson CJ, Picard Y. 2. New strategies to increase the signal-to-noise ratio in positron volume imaging. IEEE Trans Nucl Sci 1993;40(4):956–961.

66. Stodilka RZ, Glick SJ. Evaluation of geometric sensitivity for hybrid PET. J Nucl Med 2001;42(7):1116–1120.

67. Vandenberghe S, D'Asseler Y, Kolthammer J, Van de Walle R, Lemahieu I, Dierckx RA. Influence of the angle of incidence on the sensitivity of gamma camera based PET. Phys Med Biol 2002;47(2):289–303.

68. Vandenberghe S, Kolthammer JA, D'Asseler Y, et al. Influence of detector thickness on resolution in three-headed gamma camera PET. IEEE Trans Nucl Sci 2002;49(1):98–103.

69. Kijewski MF, Muller SP, Moore SC. Nonuniform collimator sensitivity: improved precision for quantitative SPECT. J Nucl Med 1997;38(1):151–156.

70. Levkovitz R, Falikman D, Zibulevsky M, Ben-Tal A, Nemirovski A. The design and implementation of COSEM, an iterative algorithm for fully 3–D listmode data. IEEE Trans Med Imaging 2001;20(7):633–642.

71. Reader AJ, Visvikis D, Erlandsson K, Ott RJ, Flower MA. Intercomparison of four reconstruction techniques for positron volume imaging with rotating planar detectors. Phys Med Biol 1998;43(4):823–834.

72. Turkington TG. Attenuation correction in hybrid positron emission tomography. Semin Nucl Med 2000;30(4):255–267.

73. Laymon CM, Turkington TG, Gilland DR, Coleman RE. Transmission scanning system for a gamma camera coincidence scanner. J Nucl Med 2000;41(4):692–699.

74. Chang LT. A method for attenuation correction in radionuclide computed tomography. IEEE Trans Nucl Sci 1978;25:638–643.

75. Karp JS, Muehllehner G, Qu H, Yan XH. Singles transmission in volume-imaging PET with a 137Cs source. Phys Med Biol 1995;40(5):929–944.

76. Dilsizian V, Bacharach SL, Khin MM, Smith MF. Fluorine-18–deoxyglucose SPECT and coincidence imaging for myocardial viability: clinical and technologic issues. J Nucl Cardiol 2001;8(1):75–88.

77. Zaidi H, Hasegawa B. Determination of the attenuation map in emission tomography. J Nucl Med 2003;44(2):291–315.

78. Zeng GL, Gullberg GT, Christian PE, Gagnon D, Chi-Hua T. Asymmetric cone-beam transmission tomography. IEEE Trans Nucl Sci 2001;48(1):124.

79. Bird NJ, Old SE, Barber RW. Gamma camera positron emission tomography. Br J Radiol 2001;74:303–306.

80. Turkington TG, Laymon CM, Schopfer KG, Coleman RE, Wainer N. Multiple point sources collimated with transaxial septa for high. IEEE Trans Nucl Sci 1999;46(6):2247–2252.

81. Kalki K, Blankespoor SC, Brown JK, et al. Myocardial perfusion imaging with a combined x-ray CT and SPECT system. J Nucl Med 1997;38(10): 1535–1540.

82. Lewitt RM, Matej S. Overview of methods for image reconstruction from projections in emission computed tomography. Proc IEEE 2003;91(10): 1588–1611.

83. Daube-Witherspoon ME, Muehllehner G. Treatment of axial data in three-dimensional PET. J Nucl Med 1987;28(11):1717–1724.

84. Vandenberghe S. Iterative Listmode Reconstruction of Coincidence Imaging. Ph.D. dissertation. Gent: University of Gent, 2002.

85. Lewittt RM, Muehllehner G, Karpt JS. Three-dimensional image reconstruction for PET by multi-slice rebinning and axial image filtering. Phys Med Biol 1994;39(3):321–339.

86. Matej S, Lewitt RM. 3D-FRP: Direct Fourier reconstruction with Fourier reprojection for fully 3–D PET. IEEE Trans Nucl Sci 2001;48(4):1378–1385.

87. Kinahan PE, Rogers JG, Harrop R, Johnson RR. Three-dimensional image reconstruction in object space. IEEE Trans Nucl Sci 1988;35:635–638.

88. Matej S, Karp JS, Lewitt RM, Becher AJ. Performance of the Fourier rebinning algorithm for PET with large acceptance angles. Phys Med Biol 1998;43(4):787–795.

89. Orlov SS. Theory of three-dimensional reconstruction: 1. Conditions of a complete set of projections. Sov Phys Crystallography 1975;20:312–314.

90. Pieper BC, Bowsher JE, Tornai MP, Archer CN, Jaszczak RJ. Parallel-beam tilted-head analytic SPECT reconstruction. In: Proceedings of IEEE Nuclear Science Symposium, 2001:1313–1317.

91. Schorr B, Townsend D. Filters for three-dimensional limited-angle tomography. Phys Med Biol 1981;26(2):305–312.

92. Tanaka E. Generalised correction functions for convolutional techniques in three-dimensional image reconstruction. Phys Med Biol 1979;24(1): 157–161.

93. Pelc NJ. A Generalized Filtered Backprojection Reconstruction Algorithm. Boston: Harvard School of Public Health, 1979.

94. Colsher JG. Fully three-dimensional positron emission tomography. Phys Med Biol 1980;25(1):103–115.

95. Ra JB, Lim CB, Cho ZH, Hilal SK, Correll J. A true three-dimensional reconstruction algorithm for the spherical positron emission tomography. Phys Med Biol 1982;27:37–50.

96. Defrise M, Clack R, Townsend DW. Solution to the 3D image reconstruction problem for 2D parallel projections. J Opt Soc Am 1993:869–877.

97. Pelc NJ. A Generalized Filtered Backprojection Reconstruction Algorithm. Sc.D. dissertation. Boston: Harvard School of Public Health, 1979.

98. Knutsson HE, Edholm P, Granlund GH, Petersson CU. Ectomography—a new radiographic reconstruction method—I. Theory and error estimates. IEEE Trans Biomed Eng 1980;27(11):640–648.

99. Harauz G, vanHeel M. Exact filters for general geometry three-dimensional reconstruction. Optik 1986;73:146–156.

100. Defrise M, Townsend DW, Clack R. FAVOR: a fast reconstruction algorithm for volume imaging in PET. IEEE Conf Record 1991:1919–1923.

101. Wessell DE. Rotating Slant-Hole Single Photon Emission Computed Tomography. Ph.D. dissertation. Durham, NC: University of North Carolina, 1999.

102. Bal G, Zeng GL, Noo F, Bal H, Clackdoyle R. Analytical reconstruction for multi-segment slant hole SPECT. In: Proceedings of IEEE Nuclear Science Symposium, Norfork, VA. Piscataway, NJ: IEEE Service Center, 2002: 1236–1240.

103. Natterer F. The Mathematics of Computerized Tomography. New York: Tuebner-Wiley, 1986.

104. Bracewell RN. Strip integration in radio astronomy. Aust J Phys 1956;9: 198–217.

105. Shepp LA, Vardi Y. Maximum likelihood reconstruction for emission tomography. IEEE Trans Med Imag 1982:113–122.

106. Lange K, Carson R. EM reconstruction algorithms for emission and transmission tomography. J Comput Assist Tomogr 1984;8(2):306–316.

107. Hudson HM, Larkin RS. Accelerated image reconstruction using ordered subsets of projection data. IEEE Trans Med Imag 1994;13(4):601–609.

108. Shao L, Nellemann P, Ye J, Koster J, Hines H. Towards quantitation for dual head coincidence cameras by using. In: Proceeding of IEEE Nuclear Science Symposium, 2000:18/2–6.

109. Panin V. Attenuation Correction in Single Photon Emission Computed Tomography Using A Priori Information. Ph.D. dissertation. Salt Lake City: University of Utah, 2000.

110. Gutman F, Gardin I, Delahaye N, et al. Optimisation of the OS-EM algorithm and comparison with FBP for image reconstruction on a dual-head camera: a phantom and a clinical 18F-FDG study. Eur J Nucl Med Mol Imaging 2003;30(11):1510–1519.

111. Parra L, Barrett HH. List-mode likelihood: EM algorithm and image quality estimation demonstrated on 2–D PET. IEEE Trans Med Imaging 1998;17(2):228–235.

112. Barrett HH, White T, Parra LC. List-mode likelihood. J Opt Soc Am A Opt Image Sci Vis 1997;14(11):2914–2923.

113. Bouwens L, van de Walle R, Koole M, et al. SPECT reconstruction from list-mode acquired data. Eur J Nucl Med 2001;28(8):969.

114. Vandenberghe S, D'Asseler Y, Koole M, Van de Walle R, Lemahieu I, Dierckx RA. Correction for detection efficiency, geometry and deadtime in gamma camera based PET list mode reconstruction. Eur J Nucl Med 2001;28(8):964–969.

115. Hillel P. Basics of gamma camera positron emission tomography. York, UK: Institute of Physics and Engineering in Medicine, 2004.

Section 2

Oncology

11

Brain Tumors

Michael J. Fisher and Peter C. Phillips

Brain tumors are the second most common malignancy of childhood, accounting for approximately 20% of all childhood cancers. The estimated incidence ranges from 2.4 to 4.1 cases per 100,000 children per year. Although nearly 60% of patients are now cured, brain tumors are still the principal cause of pediatric cancer mortality. Pediatric brain tumors are classified by histology. Medulloblastoma is the most common malignant brain tumor, and low-grade astrocytoma is the most common benign tumor.

The diagnosis and evaluation of brain tumors is directed by computed tomography (CT) and magnetic resonance imaging (MRI), which are excellent for anatomic imaging. Modern MRI, in particular, is able to identify structure with high resolution and is the standard for distinguishing abnormal tissue from normal brain. Unfortunately, these modalities are limited in their ability to differentiate benign from malignant tumors, neoplasia from inflammatory or vascular processes, postoperative changes or edema from residual tumor, and relapsed disease from radiation injury.

In contrast to CT and MRI, positron emission tomography (PET) provides functional information on a range of cellular and biologic processes including glucose metabolism, protein synthesis, DNA synthesis, membrane biosynthesis, cerebral blood flow, and hypoxia. In addition, radioligands have been developed that permit in vivo imaging of specific receptors. Positron emission tomography is useful to detect and grade tumors, delineate tumor margins, predict prognosis, and distinguish tumors from nonneoplastic processes (Fig. 11.1). It has also been used for treatment planning, guiding stereotactic biopsy, evaluating response to therapy, and for distinguishing relapse from radionecrosis. Functional PET imaging has the potential to be combined with anatomic MRI to further enhance the evaluation of these processes.

Positron emission tomography is commonly used for the evaluation of brain tumors in adults. The most common tracers are ^{18}F-fluorodeoxyglucose (FDG) and ^{11}C-methionine (MET). Although many of the adult trials include the occasional pediatric patient, there is a dearth

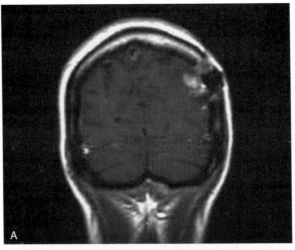

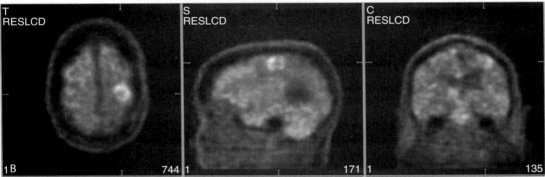

Figure 11.1. Detection of a left cortical lesion with MRI (A) and FDG-PET (B). PET shows focal uptake in this primary brain tumor. (Courtesy of Dr. P. Bhargava.)

of literature focusing on the use of PET for pediatric brain tumors. Early studies suggest that the metabolism of histologically comparable brain tumors is similar in children and adults. This chapter will therefore identify and emphasize the existing pediatric studies and use the known similarities between adult and pediatric brain tumors to expand the discussion. The focus is on FDG and MET, as they are the tracers most studied in brain tumors.

Tumor Detection

FDG-PET

FDG is the most common tracer used for PET imaging of brain tumors. It was introduced in 1976, and one of the earliest reports of its use was in the evaluation of cerebral gliomas in 1982 (1). FDG-PET imaging is based on the similarity between FDG and glucose. FDG is phosphorylated upon entering the cell; however, unlike glucose, it cannot be metabolized further and therefore accumulates. Even in the presence of oxygen, tumors rely on anaerobic glycolysis for energy. To support the energy requirement for growth, malignant cells upregulate their glucose transporters. Hence tumor FDG accumulation, like glucose, is proportional to the metabolic rate of the cell. Normal brain, however, is also dependent on glucose for its energy needs. Therefore, there is a high background of FDG signal, with uptake in the gray matter about 2.5 times that of the white matter (2).

There are various methods to analyze FDG uptake in tumors. The most quantitative methods require multiple image acquisition as well as arterial blood sampling in order to calculate the metabolic rate of glucose. This is time-consuming and invasive and therefore is of particular concern in studies of children. In addition, the calculation of the glucose metabolic rate from FDG uptake requires the use of the "lumped constant (LC)," which accounts for the differences between FDG and glucose in transport and phosphorylation. This value is based on normal brain and is assumed to be comparable with tumor; however, there is evidence that it is different for neoplastic tissue and may vary with histologic subtype (3). Given these concerns, most studies have used simple qualitative (visual scales) or semiquantitative (calculating ratios of uptake in the region of interest compared with a normal structure) approaches. Other semiquantitative approaches include calculation of the standard uptake value (SUV), which is used more often in PET imaging of the body. Numerous studies have shown that the evaluation of brain tumors with visual grading systems is at least as accurate as semiquantitative analysis (ratios of tumor to gray matter, white matter, or whole brain signal) (4,5) and SUV measurements (6). These approaches obviate the need for dynamic scanning and blood sampling, but the analysis of the "normal" comparative tissue can be confounding. Selection of the normal tissue can be difficult, particularly when the tumor is midline in location, and the uptake into normal brain may change with time and treatment, thus altering the tumor-to-normal ratio (7). Of most concern is the lack of standardization of analysis methods between studies, which makes comparison of results extremely difficult.

Since Di Chiro et al.'s (1) first report of a correlation between FDG uptake and histologic grade of glioma, numerous studies have reported the use of FDG to evaluate gliomas in adults but have also included other primary brain tumors such as ganglioglioma, dysembryoplastic neuroepithelial tumor (DNET), germ cell tumors, primitive neuroectodermal tumor (PNET), meningioma, and lymphoma. Other case reports describe the utility of FDG in the evaluation of brainstem tumors (8) and Langerhans cell histiocytosis involving the central nervous system (CNS) (9). FDG-PET has also been used to differentiate CNS lymphoma from nonmalignant processes in patients with AIDS. Both lymphoma and toxoplasmosis, a common opportunistic infection in AIDS, are contrast-enhancing by anatomic imaging, but they have very different FDG signals. Rosenfeld et al. (10) initially showed that CNS lymphomas had high FDG uptake. In addition, uptake declined with steroid treatment in a patient imaged before and 3 weeks after initiating therapy. Additional studies in patients with

AIDS confirm the high FDG accumulation in CNS lymphomas (11–15). Additionally, FDG-PET was able to distinguish between hypermetabolic lymphoma and hypometabolic toxoplasmosis lesions (11–15). In one review of 33 patients with biopsy-proven lymphoma or toxoplasmosis, all 16 lymphoma patients had high FDG uptake and all toxoplasmosis lesions were hypometabolic (16). Sensitivity is therefore high; however, the specificity of a hypermetabolic lesion is unclear. One study reported two patients with progressive multifocal leukoencephalopathy that had FDG signals indistinguishable from lymphoma (13).

FDG-PET has also been investigated for the identification of CNS metastases from non-CNS primary tumors (Fig. 11.2). Marom et al. (17)

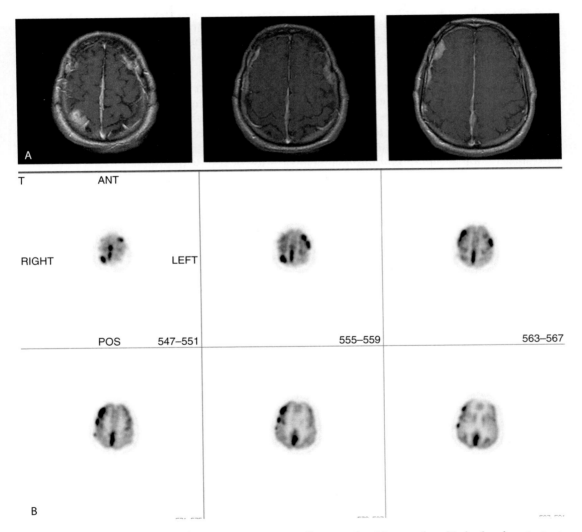

Figure 11.2. Young patient with a primary paraganglioma and evidence of multiple dural metastases visualized with MRI (A) and as very active lesions on FDG-PET (B). (Courtesy of Dr. P. Bhargava.)

evaluated FDG-PET for staging in 100 patients with newly diagnosed lung cancer and found nine patients with metastases detected by PET that were not apparent with conventional imaging. In contrast, in another study, FDG-PET identified only 68% (21 of 31) of CNS lesions in 19 patients (18). Of the 10 lesions that were missed, four had frankly decreased FDG uptake, but six may have been missed because of their small size and isointensity relative to adjacent gray matter. Soft tissue metastases usually have high glucose metabolism. Given the typical location of brain metastases at the cortical gray-white junction because of hematogenous seeding, it is not surprising that there would be difficulty in distinguishing them from adjacent cortex on FDG-PET. Larcos and Maisey (19) explored the value of routine CNS PET for detecting metastases in 273 patients with non-CNS primary tumors and detected cerebral pathology in only 2% and unsuspected metastases in only 0.7%. In addition, a blinded retrospective review evaluating FDG-PET for screening of cerebral metastases in 40 patients identified only 75% of the patients with metastases and detected only 61% of the lesions seen by MRI (20). In three patients, metastases were detected by PET that were not seen by MRI, but all three patients had other FDG-positive lesions; thus PET correctly identified them as having metastatic disease. In sum, few clinically relevant lesions were detected, and therefore Rohren et al. (20) no longer recommend routine FDG-PET imaging of the brain in patients undergoing staging with whole-body PET. Instead, they recommend anatomic imaging when indicated.

Many of the studies of FDG-PET for brain tumors include pediatric cases together with adult cases (6,8,20–27). Comparatively few studies focus exclusively on the evaluation of pediatric brain tumors (Table 11.1). Examples of tumors examined include DNET (28–30), ganglioglioma (29,30), oligodendroglioma and oligoastrocytoma (28,29), low-grade astrocytoma (28,30–33), high-grade astrocytoma (30,31,34), brainstem tumors (30,31,33,35), cerebellar medulloblastoma and supratentorial PNET (30,32,33), ependymoma (30,31,33), germ cell tumors (30,31), choroids plexus papilloma (30), craniopharyngioma (30), and pituitary adenoma (30).

Hoffman et al. (33) evaluated 17 children with posterior fossa tumors. They found the highest FDG uptake in the medulloblastomas and the lowest in the brainstem gliomas. Holthoff et al. (32) studied 15 children and found that the mean glucose metabolic rate was twice as high in medulloblastoma as in supratentorial PNET or low-grade glioma (although the latter two groups had only a few patients).

Work done at the Children's Hospital of Philadelphia described 24 patients with neurofibromatosis type 1 (NF1) with low-grade astrocytomas of the optic pathway, thalamus, or brainstem and showed that clinical outcome correlated with FDG activity (36).

Bruggers et al. (35) demonstrated that FDG-PET was useful in the management of a child with intrinsic pontine glioma. Patients with this tumor often have transient clinical and MRI worsening after radiotherapy that is believed to be due to swelling and not tumor progression. In addition, this group of patients often has clinical worsening

Table 11.1. Pediatric PET studies

Study	Year	No. of patients	Tracers	Pathology	Purpose
Mineura et al. (34)	1985	1	FDG	HGG	Detection, response to therapy
O'Tuama et al. (57)	1990	13	Met	Astr, Ep, Mbl	Detection
Hoffman et al. (33)	1992	17	FDG	Astr, BSG, CPP, Ep, JPA, Mbl	Detection, prognosis
Holthoff et al. (32)	1993	15	FDG	JPA, LGA, Mbl, PNET	Detection, response to therapy
Bruggers et al. (35)	1993	1	FDG	BSG	Detection
Plowman et al. (31)	1997	10	FDG, MET	BSG, Ep, GCT, LGG, Pc, MET	Detection, recurrence vs. radionecrosis
Duncan et al. (29)	1997	15	FDG, MET, [^{15}O]H$_2$O	DNET, Ggl, Oligo, NN	Treatment planning
Kaplan et al. (28)	1999	5	FDG, MET, [^{15}O]H$_2$O	DNET, JPA, Oligo	Treatment planning
Utriainen et al. (58)	2002	27	FDG, MET	DNET, Ep, Ggl, GCT, HGG, JPA, LGG, Mbl, Oligo	Detection, grading, prognosis
Messing-Junger et al. (140)	2002	2	FET	HGG, LGG	Directing biopsy
Pirotte et al. (92)	2003	9	FDG, MET	Ggl, HGG, LGG, Oligo, PNET, NN	Directing biopsy
Borgwardt et al. (30)	2005	38	FDG, [^{15}O]H$_2$O	BSG, CPP, Cranio, DNET, Ep, Ggl, GCT, HGG, JPA, LGG, Mbl, PNET, PitAd	Detection, grading

Astr, astrocytoma (unspecified); BSG, brainstem glioma; CPP, choroid plexus papilloma; Cranio, craniopharyngioma; DNET, dysembryoplastic neuroepithelial tumor; Ep, ependymoma; Ggl, ganglioglioma; GCT, germ cell tumor; HGG, high-grade glioma; JPA, juvenile pilocytic astrocytoma; LGG, low-grade glioma; Mbl, medulloblastoma; MET, non-CNS metastasis; NN, nonneoplasia; Oligo, oligodendroglioma/oligoastrocytoma; PNET, primitive neuroectodermal tumor; Pc, pineocytoma; PitAd, pituitary adenoma.

before MRI evidence appears. It is important, therefore, to be able to distinguish the toxicity of therapy from true tumor progression in order to make appropriate treatment decisions. In this report, the patient had worsening of symptoms in the absence of significant MRI progression 8 months after radiotherapy. The PET scan at that time showed increased FDG uptake compared with a prior PET scan 3 months earlier. Subsequent MRI (4 weeks later) showed progression, and an autopsy 3 weeks thereafter confirmed tumor progression. Although this report is anecdotal, the authors concluded that changes in PET signal may precede changes on MRI scan.

FDG metabolism can be affected by several factors unrelated to the brain tumor itself. Patients with brain tumors are often treated with corticosteroids, the impact of which on FDG uptake has been explored. Most studies have not shown an influence of steroid treatment on FDG uptake into brain tumors (37–39); however, steroids can decrease the uptake into normal cortex, thus affecting the tumor-to-background differences (37). In contrast, in the setting of high blood glucose (a common side effect of corticosteroid treatment), FDG uptake in brain tumors is decreased, but not to the same degree as the concurrent decrease in uptake into normal cortex (40). In addition, seizures can occur in the setting of a cortical brain tumor. A seizure during the time of the PET scan can markedly increase the FDG uptake and result in a false-positive scan (2), whereas PET scans performed within 24 hours after a seizure may be difficult to interpret because of "falsely" low FDG uptake.

Qualitatively, most low-grade tumors have FDG uptake less than or equal to that of normal white matter, whereas high-grade lesions have uptake greater than or equal to that of gray matter. Therefore, high-grade tumors within or adjacent to normal gray matter may be difficult to detect because of the low lesion-to-background contrast. There is a similar problem with low-grade lesions within or bordering normal white matter that has similar FDG signal. Co-registration of PET images with CT or MRI may improve evaluation of FDG uptake by helping to delineate the margins of the lesion. Borgwardt et al. (30) found that the diagnostic value of FDG-PET was improved by digital co-registration of PET and MRI in 28 of 31 pediatric cases. In particular, it improved the localization of tumor in 23 cases and the delineation of tumor margins in eight cases. In contrast, visual PET/MRI co-registration increased the diagnostic value in only three of seven cases.

Other methods to improve tumor delineation include extending the interval between FDG injection and scanning. Spence et al. (41) imaged 19 patients with supratentorial gliomas both early (0 to 90 minutes) and late (180 to 500 minutes) after injection. Compared with early imaging, delayed imaging improved the delineation of tumor relative to gray matter in 12 of the 19 patients. This was true for both high-grade gliomas (nine of 11) and progressing low-grade gliomas (three of five). It is hypothesized that degradation of FDG-6-phosphate may occur more efficiently in normal brain than in tumor tissue, accounting for this result. For the three low-grade gliomas that were subsequently shown to be stable, tumor delineation was not improved by delayed imaging.

Amino Acid PET

Because the uptake of amino acids into normal brain tissue is relatively low and appears to be less influenced by inflammation, amino acid PET imaging may have some advantages over FDG-PET in providing good contrast between tumor tissue and background (42). The higher proliferative rate of malignant cells requires an increase in protein synthesis with a consequent increased cellular need for amino acids. This results in an increased transport of amino acids into malignant cells, which is often more pronounced than the actual increase in protein synthesis (2,42). MET is the most common radiolabeled amino acid used in the imaging of brain tumors. Its uptake appears to reflect cell membrane transport more than protein synthesis (43), and its uptake in tumor is 1.2 to 3.5 times higher than in normal brain (2). There is no effect of corticosteroid treatment on MET uptake into normal brain (44) or low-grade glioma (45). MET uptake into glioblastoma is moderately decreased with steroids, but uptake persists at a level higher than low-grade gliomas (45).

Mosskin et al. (46) evaluated the uptake of MET in patients with supratentorial gliomas. In 22 of 32 cases, they found that increased MET uptake corresponded to areas of tumor on stereotactic biopsy. Five cases had tumor cells outside of the area of increased MET uptake, and five cases had MET uptake in areas without histologic evidence of tumor. Overall, in 24 cases, MET-PET was more accurate than contrast-enhanced CT in determining tumor margins. Other studies agree that tumor extent is often better determined by MET-PET than by CT or MRI (47,48); however, these studies were performed in the CT or early MRI era. Current MRI techniques represent the most sensitive means of identifying abnormal brain lesions that may be tumor, and PET may be more useful to discriminate neoplastic from nonneoplastic lesions.

In a study of 85 gliomas, De Witte et al. (49) found elevated MET uptake in 98%. Ogawa et al. (48) found a similar high MET uptake rate (97%) in high-grade gliomas, but MET uptake was only elevated in 61% of low-grade gliomas. Herholz et al. (45) studied 196 consecutive patients with suspected low-grade glioma. The authors used a MET uptake (lesion-to-contralateral normal brain) threshold of 1.47, and MET-PET distinguished tumor from nonneoplastic lesion with a sensitivity of 76% and specificity of 87%. When lesions that turned out to be malignant were excluded, sensitivity for differentiating low-grade from nonneoplastic lesions fell to 67%. Chung et al. (50) revealed a sensitivity of 89% for detecting brain tumors (31 of 35) with MET and a specificity of 100% (all 10 nonneoplastic lesions had no MET uptake). Of note, cerebrovascular lesions, such as infarction and hemorrhage, can also exhibit high MET uptake, felt to be secondary to a disrupted blood–brain barrier (51). Other ^{11}C-radiolabeled amino acids, such as [^{11}C]-tyrosine (TYR) are also useful in detecting primary brain tumors with a sensitivity of 91% and specificity of 67% (52).

Compared with FDG, MET is more sensitive for detecting tumor and delineating tumor margins. Ogawa et al. (53) evaluated 10 patients with glioma or meningioma and found MET to be superior to FDG in delineating the extent of tumor. Pirotte et al. (54) demonstrated abnormal MET uptake in 23 tumors, 11 of which had no FDG uptake or uptake equal to background. Sasaki et al. (55) found MET more useful than FDG in detecting tumor extent and in distinguishing benign from malignant astrocytomas. In a study of 54 patients with glioma, 95% were clearly visualized with MET, whereas only 51% were hypermetabolic with FDG (24). For low-grade gliomas, MET identified over 90%, but FDG identified only 21%. Chung et al. (50) showed that 22 of 24 gliomas had greater extent and degree of uptake with MET than FDG. MET-PET was also better than FDG in detecting low-grade astrocytoma and oligodendroglioma (56).

Pediatric studies have also shown the utility of MET for imaging primary brain tumors. O'Tuama et al. (57) reported that MET was useful to delineate tumor extent in 13 children. Plowman et al. (31) imaged 10 "pediatric" patients (only seven were less than 18 years old) with both FDG and MET and described PET's utility in localizing viable tumor for radiosurgery, distinguishing recurrent tumor from radiation injury, and differentiating persistent tumor from posttreatment changes when evaluating residual enhancement on MRI after surgery or radiotherapy. In a larger study of 27 children with primary brain tumors, MET-PET had a sensitivity of 96% for the detection of tumor, which was higher than that of FDG (58).

Both FDG and MET are valuable for detecting tumor and differentiating it from nonneoplastic tissue. FDG is most useful in evaluating more malignant lesions, such as high-grade glioma and lymphoma, which have particularly elevated glucose metabolism. Because of the minimal background MET uptake into normal brain, MET appears to have an advantage over FDG, particularly in detecting low-grade tumors.

Tumor Grading

FDG-PET

Most studies regarding PET grading of primary brain tumors have focused on gliomas and show a correlation between FDG uptake and histologic grade of glioma. Di Chiro and colleagues (1,59) showed that all high-grade gliomas had regions of high FDG uptake and that the mean glucose metabolic rate in high-grade gliomas was almost twice that of low-grade gliomas (7.4 versus 4.0). In addition, they reported that FDG uptake was better than contrast-enhancement on CT in predicting tumor grade (60). Delbeke et al. (61) evaluated FDG uptake in 32 high-grade and 26 low-grade brain tumors, most of which were gliomas. They defined an "optimal cut-off level" that distinguished between high-grade and low-grade tumors. Ratios of tumor-to-gray matter greater than 0.6 or tumor-to-white matter greater than 1.5 predicted high-grade pathology with a sensitivity of 94% and specificity of 77%. As gliomas are often histologically heterogeneous, Goldman et al. (62) examined 161 stereotactic PET-guided biopsy specimens from 20 patients with gliomas to see whether glucose metabolism correlated with degree of anaplasia. Glucose uptake was significantly higher in anaplastic than non-anaplastic specimens. Histologic signs of anaplasia were present in approximately 75% of samples with high FDG uptake but in only 10% of samples with low FDG uptake.

More recently, Padma et al. (63) evaluated FDG uptake in a large sample of patients with glioma scanned at various times during treatment. They found 166 patients had low uptake and 165 had high uptake. Among those with low FDG uptake, 86% were low-grade and 14% were high-grade gliomas. Of the 23 patients with high-grade glioma but low FDG uptake, all had their first PET scan after therapy, and low uptake may have been related to an effect of treatment. In contrast, 93% of the patients with high FDG uptake had high-grade gliomas, whereas only 7% had low-grade pathology. Of the latter, all 11 patients had increasing anaplasia on repeat biopsy and a rapidly declining clinical course.

One problem with the use FDG-PET to assess glioma grade is that FDG uptake may be influenced by volume averaging with adjacent tissue. For example, the apparent FDG signal of a high-grade glioma may appear artificially lower when the signal is averaged with adjacent white matter, surrounding edema, or an associated necrotic area (all regions that are inherently low in FDG uptake).

Although degree of FDG uptake is correlated with histologic grade of glioma in most cases, juvenile pilocytic astrocytomas are an exception. This is of particular importance in pediatrics, in which pilocytic astrocytomas comprise a large percentage of the brain tumor incidence. These grade I gliomas, although benign in behavior, have repeatedly been shown to have high FDG uptake, similar to that of anaplastic astrocytoma (24,33,64,65). This may be due to their very vascular nature (64) or perhaps an increased expression of glucose transporters in this tumor type (65,66). Other benign tumors that have shown high FDG uptake include choroid plexus papillomas (30,33).

FDG uptake correlated with World Health Organization (WHO) histologic grade (67) in a study of 38 children with primary brain tumors (30). Borgwardt et al. (30), using a measure of glucose metabolism called the "mean index" (based on FDG uptake in a region of interest of tumor, white matter, and gray matter), found a mean index of 4.27 in four grade IV tumors, 2.47 in four grade III tumors, 1.34 in 10 grade II tumors, and −0.31 in eight of 12 grade I tumors. Four grade I tumors (three pilocytic astrocytomas and one choroid plexus papilloma), with a mean index of 3.26, were excluded because of the known lack of association of FDG uptake and histologic grade in these tumors. Eight other patients had tumors in locations that were difficult or dangerous to biopsy (mostly brainstem) and were expected to be benign based on their appearance and subsequent clinical course. These tumors had a mean index of 1.04, consistent with low-grade histology. It is difficult to know how to interpret these results given the large number (greater than 10) of different histologies represented in this study. Although there is a known correlation between grade and prognosis for gliomas, the comparability of grading systems between different histologic subgroups of brain tumors has yet to be established. At a minimum, this report suggests a clear difference in FDG uptake between benign and malignant brain tumors.

Amino Acid PET

MET has been evaluated for grading gliomas. Derlon et al. (68) found a statistically significant relationship between MET uptake and tumor grade in 22 patients with glioma. The tumor-to-contralateral normal brain ratio was 1.04 for grade II, 1.68 for grade III, and 2.33 for grade IV lesions. The difference between grade II and the higher grade lesions was significant. In a larger study, De Witte et al. (49) found that MET uptake correlated with tumor grade in 85 patients with glioma (pilocytic astrocytomas were excluded). In addition, a tumor-to-contralateral normal brain threshold greater than 1.8 was more common for high-grade gliomas, but this dividing line did not universally distinguish between high- and low-grade lesions. Other studies have shown a correlation between MET uptake and markers of tumor proliferation in gliomas [proliferating cell nuclear antigen (69) and Ki-76 staining (50)].

In a study of 23 patients, Sasaki et al. (55) found MET to be superior to FDG in distinguishing low-grade from high-grade gliomas. Although the difference in MET uptake between grade II gliomas and higher-grade lesions was statistically significant, this was not the case for FDG. In contrast, Kaschten et al. (24) found a significant difference in FDG uptake between grade II and grade III or IV lesions, but the difference in MET uptake between grade II and III lesions did not reach significance. Ribom et al. (70) found a significant increase in MET uptake in 10 untreated low-grade gliomas from baseline to the time of progression. Of note, the tumor "hot spot" to normal cortex ratio at progression was 4.40 for patients who had developed anaplasia and 2.27 for those whose histology was unchanged.

MET may also be useful for grading oligodendrogliomas. In 47 patients, MET uptake was significantly higher in anaplastic than low-grade oligodendrogliomas (71). However, the amount of overlap was such that a threshold between anaplastic and low-grade lesions could not be identified. Although there was also a significant difference in FDG uptake between grades, this was not of the same magnitude as seen for MET. Similarly, in pediatric patients with various primary brain tumors, MET accumulation was higher in high-grade than low-grade tumors, but no clear cut-off distinguished between them (58).

With the exception of juvenile pilocytic astrocytomas, the correlation between FDG uptake and glioma grade has been repeatedly demonstrated. FDG signal thresholds can be defined that distinguish high- and low-grade tumors, but the overlap of signals does not allow complete segregation of the groups. In addition, the various methods of analysis used in different studies make between-study comparisons difficult and thus limit the generalizability of the conclusions. In sum, FDG-PET may be helpful in differentiating high- from low-grade tumors, but it is not a substitute for biopsy. MET-PET has been less extensively studied and its use for tumor grading is less clear.

Prognosis

FDG-PET

Since the earliest studies of FDG metabolism in brain tumors, it has been explored as a marker of prognosis. In a study of 45 patients with high-grade glioma, FDG uptake correlated with survival (72). Patients with high tumor glucose metabolism had a mean survival of 5 months, whereas patients with lower metabolism survived an average of 19 months. Alavi et al. (73) found that median survival of patients with hypometabolic, primary brain tumors was 33 months but only 7 months in hypermetabolic tumors. For the subgroup of patients with high-grade glioma, 1-year survival was 78% for patients with hypo-metabolic tumors and 29% for those with high glucose metabolism. Other studies of FDG-PET in gliomas, and in particular malignant gliomas, support the prognostic value of glucose metabolism (74). In addition, Schifter et al. (75) suggest that serial studies may improve the prognostic usefulness of FDG for primary brain tumors.

Given the correlation between FDG uptake and tumor grade, it is important to control for this variable when assessing the relationship between glucose metabolism and prognosis. In a study of 31 supra-tentorial high- and low-grade gliomas, Pardo et al. (76) reported that FDG uptake was at least as significant as histologic grade for progression-free and overall survival. However, this is based on univariate analysis. Padma et al. (63) suggest that FDG-PET may be better than pathology for predicting prognosis. In a study of 331 patients with benign or malignant gliomas, degree of FDG uptake was associated with survival. Although there was no difference in survival between those with tumors that had low FDG uptake and those that had no FDG uptake, there was a significant difference in survival between those with high uptake and those with low or no uptake. Specifically, patients with low-uptake tumors had a median survival of 28 months compared with only 11 months for high-uptake tumors. In addition, 94% of patients with low-uptake tumors survived greater than 1 year and 19% survived greater than 5 years. One- and 5-year survival for patients with high-uptake tumors was 29% and 0%, respectively. The 23 high-grade glioma patients with low uptake had a median survival of 20 months, and the 11 low-grade glioma patients with high FDG uptake had a median survival of 5 months. Of note, however, the authors also showed that FDG uptake correlated with tumor grade, and no clear attempt was made to distinguish PET signal as an independent variable for prognosis.

Spence et al. (77) evaluated the relationship between glucose metab-olism and prognosis using multivariate analysis in a study of 30 patients with supratentorial high-grade glioma. They found that both tumor histology and pretreatment glucose metabolism independently correlated with survival. In a larger study of 91 patients with malignant astrocytoma, those with tumor FDG uptake greater than that in the contralateral gray matter had worse prognosis than those with uptake less than that in the gray matter (78). When considered separately, glucose metabolism was predictive for glioblastoma but not anaplastic astrocytoma. As the investigators used a three-point visual scale in their evaluation, it is possible that more precise measurements of glucose uptake might have improved the delineation of survival groups. In multivariate analysis, although FDG-PET was useful in predicting the outcome for glioblastoma, histologic grading was superior.

Predicting prognosis and, in particular, clinical behavior is extremely important for low-grade gliomas. Anatomic imaging with CT or MRI does not define the aggressiveness of the lesion or the likelihood of secondary malignant transformation, and therefore does not help in directing whether a lesion can be safely observed or warrants immediate treatment. Several studies have suggested that FDG-PET may be useful for predicting both malignant transformation and prognosis in low-grade gliomas. In a study of 12 low-grade glioma patients with malignant transformation, each tumor had an area of FDG uptake similar to that seen in high-grade gliomas (79). In addition, in three patients who underwent PET scans prior to malignant degeneration, there was an increase in FDG metabolism that coincided with malignant change. Similar results were seen by De Witte et al. (23) in their study of 28 patients with low-grade gliomas. They found that tumors with higher FDG uptake were more likely to progress and result in mortality that those without high uptake. Six of the nine patients with areas of high FDG uptake died and two others had tumor recurrence. In contrast, all 19 patients with low FDG tumor uptake were alive, and only one had evidence of subsequent malignant transformation. Similar applications of FDG-PET do not apply to juvenile pilocytic astrocytomas, which, as previously noted, may have focally high FDG uptake despite excellent prognosis (64,65).

The utility of FDG-PET for tumor prognosis has been studied in other clinical scenarios and tumors. Di Chiro et al. (80) found significantly higher FDG metabolism in meningiomas that progressed or recurred than in those that did not. Barker et al. (21) evaluated FDG uptake in 55 high-grade gliomas at the time of suspected recurrence because of enlarging areas of enhancement on MRI. There was a significant difference in survival between patients with high and those with low FDG uptake (10 versus 20 months). This difference might be even more profound because most patients believed to have recurrence based on PET were offered further therapy, whereas those assessed as radiation injury were more likely to be observed or treated with steroids alone. By contrast, in a study of malignant tumors suspected of recurrence after treatment, Janus et al. (81) found that decreased FDG uptake was associated with longer survival, whereas increased FDG uptake was not predictive. Studies of patients with recurrent metasta-tic brain lesions after stereotactic irradiation have also found a signifi-cant prolongation of survival in those with low FDG uptake compared with those with high FDG uptake (82,83).

Very few reports have been published exploring the utility of FDG-PET to predict prognosis in children with primary brain tumors. Hoffman et al.'s (33) study of 17 children with primary brain tumors demonstrated no clear correlation between FDG uptake and survival. In particular, two patients with brainstem gliomas and low FDG uptake had shorter survival than two patients with higher FDG uptake. By contrast, FDG was an independent predictor of event-free survival in 21 children with newly diagnosed primary brain tumors (58). However, this study evaluated multiple different tumor types, and the small sample size limited the authors to univariate analysis.

In 24 pediatric patients with NF1 and low-grade astrocytomas of the optic pathway, thalamus, or brainstem, FDG uptake correlated with both the need for treatment and clinical outcome (36). Patients were divided into groups based on whether they required tumor therapy at some point and whether their tumors progressed or remained stable. Of patients in the no-treatment group, 93% (13 of 14) had no increase in FDG uptake, consistent with benign tumors, whereas 70% (seven of 10) in the treatment group had increased uptake consistent with more malignant pathology. When considering clinical outcome, 94% (16 of 17) of patients with stable disease had no increase in FDG uptake, but all seven patients with progressive disease had increased uptake. Overall, 96% (23 of 24) of patients had clinical outcomes that correlated with FDG activity.

Amino Acid PET

MET-PET has also been explored for predicting the prognosis of primary brain tumors. In a study of 54 low- and high-grade gliomas, a tumor-to-mean cortical MET uptake threshold of 2.1 divided patients into groups with median survival longer than 5 years (<2.1) or less than 8 months (≥2.1) (24). In comparison with FDG, the authors found MET to be slightly superior for predicting outcome. De Witte et al. (49) evaluated MET-PET in WHO grade II to IV gliomas. A tumor-to-contralateral normal brain uptake ratio greater than 2.2 was associated with poor outcome in grade II tumors. Grade III tumors had a thresh-old of 2.8 that distinguished the outcome. For grade IV tumors, there was no correlation between degree of uptake and survival (all had ele-vated uptake).

In studies of low-grade gliomas (all grade II), MET uptake correlates with clinical outcome. In 12 patients with low-grade gliomas, MET uptake distinguished patients with stable disease from those with tumor progression or death from disease (44). In addition, an SUV threshold of 3.5 differentiated aggressive from stable lesions. In a larger study of 89 patients with grade II glioma, MET uptake was inversely associated with survival for both astrocytomas and oligoden-drogliomas (84).

Only one study has attempted to evaluate MET as a predictor of survival in pediatric patients (58). In 23 children with newly diagnosed brain tumors, increased MET uptake was associated with increased likelihood of tumor progression. Furthermore, patients who died of tumor progression had significantly higher MET uptake than those who survived. As noted above, this was a mixed tumor population, and multivariate analysis was not performed.

Although some studies show a correlation between FDG uptake in brain tumors and prognosis, it is unclear as of yet whether glucose metabolism is independent of tumor grade as a risk factor. However, although FDG-PET may not offer added value for prognosis when comparing different tumor types or grades, it does appear useful for predicting prognosis in tumors with homogeneous histology and grade. Studies of MET-PET are too few to draw conclusions about its utility for assessing prognosis at this time.

Guidance for Biopsy

Brain tumors, particularly gliomas, are typically heterogeneous. There is often a variation in histologic grade within the tumor. For example, in 1000 samples from 50 supratentorial gliomas, 62% of tumors contained both high- and low-grade regions (85). Tumor behavior, response to therapy, and survival are determined by the most malignant portion of a tumor. Because of the inherent risk of sampling error, stereotactic biopsy may miss the tumor altogether or miss the most malignant portion, resulting in understaging of the tumor. This has obvious implications for selection of appropriate therapy and for subsequent survival of the patient. Efforts have been made to maximize diagnostic yield by performing multiple trajectories and using CT or MRI guidance. Usually, biopsy is directed toward contrast-enhancing areas. However, biopsies in malignant gliomas have revealed tumor cells as far as 3 cm from the area of enhancement (86). In addition, the most contrast-enhancing portion of the tumor does not always represent the most malignant area. Because MRI guidance has not been shown to reliably direct biopsy, many investigators have explored PET-directed stereotactic biopsies.

FDG-PET

Given the usefulness of FDG for detecting tumor and the correlation of FDG uptake with histologic grade, FDG may improve the diagnostic yield of stereotactic biopsy by targeting the areas of highest FDG uptake in an attempt to sample the likely most malignant area. Hanson et al. (87) manually combined anatomic imaging with visual analysis of FDG-PET images to determine the best site for stereotactic biopsy in three patients. In two of the patients, CT- or MR-guided biopsy was insufficient, but targeting to the region of high FDG uptake yielded diagnostic tissue.

Combing visual PET analysis with anatomic imaging is not sufficiently precise to direct stereotactic biopsy. Co-registration of stereotactically obtained CT images with nonstereotactically obtained PET scans can improve precision. However, obtaining both sets of images in stereotactic format by using a relocatable head frame is ideal (88). This is accomplished by fixing the head frame for both PET and CT so that the patient's head is similarly positioned for both. Using this procedure, Pirotte et al. (89) performed 78 biopsy trajectories in 38 patients. All trajectories into areas of increased FDG uptake were diagnostic, whereas six trajectories directed solely by CT were uninformative. A follow-up study from the same group used combined PET/CT to direct 90 stereotactic biopsy trajectories in 43 patients with suspected brain tumors (25). Thirty-six patients had an area of increased FDG uptake that guided at least one trajectory. If the area of FDG abnormality was smaller than the CT lesion, a biopsy was also done from a CT region that was FDG negative, and vice versa. Fifty-five trajectories were based on PET and 35 directed by CT. Only six of the 90 trajectories were nondiagnostic, and all were CT guided. Four of these trajectories were targeted to the contrast-enhancing area on CT. In all these patients, a diagnosis was subsequently made on a PET-guided biopsy. Eleven patients had a PET-guided trajectory in an area that appeared normal on CT; nine yielded tumor tissue. The biopsy in the other two patients yielded normal brain; in both cases the region was felt to be "displaced subcortical gray matter adjacent to the tumor." In patients with contrast-enhancing lesions on CT, there was a statistically significant difference in the diagnostic yield between FDG-PET- and contrast-enhanced CT-guided trajectories. In a subsequent review of PET-guided stereotactic biopsies in over 150 patients, Levivier et al. (90) suggested that PET is more accurate than CT for the selection of biopsy sites that will maximize the likelihood of obtaining tissue representative of the tumor grade. It also may allow a decrease in the number of trajectories needed and thereby a decrease in the risks, without adversely affecting the diagnostic yield.

Stereotactic PET/MRI-directed biopsies have also been performed. Massager et al. (8) performed PET and MRI in stereotactic conditions in 30 patients with a brainstem mass, and PET/MRI-directed biopsies resulted in improvement in targeting precision and in diagnostic yield. Most PET scans were performed with FDG. Early in the study, if there was a discrepancy between the PET scan and the MRI, two trajectories were done. When similar conditions arose later in the study (after the accumulation of data supporting PET-guidance), targeting was guided by PET imaging alone. A total of 37 trajectories were performed. Diagnosis was obtained in all patients and confirmed by the subsequent clinical course. Eighteen patients had a single PET-directed biopsy and the diagnostic yield was 100%. Seven patients had two different target areas due to discordance between PET and MRI; in four of these patients, PET guidance was better than MRI guidance in finding the area of highest tumor grade. Targeting in this way was very safe. There was no biopsy-related mortality and minimal morbidity (two patients had a worsening of their preoperative neurologic deficits, that resolved with time).

Amino Acid PET

MET may be better than FDG for directing stereotactic biopsies. The minimal uptake of MET into normal brain cells results in excellent tumor-to-background contrast, thus maximizing the likelihood of identifying an area of abnormal signal to direct biopsy. The increased sensitivity of MET for detecting low-grade tumors provides an advantage over FDG for guiding biopsy trajectories to regions of tumor as opposed to nonneoplastic tissue. In addition, the relatively fast kinetics and shorter half-life (20 minutes) of MET allows brief scanning times and therefore make it easier to perform multiple stereotactic studies as well as multitracer evaluations in the same day.

Co-registration of MET-PET and MR images helped guide stereotactic biopsy in a patient with a grade II oligodendroglioma (91). Biopsy from a contrast-enhancing area with low MET uptake yielded necrotic tissue, whereas tissue from a nonenhancing, hypermetabolic MET region was tumor. Pirotte et al. (54) compared MET with FDG for guiding stereotactic biopsies in 23 patients with brain tumors. There was an area of elevated MET uptake in all 23 brain tumors. Biopsy was directed by FDG in the 12 tumors with elevated FDG uptake. The other tumors had either no FDG uptake (mostly low-grade astrocytomas or oligodendrogliomas) or uptake that was indistinguishable from the adjacent gray matter and therefore required MET guidance for biopsy. All MET-guided trajectories yielded diagnostic tissue.

In a follow-up study, Pirotte and colleagues (27) performed stereotactic PET with MET and FDG and combined those images with stereotactically obtained CT or MR images in 45 patients with lesions located within or adjacent to the cortical and subcortical gray matter. All studies were performed on the same day. FDG was used to direct stereotactic biopsy if the signal was high enough to distinguish it from the background gray matter; otherwise, MET was used. Thirty-nine patients had tumors, and target selection was directed by FDG in 18 and by MET in the other 21. The six nonneoplastic lesions had no FDG or MET uptake and were biopsied under CT or MRI guidance. All 39 tumors had an area of abnormal MET uptake. All 73 trajectories in MET-positive areas yielded tumor tissue, and all 24 trajectories in areas of no MET uptake yielded nontumorous tissue. Fourteen patients had both FDG- and MET-guided biopsies; tissue from both trajectories yielded the same diagnosis. Overall, MET was superior to FDG in differentiating tumor from surrounding brain and was the only usable tracer for targeting in 21 of 39 tumors.

Pirotte et al. (92) have also used combined PET/MRI in the planning of stereotactic biopsies in nine children with infiltrative, ill-defined brain lesions. FDG was used in four, MET in two, and both tracers in three cases. Biopsy trajectories were directed to regions of high tracer uptake. For lesions located in functional areas of brain, fewer trajectories were needed without compromising the diagnostic yield. All lesions were accurately diagnosed using PET-guided biopsies.

The integration of PET into the planning of stereotactic trajectories clearly improves the diagnostic yield of biopsies compared with guidance based on anatomic imaging alone. MET appears better than FDG for identifying targets, although its shorter half-life limits its use to institutions with their own cyclotron. The use of multitracer PET may further improve the accuracy of stereotactic biopsy. In addition, the improved yield may allow a decrease in the number of trajectories required and consequently decrease the risk involved.

Treatment Response

One promising use for PET is in the evaluation of tumor response to treatment. It can be difficult at times to determine whether a given course of therapy has been effective. Low-grade tumors often do not decrease in size after therapy. However, if the tumor has responded to treatment with death of tumor cells, one would expect its level of glucose metabolism or protein synthesis to decline following therapy. Similarly, declining PET signal 3 months into a planned 12 months of therapy may indicate that the therapy is working and validate that it should be continued.

FDG-PET

Several investigators have explored the use of FDG metabolism in predicting tumor response to treatment. It is expected that tumors that respond to treatment will have a decrease in FDG uptake (Fig. 11.3). Surprisingly, several studies have found the opposite: an increase in glucose metabolism after therapy correlated with longer survival. Maruyama et al. (93) evaluated two patients with primary brain tumors and six patients with metastatic brain tumors treated with stereotactic radiosurgery. FDG-PET scans were performed before and 4 hours after treatment. Eighteen of the 19 treated tumors had a significant increase in FDG uptake (mean 29.7%) after treatment compared with eight non-irradiated tumors. For the 17 metastatic lesions, the increase in FDG uptake correlated with a subsequent decrease in tumor size. The other tumor that had an increase in FDG-PET with treatment did not significantly decrease in size, but its follow-up period was short. Of note, one patient had a second follow-up PET scan performed 2 weeks after treatment; FDG uptake had decreased to below baseline values at that time. Spence et al. (77) found similar results in 14 patients with malignant gliomas imaged with both 1-[^{11}C]glucose and FDG within 2 weeks before and within 2 weeks after external beam radiotherapy (although the exact timing for each patient is not noted). Increase in glucose metabolism after treatment correlated with prolonged survival, whereas a decrease in metabolism correlated with poorer survival. Changes in glucose metabolism with chemotherapy have also been explored (94). Ten patients with recurrent glioblastoma multiforme

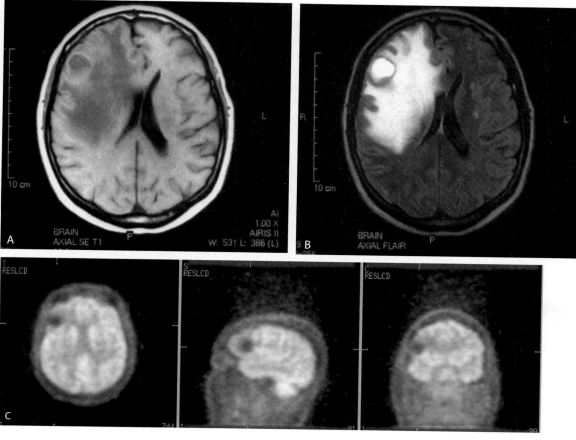

Figure 11.3. Six weeks status post radiation of a primary brain tumor, MR images (A,B) show a focal and diffuse signal abnormality. Lack of FDG uptake on PET (C) suggests that the tumor may no longer be viable. (Courtesy of Dr. P. Bhargava.)

were imaged with FDG-PET before and 24 hours after a first dose of carmustine. An increase in FDG uptake correlated with longer survival. No changes in FDG uptake were seen in normal brain tissue.

Theories to explain this seemingly paradoxical relationship between increase in glucose metabolism and survival have been reviewed by Spence et al. (95). One possibility is that the stress associated with cellular injury leads to an increase in glucose transport and thus an increase in FDG uptake. Studies show that cellular stress causes an increase in glucose transport that is associated with an increase in the amount of glucose transporters on the cell surface (96,97). Several in vitro and small-animal studies show an increase in FDG or deoxyglucose uptake shortly after treatment with chemotherapy or radiation (98–102), and this increase is associated with an increase in glucose transport (101,102). However, if the increase in FDG uptake is due to cellular stress alone, then even patients who do not respond to therapy might be expected to show an initial increase in FDG uptake, and this is not usually seen (77,94).

Another possible explanation for the increase in FDG uptake shortly after therapy is infiltration of the injured tumor with inflammatory cells, which have high glucose metabolism. In vivo studies have shown FDG uptake concentrated in the infiltrating macrophages and fibroblasts following radiation (103,104). In addition, high FDG uptake has been seen in the resection cavity walls following injection of ^{131}I-labeled antitenascin monoclonal antibody into the cavity (105). Subsequent histologic evaluation revealed infiltration of inflammatory cells into this region. Other possible mechanisms include increased energy needs for radiation injury repair (106) or apoptosis (107,108) or "uncrowding," in which the death of tumor cells with treatment allows an increase in glucose metabolism in the surviving cells (95).

Other studies suggest that this increase in glucose metabolism immediately after therapy is transient. Rozental et al. (109) evaluated FDG uptake before, 1 day, and 7 days following stereotactic radiotherapy in two patients with malignant gliomas and two patients with metastases. They found a transient increase in glucose metabolism (25% to 42%) 1 day after therapy that was not present at 7 days. In a phase II study of temozolomide for recurrent malignant glioma, Brock et al. (110) performed FDG-PET before and 14 days after treatment. A decrease in glucose metabolism of greater than 25% was associated with a response at 8 weeks. This association held true for focal regions of initial high FDG uptake but not for whole tumor uptake. Decreases in FDG uptake following treatment were also found in a study of brain tumors treated with radiation and scanned before and 1 week after completion of therapy (111).

Reports in children also show a decrease in glucose metabolism following therapy. In a child with multifocal glioblastoma multiforme, FDG uptake declined following therapy and was associated with the period of clinical improvement (34). Similarly, in seven patients with medulloblastoma/PNET who underwent follow-up FDG-PET scans at least 7 days after treatment, there was a trend toward longer duration of clinical improvement with larger decreases in tumor FDG uptake (32).

In sum, it appears that assessing tumor response by FDG-PET immediately after treatment is difficult and confounded by other variables. It is likely that change in glucose metabolism 2 weeks or so after therapy may be a more reliable indicator of response.

Amino Acid PET

There have been very few reports of the use of amino acid tracers to assess tumor response. Bustany et al. (112) showed that brain tumor MET incorporation decreased following radiotherapy in two patients. Derlon et al. (68) found a decrease in MET uptake after radiotherapy in all three glioblastoma multiforme patients studied, but not in a grade II glioma. Of six gliomas studied with MET before and 2 months following radiotherapy, three had a decrease in MET uptake (113). All three had evidence of clinical improvement, and two had a decrease in tumor size on CT. The other three patients had a rise in MET metabolism and either progression or no change in tumor size on CT. Other reports suggest no association between change in MET uptake and survival in eight patients treated with carmustine (BCNU) (95).

Studies of MET-PET in low-grade gliomas show a dose-dependent decrease in MET uptake in five patients 1 year after treatment with brachytherapy (114). Interestingly, FDG uptake did not change during that time interval. In another study of low-grade astrocytoma, many of the patients had decreasing MET uptake by serial PET scan after radiotherapy (44). As with many of the previous studies, there was no clear attempt to correlate change in PET signal over time with survival. It is interesting that three patients had higher MET uptake 3 months after treatment compared with baseline, but only one had persistent elevation at 6 months. This patient eventually progressed. Ribom et al. (70) evaluated 11 patients with low-grade glioma with MET-PET before radiotherapy and at the time of progression (1.2 to 10.7 years later). They found no significant change in MET uptake from baseline. They suggest that an initial decline in MET uptake might have been found if they had done follow-up imaging closer to the end of treatment.

MET-PET also has promise in the evaluation of response to radiotherapy in CNS lymphoma (115). Ten patients were imaged before and after radiation. The area of high MET signal declined following treatment.

TYR has been used to monitor the response to external beam radiation in 10 patients with supratentorial gliomas (three high-grade and seven low-grade) (116). At 1 to 4 months after treatment, seven patients had a decrease in tumor volume by TYR-PET. Protein synthesis rate was unchanged, however. No outcome data correlating the change in TYR volume with response or survival were available.

At present, no definitive conclusions can be drawn about the utility of PET in assessing brain tumor response to treatment. Studies are limited by the lack of outcome data as well as the wide variability in the timing of follow-up PET scans after therapy. Early imaging with FDG may yield paradoxical results, but this may be a reflection of changes in glucose metabolism in the surrounding tissue. An immediate post-therapy increase in MET signal may be less likely, as MET is not as affected by inflammation. Prospective studies evaluating both tracers should have both early and late assessment time points and should attempt to correlate changes in PET signal with survival.

Recurrence Versus Radiation Necrosis

Radiation necrosis typically refers to the late injury seen months to years after therapy. On anatomic imaging, there is usually hyperintensity on T2-weighted MRI as well as contrast enhancement on both CT and MRI. Lesions are often expansile and exert mass effect on the surrounding tissue. Given that recurrent tumor often has a similar appearance, it is typically difficult to distinguish between the two. Functional imaging with PET improves the differentiation of the two, as radionecrosis typically is hypometabolic in comparison to tumor (Fig. 11.4).

FDG-PET

FDG-PET has been studied extensively for differentiating recurrent tumor from radiation necrosis. Whereas tumor is expected to have high FDG uptake, areas of radionecrosis should have low FDG uptake. One of the earliest reports of FDG-PET in the evaluation of brain tumors was of five patients with clinical and CT findings suggestive of tumor recurrence after radiation (117). The three patients with hypermetabolic lesions were found to have recurrent tumor by biopsy or at autopsy, whereas the two patients with hypometabolic lesions had radiation necrosis. Doyle et al. (118) reported nine patients for whom there was concern about recurrent high-grade glioma. The authors had 100% accuracy in distinguishing between recurrence and radionecrosis. Seven patients had histologic confirmation of results; the other two had hypometabolic lesions and a clinical course consistent with radionecrosis.

In a larger study of 95 patients with glioma or brain metastases, both the sensitivity and specificity of FDG-PET to distinguish radionecrosis from recurrent tumor was 100% (119). Diagnosis was confirmed by histology. Similar results have been found in the evaluation of lesions after gamma knife radiosurgery (100% sensitivity and specificity) (82) and after brachytherapy (81% sensitivity, 88% specificity) (120). Overall, studies have reported a sensitivity that ranges from 81% to 100% and specificity of 40% to 100% (121). Although FDG-PET improves the diagnostic accuracy of distinguishing tumor recurrence from radionecrosis, the sensitivity for detecting recurrence can be increased by co-registering the images with MRI (122).

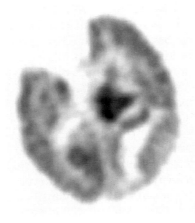

Figure 11.4. FDG-PET study of an 11-year old boy with an astrocytoma status post right frontal lobectomy and radiotherapy. High signal on FDG-PET is consistent with tumor recurrence in the deep left hemispheric white matter. (Courtesy of Dr. N. Bohnen.)

Several studies describe the impact of FDG-PET in the management of patients with suspected tumor recurrence after radiotherapy. In a study of 50 patients with suspected tumor recurrence after therapy, 30 did not undergo surgical confirmation. In the latter group, FDG-PET contributed to the treatment decisions in 80% of patients (81). In another report of 65 patients with glioma evaluated with FDG-PET to distinguish tumor recurrence from radiation necrosis, PET contributed to the management in 90% of cases (123).

One issue in many of the prior studies is selection bias; patients with negative FDG-PET scans are less likely to have a tissue diagnosis. Therefore, false-negative results might be missed. For example, in one study of 84 patients with suspected recurrent gliomas, only 31 had their lesions confirmed by biopsy. Of 11 hypometabolic lesions, only five were radiation necrosis by histology. The other six were recurrent tumor. In addition, four of 20 (20%) patients with hypermetabolic lesions were found to have radiation necrosis at biopsy (124). Reasons for false-negative scans include tumors with low histologic grade (and therefore low inherent FDG uptake), small volume of residual tumor (resulting in poor visualization after volume averaging with surrounding tissue), and tumor located within or adjacent to normal brain with similar glucose metabolism. False-positive scans can occur with inflammatory lesions and are often present acutely after radiation injury (see discussion in Treatment Response, above). In addition, some biopsy specimens from hypometabolic lesions assessed as true negatives have had viable tumor cells believed to be incapable of proliferation (95,119,120).

Amino Acid PET

Few studies have evaluated the use of MET-PET to differentiate recurrent tumor from radiation necrosis. Ogawa et al. (125) imaged 15 patients with both FDG and MET. All patients with radiation necrosis had lesions that were hypometabolic with FDG-PET. However, one patient had a lesion with low FDG uptake that was recurrent tumor. MET uptake was elevated in this lesion. The authors conclude that the combination of FDG and MET-PET improved the diagnostic accuracy. Sonoda et al. (126) used MET-PET to evaluate five patients with recurrent glioma and seven patients with radiation necrosis. MET uptake was elevated in all patients with tumor recurrence but in only one with radiation necrosis. Overall, the diagnostic accuracy of MET-PET was 92%. Co-registration of MET-PET with MRI can improve the differentiation of radionecrosis from recurrent tumor (91). In a patient with suspected recurrence 4 years after radiation, MET uptake within the region of contrast enhancement was low. However, there was another area of higher MET uptake that was not contrast enhancing. Stereotactic biopsies revealed that the contrast-enhancing area with low MET uptake was necrosis, whereas the nonenhancing region with high MET uptake was recurrent tumor.

Tsuyuguchi and colleagues have used MET-PET to differentiate tumor from radiation injury after stereotactic radiosurgery for brain metastases (127) and high-grade glioma (128). In 21 patients treated for brain metastases, only 11 underwent a surgical procedure to confirm the diagnosis; nine had recurrent tumor and two had radiation necrosis. The lesions in the other 10 patients were defined as radiation necrosis based on clinical follow-up. By visual analysis, two cases in each group would have been falsely classified. Semiquantitative analysis improved the diagnostic accuracy. Mean tumor-to-normal brain MET uptake was higher in the recurrent tumor group (1.62) than the radiation necrosis group (1.15). With a cutoff of 1.42, the sensitivity for detecting recurrent tumor was 77.8% and the specificity was 100% (127). Similar evaluation in 11 patients treated for high-grade glioma revealed a mean tumor-to-normal brain ratio of 1.87 for the relapsed tumors and 1.31 in the necrosis group. Sensitivity, specificity, and diagnostic accuracy were 100%, 60%, and 82%, respectively (128).

There are no studies of PET in children that specifically address its clinical utility in the evaluation of tumor recurrence versus radionecrosis. One case series, however, did include several children with lesions of concern on MRI scan noted sometime after the completion of radiotherapy in which FDG and MET-PET were used in the subsequent management of the patient (31).

Numerous studies demonstrate the value of FDG-PET for differentiating tumor recurrence from radiation injury. Although false negatives and false positives are clearly reported, in general there is excellent sensitivity and specificity. Furthermore, early studies with MET-PET appear promising. In sum, PET is an important modality in the evaluation of patients with suspicious MRI lesions after radiotherapy.

Treatment Planning

Positron emission tomography is helpful to define tumor margins and to identify concerning (perhaps more malignant) tumor regions. Standard external beam radiotherapy and even hyperfractionation to higher doses does not prevent all recurrences within the radiation field. PET may be useful during radiation treatment planning to define the optimal target volume and to direct higher doses to the region of tumor with the highest tracer uptake.

Nuutinen et al. (44) evaluated the feasibility of MET to define radiotherapy treatment volume in 11 patients with astrocytoma. In eight patients, the planning target volume (PTV) was larger and in one patient smaller based on CT or MRI alone. On average, the PTV was 19% smaller when planned with MET-PET assistance. In particular, MET-PET improved treatment planning for three patients whose tumor margins on MRI were inconclusive. For two patients with MET-negative tumors, MET-PET was of no use in treatment planning. In another patient, there was obvious tumor infiltration by MRI that would have been missed with MET-PET, and therefore part of the tumor would have been underdosed.

Several groups have explored PET for defining an area for radiation dose escalation. Tralins et al. (129) used FDG-PET to delineate a target boost area in 38 patients with glioblastoma multiforme. Initial PTV was determined by the T2-weighted MR signal abnormality plus a standard margin, and the initial treatment dose was 59.4 Gy. Positron emission tomography was performed when the patient was at a dose of 45 to 50.4 Gy, and the area of abnormal FDG uptake plus a 0.5-cm margin was boosted with an additional 20 Gy. Patients without abnormal FDG uptake received the standard 59.4 Gy. Twenty-seven patients were evaluable (eight had not reached their first follow-up exam and three were excluded for other reasons) and had a median actuarial time to progression of 43 weeks and survival of 70 weeks. Comparison was made between the FDG-based and theoretical gadolinium enhancement-based target boost volumes. Mean target volume based on FDG was significantly smaller than gadolinium enhancement-based volume. In addition, FDG uptake occasionally extended beyond the region of enhancement. Of note, 83% (10 of 12) of the patients who underwent an FDG-PET–based radiation boost and subsequently recurred had their first site of progression within the area of initial abnormal FDG uptake.

Solberg et al. (130) studied the feasibility of using FDG for treatment boosting in intensity modulated radiotherapy (IMRT). Treatment planning for a patient with a recurrent brain metastasis was performed using an integrated PET-CT scanner. A standard treatment plan was devised, and then an additional 20% was prescribed to the region of high FDG uptake. Evaluation of the dose distributions and dose-volume histograms show excellent coverage of the boost volume despite its irregular shape.

Levivier et al. (90) reviewed their experience using combined PET and MRI guidance in treating 34 brain tumors with gamma knife radiosurgery. The PET tracer selected depended on the tumor type. FDG was used mostly for metastases and primary malignant brain tumors, whereas MET was used primarily for benign brain tumors. The volume of increased PET signal was co-registered with the MR image. Final treatment volume was defined by MRI but modified with information from the PET scan. When the area of PET uptake extended beyond the MR margins of the tumor, it was included in the final volume (unless it was in an "unsafe" region of the brain). If the area of PET uptake was smaller and within the MR volume, then the highest spot of the delivered dose was directed to that area. Positron emission tomography contributed to the treatment plan in 31 cases (91%) and dictated an adjustment to the target volume in 25 cases (74%). No outcome data were available.

Positron emission tomography may also be useful for surgical planning. Miwa et al. (131) co-registered MR and MET-PET images in 10 patients with newly diagnosed glioblastoma multiforme. In all patients, the gadolinium-enhanced area was smaller than the area of increased MET uptake. On average, only 58.6% of the MET area was within the enhancing area, whereas 99.8% was within 3 cm outside of the enhancing region. In addition, during follow-up after treatment, a new enhancing area developed in three patients in a region that was initially unenhancing but MET positive. This implies that there were tumor cells beyond the region of gadolinium enhancement. In all cases, the MET area was smaller than the T2 hyperintense area, but it extended partially beyond the T2 hyperintense area in nine patients. Hence, the T2 hyperintense area likely contains tumor cells, and tumor may even extend beyond this area. The authors concluded that surgical resection of the gadolinium-enhancing area is insufficient and that MET uptake should be considered in surgical and radiotherapy planning.

Levivier and colleagues (90) have used PET (FDG or MET) to help direct tumor resection in 43 patients. PET and MRI were obtained stereotactically, imported and correlated with the neuronavigation software, and displayed in the eyepiece of the microscope during the surgery. The goal was to remove the entire area of abnormal tracer uptake. All tumors were maximally resected with no complications related to the technique. Because PET helps to delineate the extent of a tumor, this neurosurgical planning technique may improve the prognosis of these patients.

One of the major limitations to achieving a complete tumor resection is tumor location adjacent to eloquent areas of brain. Traditional techniques to delineate these important brain areas are not ideal (29). Wada testing for language localization is invasive, may cause complications, and may be unreliable in sedated children. Intraoperative electrical stimulation or cortical somatosensory evoked potentials require cooperation, may be unreliable, and cannot reach the medial part of the hemispheres. In addition, a craniotomy is required for placement of depth electrodes. Positron emission tomography with radiolabeled water ($[^{15}O]H_2O$) measures tissue perfusion, which is presumably increased in regions of brain that are activated. Functional imaging with $[^{15}O]H_2O$ may help to noninvasively localize important regions of cortex and improve the surgical planning to avoid these regions.

Duncan et al. (29) measured the activation of cortical regions with $[^{15}O]H_2O$ PET during motor, visual, articulation, and receptive language tasks in 15 children (aged 2 to 16 years) with seizures (7 had tumors). Thirteen patients also underwent FDG or MET-PET to help localize the seizure focus. Magnetic resonance and PET images were co-registered and directed the surgical approach. This approach helped to establish the location of eloquent cortical regions in relation to the seizure focus, determined the optimal surgical approach, and facilitated maximal resection while minimizing surgical morbidity. In addition, it helped to define the optimal timing for surgery, by providing a means to recognize when cortical reorganization is complete. (Often after cortical damage in young children, important brain functions will "relocate" to adjacent areas of cortex or even the contralateral hemisphere.)

The same group published a follow-up study using similar methods in five children (aged 3 to 13 years) with tumors adjacent to eloquent brain regions (28). In four of the patients, functional mapping altered the surgical approach to allow avoidance of speech/language or motor areas. Despite tumor location near functionally sensitive brain regions, aggressive resection was achieved without significant neurologic sequelae.

The use of PET for planning the treatment of brain tumors is one of the most exciting applications of this imaging modality. FDG and/or MET-PET can be used to help define the optimal target volume for radiotherapy as well as to identify regions for dose escalation. In addition, these tracers may improve tumor resection by helping to define tumor extent. Unfortunately, information on whether these approaches will impact patient outcome is presently lacking. Functional imaging with $[^{15}O]H_2O$ is a noninvasive method to localize eloquent regions of cortex. Preliminary studies show that multitracer PET with $[^{15}O]H_2O$ and FDG or MET assists in defining the optimal surgical approach to facilitate maximal tumor resection with minimal morbidity.

Other Agents

Although FDG and MET are the most widely used tracers, numerous other agents have been explored for PET imaging of brain tumors. These include tracers that evaluate other biologic processes including DNA synthesis, membrane biosynthesis, and hypoxia.

Amino Acid Agents with Longer Half-Life

One of the limitations of ^{11}C-labeled amino acids such as MET and TYR is that their short half-life (20 minutes) limits their use to institutions with in-house cyclotrons. Labeling tracers with ^{18}F (half-life 110 minutes) enables availability to more centers. Several forms of ^{18}F-labeled tyrosine have been synthesized, including L-2-[^{18}F]fluorotyrosine (FTyr), L-3-[^{18}F]fluoro-α-methyltyrosine (FMT), and 2-[^{18}F]fluoroethyl-L-tyrosine (FET). Preclinical studies show similar transport characteristics and tumor detection with FTyr and FET compared with MET (132). A study of FTyr in 15 brain tumors showed good tumor delineation and uptake that was associated with tumor grade (133). FMT is also useful for tumor detection, with uptake ratios that were significantly higher than with FDG (134).

   More recent studies have focused on FET. Preclinical studies report that, unlike FDG uptake, FET uptake is low in inflammatory and non-neoplastic cells (135,136). This may improve tumor delineation, particularly after surgery and radiotherapy when distinguishing between inflammatory changes and residual tumor can be difficult.

   The first clinical study of FET imaged 11 patients with gliomas (all but one malignant) and five patients with intracranial metastases from non-CNS primaries with both FET and MET (137). Fifteen of the patients had received prior surgery and/or radiotherapy, and nine were being evaluated for tumor recurrence/residual versus radiation injury or postoperative changes. Based on MET imaging, 13 of the lesions were assessed as tumors and the other three were considered to be posttreatment changes. All 13 tumors had increased FET uptake, whereas the three lesions that represented posttreatment changes had FET uptake that was significantly lower. There was close correlation between FET and MET in signal intensity and tumor extension. MET uptake was slightly higher than FET uptake in tumor, white matter, and gray matter, but the tumor-to-normal brain structure ratios were not significantly different.

Pauleit et al. (138) imaged 20 suspected primary or recurrent brain tumors with FET-PET before surgery; FET identified 14 of 16 tumors (all gliomas) for a sensitivity of 88%. Two other patients had increased FET uptake, including a patient with astrogliosis and one with a cavernoma (which was not confirmed by biopsy). Compared with 3-[^{123}I]iodo-α-methyl-L-tyrosine (IMT), an alternative tyrosine analogue used for single photon emission computed tomography (SPECT) imaging, FET was more sensitive and allowed for better differentiation of tumor from normal brain.

In addition, FET-PET has been evaluated for the grading of tumors. Weckesser et al. (139) imaged 44 suspected primary brain tumors at four 10-minute intervals following FET injection. Eleven of the lesions were in children. A diagnosis was subsequently available in 35 patients. The FET uptake was greater than normal cortex in 35 of the 44 lesions, including all 22 gliomas, three lymphomas, four other primary brain tumors, three nonneoplastic lesions, and three unbiopsied lesions. The lesions without FET uptake included one DNET, one mature teratoma, one inflammatory lesion, and six unbiopsied lesions. There was a significant difference in the ratio of FET uptake in tumor-to-contralateral normal brain between low-grade (2.0) and high-grade lesions (3.2) when imaged at 10 minutes but not 40 minutes after injection. This difference was significant between low-grade (2.0) and high-grade gliomas (3.1) as well. Of note, the uptake kinetics of FET appeared different in low-grade and high-grade lesions; FET uptake increased in low-grade and decreased in high-grade lesions from the 10- to 40-minute postinjection scan. This implies that early imaging may provide the best contrast for grading.

Messing-Junger et al. (140) co-registered FET-PET and MR images and incorporated them into a neuronavigation system to direct stereotactic biopsies in two children with bithalamic gliomas. Stereotactic biopsy, initially planned with MRI and MR spectroscopy, was redirected based on FET-PET in both cases. In one patient, the biopsy target was changed from the right thalamus to a region of FET uptake in the left thalamus. In the other patient, biopsy was redirected from a thalamic target with tumor-to-cortex FET uptake ratio of 1.7 to a hot spot (ratio of 3.8) in the left cerebellopontine angle. Whether the change in targets resulted in a change in diagnosis is unknown. In a follow-up report, the same investigators used FET to direct biopsies in 50 patients with suspected gliomas (86). Biopsies were taken from an area of increased FET uptake in FET-positive lesions. Biopsies yielded 34 gliomas and 16 nonneoplastic lesions. Of the four gliomas that did not have elevated FET, only one was high grade. Only two nonneoplastic lesions had elevated FET uptake. The sensitivity and specificity of FET for detecting tumor were both 88%. Mean tumor-to-normal brain FET uptake ratios were significantly higher for tumors (2.4) than nonneoplastic lesions (1.2). There was a trend toward higher FET uptake with increasing tumor grade, but there was substantial overlap.

Both FET and FMT are nonnatural amino acids that are not found in biologic systems. Radiolabeled, naturally occurring amino acids (like MET) are susceptible to degradation, giving rise to radiolabeled metabolites, which makes kinetic analysis of uptake complex. Many nonnatural amino acids are not metabolized and therefore may be advantageous for use in imaging brain tumors. Another radiolabeled nonnatural amino acid is 1-aminocyclobutane-1-[^{11}C]carboxylic acid (ACBC). In a comparative study with FDG, ACBC-PET identified all 19 recurrent gliomas, whereas FDG detected only 13 of 19 (141); ACBC uptake into normal brain was very low. Tumor-to-normal gray matter ACBC uptake was almost 10 times higher than FDG ratios. The better contrast between tumor and normal brain improves the ability to detect low-grade lesions. However, the investigators were unable to distinguish low-grade from high-grade lesions, and uptake did not correlate with grade or survival.

3,4-dihydroxy-6-[^{18}F]fluoro-L-phenylalanine (FDOPA) has also been explored for imaging brain tumors. It is chemically similar to L-phenylalanine, which shares amino acid transport systems with L-methionine. Prior studies have shown that MET uptake into brain is reduced by 50%, on average, after loading with L-phenylalanine (142). Becherer et al. (143) studied the feasibility of using FDOPA for imaging brain tumors. They performed FDOPA-PET in 20 patients with suspected brain lesions and MET-PET (on a separate occasion) in 19. All 19 of the brain tumors (seven low-grade gliomas, 11 high-grade gliomas, one metastatic tumor) had elevated uptake of FDOPA. For the 18 tumors in which MET was also performed, tumor-to-contralateral uptake ratios were similar and correlated between the tracers. There was one false-positive lesion (a focal demyelinating lesion) with both tracers. Five patients were imaged both 20 and 70 minutes after FDOPA injection. There was an increase in uptake of FDOPA into the basal ganglia from 20 to 70 minutes, resulting in less obvious tumor signal at that time. The authors concluded that FDOPA may be an alternative to MET for brain tumor imaging.

DNA Synthesis Agents

Tracers that measure DNA synthesis by definition should be markers of cellular proliferation and, thus, likely to be taken up into dividing tumor cells. Because normal brain cells are not dividing, excellent contrast between tumor and background normal brain should be expected. As it is the only nucleotide that is in DNA but not RNA, thymidine analogs have been the most widely studied. 2-[^{11}C]thymidine (TdR) and FDG were used to image 20 supratentorial brain tumors (144); TdR did better than FDG in detecting tumor. Increased tumor-to-cortex TdR uptake was found in 11 of 14 (79%) previously untreated tumors and in five of six (83%) recurrent tumors. TdR uptake was not correlated with tumor grade. De Reuck et al. (145) used methyl-[^{11}C]thymidine to evaluate 20 patients with brain lesions on CT or MRI. Methyl-[^{11}C]thymidine uptake was increased in eight of 10 tumors. There was no increased uptake in the 10 nontumoral lesions. Eary et al. (146) compared TdR and FDG-PET in 13 patients with primary or recurrent malignant brain tumors. Using qualitative visual analysis, uptake of TdR and FDG was similar in seven cases. In two patients, tumor recurrence was more obvious with TdR than with FDG-PET. Two tumors with high FDG but low TdR uptake had slower progression than three tumors with elevation of both tracers. Another study of 20 patients with brain tumors showed that TdR uptake increased with tumor grade (147). Although evaluation of TdR for treatment response has not been published for brain tumors, preliminary studies in non-CNS tumors suggest that it may be promising (148).

One problem with the use of TdR is its rapid metabolism yielding the labeled metabolite [^{11}C]CO$_2$. Imaging with both TdR and [^{11}C]CO$_2$ facilitates an assessment of the confounding influence of this metabolite on the interpretation of TdR imaging. Analysis that incorporates kinetic modeling using [^{11}C]CO$_2$ may further enhance the ability of TdR to delineate tumor (146,147,149). Alternatively, labeling thymidine in such a way as to limit its degradation and prolong the half-life of the label may improve its utility in evaluating brain tumors. ^{18}F-labeled tracers have a half-life of 110 minutes, whereas the half-life of ^{11}C is only 20 minutes. [^{18}F]3'-deoxy-3'-fluorothymidine (FLT) has been studied and compared with FDG in 26 patients (eight children) with brain lesions (18 were tumors).[22] Its uptake was elevated (greater than background) in all 12 patients with high-grade tumors, but FDG uptake was increased (greater than or equal to normal gray matter) in only six. Of note, however, visual grading systems were not identical. Uptake into low-grade tumors was variable for both tracers. The sensitivity of FLT for diagnosing brain tumors was 83% (15 of 18), and the specificity was 62%. All three false-negative FLT scans were low-grade astrocytomas. Using tumor-to-normal brain SUV ratios, there was a significant difference in FLT uptake between high- and low-grade tumors but not between low-grade tumors and nontumorous lesions. There was a significant correlation between FLT uptake and the degree of cellular proliferation, as measured by Ki-67 staining, in nine patients with glioma. Overall, FLT appears promising for delineating as well as grading brain tumors.

Labeling with iodine 124 (^{124}I) extends the tracer half-life even further (4.2 days) and has been used to label deoxyuridine. The long half-life allows for a "wash-out" period. Because radioactivity is retained in the tumor but over 70% of radiolabeled metabolites are excreted in the urine at 24 hours, "late" imaging improves the contrast between tumor and background (150,151). [^{124}I]Iododeoxyuridine (IUdR) has been used to image 20 patients with gliomas or meningiomas (151). All tumors had persistent labeling at 24 hours. Tumor-to-normal brain uptake ratio correlated with increasing glioma grade [grade II (2.4), grade III (3.1), grade IV (4.5)]. Uptake in meningioma was similar to low-grade glioma. The authors (151) hypothesized that image contrast would be improved even further by delaying imaging beyond 24 hours after tracer injection.

Membrane Biosynthesis Agents

In addition to increasing DNA and protein synthesis, tumors must synthesize membrane phospholipids in order to expand. Tracers explored for imaging of membrane biosynthesis include 1-[^{11}C]acetate, [^{11}C]choline, and [^{18}F]fluorocholine. Reports of 1-[^{11}C]acetate show its potential for imaging gliomas and meningiomas, with an accuracy exceeding 90%. Uptake into normal gray matter is low (95,152).

Using MR spectroscopy, choline has been shown to be elevated in malignant brain tumors. In addition, its uptake into normal cortex is low, which allows excellent contrast for tumor detection (153). [^{11}C]choline uptake into brain tumors has been reported to be elevated (154,155). Uptake into both rat glioma cells and human tumors is higher than uptake into normal brain (155). In 22 patients with suspected brain tumors, Ohtani et al. (26) found increased uptake of [^{11}C]choline in all nine high-grade gliomas and the one pilocytic astrocytoma studied. Uptake into nonpilocytic low-grade gliomas was low. There was a significant difference in tumor-to-white matter uptake ratio between high-grade and low-grade gliomas (excluding the pilocytic astrocytoma). Several other tumors had elevated [^{11}C]choline signal, including meningioma, schwannoma, craniopharyngioma, and lymphoma. [^{11}C]choline uptake into nonneoplastic lesions was low and not significantly different from low-grade gliomas. In contrast, Utriainen et al. (156) found no difference in [^{11}C]choline uptake between high-grade and low-grade gliomas.

Two ^{18}F-labeled choline tracers have been synthesized: [^{18}F]fluoromethylcholine (FCH) and [^{18}F]fluoroethylcholine (FEC). In a comparison of the two, FEC uptake into prostate cancer cells in vitro was 20% that of FCH uptake (153). In addition, the phosphorylation of FEC by choline kinase is approximately 30% lower than FCH. Case reports of FCH-PET for brain tumors reveal marked uptake in an anaplastic astrocytoma and a glioblastoma multiforme, but poor uptake in a demyelinating lesion (153,157). Good signal was achieved when imaging 5 minutes after injection, with tumor-to-normal brain uptake ratios close to 10 (153). FEC-PET was used in 12 patients with untreated gliomas and compared favorably with [^{11}C]choline (158). There was no difference in tumor signal when imaging was performed at 5 versus 20 minutes after tracer injection; however, uptake of FEC decreased in normal brain over that time, resulting in better contrast between tumor and normal brain at 20 minutes. Histology was confirmed by stereotactic biopsy targeted to the region of highest PET signal. FEC uptake (tumor-to-normal gray matter ratio) correlated with increasing tumor grade, albeit in a small sample size: grade II (0 to 4.8), grade III (12, only one case), grade IV (13.2 to 21.1). Compared with other tracers, tumor-to-normal brain ratios for glioblastoma multiforme are much higher using FEC than FDG (24,61), MET (24,49,68), or FET (137,139).

Hypoxia Agents

Most glioblastomas have regions of tumor necrosis that are hypoxic. Tissue hypoxia reduces the effectiveness of radiotherapy and potentially chemotherapy. Newer treatment strategies specifically target hypoxic tumor regions either by modifying oxygen delivery or by inducing the expression of cytotoxic compounds under hypoxic conditions. There are no structural imaging methods to evaluate tumor hypoxia. Several investigators, therefore, have explored PET tracers that bind to molecules in hypoxic cells, such as [^{18}F]fluoromisonidazole (FMISO), in order to image these tumor regions. The degree of FMISO uptake into cells is increased under hypoxic conditions (159,160). In a rat intracerebral glioma model, FMISO uptake into malignant glioma exceeded that of normal brain (161). Valk et al. (162) found FMISO uptake in three patients with malignant glioma with signals that were greater than normal cortex. Other reports of the clinical use of FMISO for imaging brain tumors have been reviewed by Spence et al. (163).

Future Studies

PET for Receptor Imaging

Ligands for receptors may be radiolabeled and used for PET imaging of brain tumors. Receptor imaging has been used before in the evaluation of pituitary adenomas. For example, [^{11}C]-L-deprenyl demonstrates specific binding to monoamine oxidase B and demonstrates high uptake in pituitary adenomas (164). Pituitary adenomas can also be imaged with [^{18}F]fluoro-ethyl-spiperone, which binds to dopamine receptors (165). Brain tumors have been imaged using tracers that bind to benzodiazepine receptors, which are elevated in some brain tumors (3). Positron emission tomography with [^{11}C]PK 1195, a benzodiazepine receptor ligand, demonstrates increased signal in gliomas relative to normal gray matter (166,167).

Using ligands directed toward receptors that are specifically increased in certain tumor types may improve the accuracy of PET imaging. The epidermal growth factor receptor (EGFR) is frequently mutated and overexpressed in malignant gliomas and has been implicated in their prognosis. 4-(3-Bromoanilino)-6,7-dimethoxyquinazoline (PD153035) is a selective EGFR tyrosine kinase inhibitor. It has been labeled with ^{11}C and evaluated using PET in vivo in rats (168). Tracer was rapidly cleared from the blood with subsequent uptake in several body organs including brain. High uptake was evident in SH-SY5Y cells (a neuroblastoma cell line that expresses EGFR) implanted subcutaneously into rats. The level of uptake was approximately 15 times that of the surrounding normal tissue. Using PET with similar tracers in patients with malignant gliomas may be useful for documenting tumor receptor expression, selecting which patients should get therapy with drugs targeting the EGFR, and monitoring the response to such therapy.

PET Imaging of Angiogenesis

Angiogenesis is the formation of new blood vessels from preexisting ones. Brain tumors, particularly gliomas, are dependent on angiogenesis for growth beyond a small size. Microvessel density has been shown to be associated with both glioma grade and prognosis. Multiple angiogenic factors have been identified, and numerous antiangiogenic drugs have been evaluated in preclinical and clinical trials (169). Positron emission tomography is being explored as a noninvasive way to image angiogenesis.

The integrin $\alpha_v\beta_3$ is a receptor expressed on activated endothelial cells and plays an important role in cell adhesion, cell migration, and angiogenesis. Because expression is low on quiescent endothelial cells, imaging of $\alpha_v\beta_3$ would be specific for angiogenic vessels. The tripeptide sequence arginine-glycine-aspartic acid (RGD) is recognized by $\alpha_v\beta_3$ integrins. Labeling of a glycosylated form of an RGD-containing peptide with ^{18}F ([^{18}F]galacto-RGD) has been explored. Imaging of mice with micro-PET allowed detection of $\alpha_v\beta_3$-positive tumors with high tumor-to-normal tissue uptake (170). A follow-up study revealed a correlation between [^{18}F]galacto-RGD uptake by PET and $\alpha_v\beta_3$ expression by subsequent Western blot analysis in subcutaneous murine models (171). Imaging of nine patients with non-CNS tumors showed tracer uptake in the majority of patients. Immunohistochemical analysis of tumor tissue after surgery showed expression of $\alpha_v\beta_3$ on tumor vessels and association of tracer uptake with the density of $\alpha_v\beta_3$-positive vessels.

An alternative tracer, N-4-[^{18}F]fluorobenzoyl-RGD ([^{18}F]FB-RGD), was taken up specifically into subcutaneous and orthotopic mouse glioma models with high tumor uptake and almost no uptake into normal brain (172). Unfortunately, tracer washout from tumor was rapid, and there was significant accumulation in the gallbladder and intestines because of hepatobiliary excretion. The same investigators introduced a polyethylene glycol formulation of the tracer ([^{18}F]FB-PEG-RGD) (173). This tracer had rapid clearance from blood with predominately renal excretion. In both subcutaneous and orthotopic mouse models, uptake into gliomas was high with very low background activity, which resulted in good contrast. There was a correlation between PET uptake and autoradiography, demonstrating that [^{18}F]FB-PEG-RGD localizes to integrin-positive tumor.

Because disease stabilization rather than tumor regression is expected from antiangiogenic agents, traditional response monitoring by anatomic imaging is insufficient. Positron emission tomography may provide an alternative for assessing response in clinical trials of these agents. $\alpha_v\beta_3$ integrin is just one of many angiogenic targets that can be selected for monitoring with PET.

PET Imaging for Assessment of Gene Therapy Protocols

Noninvasive assessment of gene expression would be useful for the evaluation of gene therapy strategies. Tjuvajev and colleagues (174) have explored the possibility of PET imaging for assessing the expression of herpes simplex virus-1 thymidine kinase (HSV1-TK) after retroviral transduction of RG2 glioma cells. Initial experiments showed 5-iodo-2′-fluoro-2′deoxy-1-beta-D-arabinofuranosyluracil (FIAU) to be a satisfactory marker substrate for measuring HSV1-TK expression (174); FIAU accumulation in transduced RG2 clones was associated with the level of HSV1-TK messenger RNA (mRNA) expression and the sensitivity of the clone to ganciclovir. Autoradiography showed that FIAU uptake was high in the TK-positive brain tumors but low in nontransduced RG2 tumors in rats. Single photon emission computed tomography showed high uptake of [^{131}I]FIAU into subcutaneous RG2 tumors and W256 mammary carcinomas that were transfected with HSV1-TK but not in nontransduced tumors (175). Tumors were produced by injecting HSV1-TK transduced and nontransduced clones into the flanks of rats. Uptake of FIAU was localized to areas of high HSV-TK protein expression using autoradiography. Once again, the degree of FIAU accumulation corresponded to the in vitro ganciclovir sensitivity of the clone used for transfection. A follow-up study using PET and [^{124}I]FIAU showed high uptake of [^{124}I]FIAU into subcutaneous RG2 and W256 tumors that had been transduced in vitro with HSV1-TK, and uptake was correlated with HSV1-TK expression (176). In addition, high [^{124}I]FIAU uptake was also seen in W256 tumors that had been transduced in vivo with HSV1-TK by direct intratumoral injection of vector into already established subcutaneous tumors. In sum, gene expression can be imaged noninvasively with PET and thus may be useful to monitor gene therapy trials in humans with brain tumors.

PET Imaging of Apoptosis

Early in apoptosis, phosphatidylserine can be found on the outer cell membrane. Annexin V binds to phosphatidylserine on the surface of apoptotic cells. Labeling of annexin V with ^{18}F may allow imaging of apoptosis. After induction of myocardial ischemia in rats, [^{18}F]annexin V accumulated in the infarcted area, where the apoptotic cells are (177). Treating rats with cycloheximide results in apoptosis in the liver. [^{18}F]Annexin V uptake in the liver of rats pretreated with cycloheximide was three to nine times that of controls (178). Subsequent analysis of the liver with terminal deoxynucleotide end-labeling (TUNEL) assays showed significant apoptosis; this correlated with [^{18}F]annexin V uptake. Toretsky et al. (179) showed an 88% increase in [^{18}F]annexin V binding to cancer cells treated with etoposide compared to untreated cells. It is anticipated that [^{18}F]annexin V or other markers of apoptosis may be used in the early assessment of response of cancer patients to therapy.

PET for Evaluation of Drug Kinetics

The pharmacokinetics of cancer drugs may be evaluated in vivo by radiolabeling the drug and imaging it with PET. By labeling temozolomide with ^{11}C, Saleem et al. (180) were able to evaluate its plasma and tissue pharmacokinetics in vivo in six patients with glioma.

[^{11}C]temozolomide was identified in the plasma and [^{11}C]CO$_2$ was the only radiolabeled metabolite identified. Because the duration of the PET scan (90 minutes) was less than the half-life of temozolomide, the pharmacokinetic parameters that could be calculated were based on the distribution and initial elimination of the drug. Both drug clearance and exposure (area under the curve, AUC) between 0 and 90 minutes were calculated. Although there was drug uptake into both tumor and normal brain tissue, the total tumor exposure was higher compared with normal gray and white matter. In addition, by labeling the drug at two different loci, the investigators were able to explore in vivo the mechanism by which temozolomide undergoes ring opening to form monomethyl triazenoimidazole carboxamide (MTIC) and subsequently the alkylating agent methyldiazonium ion.

Conclusion

Functional imaging with PET complements anatomic imaging in the evaluation of brain tumors. FDG has been shown to play a role in tumor detection, grading, and prognosis, and in the evaluation of malignant transformation. It is also useful for directing stereotactic biopsies and in differentiating tumor recurrence from radiation necrosis. MET is valuable for tumor localization and detection, particularly of low-grade tumors. It provides an advantage over FDG for directing stereotactic biopsy, and early studies are encouraging for detecting tumor recurrence. Co-registration of FDG- or MET-PET images with MRI is clearly advantageous for brain tumor evaluation. Combined PET studies using more than one tracer improve the accuracy of stereotactic biopsy (FDG and MET) and are valuable in planning tumor resections so as to minimize morbidity (FDG or MET with [^{15}O]H$_2$O). Although studies targeting brain tumors in children are sparse, the available evidence suggests a similar utility of PET in this age group. Other tracers are promising (e.g., FET, TdR, FEC), but their routine clinical use for brain tumors requires further examination. As our understanding of the molecular processes of cells improves, more specific tracers are being designed, and newer, more directed uses for PET scanning will be developed.

References

1. Di Chiro G, DeLaPaz RL, Brooks RA, et al. Glucose utilization of cerebral gliomas measured by [18F] fluorodeoxyglucose and positron emission tomography. Neurology 1982;32:1323–1329.
2. Wong TZ, van der Westhuizen GJ, Coleman RE. Positron emission tomography imaging of brain tumors. Neuroimaging Clin North Am 2002; 12:615–626.
3. Schaller B. Usefulness of positron emission tomography in diagnosis and treatment follow-up of brain tumors. Neurobiol Dis 2004;15:437–448.
4. Kim CK, Alavi JB, Alavi A, et al. New grading system of cerebral gliomas using positron emission tomography with F-18 fluorodeoxyglucose. J Neurooncol 1991;10:85–91.

5. Meyer PT, Schreckenberger M, Spetzger U, et al. Comparison of visual and ROI-based brain tumour grading using 18F-FDG PET: ROC analyses. Eur J Nucl Med 2001;28:165–174.

6. Hustinx R, Smith RJ, Benard F, et al. Can the standardized uptake value characterize primary brain tumors on FDG-PET? Eur J Nucl Med 1999; 26:1501–1509.

7. Hoekstra CJ, Paglianiti I, Hoekstra OS, et al. Monitoring response to therapy in cancer using [18F]-2–fluoro-2–deoxy-D-glucose and positron emission tomography: an overview of different analytical methods. Eur J Nucl Med 2000;27:731–743.

8. Massager N, David P, Goldman S, et al. Combined magnetic resonance imaging- and positron emission tomography-guided stereotactic biopsy in brainstem mass lesions: diagnostic yield in a series of 30 patients. J Neurosurg 2000;93:951–957.

9. Buchler T, Cervinek L, Belohlavek O, et al. Langerhans cell histiocytosis with central nervous system involvement: follow-up by FDG-PET during treatment with cladribine. Pediatr Blood Cancer 2005;44:286–288.

10. Rosenfeld SS, Hoffman JM, Coleman RE, et al. Studies of primary central nervous system lymphoma with fluorine-18–fluorodeoxyglucose positron emission tomography. J Nucl Med 1992;33:532–536.

11. Hoffman JM, Waskin HA, Schifter T, et al. FDG-PET in differentiating lymphoma from nonmalignant central nervous system lesions in patients with AIDS. J Nucl Med 1993;34:567–575.

12. Pierce MA, Johnson MD, Maciunas RJ, et al. Evaluating contrast-enhancing brain lesions in patients with AIDS by using positron emission tomography. Ann Intern Med 1995;123:594–598.

13. Heald AE, Hoffman JM, Bartlett JA, et al. Differentiation of central nervous system lesions in AIDS patients using positron emission tomography (PET). Int J STD AIDS 1996;7:337–346.

14. O'Doherty MJ, Barrington SF, Campbell M, et al. PET scanning and the human immunodeficiency virus-positive patient. J Nucl Med 1997;38: 1575–1583.

15. Villringer K, Jager H, Dichgans M, et al. Differential diagnosis of CNS lesions in AIDS patients by FDG-PET. J Comput Assist Tomogr 1995;19:532–536.

16. Roelcke U, Leenders KL. Positron emission tomography in patients with primary CNS lymphomas. J Neurooncol 1999;43:231–236.

17. Marom EM, McAdams HP, Erasmus JJ, et al. Staging non-small cell lung cancer with whole-body PET. Radiology 1999;212:803–809.

18. Griffeth LK, Rich KM, Dehdashti F, et al. Brain metastases from non-central nervous system tumors: evaluation with PET. Radiology 1993;186:37–44.

19. Larcos G, Maisey MN. FDG-PET screening for cerebral metastases in patients with suspected malignancy. Nucl Med Commun 1996;17:197–198.

20. Rohren EM, Provenzale JM, Barboriak DP, et al. Screening for cerebral metastases with FDG PET in patients undergoing whole-body staging of non-central nervous system malignancy. Radiology 2003;226:181–187.

21. Barker FG, 2nd, Chang SM, Valk PE, et al. 18–Fluorodeoxyglucose uptake and survival of patients with suspected recurrent malignant glioma. Cancer 1997;79:115–126.

22. Choi SJ, Kim JS, Kim JH, et al. [18F]3'-deoxy-3'-fluorothymidine PET for the diagnosis and grading of brain tumors. Eur J Nucl Med Mol Imaging 2005;32:653–659.

23. De Witte O, Levivier M, Violon P, et al. Prognostic value positron emission tomography with [18F]fluoro-2–deoxy-D-glucose in the low-grade glioma. Neurosurgery 1996;39:470–476; discussion 476–477.

24. Kaschten B, Stevenaert A, Sadzot B, et al. Preoperative evaluation of 54 gliomas by PET with fluorine-18–fluorodeoxyglucose and/or carbon-11–methionine. J Nucl Med 1998;39:778–785.

25. Levivier M, Goldman S, Pirotte B, et al. Diagnostic yield of stereotactic brain biopsy guided by positron emission tomography with [18F]fluorodeoxyglucose. J Neurosurg 1995;82:445–452.

26. Ohtani T, Kurihara H, Ishiuchi S, et al. Brain tumour imaging with carbon-11 choline: comparison with FDG PET and gadolinium-enhanced MR imaging. Eur J Nucl Med 2001;28:1664–1670.

27. Pirotte B, Goldman S, Massager N, et al. Combined use of 18F-fluorodeoxyglucose and 11C-methionine in 45 positron emission tomography-guided stereotactic brain biopsies. J Neurosurg 2004;101:476–483.

28. Kaplan AM, Bandy DJ, Manwaring KH, et al. Functional brain mapping using positron emission tomography scanning in preoperative neurosurgical planning for pediatric brain tumors. J Neurosurg 1999;91:797–803.

29. Duncan JD, Moss SD, Bandy DJ, et al. Use of positron emission tomography for presurgical localization of eloquent brain areas in children with seizures. Pediatr Neurosurg 1997;26:144–156.

30. Borgwardt L, Hojgaard L, Carstensen H, et al. Increased fluorine-18 2–fluoro-2–deoxy-D-glucose (FDG) uptake in childhood CNS tumors is correlated with malignancy grade: a study with FDG positron emission tomography/magnetic resonance imaging coregistration and image fusion. J Clin Oncol 2005;23:3030–3037.

31. Plowman PN, Saunders CA, Maisey M. On the usefulness of brain PET scanning to the paediatric neuro-oncologist. Br J Neurosurg 1997;11:525–532.

32. Holthoff VA, Herholz K, Berthold F, et al. In vivo metabolism of childhood posterior fossa tumors and primitive neuroectodermal tumors before and after treatment. Cancer 1993;72:1394–1403.

33. Hoffman JM, Hanson MW, Friedman HS, et al. FDG-PET in pediatric posterior fossa brain tumors. J Comput Assist Tomogr 1992;16:62–68.

34. Mineura K, Yasuda T, Kowada M, et al. Positron emission tomographic evaluations in the diagnosis and therapy of multifocal glioblastoma. Report of a pediatric case. Pediatr Neurosci 1985;12:208–212.

35. Bruggers CS, Friedman HS, Fuller GN, et al. Comparison of serial PET and MRI scans in a pediatric patient with a brainstem glioma. Med Pediatr Oncol 1993;21:301–306.

36. Molloy PT, Defeo R, Hunter J, et al. Excellent correlation of FDG-PET imaging with clinical outcome in patients with neurofibromatosis type I and low grade astrocytomas. J Nucl Med 1999;40:129P.

37. Fulham MJ, Brunetti A, Aloj L, et al. Decreased cerebral glucose metabolism in patients with brain tumors: an effect of corticosteroids. J Neurosurg 1995;83:657–664.

38. Glantz MJ, Hoffman JM, Coleman RE, et al. Identification of early recurrence of primary central nervous system tumors by [18F]fluorodeoxyglucose positron emission tomography. Ann Neurol 1991;29:347–355.

39. Roelcke U, Blasberg RG, von Ammon K, et al. Dexamethasone treatment and plasma glucose levels: relevance for fluorine-18–fluorodeoxyglucose uptake measurements in gliomas. J Nucl Med 1998;39:879–884.

40. Ishizu K, Nishizawa S, Yonekura Y, et al. Effects of hyperglycemia on FDG uptake in human brain and glioma. J Nucl Med 1994;35:1104–1109.

41. Spence AM, Muzi M, Mankoff DA, et al. 18F-FDG PET of gliomas at delayed intervals: improved distinction between tumor and normal gray matter. J Nucl Med 2004;45:1653–1659.

42. Jager PL, Vaalburg W, Pruim J, et al. Radiolabeled amino acids: basic aspects and clinical applications in oncology. J Nucl Med 2001;42:432–445.

43. Ishiwata K, Kubota K, Murakami M, et al. Re-evaluation of amino acid PET studies: can the protein synthesis rates in brain and tumor tissues be measured in vivo? J Nucl Med 1993;34:1936–1943.

44. Nuutinen J, Sonninen P, Lehikoinen P, et al. Radiotherapy treatment planning and long-term follow-up with [(11)C]methionine PET in patients with low-grade astrocytoma. Int J Radiat Oncol Biol Phys 2000;48:43–52.

45. Herholz K, Holzer T, Bauer B, et al. 11C-methionine PET for differential diagnosis of low-grade gliomas. Neurology 1998;50:1316–1322.

46. Mosskin M, Bergstrom M, Collins VP, et al. Positron emission tomography with 11C-methionine of intracranial tumours compared with histology of multiple biopsies. Acta Radiol Suppl 1986;369:157–160.

47. Bergstrom M, Collins VP, Ehrin E, et al. Discrepancies in brain tumor extent as shown by computed tomography and positron emission tomography using [68Ga]EDTA, [11C]glucose, and [11C]methionine. J Comput Assist Tomogr 1983;7:1062–1066.

48. Ogawa T, Shishido F, Kanno I, et al. Cerebral glioma: evaluation with methionine PET. Radiology 1993;186:45–53.

49. De Witte O, Goldberg I, Wikler D, et al. Positron emission tomography with injection of methionine as a prognostic factor in glioma. J Neurosurg 2001;95:746–750.

50. Chung JK, Kim YK, Kim SK, et al. Usefulness of 11C-methionine PET in the evaluation of brain lesions that are hypo- or isometabolic on 18F-FDG PET. Eur J Nucl Med Mol Imaging 2002;29:176–182.

51. Nakagawa M, Kuwabara Y, Sasaki M, et al. 11C-methionine uptake in cerebrovascular disease: a comparison with 18F-FDG PET and 99mTc-HMPAO SPECT. Ann Nucl Med 2002;16:207–211.

52. Pruim J, Willemsen AT, Molenaar WM, et al. Brain tumors: L-[1–C-11] tyrosine PET for visualization and quantification of protein synthesis rate. Radiology 1995;197:221–226.

53. Ogawa T, Inugami A, Hatazawa J, et al. Clinical positron emission tomography for brain tumors: comparison of fludeoxyglucose F 18 and L-methyl-11C-methionine. AJNR 1996;17:345–353.

54. Pirotte B, Goldman S, David P, et al. Stereotactic brain biopsy guided by positron emission tomography (PET) with [F-18]fluorodeoxyglucose and [C-11]methionine. Acta Neurochir Suppl 1997;68:133–138.

55. Sasaki M, Kuwabara Y, Yoshida T, et al. A comparative study of thallium-201 SPET, carbon-11 methionine PET and fluorine-18 fluorodeoxyglucose PET for the differentiation of astrocytic tumours. Eur J Nucl Med 1998; 25:1261–1269.

56. Derlon JM, Petit-Taboue MC, Chapon F, et al. The in vivo metabolic pattern of low-grade brain gliomas: a positron emission tomographic study using 18F-fluorodeoxyglucose and 11C-L-methylmethionine. Neurosurgery 1997;40:276–287; discussion 287–288.

57. O'Tuama LA, Phillips PC, Strauss LC, et al. Two-phase [11C]L-methionine PET in childhood brain tumors. Pediatr Neurol 1990;6:163–170.

58. Utriainen M, Metsahonkala L, Salmi TT, et al. Metabolic characterization of childhood brain tumors: comparison of 18F-fluorodeoxyglucose and 11C-methionine positron emission tomography. Cancer 2002;95: 1376–1386.

59. Di Chiro G. Positron emission tomography using [18F] fluorodeoxyglucose in brain tumors. A powerful diagnostic and prognostic tool. Invest Radiol 1987;22:360–371.

60. Patronas NJ, Brooks RA, DeLaPaz RL, et al. Glycolytic rate (PET) and contrast enhancement (CT) in human cerebral gliomas. AJNR 1983;4:533–535.

61. Delbeke D, Meyerowitz C, Lapidus RL, et al. Optimal cutoff levels of F-18 fluorodeoxyglucose uptake in the differentiation of low-grade from high-grade brain tumors with PET. Radiology 1995;195:47–52.

62. Goldman S, Levivier M, Pirotte B, et al. Regional glucose metabolism and histopathology of gliomas. A study based on positron emission tomography-guided stereotactic biopsy. Cancer 1996;78:1098–1106.

63. Padma MV, Said S, Jacobs M, et al. Prediction of pathology and survival by FDG PET in gliomas. J Neurooncol 2003;64:227–237.

64. Fulham MJ, Melisi JW, Nishimiya J, et al. Neuroimaging of juvenile pilocytic astrocytomas: an enigma. Radiology 1993;189:221–225.

65. Roelcke U, Radu EW, Hausmann O, et al. Tracer transport and metabolism in a patient with juvenile pilocytic astrocytoma. A PET study. J Neurooncol 1998;36:279–283.

66. Hustinx R, Alavi A. SPECT and PET imaging of brain tumors. Neuroimaging Clin North Am 1999;9:751–766.

67. Kleihues P, Kavanee WK. Pathology and Genetics. Tumours of the Nervous System. Lyon: IARC Press, 2000.

68. Derlon JM, Bourdet C, Bustany P, et al. [11C]L-methionine uptake in gliomas. Neurosurgery 1989;25:720–728.

69. Sato N, Suzuki M, Kuwata N, et al. Evaluation of the malignancy of glioma using 11C-methionine positron emission tomography and proliferating cell nuclear antigen staining. Neurosurg Rev 1999;22:210–214.

70. Ribom D, Engler H, Blomquist E, et al. Potential significance of (11)C-methionine PET as a marker for the radiosensitivity of low-grade gliomas. Eur J Nucl Med Mol Imaging 2002;29:632–640.

71. Derlon JM, Chapon F, Noel MH, et al. Non-invasive grading of oligodendrogliomas: correlation between in vivo metabolic pattern and histopathology. Eur J Nucl Med 2000;27:778–787.

72. Patronas NJ, Di Chiro G, Kufta C, et al. Prediction of survival in glioma patients by means of positron emission tomography. J Neurosurg 1985;62:816–822.

73. Alavi JB, Alavi A, Chawluk J, et al. Positron emission tomography in patients with glioma. A predictor of prognosis. Cancer 1988;62:1074–1078.

74. Holzer T, Herholz K, Jeske J, et al. FDG-PET as a prognostic indicator in radiochemotherapy of glioblastoma. J Comput Assist Tomogr 1993;17:681–687.

75. Schifter T, Hoffman JM, Hanson MW, et al. Serial FDG-PET studies in the prediction of survival in patients with primary brain tumors. J Comput Assist Tomogr 1993;17:509–561.

76. Pardo FS, Aronen HJ, Fitzek M, et al. Correlation of FDG-PET interpretation with survival in a cohort of glioma patients. Anticancer Res 2004;24:2359–2365.

77. Spence AM, Muzi M, Graham MM, et al. 2–[(18)F]Fluoro-2–deoxyglucose and glucose uptake in malignant gliomas before and after radiotherapy: correlation with outcome. Clin Cancer Res 2002;8:971–979.

78. De Witte O, Lefranc F, Levivier M, et al. FDG-PET as a prognostic factor in high-grade astrocytoma. J Neurooncol 2000;49:157–163.

79. Francavilla TL, Miletich RS, Di Chiro G, et al. Positron emission tomography in the detection of malignant degeneration of low-grade gliomas. Neurosurgery 1989;24:1–5.

80. Di Chiro G, Hatazawa J, Katz DA, et al. Glucose utilization by intracranial meningiomas as an index of tumor aggressivity and probability of recurrence: a PET study. Radiology 1987;164:521–526.

81. Janus TJ, Kim EE, Tilbury R, et al. Use of [18F]fluorodeoxyglucose positron emission tomography in patients with primary malignant brain tumors. Ann Neurol 1993;33:540–548.

82. Mogard J, Kihlstrom L, Ericson K, et al. Recurrent tumor vs radiation effects after gamma knife radiosurgery of intracerebral metastases: diagnosis with PET-FDG. J Comput Assist Tomogr 1994;18:177–181.

83. Ericson K, Kihlstrom L, Mogard J, et al. Positron emission tomography using 18F-fluorodeoxyglucose in patients with stereotactically irradiated brain metastases. Stereotact Funct Neurosurg 1996;66 Suppl 1:214–224.

84. Ribom D, Eriksson A, Hartman M, et al. Positron emission tomography (11)C-methionine and survival in patients with low-grade gliomas. Cancer 2001;92:1541–1549.

85. Paulus W, Peiffer J. Intratumoral histologic heterogeneity of gliomas. A quantitative study. Cancer 1989;64:442–447.

86. Floeth FW, Pauleit D, Wittsack HJ, et al. Multimodal metabolic imaging of cerebral gliomas: positron emission tomography with [18F]fluoroethyl-L-tyrosine and magnetic resonance spectroscopy. J Neurosurg 2005;102: 318–327.

87. Hanson MW, Glantz MJ, Hoffman JM, et al. FDG-PET in the selection of brain lesions for biopsy. J Comput Assist Tomogr 1991;15:796–801.

88. Thomas DG, Gill SS, Wilson CB, et al. Use of relocatable stereotactic frame to integrate positron emission tomography and computed tomography images: application in human malignant brain tumours. Stereotact Funct Neurosurg 1990;54–55:388–392.

89. Pirotte B, Goldman S, Brucher JM, et al. PET in stereotactic conditions increases the diagnostic yield of brain biopsy. Stereotact Funct Neurosurg 1994;63:144–149.

90. Levivier M, Wikler D Jr, Massager N, et al. The integration of metabolic imaging in stereotactic procedures including radiosurgery: a review. J Neurosurg 2002;97:542–550.

91. Thiel A, Pietrzyk U, Sturm V, et al. Enhanced accuracy in differential diagnosis of radiation necrosis by positron emission tomography-magnetic resonance imaging coregistration: technical case report. Neurosurgery 2000;46:232–234.

92. Pirotte B, Goldman S, Salzberg S, et al. Combined positron emission tomography and magnetic resonance imaging for the planning of stereotactic brain biopsies in children: experience in 9 cases. Pediatr Neurosurg 2003;38:146–155.

93. Maruyama I, Sadato N, Waki A, et al. Hyperacute changes in glucose metabolism of brain tumors after stereotactic radiosurgery: a PET study. J Nucl Med 1999;40:1085–1090.

94. De Witte O, Hildebrand J, Luxen A, et al. Acute effect of carmustine on glucose metabolism in brain and glioblastoma. Cancer 1994;74: 2836–2842.

95. Spence AM, Mankoff DA, Muzi M. Positron emission tomography imaging of brain tumors. Neuroimaging Clin North Am 2003;13:717–739.

96. Widnell CC, Baldwin SA, Davies A, et al. Cellular stress induces a redistribution of the glucose transporter. Faseb J 1990;4:1634–1637.

97. Sviderskaya EV, Jazrawi E, Baldwin SA, et al. Cellular stress causes accumulation of the glucose transporter at the surface of cells independently of their insulin sensitivity. J Membr Biol 1996;149:133–140.

98. Haberkorn U, Morr I, Oberdorfer F, et al. Fluorodeoxyglucose uptake in vitro: aspects of method and effects of treatment with gemcitabine. J Nucl Med 1994;35:1842–1850.

99. Haberkorn U, Oberdorfer F, Klenner T, et al. Metabolic and transcriptional changes in osteosarcoma cells treated with chemotherapeutic drugs. Nucl Med Biol 1994;21:835–845.

100. Haberkorn U, Bellemann ME, Altmann A, et al. PET 2–fluoro-2–deoxyglucose uptake in rat prostate adenocarcinoma during chemotherapy with gemcitabine. J Nucl Med 1997;38:1215–1221.

101. Fujibayashi Y, Waki A, Sakahara H, et al. Transient increase in glycolytic metabolism in cultured tumor cells immediately after exposure to ionizing radiation: from gene expression to deoxyglucose uptake. Radiat Res 1997;147:729–734.

102. Smith TA, Maisey NR, Titley JC, et al. Treatment of SW620 cells with Tomudex and oxaliplatin induces changes in 2–deoxy-D-glucose incorporation associated with modifications in glucose transport. J Nucl Med 2000;41:1753–1759.

103. Kubota R, Yamada S, Kubota K, et al. Intratumoral distribution of fluorine-18–fluorodeoxyglucose in vivo: high accumulation in macrophages and granulation tissues studied by microautoradiography. J Nucl Med 1992;33:1972–1980.

104. Reinhardt MJ, Kubota K, Yamada S, et al. Assessment of cancer recurrence in residual tumors after fractionated radiotherapy: a comparison of fluorodeoxyglucose, L-methionine and thymidine. J Nucl Med 1997;38:280–287.

105. Cokgor I, Akabani G, Kuan CT, et al. Phase I trial results of iodine-131–labeled antitenascin monoclonal antibody 81C6 treatment of patients with newly diagnosed malignant gliomas. J Clin Oncol 2000;18:3862–3872.

106. Higashi K, Clavo AC, Wahl RL. In vitro assessment of 2–fluoro-2–deoxy-D-glucose, L-methionine and thymidine as agents to monitor the early response of a human adenocarcinoma cell line to radiotherapy. J Nucl Med 1993;34:773–779.

107. Furuta M, Hasegawa M, Hayakawa K, et al. Rapid rise in FDG uptake in an irradiated human tumour xenograft. Eur J Nucl Med 1997;24:435–438.

108. Hasegawa M, Mitsuhashi N, Yamakawa M, et al. p53 protein expression and radiation-induced apoptosis in human tumors transplanted to nude mice. Radiat Med 1997;15:171–176.

109. Rozental JM, Levine RL, Mehta MP, et al. Early changes in tumor metabolism after treatment: the effects of stereotactic radiotherapy. Int J Radiat Oncol Biol Phys 1991;20:1053–1060.

110. Brock CS, Young H, O'Reilly SM, et al. Early evaluation of tumour metabolic response using [18F]fluorodeoxyglucose and positron emission tomography: a pilot study following the phase II chemotherapy schedule for temozolomide in recurrent high-grade gliomas. Br J Cancer 2000; 82:608–615.

111. Wang GJ, Volkow ND, Lau YH, et al. Glucose metabolic changes in non-tumoral brain tissue of patients with brain tumor following radiotherapy: a preliminary study. J Comput Assist Tomogr 1996;20:709–714.

112. Bustany P, Chatel M, Derlon JM, et al. Brain tumor protein synthesis and histological grades: a study by positron emission tomography (PET) with C11–L-Methionine. J Neurooncol 1986;3:397–404.

113. Mineura K, Sasajima T, Kowada M, et al. [Changes in the (11C-methyl)-L-methionine uptake index in gliomas following radiotherapy]. Gan No Rinsho 1989;35:1101–1104.

114. Wurker M, Herholz K, Voges J, et al. Glucose consumption and methionine uptake in low-grade gliomas after iodine-125 brachytherapy. Eur J Nucl Med 1996;23:583–586.

115. Ogawa T, Kanno I, Hatazawa J, et al. Methionine PET for follow-up of radiation therapy of primary lymphoma of the brain. Radiographics 1994;14:101–110.

116. Heesters MA, Go KG, Kamman RL, et al. 11C-tyrosine position emission tomography and 1H magnetic resonance spectroscopy of the response of brain gliomas to radiotherapy. Neuroradiology 1998;40:103–108.

117. Patronas NJ, Di Chiro G, Brooks RA, et al. Work in progress: [18F] fluorodeoxyglucose and positron emission tomography in the evaluation of radiation necrosis of the brain. Radiology 1982;144:885–889.

118. Doyle WK, Budinger TF, Valk PE, et al. Differentiation of cerebral radiation necrosis from tumor recurrence by [18F]FDG and 82Rb positron emission tomography. J Comput Assist Tomogr 1987;11:563–570.

119. Di Chiro G, Oldfield E, Wright DC, et al. Cerebral necrosis after radiotherapy and/or intraarterial chemotherapy for brain tumors: PET and neuropathologic studies. AJR 1988;150:189–197.

120. Valk PE, Budinger TF, Levin VA, et al. PET of malignant cerebral tumors after interstitial brachytherapy. Demonstration of metabolic activity and correlation with clinical outcome. J Neurosurg 1988;69:830–838.

121. Langleben DD, Segall GM. PET in differentiation of recurrent brain tumor from radiation injury. J Nucl Med 2000;41:1861–1867.

122. Chao ST, Suh JH, Raja S, et al. The sensitivity and specificity of FDG PET in distinguishing recurrent brain tumor from radionecrosis in patients treated with stereotactic radiosurgery. Int J Cancer 2001;96:191–197.

123. Deshmukh A, Scott JA, Palmer EL, et al. Impact of fluorodeoxyglucose positron emission tomography on the clinical management of patients with glioma. Clin Nucl Med 1996;21:720–725.

124. Ricci PE, Karis JP, Heiserman JE, et al. Differentiating recurrent tumor from radiation necrosis: time for re-evaluation of positron emission tomography? AJNR 1998;19:407–413.

125. Ogawa T, Kanno I, Shishido F, et al. Clinical value of PET with 18F-fluorodeoxyglucose and L-methyl-11C-methionine for diagnosis of recurrent brain tumor and radiation injury. Acta Radiol 1991;32:197–202.

126. Sonoda Y, Kumabe T, Takahashi T, et al. Clinical usefulness of 11C-MET PET and 201T1 SPECT for differentiation of recurrent glioma from radiation necrosis. Neurol Med Chir (Tokyo) 1998;38:342–347; discussion 347–348.

127. Tsuyuguchi N, Sunada I, Iwai Y, et al. Methionine positron emission tomography of recurrent metastatic brain tumor and radiation necrosis after stereotactic radiosurgery: is a differential diagnosis possible? J Neurosurg 2003;98:1056–1064.

128. Tsuyuguchi N, Takami T, Sunada I, et al. Methionine positron emission tomography for differentiation of recurrent brain tumor and radiation necrosis after stereotactic radiosurgery—in malignant glioma. Ann Nucl Med 2004;18:291–296.

129. Tralins KS, Douglas JG, Stelzer KJ, et al. Volumetric analysis of 18F-FDG PET in glioblastoma multiforme: prognostic information and possible role in definition of target volumes in radiation dose escalation. J Nucl Med 2002;43:1667–1673.

130. Solberg TD, Agazaryan N, Goss BW, et al. A feasibility study of 18F-fluorodeoxyglucose positron emission tomography targeting and simultaneous integrated boost for intensity-modulated radiosurgery and radiotherapy. J Neurosurg 2004;101(suppl 3):381–389.

131. Miwa K, Shinoda J, Yano H, et al. Discrepancy between lesion distributions on methionine PET and MR images in patients with glioblastoma multiforme: insight from a PET and MR fusion image study. J Neurol Neurosurg Psychiatry 2004;75:1457–1462.

132. Langen KJ, Jarosch M, Muhlensiepen H, et al. Comparison of fluorotyrosines and methionine uptake in F98 rat gliomas. Nucl Med Biol 2003; 30:501–508.

133. Wienhard K, Herholz K, Coenen HH, et al. Increased amino acid transport into brain tumors measured by PET of L-(2–18F)fluorotyrosine. J Nucl Med 1991;32:1338–1346.

134. Inoue T, Shibasaki T, Oriuchi N, et al. 18F alpha-methyl tyrosine PET studies in patients with brain tumors. J Nucl Med 1999;40:399–405.

135. Kaim AH, Weber B, Kurrer MO, et al. (18)F-FDG and (18)F-FET uptake in experimental soft tissue infection. Eur J Nucl Med Mol Imaging 2002; 29:648–654.

136. Rau FC, Weber WA, Wester HJ, et al. O-(2-[(18)F]Fluoroethyl)-L-tyrosine (FET): a tracer for differentiation of tumour from inflammation in murine lymph nodes. Eur J Nucl Med Mol Imaging 2002;29:1039–1046.

137. Weber WA, Wester HJ, Grosu AL, et al. O-(2-[18F]fluoroethyl)-L-tyrosine and L-[methyl-11C]methionine uptake in brain tumours: initial results of a comparative study. Eur J Nucl Med 2000;27:542–549.

138. Pauleit D, Floeth F, Tellmann L, et al. Comparison of O-(2-18F-fluoroethyl)-L-tyrosine PET and 3-123I-iodo-alpha-methyl-L-tyrosine SPECT in brain tumors. J Nucl Med 2004;45:374–381.

139. Weckesser M, Langen KJ, Rickert CH, et al. O-(2-[(18)F]fluorethyl)-L: -tyrosine PET in the clinical evaluation of primary brain tumours. Eur J Nucl Med Mol Imaging 2005;32:422–429.

140. Messing-Junger AM, Floeth FW, Pauleit D, et al. Multimodal target point assessment for stereotactic biopsy in children with diffuse bithalamic astrocytomas. Childs Nerv Syst 2002;18:445–449.

141. Hubner KF, Thie JA, Smith GT, et al. Positron Emission Tomography (PET) with 1–aminocyclobutane-1-[(11)C]carboxylic acid (1-[(11)C]-ACBC) for detecting recurrent brain tumors. Clin Positron Imaging 1998;1:165–173.

142. O'Tuama LA, Guilarte TR, Douglass KH, et al. Assessment of [11C]-L-methionine transport into the human brain. J Cereb Blood Flow Metab 1988;8:341–345.

143. Becherer A, Karanikas G, Szabo M, et al. Brain tumour imaging with PET: a comparison between [18F]fluorodopa and [11C]methionine. Eur J Nucl Med Mol Imaging 2003;30:1561–1567.

144. Vander Borght T, Pauwels S, Lambotte L, et al. Brain tumor imaging with PET and 2–[carbon-11]thymidine. J Nucl Med 1994;35:974–982.

145. De Reuck J, Santens P, Goethals P, et al. [Methyl-11C]thymidine positron emission tomography in tumoral and non-tumoral cerebral lesions. Acta Neurol Belg 1999;99:118–125.

146. Eary JF, Mankoff DA, Spence AM, et al. 2-[C-11]thymidine imaging of malignant brain tumors. Cancer Res 1999;59:615–621.

147. Wells JM, Mankoff DA, Eary JF, et al. Kinetic analysis of 2-[11C] thymidine PET imaging studies of malignant brain tumors: preliminary patient results. Mol Imaging 2002;1:145–150.

148. Shields AF, Mankoff DA, Link JM, et al. Carbon-11–thymidine and FDG to measure therapy response. J Nucl Med 1998;39:1757–1762.

149. Wells JM, Mankoff DA, Muzi M, et al. Kinetic analysis of 2–[11C] thymidine PET imaging studies of malignant brain tumors: compartmental model investigation and mathematical analysis. Mol Imaging 2002;1: 151–159.

150. Tjuvajev J, Muraki A, Ginos J, et al. Iododeoxyuridine uptake and retention as a measure of tumor growth. J Nucl Med 1993;34:1152–1162.

151. Blasberg RG, Roelcke U, Weinreich R, et al. Imaging brain tumor proliferative activity with [124I]iododeoxyuridine. Cancer Res 2000;60: 624–635.

152. Liu RS. 31. Clinical application of. Clin Positron Imaging 2000;3:185.

153. DeGrado TR, Baldwin SW, Wang S, et al. Synthesis and evaluation of (18)F-labeled choline analogs as oncologic PET tracers. J Nucl Med 2001; 42:1805–1814.

154. Hara T, Kosaka N, Shinoura N, et al. PET imaging of brain tumor with [methyl-11C]choline. J Nucl Med 1997;38:842–847.

155. Shinoura N, Nishijima M, Hara T, et al. Brain tumors: detection with C-11 choline PET. Radiology 1997;202:497–503.

156. Utriainen M, Komu M, Vuorinen V, et al. Evaluation of brain tumor metabolism with [11C]choline PET and 1H-MRS. J Neurooncol 2003;62: 329–338.

157. Kwee SA, Coel MN, Lim J, et al. Combined use of F-18 fluorocholine positron emission tomography and magnetic resonance spectroscopy for brain tumor evaluation. J Neuroimaging 2004;14:285–289.

158. Hara T, Kondo T, Kosaka N. Use of 18F-choline and 11C-choline as contrast agents in positron emission tomography imaging-guided stereotactic biopsy sampling of gliomas. J Neurosurg 2003;99:474–479.

159. Mathias CJ, Welch MJ, Kilbourn MR, et al. Radiolabeled hypoxic cell sensitizers: tracers for assessment of ischemia. Life Sci 1987;41:199–206.

160. Martin GV, Cerqueira MD, Caldwell JH, et al. Fluoromisonidazole. A metabolic marker of myocyte hypoxia. Circ Res 1990;67:240–244.

161. Tochon-Danguy HJ, Sachinidis JI, Chan F, et al. Imaging and quantitation of the hypoxic cell fraction of viable tumor in an animal model of intracerebral high grade glioma using [18F]fluoromisonidazole (FMISO). Nucl Med Biol 2002;29:191–197.

162. Valk PE, Mathis CA, Prados MD, et al. Hypoxia in human gliomas: demonstration by PET with fluorine-18–fluoromisonidazole. J Nucl Med 1992;33:2133–2137.

163. Spence AM, Muzi M, Krohn KA. Molecular imaging of regional brain tumor biology. J Cell Biochem Suppl 2002;39:25–35.

164. Bergstrom M, Muhr C, Jossan S, et al. Differentiation of pituitary adenoma and meningioma: visualization with positron emission tomography and [11C]-L-deprenyl. Neurosurgery 1992;30:855–861.

165. Lucignani G, Losa M, Moresco RM, et al. Differentiation of clinically non-functioning pituitary adenomas from meningiomas and craniopharyngiomas by positron emission tomography with [18F]fluoro-ethyl-spiperone. Eur J Nucl Med 1997;24:1149–1155.

166. Junck L, Olson JM, Ciliax BJ, et al. PET imaging of human gliomas with ligands for the peripheral benzodiazepine binding site. Ann Neurol 1989;26:752–758.

167. Pappata S, Cornu P, Samson Y, et al. PET study of carbon-11–PK 11195 binding to peripheral type benzodiazepine sites in glioblastoma: a case report. J Nucl Med 1991;32:1608–1610.

168. Fredriksson A, Johnstrom P, Thorell JO, et al. In vivo evaluation of the biodistribution of 11C-labeled PD153035 in rats without and with neuroblastoma implants. Life Sci 1999;65:165–174.
169. Fisher MJ, Adamson PC. Anti-angiogenic agents for the treatment of brain tumors. Neuroimaging Clin North Am 2002;12:477–499.
170. Haubner R, Wester HJ, Weber WA, et al. Noninvasive imaging of alpha(v)beta3 integrin expression using 18F-labeled RGD-containing glycopeptide and positron emission tomography. Cancer Res 2001;61:1781–1785.
171. Haubner R, Weber WA, Beer AJ, et al. Noninvasive visualization of the activated alphavbeta3 integrin in cancer patients by positron emission tomography and [(18)F]galacto-RGD. PLoS Med 2005;2:e70.
172. Chen X, Park R, Shahinian AH, et al. 18F-labeled RGD peptide: initial evaluation for imaging brain tumor angiogenesis. Nucl Med Biol 2004;31:179–189.
173. Chen X, Park R, Hou Y, et al. MicroPET imaging of brain tumor angiogenesis with 18F-labeled PEGylated RGD peptide. Eur J Nucl Med Mol Imaging 2004;31:1081–1089.
174. Tjuvajev JG, Stockhammer G, Desai R, et al. Imaging the expression of transfected genes in vivo. Cancer Res 1995;55:6126–6132.
175. Tjuvajev JG, Finn R, Watanabe K, et al. Noninvasive imaging of herpes virus thymidine kinase gene transfer and expression: a potential method for monitoring clinical gene therapy. Cancer Res 1996;56:4087–4095.
176. Tjuvajev JG, Avril N, Oku T, et al. Imaging herpes virus thymidine kinase gene transfer and expression by positron emission tomography. Cancer Res 1998;58:4333–4341.
177. Murakami Y, Takamatsu H, Taki J, et al. 18F-labelled annexin V: a PET tracer for apoptosis imaging. Eur J Nucl Med Mol Imaging 2004;31:469–474.
178. Yagle KJ, Eary JF, Tait JF, et al. Evaluation of 18F-annexin V as a PET imaging agent in an animal model of apoptosis. J Nucl Med 2005;46:658–666.
179. Toretsky J, Levenson A, Weinberg IN, et al. Preparation of F-18 labeled annexin V: a potential PET radiopharmaceutical for imaging cell death. Nucl Med Biol 2004;31:747–752.
180. Saleem A, Brown GD, Brady F, et al. Metabolic activation of temozolomide measured in vivo using positron emission tomography. Cancer Res 2003;63:2409–2415.

12

Lymphoma

Christopher J. Palestro, Josephine N. Rini, and Maria B. Tomas

In patients with lymphoma, prognosis and treatment are related to the stage of disease at diagnosis, and accurate staging, therefore, is essential for proper management. The staging procedures currently used include history and physical examination; computed tomography (CT) of the chest, abdomen, and pelvis; bone marrow biopsy; and, occasionally, staging laparotomy. Radionuclide studies, including gallium scintigraphy, bone scintigraphy, and more recently, positron emission tomography (PET) with fluorine-18 fluorodeoxyglucose (^{18}F-FDG) have been used as adjuncts for staging, follow-up, and prognosis in children with Hodgkin's disease and non-Hodgkin's lymphoma.

Hodgkin's Disease

Hodgkin's disease (HD) accounts for 13% of malignant lymphomas and less than 1% of all malignancies [1]. Although it is a relatively uncommon malignancy, HD accounts for 19% of all malignancies occurring in adolescents 15 to 19 years of age [2]. Furthermore, it is among the few potentially curable malignancies with an overall 5-year survival rate of 85% [3].

The current international staging classification of HD, the Cotswold Classification, which is a modification of the earlier Ann Arbor Classification, defines the extent of nodal involvement, extranodal disease, and systemic symptoms [4,5]. Stage I is defined as involvement of a single lymph node region or lymphoid structure. Stage II is defined as involvement of two or more lymph node regions on the same side of the diaphragm. Stage III is defined as involvement of lymph node regions or structures on both sides of the diaphragm. Stage IV is defined as extranodal involvement, such as bone or lung disease. Each stage is also classified by the presence or absence of symptoms. "A" indicates that the patient is asymptomatic; "B" indicates that the patient has weight loss, fevers, chills, and/or sweats.

Depending on the stage of disease at diagnosis, HD is treated with radiation therapy and/or chemotherapy. Because HD is not treated with surgery, and because it is impractical and unethical to biopsy all suspected sites of disease, stage is determined clinically in the majority of patients. Currently recommended staging procedures include history and physical examination; CT of the chest, abdomen, and pelvis; bone marrow biopsy; and, rarely, staging laparotomy (4).

Non-Hodgkin's Lymphoma

Non-Hodgkin's lymphoma (NHL), like HD, is a malignant neoplasm of the lymphopoietic system. This once relatively rare, but rapidly lethal, disease has increased in frequency over the past decade, and is currently the fifth most common malignancy in the United States, accounting for 4% of all cancers and 7% of cancers in children and adolescents (6).

As with HD, the prognosis and treatment of NHL are highly dependent on the histopathologic subtype and stage of disease at diagnosis. In contrast to HD, however, NHL is a heterogeneous group of pathologic entities; numerous schemes for classification have been formulated over time, specifically to guide clinicians in instituting therapy and predicting outcome. The most widely utilized classification scheme for pediatric NHL is the Revised European-American Lymphoma (REAL) classification, which emphasizes the immunophenotype of the tumor, that is, B cell or T cell (7). This classification has been further refined by the World Health Organization (WHO) classification of lymphoproliferative diseases (8). Approximately 90% of NHL is of B-cell origin and 10% is of T-cell origin. The vast majority of childhood NHLs are clinically aggressive, high-grade tumors. There are four major subtypes of pediatric NHL. Small noncleaved cell (SNCC) (Burkitt's and Burkitt's-like) accounts for about 40% of these tumors, 30% are lymphoblastic, 20% are B-large cell, and 10% are anaplastic large cell. In contrast to adults, extranodal disease is common in children with NHL. The most common sites of extranodal disease are the abdomen (31%), head and neck (29%), and thorax (26%) (9).

The initial staging of NHL is accomplished with a careful history, detailed physical examination, laboratory tests, imaging, and bone marrow biopsy. The staging strategy often used is the St. Jude Children's Research Hospital staging system, which distinguishes patients with limited disease (stages I and II) from those with extensive disease (stages III and IV). Stage I disease is defined as a single tumor or nodal area outside of the abdomen and mediastinum. Stage II disease is defined as a single tumor with regional node involvement, two or more tumors or nodal areas on one side of the diaphragm, or a primary gastrointestinal tract tumor (resected) with or without regional node involvement. Stage III disease consists of tumors or lymph node areas on both sides of the diaphragm, or any primary intrathoracic or extensive intraabdominal disease, or any paraspinal or epidural disease. Stage IV disease includes central nervous system and bone marrow involvement, with or without other sites of disease. Bone marrow involvement is defined as at least 5% malignant cells in an otherwise normal bone marrow with normal peripheral blood counts and smears (9).

^{18}F-FDG-PET in Lymphoma

Nuclear medicine, in particular gallium-67 (^{67}Ga) imaging, has long played an important part in the diagnosis, staging, and restaging of HD and NHL in children with lymphoma. ^{18}F-FDG-PET, which was approved by Medicare in July 1999, is gradually replacing gallium imaging for these indications (10,11). It has several advantages over gallium, including same-day imaging, improved spatial resolution, and a higher target-to-background ratio. The primary role of PET in patients with lymphoma, as it has been for gallium imaging, is to monitor response during therapy, to detect residual disease or relapse after treatment, and to provide prognostic information (12). Although CT is the primary imaging modality for initial staging of lymphoma, gallium and PET also play a role at the time of initial staging. Specifically, baseline studies documenting gallium or FDG-avid disease are necessary in order for posttherapy studies to be meaningful. The current Children's Oncology Group (COG) research treatment protocols for children and adolescents with newly diagnosed intermediate-risk Hodgkin's disease and advanced-stage anaplastic large-cell non-Hodgkin's lymphoma require PET or gallium imaging prior to initiation of therapy, followed by repeat imaging to assess treatment response after two cycles of chemotherapy for patients with HD, and at the end of induction chemotherapy for patients with NHL. Biopsy of PET-positive nonosseous lesions at the end of induction chemotherapy is required for patients with NHL. If the test is negative after induction chemotherapy, follow-up is recommended at the end of therapy, at relapse, and at 6 and 12 months following completion of therapy.

Because radionuclide studies provide whole-body screening, they have the potential to identify stage IV disease in a single examination (13,14). Hoh et al. (15) found that a whole-body PET-based staging algorithm may be an accurate and cost-effective method for staging lymphoma.

Physiologic Variants in Uptake of ^{18}F-FDG

Interpretation of PET scans performed for pediatric patients undergoing evaluation for lymphoma may be complicated by variable physiologic uptake of ^{18}F-FDG by the thymus gland, brown adipose tissue, skeletal muscle, and bone marrow. Recognition of normal variations in the biodistribution of ^{18}F-FDG is important in order to avoid misinterpreting normal findings as disease, as well as to avoid overlooking disease.

Thymus Uptake of FDG

The thymus gland, situated in the anterior mediastinum, is the primary site where T-cell lymphocytes differentiate and become functionally competent. The thymus gland weighs approximately 22g at birth and attains its peak weight of about 35g at puberty, after which time it decreases in size. Up to age 20, more than 80% of the gland is composed of lymphoid tissue. This tissue gradually is replaced by fatty infiltration, over time, and beyond the age of 40 only about 5% of the gland is morphologically lymphoid (16). During the first decade of life, the gland is usually quadrilateral in shape with convex lateral borders and a homogeneous appearance on CT. After age 10, the gland assumes a more triangular or arrowhead appearance. The normal thymus gradually decreases in size after puberty, becoming increasingly heterogeneous in appearance on CT because of progressive fatty infiltration (17,18).

Benign uptake of FDG may be seen in morphologically normal thymus glands as well as in thymic hyperplasia. Thymic uptake of FDG also occurs with malignancy, including lymphomatous infiltration, primary thymic neoplasms, and metastatic disease (19). Differentiating benign thymic uptake of ^{18}F-FDG from malignant infiltration is based on the intensity and configuration of tracer activity in combination with the morphologic appearance of the gland on CT (Figs. 12.1 and 12.2). Benign thymic uptake is situated in the retrosternal region and appears as an area of increased FDG activity, corresponding to the bilobed configuration of the thymus gland. The intensity of benign thymic uptake is variable. Although it tends to be mild and less than that which is seen with disease, the intensity of uptake may overlap with that of disease. For example, a maximum standard uptake value (SUV) of 3.8 was reported for physiologic thymic uptake occurring in a child following chemotherapy for osteosarcoma (20). Ferdinand et al. (19) suggest that although further research and experience are needed before identifying an upper SUV limit for physiologic thymic uptake, a maximum SUV above 4.0 may be cause to reconsider attributing anterior mediastinal uptake of ^{18}F-FDG to physiologic thymic uptake.

The incidence of benign thymic uptake is higher in younger patients with larger glands, although it may be seen well beyond puberty. One study reported that 32 of 94 patients, ranging in age from 18 to 29 years, exhibited physiologic thymic uptake of FDG (21). Benign thymic uptake of FDG is seen in children and young adults both before and after chemotherapy (22). This is in contrast to ^{67}Ga, which usually accumulates only in the thymus gland after chemotherapy and is indicative of thymic hyperplasia. In our experience with pediatric lymphoma patients, when thymic uptake of ^{18}F-FDG is seen following chemotherapy, it is identified within 2 to 12 months of chemotherapy and may persist for up to 18 months.

Brown Adipose Tissue and Skeletal Muscle Uptake of FDG

Nonpathologic, curvilinear cervical, and supraclavicular uptake of FDG, first described in 1996, originally was attributed to skeletal muscle, due to its fusiform configuration and because it usually resolved on repeat imaging after pretreatment with a muscle relaxant

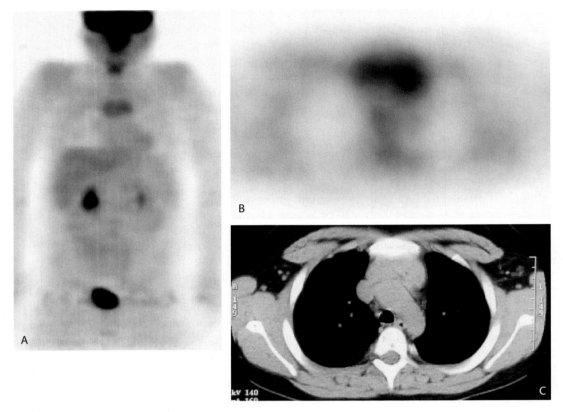

Figure 12.1. A chest x-ray (not shown) performed on a 13–year-old boy with a history of cough demonstrated a prominent mediastinum. The patient underwent positron emission tomography (PET) and computed tomography (CT) imaging with a presumptive diagnosis of lymphoma. There is mildly increased FDG uptake in the mediastinum on the PET image (A). An axial image (B) confirms the anterior location of this activity, which corresponds to a prominent but otherwise normal, thymus gland on CT (C). The child's cough resolved, and no additional workup was performed.

(diazepam) (23). With the introduction of inline hybrid PET-CT in 2001, it became apparent that bilateral curvilinear ^{18}F-FDG activity, with or without focal nodularity, extending from the neck to the supraclavicular regions and sometimes to the axillae, corresponded to adipose tissue in 2% to 4% of patients, and cervical musculature in 1% to 6% of patients studied (24–26). Benign, physiologic uptake of ^{18}F-FDG in perinephric fat, mediastinal fat, and unspecified tissue in the thoracic paravertebral region was also identified using inline hybrid PET-CT but in fewer patients and only in those patients who also demonstrated uptake in neck fat (26).

The intensity of physiologic ^{18}F-FDG uptake in adipose tissue and cervical/supraclavicular musculature is very variable with maximum standard uptake values (SUV$_{max}$) ranging from 1.9 to 20 and the average SUV$_{max}$ approximately 5 or greater, which is within the commonly accepted pathologic range (26). Adipose tissue uptake in the neck is seen predominantly in females, whereas uptake in normal musculature is more often seen in males. Of the 26 pediatric patients (<17 years old), four (15%) had fat uptake in the neck, in contrast to 16 of 837 (1.9%) adult patients who showed this pattern. Furthermore, normal muscle uptake was observed only in adult patients.

Fluorodeoxyglucose uptake by adipose tissue is attributed specifically to uptake by brown adipose tissue (BAT), which is capable of thermogenesis and is rich in mitochondria, sympathetic nerves, and adrenergic receptors. It is normally present in the neck, and near large vessels in the chest, axillae, perinephric regions, intercostal spaces along the spine, and in the paraaortic regions. It is more prominent in younger patients and in women, and it generates heat in

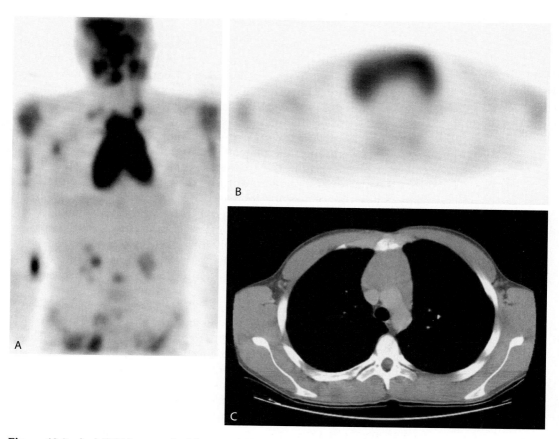

Figure 12.2. A: A PET image of a 16–year-old boy with stage IV T-cell lymphoblastic lymphoma shows numerous fluorodeoxyglucose (FDG)-avid lesions including a very large, hypermetabolic focus in the mediastinum. An axial image (B) shows the retrosternal location of this abnormality, which corresponds to lymphomatous infiltration of the thymus identified on the CT scan (C). Compare both the extent and intensity of thymic FDG uptake in this patient with lymphomatous involvement of the gland to that in the normal thymus gland in Figure 12.1.

response to cold exposure because it expresses a protein that causes uncoupling of oxidative phosphorylation in the mitochondria. This leads to the production of heat, rather than adenosine triphosphate (ATP). Thermogenesis by BAT requires increased glucose utilization (27).

Sympathetic stimulation results in increased BAT utilization of glucose. Benzodiazepines may reduce BAT uptake of FDG because they decrease anxiety, which leads to a decrease in sympathetic activity (Fig. 12.3). It also is possible that benzodiazepines have a direct action on the metabolism of BAT, as benzodiazepine receptors have been identified in BAT of rats (28,29). A recent report described resolution of benzodiazepine-resistant BAT uptake of FDG in response to temperature control, in two adolescent patients with a history of Hodgkin's lymphoma (30). In addition, a rodent study showed that propranolol and reserpine diminish BAT uptake of FDG (31).

Diffuse Bone Marrow Uptake of FDG

Diffuse bone marrow uptake of ^{18}F-FDG, regardless of intensity, usually reflects hypercellular bone marrow and not lymphomatous involvement. Nunez et al. (32) recently reviewed bone marrow and splenic uptake of FDG in 29 patients with HD, who had no evidence of marrow or splenic disease. These investigators found that there was a direct correlation between the intensity of marrow uptake and an increasing white cell count and an inverse correlation with hemoglobin and, to a lesser extent, with the platelet count; that is, the lower the hemoglobin or platelet count, the greater the marrow uptake of FDG. In all cases the marrow uptake was diffuse. The bone marrow is a metabolically active organ, and the increased FDG uptake reported by these investigators likely reflects increased metabolism and hence increased glucose consumption, by the bone marrow in response to hematologic stress. Thus the presence of diffusely increased bone marrow uptake at the time of diagnosis in patients with lymphoma should not be interpreted as evidence of marrow involvement with the disease (Fig. 12.4).

Treatment also affects bone marrow uptake of FDG, and treatment-induced metabolic changes in the bone marrow can be seen on PET studies during and after treatment for a variety of tumors. These changes do not appear to be due to chemotherapy; rather they are produced by hematopoietic cytokines, which alter the normal pattern of glucose metabolism in this organ (33). Granulocyte colony-stimulating factors (G-CSFs) and granulocyte–macrophage colony-stimulating factors (GM-CSFs) stimulate and support the proliferation of hematopoietic stem cells and mobilize stem cells into the peripheral blood. The increased proliferative activity is accompanied by increased blood flow to the bone marrow along with upregulation of glucose transport and metabolism (34). The effect of these agents on bone marrow uptake of FDG is both rapid and dramatic. In a series of 18 patients with melanoma and normal bone marrow, Yao et al. (34) reported that in patients receiving GM-CSF, the average glucose

Figure 12.3. A 9-year-old boy with newly diagnosed stage I B-cell non-Hodgkin's lymphoma (NHL). A: The initial PET scan was performed on an exceptionally cold winter day. Despite benzodiazepine (diazepam) pretreatment, there was extensive, intense FDG accumulation in the upper and lower cervical, supraclavicular, and pectoral regions bilaterally, as well as along the paravertebral regions of the thoracic spine. B: The PET scan was repeated 7 days later, using both diazepam and room temperature control. There is complete resolution of the activity seen in A. Faint anterior mediastinal activity represents thymic uptake of FDG. (No antineoplastic treatment was administered between the two studies.) Temperature control is useful in cases of benzodiazepine resistant BAT uptake of FDG.

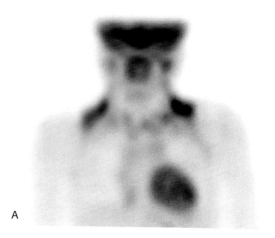

A

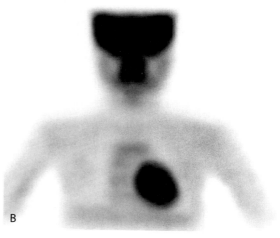

B

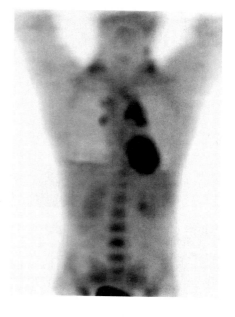

Figure 12.4. A PET image of a 14–year-old girl with stage IIIA nodular sclerosing Hodgkin's disease (HD) shows disease in the neck, mediastinum, and abdomen. There is homogeneous, prominent marrow activity. Bone marrow biopsy was negative for disease. The bone marrow is a metabolically active organ, and diffusely increased FDG uptake reflects increased metabolism, and hence increased glucose consumption, in response to hematologic stress. This pattern should not be interpreted as indicative of diffuse marrow disease.

metabolic rate on the third day of treatment was 97% above baseline, and on the 10th day of treatment was an average of 170% above baseline. Three days after completion of GM-CSF therapy, the glucose metabolic rate of the marrow had decreased to 60% above baseline but remained elevated significantly above baseline for more than 3 weeks after cessation of treatment. In contrast, the magnitude of change was more modest in patients receiving macrophage-CSF (M-CSF), perhaps because granulocytes and their precursors comprise about 60% of the marrow versus only about 2% to 5% for monocytes/macrophages. Thus, diffusely increased marrow activity soon after CSF therapy should be recognized as a manifestation of hypermetabolic bone marrow, rather than diffuse metastatic disease.

Granulocyte colony-stimulating factor exerts similar effects on splenic uptake of FDG. Sugawara et al. (35) reported substantially increased FDG uptake by the spleen during and after G-CSF treatment in patients with locally advanced breast carcinoma. This increase was less frequent and less marked, however, than the changes in the bone marrow of the same patients (Fig. 12.5).

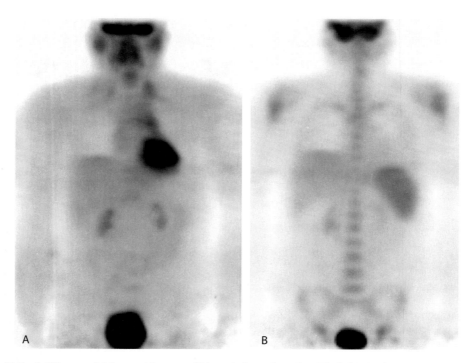

Figure 12.5. A 17-year-old boy with stage IIA nodular sclerosing Hodgkin's disease. A: Pretreatment PET demonstrates FDG uptake in the left neck and mediastinum. B: On the follow-up PET, performed after two cycles of chemotherapy, the neck and mediastinal abnormalities have resolved. There is homogeneously increased FDG activity in the bone marrow and spleen. Increased marrow and splenic activity, which is often observed after treatment in patients with lymphoma, is due to the effects of colony-stimulating factors on the hematopoietic system.

With the proliferation of cytokine use in patients with malignancies and with the increasing use of FDG-PET in oncology, hypermetabolic bone marrow is likely to be observed with increasing frequency and should not be confused with diffuse bone marrow disease. This physiologically increased bone marrow activity, unfortunately, results in increased background activity, which can potentially mask foci of disease. Thus, whenever possible, a sufficient amount of time between treatment and imaging should elapse to facilitate the differentiation of hypermetabolic from diseased marrow.

Initial Staging

Studies comparing imaging modalities in patients with lymphoma have common methodologic problems because biopsy is performed in only a small number of lymph nodes and thus histologic confirmation of results is limited. Typically, once the diagnosis is made, additional sites are biopsied only when the results of biopsy influence staging or treatment. These limitations notwithstanding, it has been shown that PET is a useful adjunct in the initial staging of lymphoma.

Nodal Staging

Newman et al. (36) compared PET and CT in thoracoabdominal lymphoma. They reported that PET identified a total of 54 sites of disease in the 16 patients studied, including all 49 sites identified by CT and five additional sites not identified on CT. In 60 patients with untreated lymphoma, Moog et al. (10) reported that both PET and CT were abnormal in 160 of the 740 sites evaluated. Seven of 25 additional sites detected only on PET were confirmed to be disease. There were two false-positive sites and 16 unresolved sites. Of six sites detected only on CT, three were false positives and three were unresolved. In this series, PET was more sensitive and specific than CT. Jerusalem et al. (37) compared PET and conventional nodal staging results in 60 patients. In this series PET identified additional nodal disease sites in 15 patients, including 10 with high-grade lymphoma. Conventional staging methods, CT, and physical examination detected PET-negative sites in 11 patients, seven of whom had low-grade lymphoma. These investigators concluded that PET is complementary to, and not a substitute for, conventional staging methods.

Recently, Rini et al. (38) compared PET and gallium imaging in children and young adults, 5 to 23 years old, with newly diagnosed, untreated HD. The PET studies were performed using a coincidence detection system with measured attenuation correction. Gallium imaging included planar whole-body imaging and single photon emission computed tomography (SPECT) from the top of the ears to the mid-thighs. There were 118 sites of nodal disease in this population, 105 (89%) of which were supradiaphragmatic. Positron emission tomography was slightly more sensitive overall (89%) than gallium (86%). Both tests were equally sensitive (89%) for supradiaphragmatic nodal disease. Not surprisingly, PET was more sensitive (77%, 10/13) than gallium (54%, 7/13) for infradiaphragmatic disease (Fig. 12.6).

Extranodal Staging

Moog et al. (39) compared PET and CT for detecting extranodal disease in 81 patients. The studies detected 42 extranodal sites; PET identified 19 sites that were not identified on CT. Fourteen of the sites were subsequently confirmed to be lymphoma: bone marrow (nine), spleen (three), other (two). There were seven extranodal lesions seen only on CT, only one of which proved to be diseased. There were five false-positive lesions, and one was not resolved. Jerusalem et al. (37) found a high rate of agreement between PET and CT in the liver, spleen, and digestive tract. In 30 patients with Hodgkin's disease, Rini et al. (38) found that PET detected 15 (75%) of 20 extranodal sites of disease, whereas gallium detected only seven (35%). Although the sensitivity of both tests was similar for lung and bone disease, PET was significantly more sensitive than gallium for detecting splenic disease (Fig. 12.6).

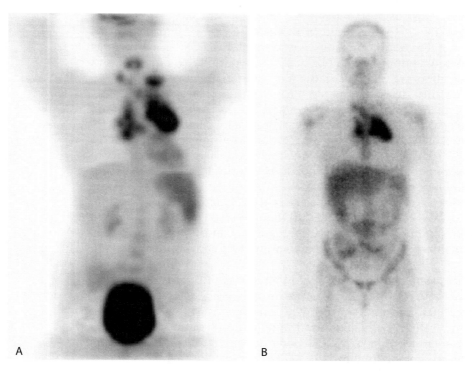

A   B

Figure 12.6. A 16-year-old girl with stage IVB nodular sclerosing HD and laparoscopically confirmed splenic disease. PET (A) shows extensive supraclavicular and mediastinal disease that also is well seen on gallium (B). Splenic disease is clearly seen on PET but not on gallium.

Based on available data, PET is superior to bone scintigraphy for detecting lymphomatous involvement of the bone. Moog et al. (40) studied 56 patients with both PET and bone scintigraphy. Skeletal involvement was detected by both methods in 12 patients. Positron emission tomography identified disease in an additional three patients with negative bone scans. Bone scintigraphy, in contrast, failed to detect any patients with osseous involvement who were not identified with PET (Fig. 12.7).

The results of PET for detecting lymphomatous involvement of the marrow have been variable. In one series, PET correctly identified only 13 of 21 (62% sensitivity) patients with biopsy-proven marrow involvement. Three patients with positive PET studies had negative biopsies (37). In another investigation, PET results agreed with marrow biopsy results in 39 of 50 (78%) patients. There were eight false-positive and three false- negative PET studies (41). In yet another series, PET and marrow biopsies were concordant in 64 (82%) of 78 patients, concordant and positive in seven patients, and concordant and negative in 57 patients. The two tests were discordant in 14 (18%) patients. Among the discordant results, PET was false negative in four patients and true positive in eight patients. In two patients, the discordant results were unresolved. Among the eight patients with true-positive PET/false-negative marrow biopsies, the abnormalities on the radionuclide study were focal and remote from the biopsy site (42). Thus, at the present time, PET is complementary to, but not a substitute for, marrow biopsy. Biopsy is probably more sensitive for diffuse marrow disease, whereas the radionuclide test is useful for identifying focal disease remote from the biopsy site.

Lymphomatous involvement of the spleen is characterized by one or more tumor nodules, often less than 1cm in diameter. Although marked splenomegaly almost always indicates tumor involvement, lymphomatous spleens frequently are normal in size, and modestly enlarged spleens often do not contain tumor (43). Computed tomography, which traditionally has been used to evaluate the spleen, is associated with large numbers of false-positive and false-negative results, with reported accuracies ranging from 37% to 91% (44,45). Aygun et al. (46) reported that in 17 patients with HD who underwent staging laparotomy, the sensitivity and specificity of the CT-derived splenic index, for detecting splenic disease, were 50% and 66%, respectively. The positive and negative predictive values of the test were 57% and 60%, respectively. Indeed, for patients with lymphoma, in whom therapy would be altered if splenic disease were encountered, surgical evaluation of the spleen may be required. Because of the morbidity and potential complications associated with surgery, a noninvasive technique capable of reliably assessing the spleen in these patients would be of considerable value.

Recent studies have shown that PET accurately characterizes the spleen in patients undergoing initial staging of lymphoma. For patients with newly diagnosed, untreated HD or NHL, the presence of diffuse or focal splenic uptake of FDG more intense than hepatic uptake sug-

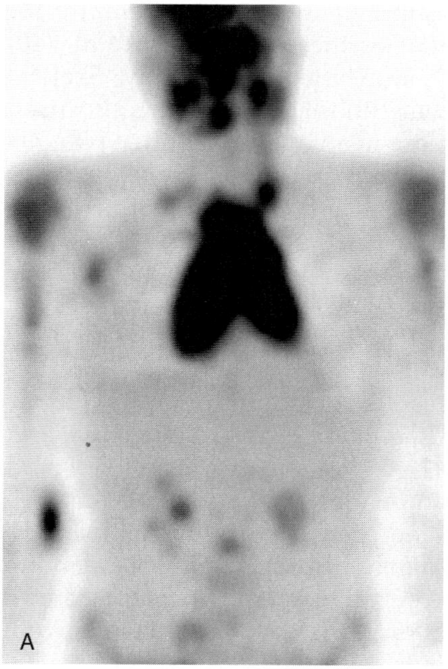

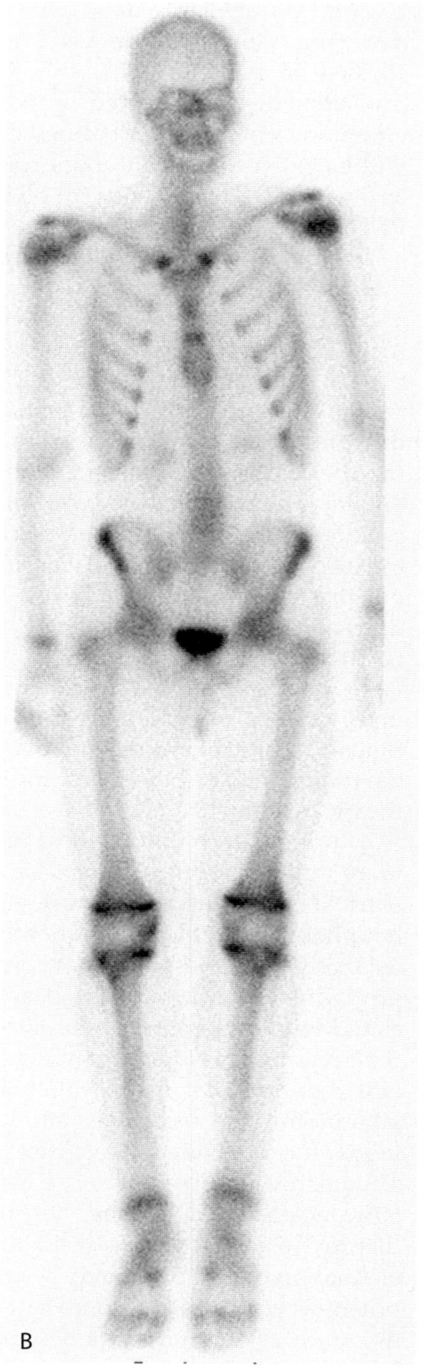

Figure 12.7. A 16-year-old boy with stage IV T-cell lymphoblastic lymphoma (same patient illustrated in Fig. 12.2). A: In addition to the FDG-avid soft tissue lesions on the PET scan, there are numerous bony lesions in the humeri, mid-lumbar spine and the pelvis. B: On the bone scan, however, only the proximal left humeral lesion is identified.

gests lymphomatous involvement (47,48). Application of these criteria to PET studies performed in children and adults with recently diagnosed HD or NHL yielded overall accuracies of 97% and 100% (47,48). Positron emission tomography was more accurate than CT (100% versus 57%) using a positive CT-derived splenic index or splenic hypodensities as the criterion for a positive CT scan (48). Positron emission tomography also was more accurate than gallium (97% versus 78%), with the criterion for a positive gallium study being splenic uptake of gallium at least as intense as hepatic uptake (47). In a series of 30 children and young adults with newly diagnosed HD, Rini et al. (38) reported that PET was significantly more accurate than gallium (93% versus 67%) for detecting splenic disease. Among four patients who underwent surgical staging (two with splenic disease and two without), the accuracy of PET was 100%. Gallium was negative in all four patients including both with splenic disease, for an accuracy of 50%. The CT-derived splenic index was correct in only one patient (25% accuracy). Computed tomography was false negative in one patient with disease and false positive in two patients without disease (Figs. 12.8 and 12.9).

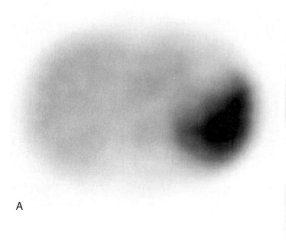

A

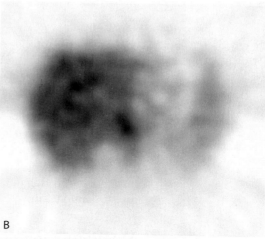

B

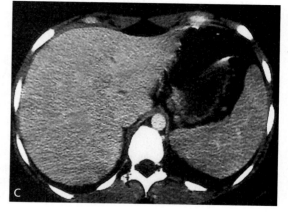

C

Figure 12.8. A 16-year-old girl with stage IVB nodular sclerosing HD and laparoscopically confirmed splenic disease (same patient illustrated in Fig. 12.6). A: On the PET image, the intense splenic uptake of FDG exceeds that of the liver. B: On the gallium scan, splenic uptake is less intense than hepatic uptake, that is, normal. C: On the CT scan, the spleen is normal in size with homogeneous parenchyma. The splenic index was 780 mL (normal for age ≤ 820 mL). [*Source:* Rini et al. (47), with permission of *Clinical Nuclear Medicine.*]

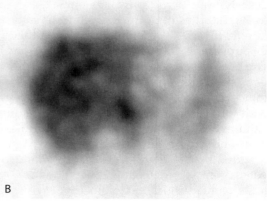

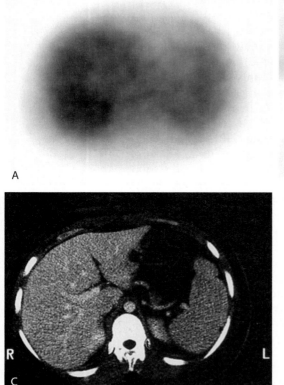

Figure 12.9. A 17-year-old boy with stage IIA nodular sclerosing HD. PET (A) and gallium (B) studies are negative for splenic disease. On the CT scan (C), the spleen is enlarged. The splenic index was 1250 mL (normal ≤ 840 mL). [*Source:* Rini et al. (47), with permission of *Clinical Nuclear Medicine.*]

With the development of increasingly sophisticated noninvasive diagnostic techniques, the need for surgical staging of lymphoma has decreased steadily. The use of PET to evaluate the spleen in patients undergoing initial staging of lymphoma may further reduce the need for surgical staging.

Monitoring the Response to Therapy

Response to Treatment after Completion of Therapy

Evaluation of the treatment response is an important part of the management of lymphoma. Accurate identification of residual viable tumor following completion of therapy facilitates the initiation of salvage therapy earlier in the course of the disease, rather than waiting for clinical evidence of disease relapse. Incomplete resolution of a lymphomatous mass after treatment is a significant problem in the patient with lymphoma. Although residual abnormalities occur in more than 60% of patients with lymphoma, viable tumor is present in less than 20% of these masses (49). There are no reliable CT or magnetic resonance imaging (MRI) criteria for differentiating residual disease from fibrosis or necrosis. Gallium imaging has for many years been the standard imaging test for posttreatment evaluation of patients with lymphoma. There are data that suggest that PET may be superior to gallium for the posttreatment assessment of patients with lymphoma. The positive and negative predictive values of the test range between 70% and 100% and 83% and 100%, respectively. Cremerius et al. (50), in a study of 27 patients, found that PET correctly identified all 15 patients with residual disease or relapse, and 11 of 12 patients who remained disease-free; PET was significantly more accurate than CT in this population (Fig. 12.10).

Spaepen et al. (51) evaluated 93 patients with NHL after treatment. Nine patients with negative PET scans received additional therapy based on abnormal CT results. Fifty-eight patients with negative PET scans remained in complete remission during a median follow-up period of 21 months. Twenty-six patients had persistently abnormal PET scans at the end of treatment and all of them relapsed. It is important to note that in 14 (54%) of these 26 patients only PET demonstrated evidence of disease.

Jerusalem et al. (52) compared FDG-PET and CT in the posttreatment evaluation of patients with lymphoma. Residual masses were present on CT in 24 (44%) of 54 patients. All six patients in whom both PET and CT were abnormal relapsed, whereas only five of 19 patients with abnormal CT and normal PET scans relapsed. Three of 29 patients in whom CT and PET were both normal relapsed. The positive predictive values for relapse of PET and CT were 100% and 42%, respectively. These investigators also found that a positive PET scan after treatment was associated with poor survival. The 1-year progression-free survival of patients with positive PET studies after treatment was 0%, whereas the 1-year progression-free survival of patients with negative PET studies after treatment was 86%.

Guay et al. (53) reviewed the prognostic value of posttreatment PET in 48 patients with HD. These investigators found that the sensitivity and specificity of PET to predict relapse in the population studied were 79% and 97%, respectively, and the positive and negative predictive values of the test both were 92%. The 92% diagnostic accuracy of PET was significantly higher than the 56% diagnostic accuracy of CT.

Depas et al. (54) evaluated 16 children with lymphoma after completion of treatment. The PET studies were true negative in 15 patients and false positive in one patient (94% specificity). In contrast, conventional methods were false positive in seven patients (56% specificity).

Zinzani et al. (55) reviewed the results of 44 patients with abdominal lymphoma at the end of treatment. In this investigation, none of the seven patients with negative PET and negative CT scans relapsed. Twenty-four patients had abnormal CT scans and normal PET scans; only one relapsed. All 13 patients in whom both PET *and* CT scans were abnormal relapsed.

The results of these investigations illustrate the importance of including PET studies in the evaluation of patients following treatment of lymphoma. These data also suggest that it may be possible, on the basis of the combined results of PET and CT, to stratify patients into risk

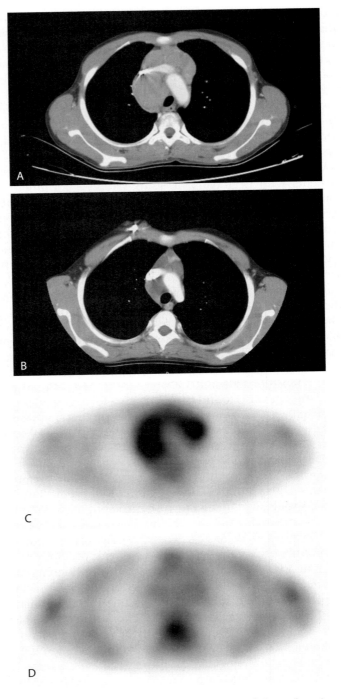

Figure 12.10. A 14-year-old boy with stage IIIB nodular sclerosing HD. A: Extensive mediastinal lymphadenopathy is present on the pretreatment CT scan. B: There is residual lymphadenopathy on the posttreatment CT scan, and it is not possible to differentiate persistent disease from fibrosis. C: There is extensive metabolically active disease on the pretreatment PET scan. D: There is complete resolution of the mediastinal activity on the posttreatment PET scan, however, confirming that the residual adenopathy present on the post-treatment CT scan did not contain viable tumor.

groups for relapse. Patients in whom both studies are abnormal would be at highest risk, whereas those in whom both studies were negative would be at lowest risk for relapse.

Neither PET nor any other currently available imaging technique can exclude the possibility of subsequent relapse, because of an inherent inability to detect microscopic foci of disease. Although the ability of PET to detect residual disease is now well documented, the benefits of additional therapies given on the basis of the PET findings remain to be determined. Finally, the effectiveness of FDG-PET to detect residual disease in the various subgroups of HD and NHL must also be determined.

Predicting Response During Therapy

Early recognition of ineffective treatment would allow prompt initiation of a potentially more effective therapeutic regimen. Initial studies indicate that, in patients with lymphoma, PET can distinguish responders from nonresponders early in the course of treatment (Fig. 12.11). Jerusalem et al. (56) evaluated patients after a median three courses of chemotherapy and found that all patients who had negative PET scans went into complete remission, whereas only one of five patients with persistent abnormal activity on PET scans went into complete remission. Hoekstra et al. (57) reported that PET scans were normal after two cycles of chemotherapy in patients who eventually achieved complete remission. Treatment failures, in contrast, were associated with high uptake on the PET scans, and a variable outcome was associated with low-level uptake. Although Romer et al. (58) observed markedly decreased tumor uptake as early as 7 days after commencement of chemotherapy, these investigators found that uptake at 42 days, just before the third cycle of chemotherapy, was a better predictor of long-term outcome than FDG uptake at 7 days. Kostakoglu et al. (59) reported that PET has a high prognostic value for evaluation of response after one cycle of therapy in aggressive NHL and HD. Ninety percent of patients with abnormal PET studies after one cycle of treatment had relapse of their disease, with a median progression-free survival of 5 months. Eighty-five patients with negative FDG-PET studies after one cycle remained in complete remission for at least 18 months. All but one patient who had abnormal PET scans after one cycle and after completion of therapy relapsed. Finally, in this investigation the relapse rate for patients with negative PET scans after completion of treatment was 35%, whereas in patients with negative PET scans after one cycle, the relapse rate was 15%.

Depas et al. (54) performed PET scans on 19 children at various times during treatment; PET was negative in all 19 patients. Three patients had an incomplete response to treatment, and PET failed to identify any of them.

In summary, in patients with lymphoma, PET is predictive of response to therapy after, as well as during, treatment. A negative PET result early in the course of treatment suggests that these patients could probably complete a full course of their first-line treatment. Patients

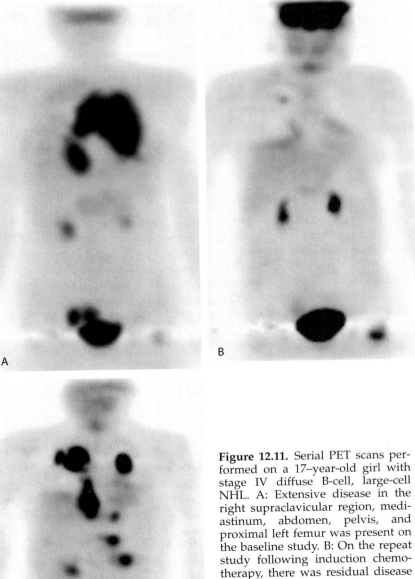

Figure 12.11. Serial PET scans performed on a 17–year-old girl with stage IV diffuse B-cell, large-cell NHL. A: Extensive disease in the right supraclavicular region, mediastinum, abdomen, pelvis, and proximal left femur was present on the baseline study. B: On the repeat study following induction chemotherapy, there was residual disease in the chest pelvis, and left femur. The finding on PET of an incomplete response to treatment suggests that more aggressive treatment is needed and is indicative of a poor prognosis. Based on the PET results, therapy was changed in this patient. C: A subsequent PET scan, unfortunately, demonstrated progression of disease to which the patient eventually succumbed.

with positive PET results during treatment have a less favorable prognosis and could be switched to more aggressive therapy, including stem cell transplantation, sooner, with the hope of achieving a more favorable outcome.

Routine Follow-Up in Asymptomatic Patients

Few data are available on the role of PET in the routine follow-up of asymptomatic patients after treatment. Depas et al. (54) reviewed the results of 59 PET scans performed in 19 children with lymphoma who were in long-term remission. Fifty-six of the 59 studies were true negative, and three were false positive: atrial uptake, asymmetric thymic uptake, and axillary adenitis. In contrast there were 20 false-positive results using conventional methods.

In a series of 36 patients with HD, patients were imaged at 4- to 6-month intervals for up to 3 years after completion of therapy (60). Patients who demonstrated abnormal FDG accumulation underwent repeat PET imaging 4 to 6 weeks later. One patient had residual disease and four patients relapsed. All five were detected with PET prior to their detection with clinical examination, laboratory tests, or CT. Six patients had false-positive PET scans, but the confirmatory PET scan was always negative. These investigators concluded that PET could help identify patients needing salvage chemotherapy prior to the appearance of clinically overt disease.

Conclusion

Fluorodeoxyglucose-PET is a powerful new tool in the management of children with lymphoma. It is complementary to conventional imaging studies in the staging of the disease, and it is extremely useful for monitoring response to therapy. Although more investigation is needed, this technique at the end of therapy can, together with CT, potentially stratify patients into risk groups for relapse. Equally exciting is the potential ability of FDG-PET to identify nonresponders early in the course of their treatment, facilitating a change in their management sooner rather than later, with the anticipation of improved survival.

References

1. Jemal A, Tiwari RC, Murray T, et al. Cancer statistics, 2004. CA Cancer J Clin 2004;54:8–25.
2. Bleyer A. Older adolescents with cancer in North America: deficits in outcome and research. Pediatr Clin North Am 2004;49:1027–1042.
3. Kennedy BJ, Fremgen AM, Menck HR. Hodgkin's disease survival by stage and age. J Am Geriatr Soc 2000;48:315–317.
4. Lister TA, Crowther D, Sutcliffe SB, et al. Report of a committee convened to discuss the evaluation and staging of patients with Hodgkin's Disease: Cotswolds Meeting. J Clin Oncol 1989;7:1630–1636.
5. Moog F, Bangerter M, Diederichs CG, et al. Lymphoma: role of whole-body 2–deoxy-2–[F-18]fluoro-D-glucose (FDG) PET in nodal staging. Radiology 1997;203:795–800.

6. Percy CL, Smith MA, Linet M, et al. Lymphoma and reticuloendothelial neoplasms, In: Ries LA, Smith MA, Gurney JG, et al., eds. Cancer Incidence and Survival Among Children and Adolescents: US SEER Program 1975–1995. NIH Publication No. 99–4649. Bethesda, MD: National Cancer Institute, 1999:35–50.

7. Harris N, Jaffe E, Stein H, et al. A revised European-American classification of lymphoid neoplasms: a proposal from the International Study Group. Blood 1994;84:1361–1392.

8. Harris N, Jaffe E, Diebold J, et al. World Health Organization classification of neoplastic diseases of the hematopoietic and lymphoid tissues: report of the clinical advisory committee meeting—Airlie House, Virginia, November 1997. J Clin Oncol 1999;17:3835–3849.

9. Murphy SB, Fairclough DL, Hutchison RE, et al: Non-Hodgkin's lymphomas of childhood: an analysis of the histology, staging, and response to treatment of 338 cases at a single institution. J Clin Oncol 1989;7:186–193.

10. Moog F, Bangerter M, Diederichs CG, et al. Lymphoma: role of whole-body 2–deoxy-2–[F-18]fluoro-D-glucose (FDG) PET in nodal staging. Radiology 1997;203:795–800.

11. Kostakoglu L, Goldsmith SJ. Fluorine-18 fluorodeoxyglucose positron emission tomography in the staging and follow-up of lymphoma: is it time to shift gears? Eur J Nucl Med 2000;27:1564–1578.

12. Rehm PK. Radionuclide evaluation of patients with lymphoma. Radiol Clin North Am 2001;39:957–978.

13. Parkhurst JB, Foster P, Johnson SF, et al. Upstaging of non-Hodgkin's lymphoma in a child based on 67 gallium scintigraphy. J Pediatr Hematol Oncol 1998;20:174–176.

14. Anderson KC, Leonard RC, Canellos GP, et al. High-dose gallium imaging in lymphoma. Am J Med 1983;75:327–331.

15. Hoh CK, Glaspy J, Rosen P, et al. Whole-body FDG-PET imaging for staging of Hodgkin's disease and Lymphoma. J Nucl Med 1997;38:343–348.

16. Parslow TG. Lymphocytes and lymphoid tissue. In: Sites DP, Terr AI, Parslow TG, eds. Basic and Clinical Immunology. Norwalk, CT: Appleton and Lange, 1994:22–40.

17. Francis IR, Glazer GM, Bookstein FL, et al. The thymus: reexamination of age-related changes in size and shape. AJR 1984;145:249–254.

18. Baron RL, Lee JKT, Sagel SS, et al. Computed tomography of the normal thymus. Radiology 1982;142:121–125.

19. Ferdinand B, Gupta P, Kramer EL. Spectrum of thymic uptake at 18F-FDG PET. RadioGraphics 2004;24:1611–1616.

20. Brink I, Reinhardt MJ, Hoegerle S, et al. Increased metabolic activity in the thymus studied with FDG PET: age dependency and frequency after chemotherapy. J Nucl Med 2001;42:591–595.

21. Nakahara T, Fujii H, Ide M, et al. FDG uptake in the morphologically normal thymus: comparison of FDG positron emission tomography and CT. Br J Radiol 2001;74:821–824.

22. Rini JN, Leonidas JC, Tomas MB, Chen B, Karaylcin G, Palestro CJ. ^{18}F-FDG uptake in the anterior mediastinum: Physiologic thymic uptake or disease? Clin Positron Imaging 2000;3:115–125.

23. Barrington SF, Maisey MN. Skeletal muscle uptake of fluorine-18–FDG: effect of oral diazepam. J Nucl Med 1996;37:1127–1129.

24. Cohade C, Osman M, Pannu HK, et al. Uptake in supraclavicular area fat ("USA-Fat"): description on 18F-FDG PET/CT. J Nucl Med 2003;44:170–176.

25. Hany T, Gharehpapagh E, Kamel E, et al. Brown adipose tissue: a factor to consider in symmetrical tracer uptake in the neck and upper chest region. Eur J Nucl Med Mol Imaging 2002;29:1393–1398.

26. Yeung HWD, Grewal RK, Gonen M, et al. Patterns of 18F-FDG uptake in adipose tissue and muscle: a potential source of false-positives for PET. J Nucl Med 2003;44:1789–1796.

27. Himms-Hagen J. Thermogenesis in brown adipose tissue as an energy buffer. N Engl J Med 1984;311:1549–1558.

28. Anholt R, de Souza E, Oster-Granite M, Snyder S. Peripheral-type benzodiazepine receptors: autoradiographics localization in whole-body sections of neonatal rats. J Pharmacol Exp Ther 1985;233:517–526.

29. Hirsch J. Pharmacological and physiological properties of benzodiazepine binding sites in rodent brown adipose tissue. Comp Biochem Physiol [C] 1984;77:339–343.

30. Garcia CA, Van Nostrand D, Majd M, et al. Benzodiazepine-resistant "brown fat" pattern in positron emission tomography: two case reports of resolution with temperature control. Mol Imaging Biol 2004;6:368–372.

31. Tatsumi M, Engles JM, Ishimori T, et al. Intense ^{18}F-FDG uptake in brown fat can be reduced pharmacologically. J Nucl Med 2004;45:1189–1193.

32. Nunez RF, Rini JN, Tronco GG, et al. Correlacion de los parametros hematologicos con la captacion de FDG en medula osea y bazo en la PET. Rev Esp Med Nucl 2005;24:107–112.

33. Sugawara Y, Fisher SJ, Zasadny KR, et al. Preclinical and clinical studies of bone marrow uptake of fluorine-1–fluorodeoxyglucose with or without granulocyte colony-stimulating factor during chemotherapy. J Clin Oncol 1998;16:173–180.

34. Yao W-J, Hoh CK, Hawkins RA, et al. Quantitative PET imaging of bone marrow glucose metabolic response to hematopoietic cytokines. J Nucl Med 1995;36:794–799.

35. Sugawara Y, Zasadny KR, Kison PV, et al. Splenic fluorodeoxyglucose uptake increased by granulocyte colony-stimulating factor therapy: PET imaging results. J Nucl Med 1999;40:1456–1462.

36. Newman JS, Francis IR, Kaminski MS, et al. Imaging of lymphoma with PET with 2–[F-18]-fluoro-2–deoxy-D-glucose: correlation with CT. Radiology 1994;190:111–116.

37. Jerusalem G, Warland V, Najjar F, et al. Whole-body 18F-FDG PET for the evaluation of patients with Hodgkin's disease and non-Hodgkin's lymphoma. Nucl Med Commun 1999;20:13–20.

38. Rini JN, Nunez R., Nichols K, et al. Coincidence-detection FDG-PET versus gallium in children and young adults with newly diagnosed Hodgkin's Disease. Pediatr Radiol 2005;35:169–178.

39. Moog F, Bangerter M, Diederichs CG, et al. Extranodal malignant lymphoma: detection with FDG PET versus CT. Radiology 1998;206:475–481.

40. Moog F, Kotzerke J, Reske SN. FDG PET can replace bone scintigraphy in primary staging of malignant lymphoma. J Nucl Med 1999;40:1407–1413.

41. Carr R, Barrington SF, Madan B, et al. Detection of lymphoma in bone marrow by whole-body positron emission tomography. Blood 1998;91:3340–3346.

42. Moog F, Bangerter M, Kotzerke J, et al. 18–F-fluorodeoxyglucose-positron emission tomography as a new approach to detect lymphomatous bone marrow. J Clin Oncol 1998;16:603–609.

43. Castellino RA. Hodgkin disease: practical concepts for the diagnostic radiologist. Radiology 1986;159:305–310.

44. Strijk SP, Wagener DJ, Bogman MJ, et al. The spleen in Hodgkin disease: diagnostic value of CT. Radiology 1985;154:753–757.

45. Munker R, Stengel A, Stabler A, Hiller E, Brehm G. Diagnostic accuracy of ultrasound and computed tomography in the staging of Hodgkin's disease. Verification by laparotomy in 100 cases. Cancer 1995;76:1460–1466.

46. Aygun B, Karakas SP, Leonidas J, et al. Reliability of splenic index to assess splenic involvement in pediatric Hodgkin's Disease. J Pediatr Hematol Oncol 2004;26:74–76.

47. Rini JN, Manalili EY, Hoffman MA, et al. The utility of 18FDG and 67Ga for the detection of splenic involvement in Hodgkin's disease. Clin Nucl Med 2002;27:572–577.

48. Rini JN, Leonidas JC, Tomas MB, et al. FDG PET versus CT for evaluating the spleen during initial staging of lymphoma. J Nucl Med 2003;44: 1072–1074.

49. Kostakoglu L, Goldsmith SJ. 18F-FDG PET for evaluation of the response to therapy for lymphoma, and for breast, lung, and colorectal carcinoma. J Nucl Med 2003;44:224–239.

50. Cremerius U, Fabry U, Neuerburg J, et al. Positron emission tomography with 18F-FDG to detect residual disease after therapy for malignant lymphoma. Nucl Med Commun 1998;19:1055–1063.

51. Spaepen K, Stroobants S, Dupont P, et al. Prognostic value of positron emission tomography (PET) with fluorine-18 fluorodeoxyglucose ([18F]FDG) after first-line chemotherapy in non-Hodgkin's lymphoma: is [18F]FDG-PET a valid alternative to conventional diagnostic methods? J Clin Oncol 2001;19:414–419.

52. Jerusalem G, Beguin Y, Fassotte MF, et al. Whole-body positron emission tomography using 18F-fluorodeoxyglucose for posttreatment evaluation in Hodgkin's disease and non-Hodgkin's lymphoma has higher diagnostic and prognostic value than classical computed tomography scan imaging. Blood 1999;94:429–433.

53. Guay C, Lepine M, Verreault J, et al. Prognostic value of PET using 18F-FDG in Hodgkin's disease for posttreatment evaluation. J Nucl Med 2003;44(8):1225–1231.

54. Depas G, De Barsy C, Jerusalem G, et al. 18F-FDG PET in children with lymphomas. Eur J Nucl Med Mol Imaging 2005;32:31–38.

55. Zinzani PL, Magagnoli M, Chierichetti F, et al. The role of positron emission tomography (PET) in the management of lymphoma patients. Ann Oncol 1999;10:1181–1184.

56. Jerusalem G, Beguin Y, Fassotte MF, et al. Persistent tumor 18F-FDG uptake after a few cycles of polychemotherapy is predictive of treatment failure in non-Hodgkin's lymphoma. Haematologica 2000;85:613–618.

57. Hoekstra OS, Ossenkoppele GJ, Golding R, et al. Early treatment response in malignant lymphoma, as determined by planar fluorine-18–fluorodeoxyglucose scintigraphy. J Nucl Med 1993;34:1706–1710.

58. Romer W, Hanauske AR, Ziegler S, et al. Positron emission tomography in non-Hodgkin's lymphoma: assessment of chemotherapy with fluorodeoxyglucose. Blood 1998;91:4464–4471.

59. Kostakoglu L, Coleman M, Leonard JP, et al. PET predicts prognosis after 1 cycle of chemotherapy in aggressive lymphoma and Hodgkin's disease. J Nucl Med 2002;43:1018–1027.

60. Jerusalem G, Beguin Y, Fassotte MF, et al. Early detection of relapse by whole-body positron emission tomography in the follow-up of patients with Hodgkin's disease. Ann Oncol 2003;14:123–130.

13

Neuroblastoma

Barry L. Shulkin

Neuroblastoma is the most common extracranial solid tumor of childhood. It comprises 8% to 10% of all childhood neoplasms. Neuroblastoma is derived from primordial neural crest cells that normally differentiate into the sympathetic nervous system. The prevalence is about 1 case per 7000 newborns. There are about 600 new cases in the United States per year, and over 90% occur in children less than 6 years old. The median age is 22 months. Most primary tumors occur within the abdomen, especially the adrenal gland, although they may arise from any site along the course of the sympathetic nervous system. Other common sites are paraspinal ganglia of the posterior mediastinum and abdomen. About 60% of patients have widely metastatic osseous disease at presentation.

Related to their origin from precursor cells of the sympathetic nervous system, most of these tumors are associated with high urinary levels of catecholamine metabolites, such as vanillylmandelic acid formed from norepinephrine, homovanillic acid formed from dopamine, or dopamine. Occasionally the tumor may cause hypertension (1).

The prognosis of patients with neuroblastoma depends on the histopathologic system developed by Shimada et al. (2). This incorporates the patient's age, the presence or absence of Schwann cell stroma, the degree of differentiation, and the mitosis-karyorrhexis index (number of mitoses and ruptured cell nuclei).

Staging is based on the International Neuroblastoma Staging System (INSS) (3). In general, stage 1 is a localized tumor without regional lymph node involvement, stage 2 is a unilateral tumor with either incomplete gross resection or ipsilateral nodal involvement, stage 3 is tumor that crosses the midline or has contralateral nodal involvement, and stage 4 is tumor disseminated to distant nodes, bone, bone marrow, liver, etc. Stage 4s is a special category of infants less than 1 year of age with a localized primary tumor and dissemination only to liver, skin, or bone marrow.

Meta-Iodobenzylguanidine (mIBG)

Any discussion of functional imaging of neuroblastoma is incomplete without reference to meta-iodobenzylguanidine (mIBG). This is the conventional agent for functional imaging of neuroblastoma. This agent was originally applied to the localization of pheochromocytoma. Sisson and colleagues (4) demonstrated its utility in the management of patients with pheochromocytoma. Its use in neuroblastoma followed shortly (5,6). This agent requires the presence of a functional type 1 catecholamine uptake system. Within the sympathetic nervous system, type 1 catecholamine uptake transports the neurotransmitter norepinephrine from the synaptic cleft back into the presynaptic nerve terminal. This serves to terminate neurotransmission until norepinephrine is once again released into the synaptic cleft. Functional imaging with mIBG takes advantage of the adrenergic origin of neuroblastoma. mIBG is taken up by and concentrated within most neuroblastomas both in vivo and in vitro. mIBG exists within both the cytoplasm and specialized norepinephrine storage granules. Most of the agents we will discuss also depend on type 1 catecholamine uptake for transport into neuroblastoma cells. mIBG can be labeled with the various isotopes of iodine. Iodine-131 (^{131}I) mIBG was the first agent developed by Wieland and colleagues (7). Its use in the imaging of pheochromocytoma was reported by Sisson. mIBG was soon labeled with ^{123}I. For many years, only ^{131}I mIBG was available commercially in the United States although ^{123}I mIBG was available in Europe. However, many pediatric centers in the United States used ^{123}I mIBG, which was synthesized on site for local use only. Now ^{123}I mIBG is available widely within the United States, and it is expected that it will soon be approved by the Food and Drug Administration (FDA) for use in children.

High-quality images can be obtained using ^{131}I mIBG with careful attention to detail (8). Serial images are usually obtained 24, 48, and sometimes 72 hours after injection of 0.5 to 1 mCi reduced by child weight or body surface area. Images of the entire body are recommended at 20 minutes per bed position using a high-energy collimator. The dose of ^{131}I mIBG is limited due to the relatively long half-life of the ^{131}I label (8 days), the presence of the beta particle that adds to the radiation dose but does not contribute to imaging, and the high-energy photon. Higher doses of ^{123}I mIBG can be given for the same radiation exposure, resulting in much higher quality images (Fig. 13.1). About 10 times as many counts are obtained using ^{123}I mIBG as with ^{131}I mIBG. ^{123}I mIBG has advantages of shorter half-life (13 hours), ideal energy of the photon imaged (159 keV), and lack of beta particle. The sensitivity of mIBG in the detection of neuroblastoma is about 90% and specificity nearly 100%.

Meta-iodobenzylguanidine has also been labeled with ^{124}I, which decays by both electron capture (75%) and positron emission (25%). The electron capture mode of decay results in multiple high-energy single photons that add to the radiation burden and increase the background of the PET image due to scatter and detection of random coin-

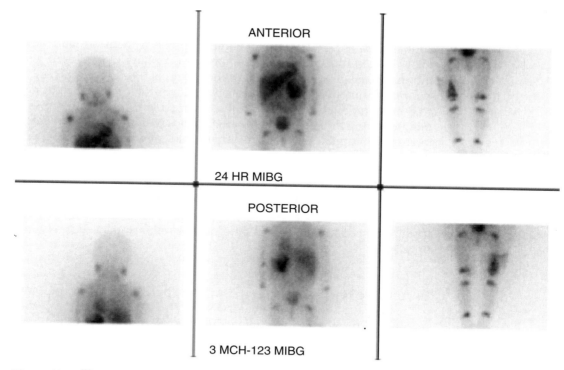

Figure 13.1. ^{123}I–meta-iodobenzylguanidine (mIBG) images of a 16–month-old girl who presented with a pathologic fracture of the right femur. Top row: anterior images; bottom row: posterior images; left panel: head, neck, chest; middle panel: chest, abdomen, pelvis; right panel: lower extremities. Abnormal areas of uptake of mIBG, representing deposits of neuroblastoma, are seen in both humeral heads, wrists, femoral heads, knees, and ankles. The primary tumor is seen in the left upper abdomen, representing a large left adrenal neuroblastoma. Tumor involvement of the right distal femur was responsible for the pathologic fracture.

cidence events. The half-life of [124]124 is 4.2 days. This allows imaging over several days, but the long half-life and electron capture method of decay limit the dose that can be given. Ott and colleagues (9) have described its use for planning treatment with ^{131}I-mIBG in a 43-year-old man with neuroblastoma, and a 62-year-old with pheochromocytoma. The injected doses were only about 0.5 mCi and 1.0 mCi of [124]I-mIBG, and images of 18 to 24 minutes duration were obtained at 24 and 48 hours. Uptake in both the tumors and surrounding tissues was shown. From calculations of the distribution of [124]I-mIBG, the authors calculated that 300 mCi of ^{131}I-mIBG, the dose given to the patient with neuroblastoma, was subtherapeutic.

Since the introduction of mIBG, there has been much research involving the catecholamine reuptake transporter. The amino acid sequence of the receptor was described in 1991 (10). The gene for the protein is located on chromosome 16. The protein structure consists of 617 amino acids with 12 membrane-spanning domains. There is considerable homology among the norepinephrine, dopamine, and serotonin transporters. It is sodium and chloride dependent and appears to involve sequential binding of sodium, chloride, and catecholamine. Type 1 uptake is blocked by a number of agents, including cocaine, tricyclic antidepressants, phenylpropanolamine, pseudoephedrine, and labetolol (11). Administration of these agents is unlikely in children with the exception of pseudoephedrine and labetolol. Pseudoephedrine is a sympathomimetic amine found in many over-the-counter cough and cold preparations. Labetolol is a β-adrenergic antagonist that appears unique among these agents in its interference with type 1 uptake. Interference with uptake is recognized by the lack of normal salivary gland and cardiac uptake of tracer, and by prominent muscle deposition. Although we have seen some uptake in neuroblastomas, the extent of disease may be underestimated in the presence of interfering substances. Although not tested, we expect that these agents, via interference with type 1 uptake, would also interfere with the uptake of other tracers (described below) that enter the neuroblastoma cell via type 1 uptake.

Fluorodeoxyglucose

In contrast to mIBG, fluorodeoxyglucose (FDG) is concentrated by a different mechanism—the glucose transporter. Fluorodeoxyglucose is an analog of the naturally occurring sugar glucose. Because most tumors preferentially use glucose for energy, FDG is concentrated within most tumors. Many tumors found in adults, such as lung cancer, head and neck tumors, melanoma, breast cancer, esophageal cancer, and colorectal cancer, are usually well depicted by FDG–positron emission tomography (PET), and FDG-PET has become well established as an important tool for the management of patients with these diseases.

Our initial experience with neuroblastoma occurred over 10 years ago (12). We studied 17 patients (20 scans) with neuroblastoma using FDG. Comparison was made with mIBG scintigraphy. At that time, FDG-PET imaging was much more challenging than it is today. Scanning required choosing the area of interest prior to injection and performing transmission attenuation correction scans before injection. Patients needed to lie still for the next 50 minutes or so while uptake occurred. At that point, tumor to nontumor concentration was usually adequate for tumor imaging. Non–attenuation-corrected views of various sections of the body might next be obtained as a screening measure. Images were constructed with filtered backprojection. In 16 of 17 patients, tumor uptake of FDG was readily identified.

In patients studied prior to initiation of therapy, uptake of FDG was usually quite intense. In each of seven patients, the primary tumor was readily visualized. Standard uptake values (SUVs) ranged from 2.0 to 4.0 (mean 2.8 ± 0.7). For depiction of the primary tumor, FDG was better than mIBG in two, mIBG was better than FDG in three, and the scans were equal in two. Six of seven patients had diffuse bone marrow uptake of FDG and mIBG, and bone marrow involvement was confirmed by bone marrow biopsy. Overall, FDG compared quite favorably with mIBG. In two of these patients, FDG scans were considered superior to mIBG scans, in three patients mIBG scans were considered superior to FDG, and in two patients the scans were equivalent.

Ten patients (13 scans) were studied during or following therapy when residual or recurrent disease was suspected clinically. Fluorodeoxyglucose uptake was found in tumor sites of nine of 10 patients. However, mIBG scans were rated as superior to FDG-PET scans in eight of 11 scans, FDG-PET superior to mIBG in two, and FDG and mIBG equivalent in one. One patient had a neuroblastoma that did not concentrate mIBG. In this patient, FDG clearly defined sites of tumor in the bones and abdomen (Fig. 13.2). We concluded that the majority of neuroblastomas are metabolically active and can be detected using FDG-PET (Fig. 13.3, see color insert). For the most part, mIBG imaging was superior to FDG-PET for evaluating patients with neuroblastoma. Evaluation of patients with neuroblastoma using FDG-PET is most beneficial in tumors that either fail to concentrate or only weakly accumulate mIBG.

Kushner et al. (13) have utilized FDG-PET scans as a means of monitoring treatment effects and disease status. Fifty-one patients who underwent 92 FDG-PET scans were reported. In patients who

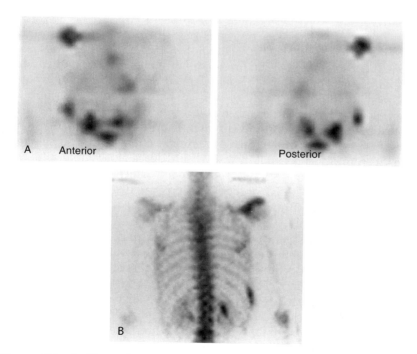

Figure 13.2. A: Fluorodeoxyglucose (FDG) projection images (anterior left, posterior right) of a 19-year-old with esthesioneuroblastoma that did not accumulate mIBG. The images cover 40 cm in the z-axis from the shoulders to the mid-abdomen. Abnormal uptake in seen in the right shoulder, a right lower rib, and a midline focus at the edge of the images inferior to the kidneys. B: Bone scan (posterior image) shows abnormal uptake in the right shoulder and a right lower rib corresponding with the osseous uptake of FDG.

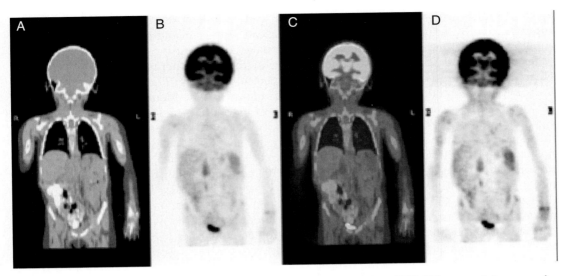

Figure 13.3. Positron emission tomography–computed tomography (PET-CT) coronal images of a 4-year-old girl with refractory neuroblastoma following bone marrow transplantation. A: CT scan. B: FDG-PET scan with attenuation correction. C: Fusion image of CT scan and FDG-PET scan with attenuation correction. D: FDG-PET scan without attenuation correction. Abnormal uptake of FDG in the abdomen is seen to the right of the midline medial to the liver, representing residual neuroblastoma. (See color insert.)

underwent multiple staging evaluations using FDG-PET, scans documented complete and partial remissions, stable disease, and progressive disease. In patients with soft tissue lesions, SUVs ranged from 1.8 to 8.4, median 5.3. In four newly diagnosed patients, FDG and ^{131}I-mIBG scans showed similar results in three. In a single patient, FDG-PET showed more extensive disease. The authors found that serial FDG-PET scans accurately depict treatment effects and disease evolution. Scan findings correlated well with disease status determined by conventional imaging studies and urinary catecholamine metabolite excretion. Both FDG-PET and mIBG depict widespread bone metastases, but FDG-PET may be better than mIBG for the detection of hepatic involvement.

Kushner et al. (13) speculate that FDG-PET might provide clinically useful information about the proliferative activity of a lesion that could influence treatment decisions. For example, a considerable decrease in activity during therapy could indicate a good response that justifies continuation of the current regimen. However, residual uptake in a neoplasm may be due to tumor inflammation rather than neoplasm. We believe it is unlikely that FDG-PET will replace mIBG scanning in the management of patients with neuroblastoma.

In patients with neuroblastoma, there are foci of FDG uptake that are not due to neuroblastoma. These include bowel, urinary tract, thymus, and bone marrow. Pathologic sites of uptake not due to neuroblastoma were skin, pleura, and lungs due to radiotherapy. Trauma and inflammation are additional causes of abnormal uptake that we have encountered.

Other Catecholamine or Catecholamine-Like Tracers

Several other positron-emitting tracers have been or may be applied to the study of neuroblastoma. Positron-emitting tracers have several potential advantages over conventional tracers. Positron emission tomography offers improved resolution compared to single photon emission computed tomography (SPECT): the ability to accurately quantify uptake, the use of multiple short-acting tracers to characterize a tumor in a single setting, and the likelihood of completing the study within a couple of hours following injection.

Carbon-11 hydroxyephedrine (HED) was developed for imaging the sympathetic nervous system, in particular cardiac sympathetic innervation. It is synthesized by direct *N*-methylation of metaraminol. The aromatic component of HED is less lipophilic than that of mIBG. Hydroxyephedrine bears closer structural similarity to norepinephrine, but unlike norepinephrine, HED is not metabolized. After finding that HED was highly concentrated into deposits of pheochromocytoma, we examined its uptake in neuroblastoma and compared it with mIBG (14). In each of seven patients studied, there was uptake of HED into sites of neuroblastoma identified by mIBG scanning (Fig. 13.4). The uptake was quite rapid. By 2 minutes, 80% of the mean maximal uptake had occurred. In most patients, retention of HED was also quite high. Raffel and Wieland (15) have shown that in cardiac cells, the retention of HED is dependent on active transport of tracer into the cell. Once in the cell, HED is present in both catecholamine storage vesicles and free within the cytoplasm. Hydroxyephedrine passively exits the cell and is rapidly taken up again through the catecholamine reuptake system. Although the concentration of HED appears fixed, this equilibrium is a result of a dynamic system of egress and entrance.

With HED, hepatic and renal activity is prominent early (Fig. 13.5). As a result, tumor-to-liver ratios increase during the duration of the study as the liver activity declines and the tumor concentration remains relatively fixed. There is excellent clearance of mIBG from the soft tissues in the first 24 hours, and very high quality images can be acquired using ^{123}I-mIBG and SPECT. Because of the limited availability of ^{11}C-HED and the need for a cyclotron and PET chemistry expertise for its synthesis, it is unlikely that this agent will have a major role in the evaluation of patients with neuroblastoma.

[11]C-epinephrine has also been studied in both pheochromocytoma and neuroblastoma (16,17). Epinephrine is a catecholamine product of the adrenal medulla, synthesized by methylation of norepinephrine. In vivo, epinephrine has many physiologic effects. These include cardiac stimulation, bronchodilation, and vasodilation. Like norepinephrine, one of the processes through which the effects of epinephrine are regulated is reuptake into the presynaptic neuron via the catecholamine reuptake system.

[11]C-epinephrine was developed to investigate the sympathetic innervation of the heart. We showed that it was concentrated by pheochromocytomas and thus undertook to evaluate it as a potential imaging agent for neuroblastoma. In the presynaptic neuron of the sympathetic

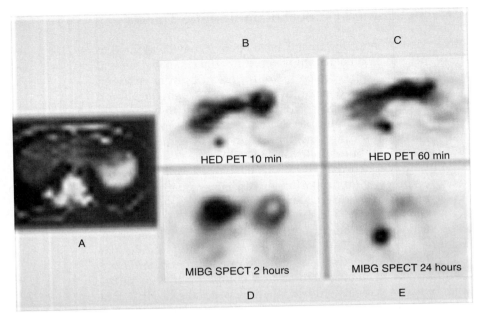

Figure 13.4. A: T2-weighted transverse magnetic resonance imaging of the lower chest and upper abdomen. A mass with high signal intensity is seen in the posterior right lung field. B: The first hydroxyephedrine (HED) PET scan at the same level was acquired 10 minutes postinjection, and it shows there is intense uptake within the right posterior lung mass. C: The second HED-PET image was acquired 60 minutes postadministration, and it shows that good uptake remains within the mass, demonstrating the high retention of HED. D: The first mIBG-SPECT scan was acquired 2 hours postinjection, and it shows no definite uptake within the mass. E: The second mIBG-SPECT examination was acquired at 24 hours, and it shows clear accumulation of mIBG within the tumor, confirming its adrenergic nature. The tumor was removed surgically and shown to be a neuroblastoma. [*Source:* Shulkin et al. (14), with permission.]

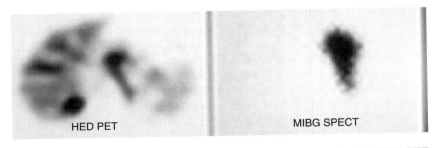

Figure 13.5. A 9-year-old boy with refractory neuroblastoma. Left: A HED-PET scan of the mid-abdomen 30 minutes postinjection. There is accumulation of HED to the left of the liver as well as excretion of HED through the right kidney. Right: An mIBG-SPECT scan at 24 hours shows excellent uptake within the neuroblastoma. There is little remaining liver and kidney activity, and thus the tumor appears quite prominent. [*Source:* Shulkin et al. (14), with permission.]

Figure 13.6. Anterior projection image of ^{11}C-epinephrine PET scan of a 29-year-old woman with widespread neuroblastoma. Abnormal uptake is seen in both shoulders, in a very large abdominal mass with decreased uptake in the center, representing necrosis, and in the pelvic bones and femurs bilaterally. The PET scan identified the same areas of disease as the mIBG scan (not shown).

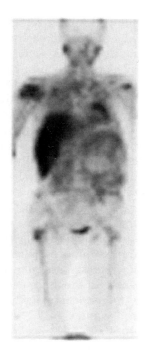

nervous system, after transport intracellularly, norepinephrine and epinephrine are stored in granules that protect catecholamines from intracellular degradation by the enzyme monoamine oxidase. Because neuroblastomas have relatively few catecholamine storage granules compared to pheochromocytomas, it was not clear that ^{11}C-epinephrine would be retained intact in the neuroblastoma cell in sufficient quantity and over sufficient time to generate a detectable signal.

We have studied over 20 patients with neuroblastoma using PET and ^{11}C-epinephrine (Figs. 13.6 and 13.7). Between one half and two thirds

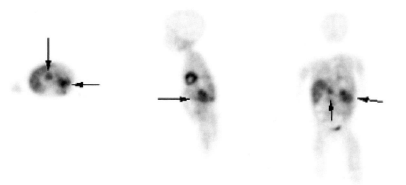

Figure 13.7. ^{11}C-epinephrine PET images of a 4-year-old girl with ganglioneuroblastoma. Left: transverse image; middle: sagittal image; right: coronal image. The arrows point to two areas of abnormal uptake within the abdomen, which were also identified on mIBG and CT scanning.

showed uptake of ^{11}C-epinephrine within the tumor(s); mIBG uptake was present in each of the tumors studied. Positron emission tomography studies were performed dynamically immediately following injection. The first-pass extraction for those tumors that did show uptake was very high, as these neuroblastomas were distinguishable from background activity within 2 minutes following injection. The retention of ^{11}C-epinephrine was also quite good, foci of neuroblastoma generally appearing more intense as background activity declines. It is unclear why only some neuroblastomas that concentrate mIBG concentrate ^{11}C-epinephrine. Smets and colleagues have shown that mIBG in neuroblastomas is less dependent on granular storage than mIBG in pheochromocytomas and that a substantial portion of mIBG exists freely within the cytoplasm of neuroblastoma cells (18). It is possible that ^{11}C-epinephrine is retained only in those tumors with substantial quantities of storage granules to protect catecholamines, whereas in those tumors that are not visualized with ^{11}C-epinephrine, there are too few storage granules to protect the tracer from intracellular degradation and thus the prompt loss of signal.

Other agents may soon be applied to the functional imaging of neuroblastoma. 4-[^{18}F]-fluoro-3-iodobenzylguanidine (FIBG) has been synthesized and shown in vitro to bind to human neuroblastoma cells (19). Additionally, high uptake was noted in the mouse heart and adrenal glands. This agent might be a good positron-emitting analog of mIBG. P-[^{18}F]fluorobenzylguanidine (PFBG) has been shown to image myocardial sympathetic innervation and neuroendocrine tissues. It was administered to two dogs with pheochromocytomas (20). Rapid uptake was found with blood pool clearance within 10 minutes. There was also high uptake within the myocardium. The SUVs were greater than 25 by 10 minutes. Although not yet used in human pheochromocytomas or neuroblastomas, these agents should accumulate in these neuroendocrine tumors that possess active type 1 catecholamine transport mechanisms.

6-[^{18}F]-Fluorodopamine (^{18}F-DA) has been successfully used to localize sites of pheochromocytoma in patients with metastatic pheochromocytoma (21). The rationale for its use is that dopamine is a better substrate for norepinephrine transport mechanism than is norepinephrine. ^{18}F-DA was studied in 16 patients at the National Institutes of Health, where 1.0 mCi of ^{18}F-DA was administered intravenously and imaging was begun immediately. Fifteen of 16 patients had abnormal ^{18}F-DA scans, whereas only nine of 16 had abnormal ^{131}I-mIBG scans; 38 foci of uptake were found by both agents, 90 by ^{18}F-DA alone, and 10 by ^{131}I-mIBG alone. In each of the seven patients with negative ^{131}I-mIBG studies, ^{18}F-DA scans demonstrated one to four lesions, and most of these were documented by computed tomography or magnetic resonance imaging studies. It is also likely that this agent will be concentrated in neuroblastomas that possess active type 1 catecholamine transport systems.

[18]F-dihydroxyphenylalanine (DOPA) has also been shown to be concentrated in pheochromocytomas (22). Its uptake is said to represent the capability of neuroendocrine tumors to concentrate decarboxylate

and store amino acids and their biogenic amines. In vitro studies (by Shulkin, unpublished) suggest that type 1 catecholamine uptake is involved as well. Because neuroblastomas often excrete dopamine metabolites, it is likely that ^{18}F-DOPA would also be concentrated within neuroblastomas.

Tracers of the Future

We have studied a variety of tracers in vitro to assess their potential for imaging of neuroblastoma in vivo (23). These include amino acids, nucleosides, and a variety of others. Many of the compounds showed uptake greater than that of mIBG. The compounds with the highest uptake were the essential amino acids threonine and methionine. Although it is promising in vitro, experiments in vivo using animal tumor models or human patients will be needed to assess the clinical utility of these agents. It is certainly possible that liver, renal, or bone marrow activity will be excessively high to distinguish tumor from background. Other promising agents are radiolabeled thymidine or its analog, fluorothymidine, to assess cellular proliferation. This agent could be especially useful in determining the response of tumors to antineoplastic therapy.

Conclusion

Neuroblastoma has been studied using multiple positron-emitting tracers. Because of its derivation from tissues related to the sympathetic nervous system, neuroblastomas are commonly evaluated using functional imaging with the conventional nuclear medicine tracer radiolabeled mIBG, which is concentrated by the uptake one mechanism. Tracers that reflect activity of the norepinephrine transport mechanism of tissues of the sympathetic nervous system labeled with positron-emitting radionuclides have also been utilized. These include ^{11}C-hydroxyephedrine and ^{11}C-epinephrine. Other related tracers, such as ^{18}F-fluorodopamine, are expected to also show uptake in neuroblastomas. Because of the malignant nature of neuroblastoma and the tendencies for malignancies to preferentially utilize glucose for metabolism, neuroblastomas have also been imaged using the positron-emitting glucose analog, ^{18}F-FDG. We expect that tracers that reflect other physiologic and pathophysiologic mechanisms, including amino acid uptake and cellular proliferation, will soon be studied for their ability to reveal additional information about this often-fatal malignancy of childhood.

References

1. Brodeur GM, Castleberry RP. Neuroblastoma. In: Pizzo PA, Poplack DG, eds. Principles and Practice of Pediatric Oncology, 3rd ed. Philadelphia: Lippincott-Raven, 1997:761–797.

2. Shimada H, Chatten J, Newton WA Jr, et al. Histopathologic prognostic factors in neuroblastic tumors: definition of subtypes of ganglioneuroblastoma and an age-linked classification of neuroblastomas. J Natl Cancer Inst 1984;73:405.

3. Brodeur GM, Pritchard J, Berthold F, et al. Revisions in the international criteria for neuroblastoma diagnosis, staging, and response to treatment. J Clin Oncol 1993;11:1466.

4. Sisson JC, Frager MS, Valk TW, et al. Scintigraphic localization of pheochromocytoma. N Engl J Med 1981;305(1):12–17.

5. Treuner J, Feine U, Niethammer D, et al. Scintigraphic imaging of neuroblastoma with [131–I]iodobenzylguanidine. [Letter] Lancet 1984;1(8372): 333–334.

6. Sisson JC, Shulkin BL. Nuclear medicine imaging of pheochromocytoma and neuroblastoma. Q J Nucl Med 1999;43(3):217–223.

7. Wieland DM, Wu J, Brown LE, Mangner TJ, Swanson DP, Beierwaltes WH. Radiolabeled adrenergic neuron-blocking agents: adrenomedullary imaging with [131I]iodobenzylguanidine. J Nucl Med 1980;21(4): 349–353.

8. Shulkin BL, Shapiro B. Current concepts on the diagnostic use of MIBG in children. J Nucl Med 1998;39(4):679–688.

9. Ott FJ, Tait D, Flower MA, Babich JS, Lambrecht M. Treatment planning for 131I-mIBG radiotherapy of neural crest tumours using 124I-mIBG positron emission tomography. Br J Radiol 1992;65:787–791.

10. Runkel F, Bruss M, Nothen MM, Stober G. Propping P, Bonisch H. Pharmacological properties of naturally occurring variants of the human norepinephrine transporter. Pharmacogenetics 2000;10(5):397–405.

11. Khafagi FA, Shapiro B, Fig LM, Mallette S, Sisson JC. Labetalol reduces iodine-131 MIBG uptake by pheochromocytoma and normal tissues. J Nucl Med 1989;30(4):481–489.

12. Shulkin BL, Hutchinson RJ, Castle VP, Yanik GA, Shapiro B, Sisson JC. Neuroblastoma: positron emission tomography with 2-[fluorine-18]-fluoro2–deoxy-D-glucose compared with metaiodobenzylguanidine scintigraphy. Radiology 1996;199:743–750.

13. Kushner BH, Yeung HWD, Larson SM, Kramer K, Cheung N-K V. Extending positron emission tomography scan utility to high-risk neuroblastoma: fluorine-18 fluorodeoxyglucose positron emission tomography as sole imaging modality in follow-up of patients. J Clin Oncol 2001;19(14): 3397–3405.

14. Shulkin BL, Wieland DM, Baro ME, et al. PET hydroxyephedrine imaging of neuroblastoma. J Nucl Med 1996;37(1):16–21.

15. Raffel DM, Wieland DM. Influence of vesicular storage and monoamine oxidase activity on [11C]phenylephrine kinetics: studies in isolated rat heart. J Nucl Med 1999;40(2):323–330.

16. Shulkin BL, Wieland DM, Sisson JC. PET studies of pheochromocytoma with C-11 epinephrine. Radiology 1994;193:273.

17. Shulkin BL, Wieland DM, Castle VP, Hutchinson RJ, Sisson JC. Carbon-11 epinephrine PET imaging of neuroblastoma. J Nucl Med 1999;40(5): 129.

18. Smets LA, Janssen M, Metwally E, Loesberg C. Extragranular storage of the neuron blocking agent meta-iodobenzylguanidine (MIBG) in human neuroblastoma cells. Biochemical Pharmacology 1990;39(12):1959–1964.

19. Vaidyanathan G, Affleck DJ, Zalutsky MR. 4–[18F]fluoro-3–iodobenzyl guanidine, a potential MIBG analogue for positron emission tomography. J Med Chem 1994;37(21):3655–3662.

20. Berry CR, DeGrado TR, Nutter F, et al. Imaging of pheochromocytoma in 2 dogs using p-[18F] fluorobenzylguanidine. Vet Radiol Ultrasound 2002;43(2):183–186.

21. Ilias I, Yu J, Carrasquillo JA, et al. Superiority of 6–[18F]-fluorodopamine positron emission tomography versus [131I]-metaiodobenzylguanidine scintigraphy in the localization of metastatic pheochromocytoma. J Clin Endocrinol Metab 2003;88(9):4083–4087.

22. Hoegerle S, Ghanem N, Altehoefer C, et al. Pheochromocytomas: detection with 18F DOPA whole body PET—initial results. Radiology 2002;222(2): 507–512.

23. Goodwill T, Shulkin BL, Schumacher K, Devooght J, Castle V. Metabolic characterization of neuroblastoma. J Nucl Med 2002;43(5):36.

14

Wilms' Tumor

Sue C. Kaste and Jeffrey S. Dome

The clinical applications of fluorine-18 fluorodeoxyglucose–positron emission tomography (^{18}F-FDG-PET) imaging in adults have grown rapidly. However, only recently has this technology and the merged technology of PET and computed tomography (PET-CT) been extended to children and adolescents. Thus, information about the indications and utility of PET-CT in pediatric oncology is limited. This chapter discusses the initial experience with PET and PET-CT imaging of patients with Wilms' tumor.

Epidemiology of Wilms' Tumor

Wilms' tumor is the most common malignant pediatric renal tumor and accounts for 6% of all cases of childhood cancer in the United States each year. Approximately eight cases are identified annually per million children under the age of 15 years; the annual number of new cases in the United States is estimated to be 500 (1). The frequency of Wilms' tumor is slightly higher in blacks than in whites but is considerably lower in Asians than in whites. In the United States, the incidence of Wilms' tumor (either unilateral or bilateral) is slightly less in boys than in girls (2).

The association between Wilms' tumor and genetic malformation syndromes is well known, although these syndromes are present in only a small number of patients with Wilms' tumor. The syndromes most commonly associated with Wilms' tumor are WAGR (*W*ilms' tumor, *a*niridia, *g*enitourinary malformation, mental *r*etardation) syndrome, Denys-Drash syndrome (pseudohermaphroditism, glomerulopathy, renal failure, and Wilms' tumor), and Beckwith-Wiedemann syndrome (macroglossia, omphalocele, visceromegaly, hemihypertrophy, Wilms' tumor, and other cancers) (3).

Pathology

Classical Wilms' tumor contains blastemal, epithelial, and stromal cells, although many tumors do not contain all three types of cells (4). About 7% of tumors contain anaplasia, which is defined by cells with enlarged nuclei, hyperchromasia, and irregular mitotic figures (5). When present, anaplasia usually occurs diffusely throughout a tumor but also may be focal (6). Patients whose tumors contain focal anaplasia have better outcomes than those whose tumors contain diffuse anaplasia (7). Tumors that are not anaplastic at all are associated with the best prognosis and are thus designated as having "favorable histology." Less common renal tumors of childhood include clear cell sarcoma of the kidney, malignant rhabdoid tumor, congenital mesoblastic nephroma, and renal cell carcinoma.

Nephrogenic rests are precursors of Wilms' tumor; these are clusters of embryonal nephroblastic cells that persist abnormally into childhood (8). Nephrogenic rests are found in about 40% of patients with unilateral Wilms' tumor and in nearly all patients with bilateral Wilms' tumor (8). Nephrogenic rests are classified as nascent/dormant, maturing/sclerosing, or hyperplastic. Hyperplastic nephrogenic rests can be quite large and are often difficult to distinguish from Wilms' tumor (8).

Prognostic Factors

The most powerful prognostic factors for patients with Wilms' tumor are tumor histology and stage. Anaplastic histology predicts a markedly higher risk of recurrence than does favorable histology. Likewise, advanced tumor stage is associated with increased risk of recurrence. Other adverse prognostic factors include older patient age (9,10), blastemal-predominant histology after chemotherapy (11), loss of heterozygosity on chromosome arms 1p and 16q (12,13), gain of chromosome arm 1q (14), and a high level of telomerase expression (15,16). Ongoing biology studies are likely to identify additional molecular prognostic factors.

Treatment

The treatment of Wilms' tumor involves surgery, chemotherapy, and, in some cases, radiation therapy. The longstanding approach used by the National Wilms' Tumor Study Group (NWTSG) has been a nephrectomy at the time of diagnosis, with subsequent chemotherapy and radiation therapy (17). The approach used by the International Society of Pediatric Oncology (SIOP) has been to administer several weeks of chemotherapy before nephrectomy (18). Each approach has distinct advantages, and the outcomes are similar. Table 14.1 lists the outcomes of patients treated on the most recently reported NWTSG studies. Given the excellent overall survival rates of patients with Wilms' tumor, a priority of recent clinical trials has been to limit therapy, and its associated toxicity, in patients who are at low risk of disease recurrence.

Table 14.1. Outcomes of patients treated on the National Wilms' Tumor Study Group (NWTSG) studies NWTS-3 and -4 (Data from 7, 19)

Tumor histology and stage	4-Year relapse-free survival (%)	4-Year overall survival (%)
Favorable histology		
Stage I	89.0	95.6
II	87.4	91.1
III	82.0	90.9
IV	79.0	80.9
V (bilateral)	–	81.7
Diffuse anaplasia		
Stage I	93.8	93.3
II	71.6	70.1
III	58.7	56.3
IV	16.7	16.7

Potential Applications of PET/PET-CT Imaging to Wilms' Tumor

Functional imaging studies such as PET or PET-CT may increase the accuracy of tumor staging, distinguish between benign and malignant lesions, and assess the early response to treatment in patients with measurable tumors. Although experience with ^{18}F-FDG-PET/PET-CT imaging in Wilms' tumor is limited, preliminary reports (20) and our experience suggest that Wilms' tumors are often ^{18}F-FDG–avid.

Tumor Staging

Diagnostic imaging studies play a key role in the staging of primary Wilms' tumor. Imaging studies delineate the local extent of the tumor and detect the presence of metastatic disease (Fig. 14.1). The most common sites of metastasis are the lungs, regional lymph nodes, and liver. Approximately 10% of patients have lung metastases at diagnosis (21), and 47% have pulmonary metastases at the time of relapse (22).

Chest radiography and chest CT are routinely used to detect pulmonary metastatic disease (23,24). Chest radiographs are limited by resolution and sensitivity; CT imaging is complicated by inter- and intraobserver discordance in interpreting the presence and significance of pulmonary nodules (25). A common dilemma faced by clinicians is the management of patients with small pulmonary nodules. The NWTSG reported that 17% of lung nodules in patients with newly diagnosed Wilms' tumor were found on biopsy to be benign (26). Therefore, the management of such lesions is particularly problematic unless biopsy is performed. Although several studies have shown an increased risk of pulmonary relapse in patients with CT-identified pulmonary nodules, intensified chemotherapy and pulmonary irradiation are not without toxic effects (25–27). As with other pediatric malignancies, pulmonary metastases of Wilms' tumor can differentiate into benign mature tumor cells, further complicating the interpretation of follow-up imaging examinations on the basis of anatomic appearance (27–29).

^{18}F-FDG has the potential ability to differentiate metabolically hyperactive nodules from quiescent and metabolically hypoactive nodules (30,31). Because both malignant and inflammatory diseases can involve glucose hypermetabolism, ^{18}F-FDG-PET/PET-CT is unlikely to differentiate benign from malignant nodules with absolute specificity. However, with refinement of PET techniques, including quantitative techniques and delayed imaging, characteristics that differentiate benign from malignant lesions may be discerned. Even with the currently available techniques, hypermetabolic pulmonary lesions would be more likely to be malignant and therefore could be preferentially biopsied.

Accurate staging of recurrent Wilms' tumor facilitates the design of multidisciplinary regimens to treat all sites of disease. ^{18}F-FDG-PET/PET-CT provides sensitive detection of metabolically active sites of disease, some of which are undetected by other imaging modalities (Fig. 14.2). A patient treated for recurrent anaplastic Wilms' tumor at St. Jude Children's Research Hospital, Memphis, TN, had persistent pulmonary nodules in the right middle lobe after chemotherapy. Surgical removal of the affected area of the lung was considered, and a PET-CT scan was performed to detect other possible sites of disease. The PET-CT scan revealed FDG avidity in the right pulmonary hilum

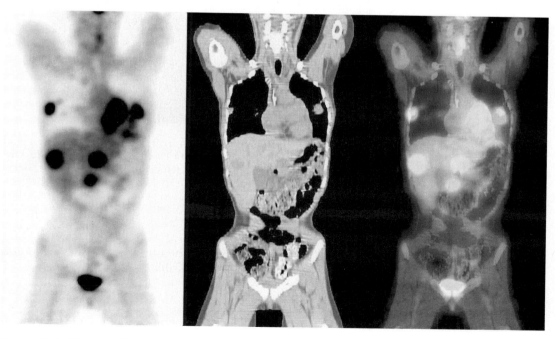

Figure 14.1. Fluorine-18 fluorodeoxyglucose–positron emission tomography (^{18}F-FDG-PET)–computed tomography (CT) images of a 10-year-old girl with recurrent Wilms' tumor. PET-CT imaging was performed to determine the extent of disease. Note numerous sites of ^{18}F-FDG avidity. (Courtesy of Dr. Barry Shulkin.)

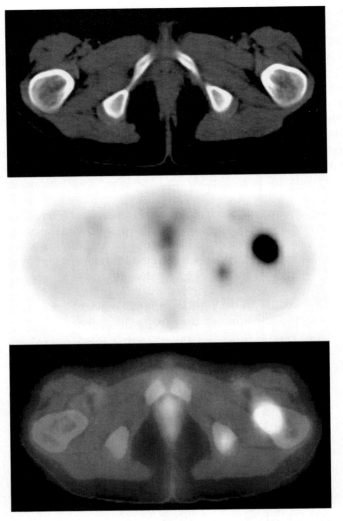

Figure 14.2. Intensely ^{18}F-FDG-avid lesions in the left proximal femur and ischium of this patient (also shown in Fig. 14.1) were not evident on the corresponding CT images captured with bone windows. (Courtesy of Dr. Barry Shulkin.)

and upper right chest, suggesting that the tumor was widespread and that complete resection would be impossible (Fig. 14.3).

Bilateral Wilms' Tumor

The treatment of bilateral Wilms' tumor is challenging. The goal of treatment is to eradicate tumor cells while preserving as much renal parenchyma as possible. Patients typically receive preoperative chemotherapy, thereby reducing tumor burden and facilitating surgery. Approximately 40% of tumors are reduced more than 50% in size by chemotherapy (32). Failure to respond can signify that the tumor cells are anaplastic or otherwise resistant to treatment, requiring augmentation of therapy and perhaps nephrectomy. However, tumors with extensive rhabdomyomatous differentiation or necrosis may also fail to respond, and augmentation of chemotherapy is not indicated for these cases. Positron emission tomography scanning has been reported to differentiate viable germ cell tumor from mature teratoma and tissue necrosis (33), and therefore it may also help in distinguishing between proliferating and nonproliferating bilateral Wilms' tumor.

A theoretical obstacle to the use of PET scanning to image bilateral Wilms' tumor is the possibility that clearance of ^{18}F-FDG through the genitourinary tract could mask an intrarenal tumor. However, active tumors can be visualized within the renal parenchyma due to

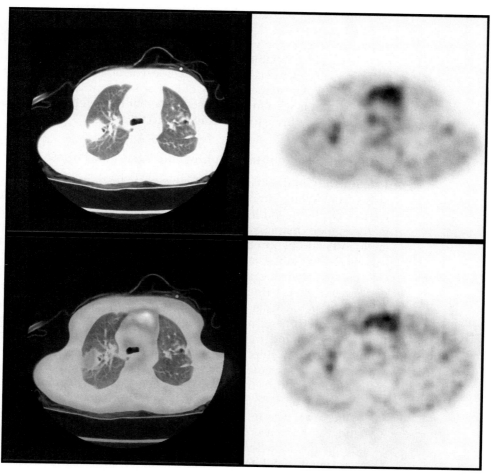

Figure 14.3. A patient treated for recurrent anaplastic Wilms' tumor underwent PET-CT imaging to detect other possible sites of disease before undergoing a possible right middle lobectomy for pulmonary nodules that persisted after chemotherapy. ^{18}F-FDG avidity in the right pulmonary hilum and upper right chest indicated widespread metastatic disease that precluded complete resection.

higher uptake by tumor than by normal kidney (20,34). Shulkin and colleagues (20) reported two patients with bilateral Wilms' tumor who underwent PET scans to guide clinical management. One patient with bilateral multifocal Wilms' tumor had an initial response to therapy during the first 2 months of treatment, but then had stable disease. A PET scan showed persistent ^{18}F-FDG avidity in one of the right-kidney tumors, which was confirmed by biopsy to be Wilms' tumor. Interestingly, the left kidney, which was not FDG-avid, also contained Wilms' tumor with areas of nephroblastomatosis. It would be informative to know whether the difference in FDG avidity reflected residual Wilms' tumor in the right kidney that was less differentiated and proliferative than that in the left kidney.

The second patient underwent bilateral open biopsy of bilateral renal masses that showed favorable-histology Wilms' tumor in the right kidney and anaplastic Wilms' tumor in the left kidney. She underwent ^{18}F-FDG imaging after the left renal mass failed to decrease in size to the same extent as the right renal mass in response to chemotherapy. The PET scan revealed ^{18}F-FDG avidity in the rim of the left renal mass but no uptake in the right renal mass. Bilateral partial nephrectomy revealed residual viable tumor in the left kidney but necrotic tumor without viable elements on the right side, correlating well with the PET findings (20). A systematic study of PET scans in patients with bilateral Wilms' tumor is warranted to assess whether the level of ^{18}F-FDG activity correlates with histologic response to therapy.

Differentiating Between Nephrogenic Rests and Wilms' Tumor

The difficulty of distinguishing nephrogenic rests and nephroblastomatosis from Wilms' tumor can create a diagnostic dilemma. Although the two entities—and the spectrum between them—have some distinct features, their imaging characteristics can be similar. Typically, nephrogenic rests and nephroblastomatosis are multifocal or diffuse bilateral lesions located in the subcapsular portion of the kidneys. They may be classified by their location as intralobar and perilobar, with perilobar nephrogenic rests being more common. On ultrasonography (US) and CT, nephrogenic rests appear as homogeneous, hypodense, poorly enhancing peripheral nodules. As with Wilms' tumor, they are hypointense on T1- and hyperintense on T2-weighted sequences (35). A Wilms' tumor is a hypervascular intrarenal mass that is usually large and may be associated with vascular invasion. Unlike nephrogenic rests, Wilms' tumor is usually an inhomogeneous echogenic solid mass on ultrasound and CT (particularly contrast-enhanced CT) studies. On magnetic resonance imaging (MRI), Wilms' tumor is hypointense on T1- and hyperintense on T2-weighted sequences (35) and enhances inhomogeneously when intravenous contrast medium is used (36–38). Contrast-enhanced MRI improves the imaging distinction of Wilms' tumor from nephrogenic rests, achieving an overall sensitivity of 57% for detection of the lesion and an overall accuracy of 65%. Although better than those of excretory urography and ultrasound, these values are far from ideal. Further, small nephrogenic rests less than 4mm in size and those intermixed with Wilms' tumor may be overlooked by MRI (36). Rohrschneider et al. (39) found that the homogeneity of nephrogenic rests is the imaging feature that best differentiates them from Wilms' tumor. The authors also reported US to be less sensitive than CT or MRI in detecting small nephrogenic rests.

^{18}F-FDG-PET/PET-CT imaging has the potential to distinguish between benign nephrogenic rests and nephroblastomatosis and to identify their potential evolution into Wilms' tumor. Shulkin et al. (20) described a case in which FDG uptake was observed in active sites of Wilms' tumor but absent in benign nephrogenic rests. It is likely that FDG avidity varies according to the subtype of nephrogenic rest (sclerotic vs. hyperplastic). Lesions smaller than 4 or 5 mm might still be overlooked because of the limitations of PET/PET-CT resolution, unless they are very hypermetabolic. It would be worthwhile to prospectively compare ^{18}F-FDG avidity with histology in patients with bilateral or multifocal kidney lesions.

Differentiation of Residual Tumor from Other Entities

Residual imaging abnormalities observed after treatment of unresectable or metastatic Wilms' tumor may not indicate viable tumor. It can be difficult to distinguish active or recurrent disease from nonmalignant abnormalities such as postoperative changes, scarring, or abscess formation. Although ^{18}F-FDG avidity is not a specific indicator of malignancy, increased avidity can identify a site of potential residual or recurrent disease and direct biopsy to the area (20). Figure 14.4 illustrates this application. It shows the PET-CT scan of a patient with stage IV Wilms' tumor with favorable histology who presented with very extensive lung disease. After several months of treatment with

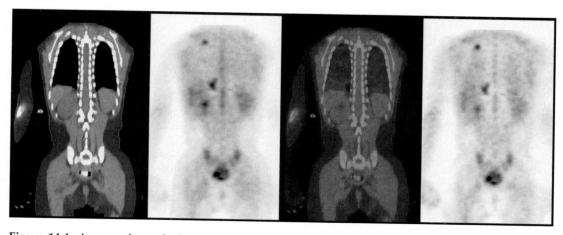

Figure 14.4. A young boy who had experienced multiple recurrences of Wilms' tumor had extensive pulmonary scarring caused by multiple thoracotomies for excision of metastatic tumor. Biopsy of the right upper-lobe mass, directed by ^{18}F-FDG-avidity, demonstrated Wilms' tumor with rhabdomyomatous differentiation, containing predominant stromal cells and a few glandular elements. Interestingly, the mass was FDG-avid, although it was not actively proliferating. This observation raises the question of whether tumors with rhabdomyomatous differentiation may be FDG-avid.

different chemotherapy agents, the patient had progressive pulmonary disease and received lung radiation and more chemotherapy. Therapy was stopped after several more months, although CT of the chest continued to show multiple lesions, some of which were consistent with scar tissue on biopsy. Six months after the completion of therapy, CT scan showed an increase in the size of a right upper lobe nodule. A PET-CT scan was done to evaluate sites of potentially viable tumor within the markedly abnormal-appearing lungs. ^{18}F-FDG uptake was observed in the growing right lung nodule and the right pulmonary hilum (Fig. 14.4) but not in other abnormal areas. Computed tomography–guided biopsy of the ^{18}F-FDG-avid nodule revealed a cellular metastatic Wilms' tumor consisting mostly of mature fibrous stroma.

Conclusion

Although its application in staging Wilms' tumor and monitoring response to treatment is not yet extensive, ^{18}F-FDG-PET/PET-CT shows promise for identifying metastatic disease, differentiating benign nephrogenic rests and nephroblastomatosis from Wilms' tumor, directing biopsy sites, and contributing to surgical planning. However, large prospective studies are needed to determine the impact of this modality on staging, assessment of treatment response, and ultimate patient outcome.

Acknowledgments

The authors thank Ms. Sandra Gaither and Ms. Melissa Mills for manuscript preparation and Ms. Sharon Naron for editing.

References

1. Ries LAG, Eisner MP, Kosary CL, et al. SEER Cancer Statistics Review, 1975–2000. Bethesda, MD: National Cancer Institute, 2003. http://seer.cancer.gov/csr/1975_2000/index.html.
2. Breslow N, Olshan A, Beckwith JB, et al. Epidemiology of Wilms tumor. Med Pediatr Oncol 1993;21(3):172–181.
3. Dome JS, Coppes MJ. Recent advances in Wilms tumor genetics. Curr Opin Pediatr 2002;14(1):5–11.
4. Qualman SJ, Bowen J, Amin MB, et al. Protocol for the examination of specimens from patients with Wilms tumor (nephroblastoma) or other renal tumors of childhood. Arch Pathol Lab Med 2003;127(10):1280–1289.
5. Bonadio JF, Storer B, Norkool P, et al. Anaplastic Wilms' tumor: clinical and pathologic studies. J Clin Oncol 1985;3(4):513–520.
6. Faria P, Beckwith B, Mishra K, et al. Focal versus diffuse anaplasia in Wilms tumor-new definitions with prognostic significance. Am J Surg Pathol 1996;20:909–920.
7. Green DM, Beckwith JB, Breslow NE, et al. Treatment of children with stages II to IV anaplastic Wilms' tumor: a report from the National Wilms' Tumor Study Group. J Clin Oncol 1994;12(10):2126–2131.

8. Beckwith JB, Kiviat NB, Bonadio JF. Nephrogenic rests, nephroblastomatosis, and the pathogenesis of Wilms' tumor. Pediatr Pathol 1990;10(1–2): 1–36.

9. Breslow N, Sharples K, Beckwith JB, et al. Prognostic factors for Wilms' tumor patients with nonmetastatic disease at diagnosis-results of the third National Wilms' Tumor Study. Cancer 1991;68:2345–2353.

10. Pritchard-Jones K, Kelsey A, Vujanic G, et al. Older age is an adverse prognostic factor in stage I, favorable histology Wilms' tumor treated with vincristine monochemotherapy: a study by the United Kingdom Children's Cancer Study Group, Wilms' Tumor Working Group. J Clin Oncol 2003; 21(17):3269–3275.

11. Weirich A, Leuschner I, Harms D, et al. Clinical impact of histologic subtypes in localized non-anaplastic nephroblastoma treated according to the trial and study SIOP-9/GPOH. Ann Oncol 2001;12(3):311–319.

12. Grundy PE, Telzerow PE, Breslow N, et al. Loss of heterozygosity for chromosomes 16q and 1p in Wilms' tumors predicts an adverse outcome. Cancer Res 1994;54(9):2331–2333.

13. Grundy RG, Pritchard J, Scambler P, et al. Loss of heterozygosity on chromosome 16 in sporadic Wilms' tumour. Br J Cancer 1998;78(9):1181–1187.

14. Hing S, Lu YJ, Summersgill B, et al. Gain of 1q is associated with adverse outcome in favorable histology Wilms' tumors. Am J Pathol 2001;158(2): 393–398.

15. Dome JS, Chung S, Bergemann T, et al. High telomerase reverse transcriptase (hTERT) messenger RNA level correlates with tumor recurrence in patients with favorable histology Wilms' tumor. Cancer Res 1999;59: 4301–4307.

16. Dome JS, Bockhold CA, Li SM, et al. Telomerase RNA expression as a prognostic marker in patients with favorable histology Wilms tumor. Proc Am Soc Clin Oncol 2004;23:799.

17. Grundy PE, Green DM, Coppes MJ, et al. Renal tumors. In: Pizzo PA, Poplack DG, eds. Principles and Practice of Pediatric Oncology. Philadelphia: Lippincott Williams & Wilkins, 2002:865–893.

18. Tournade MF, Com-Nougue C, de Kraker J, et al. Optimal duration of preoperative therapy in unilateral and nonmetastatic Wilms' tumor in children older than 6 months: results of the Ninth International Society of Pediatric Oncology Wilms' Tumor Trial and Study. J Clin Oncol 2001;19(2):488–500.

19. Green DM, Breslow NE, Beckwith JB, et al. Comparison between single-dose and divided-dose administration of dactinomycin and doxorubicin for patients with Wilms' tumor: a report from the National Wilms' Tumor Study Group. J Clin Oncol 1998;16(1):237–245.

20. Shulkin BL, Chang E, Strouse PJ, et al. PET FDG studies of Wilms tumors. J Pediatr Hematol Oncol 1997;19(4):334–338.

21. D'Angio GJ, Rosenberg H, Sharples K, et al. Position paper: imaging methods for primary renal tumors of childhood: costs versus benefits [published erratum appears in Med Pediatr Oncol 1993;21(9):695]. Med Pediatr Oncol 1993;21(3):205–212.

22. D'Angio GJ, Breslow N, Beckwith JB, et al. Treatment of Wilms' tumor. Results of the Third National Wilms' Tumor Study. Cancer 1989;64(2): 349–360.

23. Wootton-Gorges SL, Albano EA, Riggs JM, et al. Chest radiography versus chest CT in the evaluation for pulmonary metastases in patients with Wilms' tumor: a retrospective review. Pediatr Radiol 2000;30(8):533–537.

24. Owens CM, Veys PA, Pritchard J, et al. Role of chest computed tomography at diagnosis in the management of Wilms' tumor: a study by the

United Kingdom Children's Cancer Study Group. J Clin Oncol 2002; 20(12):2768–2773.

25. Wilimas JA, Kaste SC, Kauffman WM, et al. Use of chest computed tomography in the staging of pediatric Wilms' tumor: interobserver variability and prognostic significance. J Clin Oncol 1997;15(7):2631–2635.

26. Meisel JA, Guthrie KA, Breslow NE, et al. Significance and management of computed tomography detected pulmonary nodules: a report from the National Wilms Tumor Study Group. Int J Radiat Oncol Biol Phys 1999;44(3):579–585.

27. Kodish E, Shina D, Morrison S, et al. Wilms' tumor with pulmonary nodules persisting after chemotherapy and radiation. Med Pediatr Oncol 1995;25(5):414–419.

28. Shimmoto K, Ushigome S, Nikaido T, et al. Maturation of pulmonary metastases of Wilms' tumor after therapy: a case report. Pediatr Hematol Oncol 1991;8(2):147–157.

29. Silvan AAM, del Castillo G, Caro AM, et al. Maturation of Wilms' tumor pulmonary metastases to benign fibromas after therapy. Med Pediatr Oncol 1984;12:218–220.

30. Agress H Jr, Cooper BZ. Detection of clinically unexpected malignant and premalignant tumors with whole-body FDG PET: histopathologic comparison. Radiology 2004;230(2):417–422.

31. Shulkin BL, Mitchell DS, Ungar DR, et al. Neoplasms in a pediatric population: 2–[F-18]-fluoro-2-deoxy-D-glucose PET studies. Radiology 1995; 194(2):495–500.

32. Horwitz JR, Ritchey ML, Moksness J, et al. Renal salvage procedures in patients with synchronous bilateral Wilms' tumors: a report from the National Wilms' Tumor Study Group. J Pediatr Surg 1996;31(8):1020–1025.

33. Sugawara Y, Zasadny KR, Grossman HB, et al. Germ cell tumor: differentiation of viable tumor, mature teratoma, and necrotic tissue with FDG PET and kinetic modeling. Radiology 1999;211(1):249–256.

34. Wahl RL, Harney J, Hutchins G, et al. Imaging of renal cancer using positron emission tomography with 2-deoxy-2-(18F)-fluoro-D-glucose: pilot animal and human studies. J Urol 1991;146(6):1470–1474.

35. Lowe LH, Isuani BH, Heller RM, et al. Pediatric renal masses: Wilms tumor and beyond. Radiographics 2000;20(6):1585–1603.

36. Gylys-Morin V, Hoffer FA, Kozakewich H, et al. Wilms tumor and nephroblastomatosis: imaging characteristics at gadolinium-enhanced MR imaging. Radiology 1993;188(2):517–521.

37. White KS, Kirks DR, Bove KE. Imaging of nephroblastomatosis: an overview. Radiology 1992;182(1):1–5.

38. Antall PM, Myers MT, Dahms B, et al. Growth of a new intrarenal lesion in the remaining kidney of a patient with bilateral nephroblastomatosis and a previous nephrectomy for Wilms tumor. Med Pediatr Oncol 2000; 35(1):66–72.

39. Rohrschneider WK, Weirich A, Rieden K, et al. US, CT and MR imaging characteristics of nephroblastomatosis. Pediatr Radiol 1998;28(6):435–443.

15

Primary Bone Tumors

Robert Howman-Giles, Rodney J. Hicks, Geoffrey McCowage, and David K. Chung

Musculoskeletal sarcomas represent a heterogeneous group of malignancies involving bone and soft tissue with a highly variable natural history and a correspondingly diverse range of potential therapeutic strategies. The choice of treatment is largely driven by prognostic factors but is also dependent on local expertise, resources, and philosophies and the particular clinical circumstances of individual patients. Important considerations include the type, grade, extent, and location of the tumor. Curative treatment approaches in osteogenic sarcoma combine surgery and chemotherapy. In Ewing sarcoma, chemotherapy is used, and local control is achieved by surgery, radiotherapy, or a combination of both (1–3).

This chapter focuses on primary bone tumors in the pediatric population with an emphasis on the two most common forms: osteogenic sarcoma (OS) and Ewing sarcoma (ES). An initial general clinical summary provides the setting for understanding the role of diagnostic imaging in their assessment and management. The current contribution of positron emission tomography (PET) is summarized with an outline of likely future developments that promise to expand its range of applications.

Epidemiology

Primary bone tumors make up 5% to 6% of childhood malignancy, and the overwhelming majority of cases consist of either OS or ES (4–7). Other conditions more common in the pediatric than the adult population are Langerhans cell histiocytosis and primary bone lymphoma; however, collectively these account for a small percentage of primary malignant bone tumors. A smaller number of patients have other diagnoses such as malignant fibrous histiocytoma, angiosarcoma, and chondrosarcoma, but these conditions are very rare in the pediatric age group. The age distribution of patients with bone tumors is different from most other forms of childhood cancer. Childhood leukemia and solid tumors such as neuroblastoma, Wilms' tumor, and soft tissue sarcomas have their peak incidence during the first decade. In contrast, both OS and ES are more common in the second and third decades, a period in life also associated with accelerated normal bone growth.

Osteogenic sarcoma is a rare cancer arising from bone matrix and affecting children and adolescents. There is no sex or race predilection; in the United States the incidence is estimated to be 2 to 3 per million people. Most cases of OS (approximately 80%) occur between the ages of 5 and 25 years. Primary OS characteristically occurs in the metaphyseal regions of the long bones of the extremities, most frequently the distal femur, proximal tibia, and proximal humerus. Approximately 55% arise near the knee, but any bone can be affected including the flat bones and axial skeleton (4,6). Osteogenic sarcoma is usually a primary bone malignancy, but secondary forms may arise from Paget's disease, fibrous dysplasia, and multiple chondromas. These secondary forms are generally confined to older individuals and are not relevant to the pediatric population. There is also an association with previous radiation therapy, with the majority of cases in this group appearing within 7 to 15 years after the therapy. Again, this is usually beyond the pediatric period. There is, however, an association with bilateral retinoblastoma that is relevant to pediatric patients. Outcome is usually poor in all these secondary forms of OS (6).

Ewing sarcoma is a rare tumor arising from mesenchymal origin. It is the second most common malignant bone tumor after OS. It most commonly occurs in the second decade, with a peak age range from 4 to 15 years. The frequency in the United States ranges from 0.3 per million for children <3 years to 4.6 per million in patients aged from 15 to 19 years. Males are affected more frequently than females with a ratio of 1.5:1. Ewing sarcoma is most common in the white population and is rare in black and Chinese children. It most frequently involves the pelvis (25%), femur, tibia and fibula, spine, ribs, and humerus. Any bone may be involved (5,7).

Presentation

The most common presenting symptom for primary bone tumors is a painful swelling arising in bone. Pain is often initially attributed to trauma or physical exercise; symptoms may be present for several weeks or even months before diagnosis. The pain may be intermittent and severe, usually with a palpable mass, which is rapidly growing and often tender. There may be referred pain to the limbs if the primary is in the axial skeleton or pelvis. There may also be pain related to nerve root or cord compression if there is spinal involvement. Occasionally the patient may present with a pathologic fracture. The presentation may be similar to acute or chronic osteomyelitis with systemic symptoms of fever, malaise, weight loss, and leukocytosis. The majority of patients do not have clinical evidence of metastatic disease, but most are thought to have microscopic metastases, undetectable by conventional imaging techniques, at the time of presentation. Approximately 15% to 20% of patients have clinically evident metastatic disease at diagnosis. The lungs are the most common site of metastases, followed by bone and bone marrow (4,5).

Although imaging studies may be highly suggestive of the diagnosis of primary bone tumors, they cannot reliably differentiate among the various types of malignant bone tumor and occasionally cannot differentiate between malignant and benign conditions. Histopathologic confirmation, therefore, is required. Other differential diagnoses based on radiologic appearances can include infection (particularly destructive osteomyelitis), which may be very difficult to differentiate from malignancy, particularly in some areas such as the sacroiliac joint and vertebrae, and other bone malignancies including bone metastases and primary lymphoma of bone (4–8).

The treatments for OS and ES have much in common, in particular the routine use of neoadjuvant chemotherapy and the role of surgery. Radiotherapy has an important role in ES, particularly if the primary tumor cannot be surgically resected. There are, however, important differences in the approach to management of these two tumors. Knowledge of tumor histology, grade, and the presence or absence of metastases are the main prerequisites for allowing appropriate treatment selection. The other major factor that influences treatment and prognosis is the tumor response to therapy (9–11).

As these tumors are very heterogeneous in nature, the sites for biopsy are critical for accurate histologic staging. Biopsy of a small site of a tumor may not represent the overall character of the tumor and has the potential to miss high-grade areas (12). The implications of this are errors in diagnosis and grading that could influence the type of treatment given (13–15). Nondiagnostic biopsies may also occur, necessitating repeat biopsy. This may increase the risk of biopsy track seeding and may complicate the subsequent surgical technique. Open biopsy yields larger tissue samples for analysis and is generally preferable to core-needle biopsy. However, in experienced units, core biopsy can be a reliable technique and can expedite diagnosis because operating room time is not required. When planning biopsy, the nature of planned subsequent definitive surgery needs to be considered so that the biopsy site and tract can be included in the final resection. Resection at diagnosis is rarely performed, as delayed resection after neoadjuvant chemotherapy is now routine initial management of primary bone tumors (8).

Metastatic spread is mainly hematogenous initially to the lungs and later skeleton and bone marrow, although spread via the lymphatic system may occur. If local recurrence occurs, it is often difficult to diagnose as there is disturbance of the normal anatomic structures due to previous surgery or radiotherapy and imaging can be difficult to interpret due to artifacts from limb prostheses (8,13).

Histopathology

The diagnosis of malignancy involving bone requires histopathologic confirmation. Histopathology of OS reveals malignant sarcomatous tissue composed of pleomorphic spindle cells admixed with an extracellular matrix composed primarily of osteoid and bone. Such osteoid is an absolute requirement for the diagnosis of OS to be made, although occasionally osteoid is present only in small amounts, making the diagnosis difficult. Conversely, in the presence of pathologic fracture, immature osteoid can mimic OS. A number of histologic subtypes of OS exist, each with characteristic pathologic features. The most common subgroup is conventional OS, which is further divided into osteoblastic, chondroblastic, or fibroblastic variants, depending on the dominant pattern of differentiation of tumor cells. Other subgroups are telangiectatic, small cell, multifocal, periosteal, and parosteal OS. Most of these subtypes have similar clinical behavior, and management is similar except for the parosteal variant, which is more common in older patients, is typically of low histopathologic grade, and is associated with a more indolent clinical course (4,6).

Ewing sarcoma, peripheral neuroepithelioma, and primitive neuroectodermal tumor (PNET) belong to the Ewing family of tumors. Ewing sarcoma derives from a primitive neuroectodermal cell with variable differentiation. It is a poorly differentiated small, round, blue cell tumor where PNET shows discernible differentiation. All these tumors show some neural differentiation and have neural features, including expression of neuron specific enolase and S-100 protein. Both show a characteristic chromosomal translocation t(11; 22) or a variation within the tumor cell (5,7).

Diagnostic Imaging of Primary Bone Tumors

Anatomic imaging techniques including radiography, ultrasound, computed tomography (CT), and magnetic resonance imaging (MRI) currently play a dominant role in the evaluation of suspected and known sarcomas of both soft tissue and bone. Nuclear medicine techniques such as bone scintigraphy, thallium-201 (^{201}TI), and gallium-67 (^{67}GA) imaging have all been used in the assessment of primary bone tumors. However, PET is becoming the most important modality for assessing biologic characteristics of the tumor, for primary staging, and for determining response to treatment (13,16–18).

The diagnosis of primary bone tumor is usually made on a plain radiograph but may be suspected based on clinical examination findings. Osteogenic sarcoma is usually seen as an expansile, destructive lesion but may be sclerotic, lytic, or a combination of both. There is usually a significant degree of new bone formation. Often bone spicules are present running perpendicularly to the surface or arranged radially as a "sunburst" pattern. This is typical of the most common osteoblastic form of OS. There is usually a poorly defined zone of transition to normal bone that may be associated with a soft tissue mass. Lifting of the bone's normal periosteum by tumor may lead to the formation of Codman's triangle (6,19). The local extent, intramedullary spread, and relationship to soft tissue structures, particularly the neurovascular bundle, is best detected by cross-sectional imaging, in particular, by MRI.

In ES conventional radiology shows an aggressive destructive tumor with a permeated or moth-eaten appearance—a predominantly lytic lesion with poorly defined margins. The lesion is usually diaphyseal or metaphyseal with a soft tissue mass. There may be saucerization of the bone and a lamellated periosteal reaction with an onionskin pattern. There may be a spiculated pattern of new bone formation, which can be confused with the more common OS. Sclerotic lesions occur in approximately 25% of cases. There may be invasion of cortical bone, or the cancer may traverse the Haversian system and cause a large soft tissue mass in the absence of significant bone destruction. Based on the variable patterns observed radiologically, the differential diagnosis can include infection, OS, chondrosarcoma, fibrosarcoma, soft tissue sarcoma, and Langerhans cell histiocytosis. Lymphoma and leukemia may also mimic ES radiologically (7,19).

Magnetic resonance imaging and CT scanning allow definition of intralesional structural characteristics and of the relationship between tumor boundaries and adjacent normal tissues, including bone and neurovascular structures. For this purpose, MRI is now the major diagnostic tool (19,20). Regional anatomic information is important to determine the need for and approach to biopsy and to guide subsequent locoregional therapies, including radiotherapy and surgery. Tissue heterogeneity can make problematic the selection of the most appropriate biopsy site and the interpretation of anatomic imaging results following therapy. This is an important potential limitation because the behavior of sarcomas, their prognosis, and determination of the most appropriate management are influenced by the highest histologic grade of tumor that is present (12,21,22). Furthermore, for staging purposes, sensitive and specific whole-body screening capability is required.

Metastatic spread usually occurs first to the lungs and then to the skeleton. Computed tomography scan of the thorax is the main imaging modality for detection of pulmonary metastases, and the radionuclide bone scan is currently the primary investigation to detect skeletal metastases (4,5). Combined PET/CT imaging, however, is becoming the preferred modality for the detection of metastatic spread because of its ability to detect both soft tissue and bone sites of disease (Fig. 15.1), whereas the contemporaneous CT maintains good sensitivity for small lung metastases.

Treatment

The overall plan of management for localized primary bone tumor generally involves administration of preoperative neoadjuvant chemotherapy, delayed tumor resection and/or radiotherapy, and then further chemotherapy (8). The choice of postoperative chemotherapy is often dependent on the degree of tumor necrosis documented in the resection specimen on comprehensive histopathologic examination (11,13). Neoadjuvant chemotherapy is routinely used for several reasons:

- Chemotherapy treats micrometastatic disease, which is believed to be present but undetectable in many cases.

Figure 15.1. Pelvic Ewing sarcoma with bone metastases. A: A 13-year-old boy presented with a painful right hip. Magnetic resonance imaging (MRI) [short time inversion recovery (STIR) sequence coronal views] shows a primary pelvic tumor in the right iliac wing with a large soft tissue mass. B: Technetium-99m (^{99m}Tc) methylene diphosphonate (MDP) total bone scan shows a right pelvic primary tumor with marked osteoblastic reaction and metastatic sites in left mid-femur and sacrum. No other sites were detected. C: Fluorine-18 fluorodeoxyglucose (^{18}F-FDG) scan shows primary tumor and multiple metastases in the bone and marrow, particularly in the spine and pelvis. The patient initially responded to chemotherapy and radiotherapy to the primary tumor. Follow-up positron emission tomography (PET) showed good response with only a mild uptake of FDG in the primary site. The patient subsequently relapsed with metastases in the bone on PET (not shown).

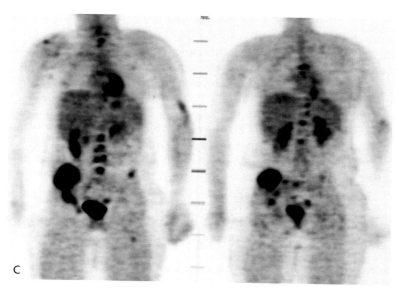

C

Figure 15.1. *Continued.*

- Resolution of soft tissue masses using chemotherapy may facilitate subsequent surgery.
- The period of some weeks between diagnosis and surgery allows for the ordering of customized orthopedic components such as prostheses or bone allografts that will be used at the time of surgical resection and limb reconstruction.
- Valuable information is obtained regarding the sensitivity of the tumor to the neoadjuvant chemotherapy agents. Patients with tumors that have a good histopathologic response to these drugs are given similar therapy postoperatively, whereas alternate agents and external beam radiotherapy may be considered if the tumor response has been poor.

After neoadjuvant chemotherapy but prior to surgery, imaging studies are repeated to evaluate tumor response and to exclude the development of new metastatic disease that might make aggressive surgery inappropriate. In particular, detection of metastases significantly reduces the chance of disease-free survival and usually argues against aggressive surgery on the primary unless the number of metastatic sites is small and also amenable to surgical resection.

Surgery in OS generally takes the form of a limb salvage procedure (4,23,24). The data show that the overall survival rate with such procedures approximates that obtained using amputation, but the functional outcome is superior. There is a higher risk of local recurrence (13,25,26), so effective multidrug chemotherapy is mandatory to prevent it. Similarly, in ES where historically radiotherapy was used for local control and surgery was used primarily for expendable bones, limb salvage surgery following chemotherapy is now the treatment of choice if the tumor can be completely removed and the function after surgery is predicted to be reasonable. The preference for surgery when possible in ES is largely due to the late effects of radiotherapy, especially second malignancy. In both cancers, radical tumor resection is performed if possible, followed by some form of reconstructive procedure using a prosthetic component, bone autograft or allograft, or more complex procedures, for example, rotation arthroplasty.

Histopathologic response is particularly important in primary bone tumors because lower "cell kill" is associated with an inferior prognosis (25). Alternate chemotherapy agents may be applied in such settings. Where there has been a good histologic response, similar agents are used postoperatively as were used at diagnosis, for a total treatment duration of 5 to 12 months (8).

Following completion of chemotherapy, most patients undergo some form of periodic screening for detection of recurrence and metastatic disease. Protocols vary but usually include chest x-ray, chest CT, imaging of the primary site with MRI or CT, and radionuclide bone scan. Fluorodeoxyglucose (FDG)-PET is having increasing application in this area.

Recurrent disease following therapy is a grave development, and only a small minority of such patients survive their disease. Restaging by imaging may be vital in facilitating timely diagnosis of recurrence and thereby improving the poor prognosis of such patients. Positron emission tomography has a major role in restaging. Therapeutic options for recurrent sarcoma include surgery, further chemotherapy, and palliative radiation therapy. Patients who develop isolated pulmonary metastases may be candidates for thoracotomy and metastasectomy; occasionally multiple such procedures can provide prolonged disease control. Recurrence at the primary site may require amputation. Further chemotherapy options may be limited because recurrence implies that there is drug resistance to the original agents. Such patients are candidates for experimental drug trials using novel agents.

Prognosis

The best predictor of outcome for patients with primary bone tumors without evidence of metastatic disease is the histologic response to induction chemotherapy (Figs. 15.2 and 15.3). This assessment is usually made at the time of surgery after neoadjuvant chemotherapy (4,5,25). A method to noninvasively assess treatment response would be very useful, as nonresponding tumors may require alternative or additional chemotherapy prior to their definitive surgery. Patients with OS that is localized at diagnosis have a relatively good prognosis: approximately 55% to 75% of such patients can be expected to be cured permanently. Patients with metastatic disease have an event-free survival below 20% (4). For ES, the European Intergroup Cooperative Ewing's Sarcoma Study (EICESS) reported the 3-year event-free survival rate was 66% in patients with localized tumors, 43% in those with lung metastases at initial diagnosis, and 29% in those with other metastases. A large tumor volume and a tumor primarily localized to the pelvic area were also negative prognostic factors (5).

Positron Emission Tomography

Positron emission tomography (PET) is an exciting technology for cancer evaluation, combining relatively high spatial resolution with high lesion contrast and the ability to assay biologic processes throughout the body. The commonest PET tracer used is fluorine-18 fluorodeoxyglucose (FDG). New hybrid PET-CT devices provide further enhancement of the potential of this modality by allowing accurate co-registration of functional and anatomic information, improving the localizing ability of PET (27).

The improved management and outcomes for primary bone tumors relate to improved diagnostic methods and to more reliable staging of the disease, which allows more appropriate treatment with both neoadjuvant chemotherapy and more patient-specific surgical procedures. Positron emission tomography is having increasing application as an additional modality to conventional imaging for more accurate tumor staging and restaging. This relates to primary tumor localization and extent, including soft tissue local disease, intramedullary extension, and detection of metastatic disease. It is also becoming the preferred modality to determine tumor response to neoadjuvant therapy. Therefore, PET has a major impact on the selection of appropriate chemotherapy regimens, surgical procedures, and prognosis (13,17,18).

Positron emission tomography imaging entails not only improved sensitivity for detecting malignant lesions but also quantitative procedures to be applied in the evaluation of primary bone tumors. The usual methods for quantitation are standard uptake value (SUV), tumor-to-background ratios (T/BG), graphical analysis, and nonlinear regression analysis based on a three-compartment model (13). These methods can generally be applied in the evaluation of primary bone tumors. In some cases, lack of significant blood pool–containing structures in the imaging field of view limits image-based evaluation of the arterial input function of radiotracer and may require arterial blood sampling. For practical reasons, most clinical studies have utilized SUV calculation rather than compartmental modeling or other quantitative approaches.

Initial Imaging of Primary Tumor

Tumor Grading

Many publications indicate that as the degree of FDG uptake is a measure of metabolic activity, it is indicative of tumor grade, that is, aggressiveness. The early studies using PET in musculoskeletal tumors in primarily adult populations showed increased uptake of FDG. The highest uptake of FDG was found in high-grade tumors, both soft tissue sarcomas and OS, when compared to low-grade or benign tumors (28–30). Subsequent publications have confirmed this finding. There is a significant correlation of histologic grading or tumor aggressiveness with FDG uptake measured by T/BG ratio, SUV, or kinetic modeling techniques (Table 15.1). Eary et al. (12) reported that tumor FDG uptake expressed as maximum SUV (SUV_{max}) has a high

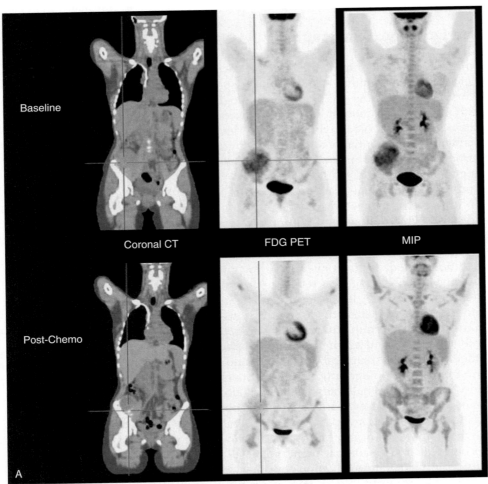

Figure 15.2. A good response to treatment. A: Ewing sarcoma. Images obtained on a combined PET–computed tomography (CT) of a large Ewing sarcoma of the pelvis with an extensive soft tissue mass at baseline (above) and after three cycles of chemotherapy (below). CT demonstrated negligible change, but a significant reduction in metabolic signal was apparent in both the osseous and soft tissue components, indicating a favorable response to treatment. The maximum intensity projection (MIP) images demonstrate relatively increased bone marrow activity following treatment. This is a common finding following chemotherapy and is thought to represent activated bone marrow. The changes are more pronounced with the use of growth factor (e.g., granulocyte colony-stimulating factor, G-CSF) support, but in children they can be very prominent even without this growth factor. B: Osteogenic sarcoma. Sequential coronal planes at baseline (above) and following completion of chemotherapy (below) demonstrate normal physiologic uptake of radiotracer in the epiphyseal growth plates of the right knee. A slightly heterogenous lesion with high FDG avidity is present on the baseline study in distal left femur that clearly crosses the growth plate to involve the epiphysis. On the posttreatment scan there is only low-grade peripheral uptake and no residual FDG uptake epi-centered on the initial sites of tumoral involvement. This was classified as a complete metabolic response and had >98% necrosis on the excision pathology specimen. C: From the same case displayed in B, MIP images demonstrate the change in biodistribution of FDG at baseline (left) and after chemotherapy (right). Normalizing the images to liver, which generally has the highest basal utilization of glucose of normal soft tissues under fasting conditions, demonstrates a marked reduction in uptake in the primary tumor but a marked increase in bone marrow activity. The posttreatment scan (performed during winter) also demonstrated significant uptake in cervical, axillary, paravertebral, and peridiaphragmatic brown fat. Despite the lack of significant CT response, the transaxial reference images (below) demonstrate a very significant reduction in tumoral FDG uptake. In the posttreatment setting, it is common to have a very homogeneous rim of low-grade uptake around the periphery of the initial tumoral site. This correlates with the development of an inflammatory pseudocapsule. We do not interpret this as residual tumor and classified this as a complete metabolic response. Partial metabolic responses are usually characterized by residual FDG that is epi-centered within areas of previous tumoral uptake rather than being peripheral to them.

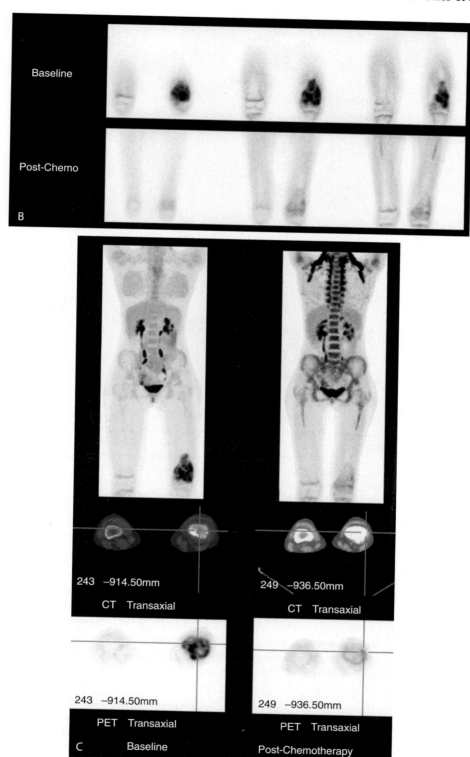

Figure 15.2. *Continued.*

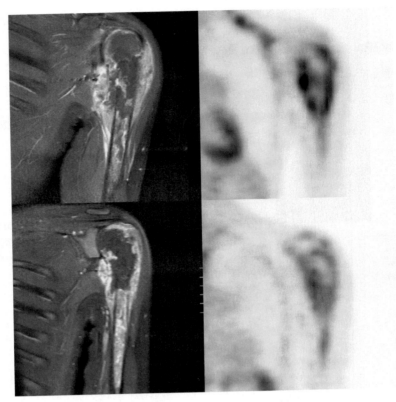

Figure 15.3. A poor response to treatment. Osteogenic sarcoma of the proximal left humerus in a 14-year-old girl. Top row shows pretherapy MRI (T1 post-gadolinium) and ^{18}F-FDG study. The MRI shows marked destruction of the proximal humerus with tumor crossing the growth plate, central bone necrosis, and extensive soft tissue tumor mass. The PET study shows marked heterogeneous distribution of FDG in the proximal humerus with focal increased metabolism seen peripherally and central necrosis. This scan indicates more specific biopsy sites in the most metabolic areas. This patient was a poor responder to neoadjuvant therapy (bottom row), with the MRI showing significant enhancement and the PET study persisting increased uptake. The post-surgical resection specimen showed <5% necrosis confirming poor response. Subsequently, this patient developed pulmonary metastases.

correlation with tumor grade in a series of 42 patients with soft tissue and bone sarcoma. Specific types of bone tumor were not detailed. The same group reported that the median SUV_{max} was significantly different for each histologic grade of tumor when divided into high-, intermediate-, and low-grade tumors. Looking at other markers of tumor aggressiveness, such as increased tumor cellularity, mitosis, and level of Ki-67 (proliferation of a specific nuclear antigen detected by immunohistochemical staining which correlates with growth fraction of tumors) proliferative index, there was also a significant correlation found with SUV_{max}. These researchers and others have also found moderate correlation with tissue levels of the cell growth regulation product p53 (31,32). These parameters have been correlated with a poorer outcome for higher tumor grades, shorter survival, and development of distant metastatic disease.

Table 15.1. Summary of studies of histologic grading or tumor aggressiveness and measures of fluorodeoxyglucose uptake

Study	No. of patients and tumor type	Histologic grade good	Overlap malignant vs benign	SUV T/NT	SUV malignant	SUV benign	Mit cell Ki-67	Sensitivity	Specifity	Accuracy	Survival SUV high
Eary et al. (12)	70 ST and BS	Yes									Yes
Schulte et al. (33)	202; 44 OS, 14 ES	Yes	Yes	T/NT >3.0	T/BG 3.3–73* T/BG 1.4–31.0**	T/BG 3.0–35.0		93%	67%	82%	
Feldman et al. (34)	45 ST and BS, 24 BS, 3 OS, 1 ES	Yes	Yes	SUV$_{max}$ >2.0	SUV$_{max}$ 3.74–9.23	SUV$_{max}$ 0.81–1.74		92%	100%	92%	
Dimitrakopoulou-Strauss et al. (35)	83; 9 OS, 8 ES	Yes		SUV + dynamic indices	SUV$_{max}$ 3.7 (0.4–12.3)	SUV$_{max}$ 1.1 (0.4–3.5)		SUV 54% SUV + dynamic 76%	91% 97%	75% 88%	
Aoki et al. (36)	52; 6 OS, 2 ES	Yes	Yes	SUV$_{mean}$	SUV 4.34 ± 3.19	SUV$_{mean}$ 2.18 ±1.52					
Kole et al. (38)	26; 5 OS, 2 ES	No	Yes large	SUV$_{av}$ MRFDG SUV$_{max}$	SUV$_{av}$ 3.2 (0.74–7.64) SUV$_{max}$ 7.07 (2.23–16.06)	SUV$_{av}$ 0.53 (0.22–1.07)					
Eary et al. (31)	209; 52 BS	Yes					Yes				Poor
Franzius et al. (39)	29 OS	Yes		T/NT$_{avg}$ 4.5 T/NT$_{max}$ 12.6	SUV$_{max}$ 1.4–60.0						T/NT$_{max}$ poor
Folpe et al. (32)	89 ST and BS	Yes					Yes				Poor

*High grade sarcoma
**Low grade sarcoma

BS = Bone sarcoma; ES = Ewing sarcoma; Mit Cell Ki67 = correlation SUV with indices of tumor aggressiveness (i.e. mitotic activity, cellularity, Ki67); OS = osteogenic sarcoma; Overlap = between malignant and benign. Some benign may have high uptake; ST = soft tissue; SUV$_{av}$ = SuVaverage; T/NT = Tumor uptake/Nontumor uptake.

Schulte et al. (33) used T/BG ratios in their series of 202 patients, including 44 patients with OS and 14 with ES. Among the bone sarcomas, OS had a tendency to higher T/BG ratios than did ES. Glucose metabolism was greater for high-grade malignant lesions than for low-grade tumors. Using a T/BG ratio of >3.0 for malignancy, the sensitivity was 93%, specificity 66.7%, and accuracy 81.7%. Other authors have used cutoff values of SUV to help differentiate between malignant and benign bone lesions. Feldman et al. (34) reported using a SUV_{max} cutoff of 2.0 for differentiating malignant from benign osseous and nonosseous lesions. They reported a sensitivity of 91.7%, specificity of 100%, and accuracy of 91.7%. All aggressive lesions had a SUV_{max} of >2.0. The differentiation was significant statistically. Dimitrakopoulou-Strauss et al. (35) reported dynamic quantitative FDG-PET in 9 OS and 8 ES patients in a group of 83 patients. Malignant tumors showed enhanced uptake, but there was visually an overlap with some benign lesions. The mean SUV was 3.7 (range 0.4–12.3) for malignant tumors compared to 1.1 (range 0.4–3.5) for benign lesions. Two grade I OS, one grade I ES, and a neuroectodermal tumor did not show enhanced FDG uptake. The authors used other parameters that also showed higher values in malignant tumors compared to benign lesions, but there was some overlap. They reported a sensitivity of 76%, specificity of 97%, and accuracy of 88%. Aoki et al. (36) in 52 patients showed a significant difference in the mean SUV between benign and malignant bone conditions. Although OS had high SUV, there were several other conditions, in particular giant cell tumors, fibrous dysplasia, sarcoidosis, and Langerhans cell histiocytosis, that also had high values. A cutoff level for differentiating OS could not be applied. Other benign or nonmalignant conditions that may have high FDG uptake and high SUV values are infective or inflammatory conditions such as osteomyelitis. Watanabe et al. (37) could not differentiate between osteomyelitis and malignant bone tumors. Also of note in their group of patients was that skeletal metastases tended to have higher SUV values than primary OS.

Only one publication reported no correlation between metabolic rate of glucose metabolism and biologic aggressiveness of bone tumors. Kole et al. (38) described 19 malignant and seven benign tumors. All lesions were clearly visualized by FDG-PET except for an infarct in a humerus. When SUV and Patlak derived metabolic rates were used to try to differentiate between benign and malignant tumors, there was a wide overlap between patients. The authors also commented that patients with low metabolic rates had a poor response to chemotherapy, and one patient with high rate responded well. They also observed that malignant fibrous histiocytoma and lymphoma had high rates compared to OS.

Indication of Prognosis

The prognostic value of PET may be even more important than its ability to define histopathologic grade. Eary et al. (31) analyzed SUV_{max} for the ability to predict patient survival and disease-free survival. In a retrospective analysis of 209 patients with sarcoma (52 primary bone tumors) who had FDG-PET, a multivariate Cox regression analysis was applied to SUV_{max} in predicting time to death or disease progression. The authors stated that SUV_{max} is a significant independent predictor of patient survival and disease progression. Tumors with higher SUV_{max} had a significantly poorer prognosis. Also, SUV_{max} had better correlation for histologic tumor grades with a higher significance of baseline SUV for prediction of outcome compared to conventional tumor imaging. Franzius et al. (39) evaluated 29 patients with primary OS. Using the average and maximum tumor-to-nontumor ratios (T/NT), they determined there were prognostic implications for OS based on the degree of FDG uptake. After chemotherapy, the patients underwent surgery, and response was determined histologically. Both overall and event-free survival were significantly better in patients with low T/NT_{max} than in patients with high T/NT_{max}. It was concluded that the initial glucose metabolism of primary OS, as measured by FDG T/NT_{max}, clearly discriminated between those patients with a high probability of overall and event-free survival versus OS patients with a poor prognosis. Of note was the fact that no significant difference was found between the various OS histology subtypes or the different regression grades. There was also no significant difference between the size of the primary tumor and uptake values. The fact that high FDG uptake correlates strongly with a poor outcome despite imperfect correlation with other known prognostic factors suggests that it may reflect a number of disparate adverse biologic characteristics.

Local Extent of Primary Tumor

Conventional cross-sectional radiographic imaging, that is, MRI and CT, are routinely used to define both the intraosseous and extraosseous extent of the primary tumor (Figs. 15.1 and 15.2). However, PET adds further information to these cross-sectional techniques, particularly with respect to intramedullary extension and skip lesions. Magnetic resonance imaging may overestimate tumor extension due to signal abnormalities of peritumoral edema. Also changes within the marrow cavity may be considered abnormal in children but may be due to physiologic red blood marrow distribution (40). Other changes such as necrosis or fibrosis within the tumor can be characterized better with PET.

Biopsy and Sampling Error

Histopathologic classification is a vital step in the management of suspected sarcomas. Tumor grade determined from biopsy has significant prognostic and management implications. The ability of PET to determine the biologic aggressiveness of tumors is very useful in indicating which sites in a tumor should be biopsied. There is usually marked heterogeneity of FDG uptake in sarcomatous tumors, and the accuracy of tumor diagnosis and the histologic grading may suffer from poor sampling. The areas of high metabolic activity are often seen in the peripheral regions of the tumor mass, particularly in large heterogeneous tumors within which there may be large areas of necrosis. False tumor grading, particularly an erroneous assessment of low grade, could have a significant impact on appropriate chemotherapeutic options. Folpe et al. (32) reported a good differentiation between levels of tumor grading by PET but could not distinguish between grade II and grade III tumors. Also, other tumors and some benign tumors may have high SUV values. Currently the published data do not support the idea that biopsy can be avoided as there are different histologic types of bone tumors that will determine specific treatments and there can be an overlap of some benign conditions. As the higher grades of tumor determine the overall histologic tumor grade and therefore predict outcome, the application of PET to indicate the most metabolically active sites of the tumor (Fig. 15.3) should allow better and more accurate sampling of the tumor (13,18).

False Positives

Fluorodeoxyglucose-PET has been reported to show increased accumulation in other malignant tumors, and in benign, inflammatory, and infective lesions. These include giant cell tumor, fibrous dysplasia, Langerhans cell histiocytosis, chondroblastoma, chondromyxoid fibroma, desmoplastic fibroma, aneurysmal bone cyst, nonossifying fibroma, fracture (Fig. 15.4), simple bone cyst with fracture, acute and chronic osteomyelitis, and renal osteopathy (13,33). These conditions generally require a positive diagnosis, if only for purposes of reassur-

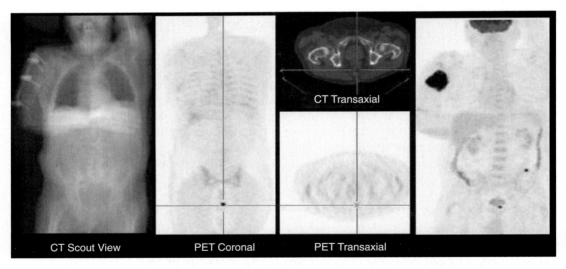

Figure 15.4. False-positive PET from a pathologic fracture. Although not a pediatric case, this figure illustrates the difficulty that can arise in differentiating between a pathologic fracture and primary osteosarcoma of bone. Based on clinical presentation and a biopsy taken at the time of internal fixation, this patient was believed to have an osteosarcoma of the right humerus. A staging PET scan demonstrated focal uptake in the prostate, and metastatic prostate cancer was subsequently confirmed on further immunohistochemistry of the initial biopsy specimen.

ance, and may have specific treatment that can be delivered once a diagnosis has been reached. Accordingly, these false-positive results need to be considered in the clinical context in which they occur. Certainly, if they were to lead to unnecessary or inappropriate surgery or chemotherapy, these results would be considered undesirable, but if they help to guide biopsy or exclude additional sites of disease, they can make a valuable contribution to patient management.

Metastatic Disease

In approximately 20% of cases there are clinically detectable metastases at diagnosis.

Pulmonary

As the main metastatic spread is to the lungs initially, high-resolution spiral CT (HRCT) is the recommended investigation. Since the implementation of the HRCT technique, there has been a doubling of detection of pulmonary metastases (10,13). Localized areas of pulmonary metastatic disease may be amenable to surgical removal. Positron emission tomography scans are useful to exclude additional macroscopic disease beyond the lungs. In some cases PET can also reliably identify false-positive results on CT and thereby spare patients unnecessary thoracotomy.

Schulte et al. (41) performed a comparison of CT and PET in detecting pulmonary metastases but did not show any significant difference for the number of lesions. Other studies have reported similar findings in soft tissue sarcoma. However, Franzius et al. (42) reported a comparison of CT and PET for pulmonary metastases in 32 patients who had 49 PET scans. The sensitivity, specificity, and accuracy of FDG-PET were 50%, 100%, and 92%, respectively. The metastases missed by PET were small (<9 mm). However, additional lesions were detected that were not seen by CT. Lucas et al. (43) also reported, in soft tissue sarcomas, metastatic spread outside the lungs, which was not seen by CT or MRI.

In summary, HRCT is the recommended modality for the detection of pulmonary metastases, particularly for <1 cm lesions; however, PET may add further information on whether these are malignant and may detect extrapulmonary metastases. Because benign pulmonary nodules are relatively common, particularly with newer helical CT scanners, not all lesions seen in the lungs in the context of primary osseous tumors are malignant. In the clinical situation where no previous investigations are available to determine the appearance or growth of lung nodules, PET can provide complementary information regarding the likelihood of malignancy. Those nodules that have intense FDG uptake are highly likely to represent metastases. Less intense FDG uptake should also be considered suspicious if the size of the nodule in question is less than twice the reconstructed spatial resolution of the PET scanner being used, because partial-volume effects significantly degrade count recovery for small lesions (44). For most modern PET scanners, this would

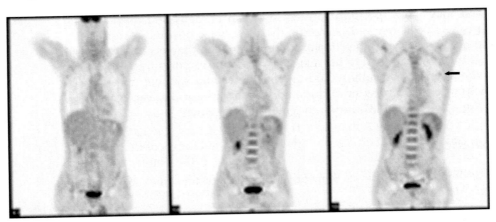

Figure 15.5. Pulmonary metastases. This patient with multifocal local recurrence related to osteosarcoma of the right lower leg (not shown) had multiple new lung nodules on CT scanning. Only the largest of these, a 9-mm left upper lobe lesion was clearly abnormal on FDG-PET (right coronal plane image). Nevertheless, the presence of metabolic abnormality in any nodules that are sufficiently large to be relatively unaffected by partial volume effects increases the likelihood that any other nonvisualized but smaller nodules are also malignant.

equate to lesions less than 10 mm in diameter. Respiratory excursion can also lead to partial volume effects, and one would generally expect somewhat lower FDG uptake in basal than apical lung nodules of comparable size due to greater respiratory blurring in the former. Finally, the avidity of the primary tumor is usually reflected in the intensity of uptake in metastatic sites. Accordingly, absence of FDG uptake in a lesion of 10 mm in the apex of the lung of a patient with an OS with a SUV_{max} of 25 is much more likely benign than malignant, whereas a lesion of the same size in the lung base of a patient with an ES with a SUV_{max} of 3.5 has a higher likelihood of malignancy on technical considerations alone. Of course, the radiologic features of the nodule, other clinical details, and the prevalence of benign lung nodules in the general population of the case in question also influence the likelihood of malignancy (Fig. 15.5).

Skeleton

The second most common area of metastatic disease is the skeleton, which occurs in 10% to 20% of patients with metastatic disease. Franzius et al. (45) looked at 70 patients with primary bone tumors (32 OS, 38 ES) for metastatic disease. The reference methods for imaging modalities were histopathologic analysis and conventional imaging with follow-up for 6 to 64 months. In 21 examinations, 54 osseous metastases were detected (5 OS, 49 ES). Fluorodeoxyglucose-PET had sensitivity, specificity, and accuracy of 90%, 96%, and 95%, respectively, compared to the radionuclide bone scan using technetium-99m (^{99m}Tc)-MDP [methylene diposphonate], which had 71%, 92%, and 88%, respectively. Interestingly, when the OS and ES were compared, the performance of PET relative to bone scanning differed. For ES, the sensitivity, specificity, and accuracy of PET were 100%, 96%, and 97%, respectively, compared to bone scintigraphy of 68%, 87%, and 82%, respectively. However, none of the five OS osseous metastases were detected by FDG but were true positive on the bone scan. In a more recent publication by the same group, the authors reported 100% detection by FDG-PET in six sites of bony metastatic disease from OS (46). These differences may relate to the contrast resolution of the respective modalities. Very high osteoblastic activity in metastatic OS sites may improve lesion sensitivity even though the spatial resolution of planar and SPECT bone scanning is less than that of PET. Conversely, improvements in PET instrumentation including improved scanner resolution and better attenuation correction methods could also improve lesion sensitivity.

Daldrup-Link et al. (47) compared FDG-PET, bone scintigraphy, and whole-body MRI for detection of bone metastases from multiple types of malignancies. They looked at 39 children and young adults with various metastases including 20 patients with ES and three with OS. Of 51 bone metastases, the overall sensitivity for FDG-PET, whole-body MRI, and bone scintigraphy were 90%, 82%, and 71%, respectively. False-negative sites were different for the three modalities. In one patient with osteogenic sarcoma, a single metastasis was diagnosed with bone scintigraphy and MRI but was negative on FDG-PET. Most false-negative findings for PET were in the skull; for MRI in flat and small bones, the skull, carpal bones, and radius; and for bone scintigraphy in the spine. The number of skeletal metastases was inversely related to lesion size. Large lesions >5 cm were correctly diagnosed with FDG-PET and MRI in 100% of patients, but skeletal scintigraphy had a sensitivity of 93%. Sensitivity for smaller lesions of 1 to 5 cm for FDG-PET was 86%, MRI 79%, and skeletal scintigraphy 62%. For bone metastases <1 cm, FDG-PET showed a sensitivity of 86%, MRI 57%, and skeletal scintigraphy 57%. More false positives, however, were found with PET; they were, in this series, a simple bone cyst, an enchondroma, and an osteoma. The latter two were diagnosed with plain radiography. Increased sensitivities for detection of lesions were found by combining the modalities: for skeletal scintigraphy and MRI, 90%; for skeletal scintigraphy and FDG-PET, 96%; and for MRI and FDG-PET, 96%. Thus the sensitivities of skeletal scintigraphy and MRI alone were significantly increased either in combination with each other or with PET. But the sensitivity of PET was not increased significantly by combining with one of the other modalities. In clinical practice, as opposed to technical validation studies, PET should always be interpreted in the clinical context and with careful correlation of all the imaging results available in a given patient. The choice and order in which imaging studies are performed will also likely be determined by a multitude of factors including cost, convenience, and availability. Although bone scanning is relatively inexpensive and widely available, it is probably worthwhile in most cases of OS, but its role in ES and other sarcomas must be questioned if PET is available.

In the future there may be a role for ^{18}F-PET scans. Initial evaluation indicates a high detection rate for skeletal metastases. Accordingly, this may enhance the sensitivity for metastases in OS compared to FDG-PET by virtue of higher lesion avidity and compared to bone scintigraphy by virtue of superior spatial resolution (13).

Other Secondary Sites

Metastases to other areas, for example, lymph nodes, brain, and soft tissue, are uncommon but can be detected by PET. There are no data comparing conventional radiology techniques with PET for this role. The ability of PET, however, to screen the whole body is a significant advantage (13,41,43).

Assessment of Response to Treatment

Response to preoperative adjuvant chemotherapy has been shown to be the most important prognostic factor in the management of OS and ES, as the degree of tumor necrosis from the therapy is highly correlated with disease-free survival after therapy (8,21,22). Due to the surgical and prognostic implications relating to an adequate response to neoadjuvant therapy, a noninvasive marker for assessing histologic response would be very clinically useful. Tumor necrosis can exist in the primary tumor and is itself a manifestation of large or aggressive tumors. It can be difficult to know on the basis of a small pretreatment biopsy the proportion of viable and nonviable tumor and therefore compare relative change in this parameter when confronted by a large excisional specimen posttreatment. Evaluation of early response to chemotherapy in primary bone tumors after 3 to 6 weeks of therapy may be highly predictive of tumor necrosis; whether PET is valid for this purpose requires further study. In this way, noninvasive assessment of chemotherapy response by PET may significantly alter patient management (Figs. 15.2 and 15.3). For instance, limb-sparing surgery is more likely to be considered if there is a favorable response to chemotherapy. There may be an alteration in surgical approach. Also if there is an unfavorable response several investigators recommend a change in chemotherapeutic regimen. The earlier that this can be detected, the earlier the change can be made (4,5,8,13).

Radiologic methods such as radiography, CT, and MRI are poorly suited for discriminating adequately between responding and nonresponding osseous tumors. The tumors frequently do not change in size, or there may be some minor change in the soft tissue mass around the osseous component. The response of the tumor detected by using these conventional methods does not reflect the quantity of residual viable tumor. New techniques using dynamic contrast-enhanced MRI have been shown to improve the differentiation of viable sarcoma tissue from tumor necrosis as an early indicator of recurrence. This technique is promising and needs further evaluation (18,48,49).

Functional nuclear medicine biological methods such as thallium 201 (^{201}Tl), ^{99m}Tc sestamibi, and FDG-PET have been shown to be effective response markers for chemotherapy assessment in primary bone tumors (17). ^{201}Tl and ^{99m}Tc sestamibi have been used to determine grade and response to chemotherapy. A negative ^{201}Tl or ^{99m}Tc sestamibi scan after therapy reflected a grade III to IV response with >90% necrosis of tumor cells. Kostakoglu et al. (50) reported for ^{201}Tl a sensitivity of 100%, specificity of 87.5%, and accuracy of 96.5% compared to sensitivities of 95%, 50%, and 82.7%, respectively, for CT, MRI, and angiography in bone and soft tissue sarcomas. However, FDG-PET with its uptake quantifiable by using SUV or T/BG ratios adds further information and is recommended if available.

Jones et al. (51) were one of the first groups to report the impact of FDG-PET in the monitoring of treatment in patients with musculoskeletal sarcoma, 3 of whom had OS. The authors observed a 25% to 50% reduction of the peak and average SUV, 1 to 3 weeks after chemotherapy was instituted; this correlated with >90% tumor cell necrosis. They also reported that there was increased FDG uptake seen in granulation tissue and in the pseudofibrous capsule in treated cancers. This indicates that there is FDG uptake in both the viable tumor and some benign reactive tissues (Fig. 15.2C). This has the potential to overestimate the presence of OS. Other groups have reported changes in response to treatment in a significant number of patients with primary bone tumors by using PET and showed good correlation with histopathologic changes after treatment (Table 15.2) (41, 52, 53).

Franzius et al. (52) reported good correlation in 17 patients between T/NT ratios and primary bone tumors (11 OS, 6 ES). The mean T/NT was 5.2 (range 2.2–13.6) for all 17 patients with posttherapy values of 2.3 (0.9–11.9). For OS pretherapy T/NT was 5.5 (2.3–13.6) and posttherapy 2.8 (0.9–11.9); for ES the pretherapy was 5.3 (2.2–11.9) and posttherapy 1.4 (1.0–1.9). There was good correlation with tumor necrosis on histopathology in 15 of 17 overall, in 9 of 11 patients with OS, and in all 6 of the patients with ES. The authors found that a threshold of a 30% decrease in the ratio represented good responders (<10% viable tumor cells) and could distinguish these patients from poor responders in all cases.

Hawkins et al. (53) looked at SUV values of FDG-PET uptake in 14 OS and 14 ES patients. They used SUV$_{max}$ values in tumors pre-(SUV1) and post-(SUV2) chemotherapy. They demonstrated that a reduction in tumor FDG uptake, measured by SUV2$_{max}$ and the ratio of SUV2/SUV1, correlated with chemotherapy response as quantified by percent necrosis after surgical resection. In OS SUV1 was 8.2 (2.5–24.1) and decreased to SUV2 of 3.3 (1.6–12.8) after chemotherapy; SUV2 was particularly accurate in identifying OS patients with unfavorable response. In the ES group, the SUV1 was 5.3 (range 2.3–11.8) and decreased to SUV2 of 1.5 (0–2.4) posttherapy. The mean percent necrosis of the OS group was lower than the ES group; only 28% of OS tumors responded adequately with a mean percent necrosis of >90%. However, the authors report that both the SUV2 and SUV2/SUV1 ratio are imperfect at distinguishing favorable from unfavorable responses. Using a cutoff point of <2 for SUV2 to predict favorable response was incorrect in 16% and using a cutoff point of <0.5 for SUV2/SUV1 for a favorable response was incorrect in 27% of patients. The most likely

Table 15.2. Changes in response to treatment in patients with primary bone tumors

Study	Pathology	Pretherapy SUV1, T/NT1, T/BG1,	Posttherapy SUV2, T/NT2, T/BG2	Response	Correlation with necrosis
Franzius et al. (52)	17 BS	T/NT mean 5.2 (2.2–13.6)	T/NT mean 2.3 (0.9–11.9)	15/17 good	Yes
	11 OS	T/NT 5.5 (2.3–13.6)	T/NT 2.8 (0.9–11.9)	9/11 good	Yes
	6 ES	T/NT 5.3 (2.2–11.9)	T/NT 1.4 (1.0–1.9)	6/6 good	Yes
Hawkins et al. (53)	18 OS	SUV_{mean} 8.2 (2.5–24.1)	SUV_{mean} 3.3 (1.6–12.8)	Yes	Mean 66% (0–98%)
	15 ES	SUV 5.3 (2.3–11.8)	SUV_{mean} (0–2.4)	Yes	Mean 98% (90–100%)
			OS SUV2/SUV1 0.55 (0.12–1.1) ES SUV2/SUV1 0.35 (0.16–0.73)		
Schulte et al. (41)	27 OS	T/BG 10.3 (3.3–33.2)			
	Responder	T/BG 10.34 (3.89–33.2)	T/BG 2.27 (0.32–17.5)	Good	Yes
	Nonresponder	T/BG 9.64 (3.26–22.2)	T/BG 6.37 (2.24–20.33)	Poor	Yes
Jones et al. (51)	9 ST and BS	SUV_{max} 5.8 (2.0–12.0) 6/9 high grade SUV_{mean} 3.6 (1.7–6.1)	SUV_{max} 3.3 (2.3–4.3) 2/9 SUV_{mean} 2.1 (1.8–2.3) 2/9	3 OS Yes	>90% Yes

BS = Bone sarcoma; ES = Ewing sarcoma; OS = steogenic sarcoma; ST = Soft Tissue Sarcoma; SUVm = SUVmean; T/BG = Tumor/Background; T/NT = Tumor/Nontumor.

explanation was due to increased FDG uptake in inflammatory infiltrates or reactive fibrosis within the tumor as a response to chemotherapy. Other reasons are that the histopathologic evaluation averages the percentage of necrosis across the entire resected tumor specimen, whereas the SUV technique is based on the maximum value within the tumor. Stated another way, a specimen that is extensively necrotic but with isolated foci of viable tumor would be classified as favorable, but the maximum SUV may remain elevated reflecting the focal viable tumor. A method similar to that proposed by Larson et al. (54)

that integrates the extent and intensity of metabolic activity may be useful in such situations. The methodology to define the volume of abnormal voxels—whether single or multiple voxels should be used—for determination of the degree of SUV abnormality remains to be established (18).

Schulte et al. (41), studying 27 patients with OS using T/BG ratios, found a reduction in T/BG of >40% represented responders to chemotherapy with an accuracy of 92.6%. The T/BG before therapy in all patients ranged from 3.3 to 33.2 (median 10.3). In the responder group, the pretherapy T/BG was 10.34 (3.89–33.2) and in nonresponders 9.64 (3.26–22.2). The posttherapy T/BG was for responders 2.27 (0.32–17.5) and nonresponders 6.37 (2.24–20.33). The posttherapeutic values differed significantly between the responders and nonresponders. The extent of T/BG reduction, however, did not precisely predict the quantitative amount of tumor necrosis. They did not report any false-positive cases where they classified a responder as a nonresponder due to benign reactive uptake as described by Jones et al. (51).

Serial assessments to monitor chemotherapeutic response were also discussed by Nair et al. (55). They looked at 16 patients with OS. The percentage change in tumor to background ratio (T/BR) did not predict a 90% or higher rate of tumor necrosis. Visual assessment and T/BR values, however, were predictive in 15 of 16 patients.

Further evaluation of the optimal quantitative method to assess response should be undertaken, but the present data indicate that FDG-PET is a relatively accurate indicator of tumor response to neoadjuvant therapy.

Local Tumor Recurrence

The ability to detect residual viable tumor after therapy and to detect local recurrence of tumor as early as possible is vital for improvement in survival. It is also one of the most difficult areas of management. Conventional imaging has significant limitations because of changes in normal anatomy, distortion of tissue planes, and lack of distinction between tumor and postoperative tissue, and image artifacts from metallic limb prostheses. Differentiation from fibrosis, posttherapeutic changes, and inflammatory tissue changes can be extremely difficult. Magnetic resonance imaging with gadolinium enhancement may also show increased enhancement in immature scar tissue and nonmalignant reactive tissue (56). Most of the comparisons of MRI and FDG-PET for the assessment of residual viable tumor and local recurrence relate to soft tissue sarcomas, presumably due to the inherent difficulties in evaluating periprosthetic sites. Garcia et al. (57) reported FDG was helpful in differentiating active musculoskeletal sarcomas from posttreatment changes in 48 patients. There were 18 patients with OS. The diagnosis was confirmed by histology, and the sensitivity and specificity were 98% and 90%, respectively. Similar results were found by el-Zeftawy et al. (58) in 20 patients with both bone and soft tissue tumors. The authors' conclusion was that FDG added important information to CT and MRI to help differentiate postoperative change from local recurrence (Fig. 15.6). Franzius et al. (46) also reported detection of local recurrence in 6 patients with OS but had 1 false-negative study. In the same group of patients, the MRI detected all 6 recurrences, but there were 2 false-positive studies. In another group, Lucas et al. (43) found that MRI had a higher sensitivity of 88.2% compared to PET of 73.7% for the detection of local recurrence of soft tissue sarcomas after amputation. There are, however, significant difficulties with CT and MRI in patients with implantation of metallic prostheses (59). Hains et al. (60) described the limitations of FDG-PET in detecting local recurrence in amputation stumps. In their study, focal areas of FDG were seen in known pressure areas and skin breakdown for up to 18 months after surgery. However, in the absence of localized clinical changes in the stump, any uptake may represent recurrence and should be biopsied (Fig. 15.7). The co-registration of PET with CT or MRI should help significantly in these cases.

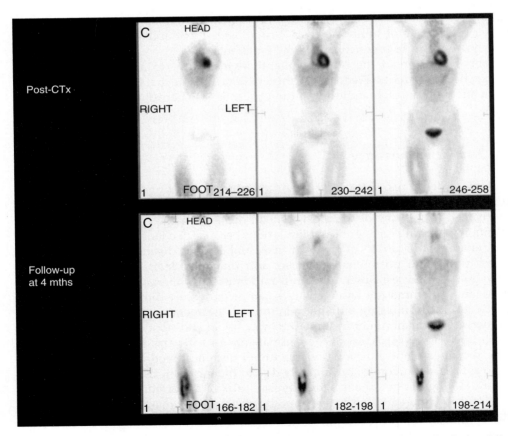

Figure 15.6. Recurrence. This patient had undergone chemotherapy for a distal right femoral Ewing sarcoma. The posttherapy PET scan demonstrated a very good but partial metabolic response with mildly increased activity inferomedially in the femur. A follow-up scan (below) performed 4 months later demonstrates extensive local recurrence. Note normal thymic uptake in an adolescent.

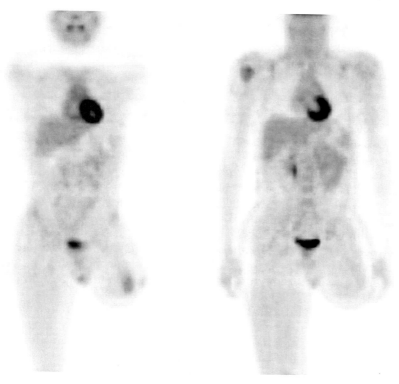

Figure 15.7. Recurrence of osteogenic sarcoma in amputation stump and development of skeletal metastases. This patient had a primary osteogenic sarcoma (OS) of the left femur removed 2 years previously. The PET study shows recurrence in the amputation stump and a metastatic deposit in the proximal right humerus. The patient developed multiple skeletal metastases over the following 6 months and died.

Other PET Radiopharmaceutical Agents

Fluorine-18 Fluoride

Unchelated fluorine-18 fluoride (^{18}F) was introduced as a bone imaging agent in 1962 (61). It became the standard for bone scanning until the introduction of ^{99m}Tc–labeled diphosphonates. It has a similar mechanism of uptake to the latter, depending on local blood flow for tracer delivery, diffusion through extracellular fluid to the bone mineral interface, and adsorption to the hydroxyapatite crystal to form fluoroapatite (62). Therefore, uptake reflects osteoblastic activity.

Inevitable comparisons have been made with ^{99m}Tc diphosphonate bone scans. One cited advantage of ^{18}F is superior pharmacokinetics. ^{18}F has a higher extraction rate and faster blood clearance, allowing imaging to commence as early as 1 hour after intravenous administration (63). Other advantages arise in combination with current generation PET or PET-CT scanners, allowing dynamic quantitation and superior spatial and contrast resolution. One main drawback is the higher cost of ^{18}F compared to the more widely available diphospho-nate radiopharmaceuticals. However, as FDG production increases, ^{18}F fluoride production as a by-product could become more efficient and decrease radiotracer costs.

To date there has been little published experience with ^{18}F-PET in primary bone tumors and even less for the pediatric population. One early series was from Hoh et al. (63), who reported their experience in 19 adult patients with a mix of benign and malignant bone patholo-gies. Using visual and a semiquantitative assessment (uptake ratio of lesion-to-contralateral bone), it was not possible to differentiate benign from malignant lesions. Of interest, there were 4 patients with OS in the group. The three patients who had no prior treatment had primary tumors with the highest uptake ratios in the study. The other patient's scan followed systemic therapy; the uptake here was lower than the other three, suggesting a potential role for ^{18}F-PET in therapeutic mon-itoring. Three of these 4 patients had multiple scan lesions, indicating that metastases were also visualized, both skeletal and pulmonary. One patient was specifically mentioned with uptake in multiple pulmonary nodules.

Going further than the above study, would formal dynamic ^{18}F-PET quantitation with blood sampling improve either the differentiation between benign and malignant lesions or be incorporated into thera-peutic monitoring of primary bone tumors? As yet no studies have addressed this question. However, we can look at the experience with ^{99m}Tc diphosphonates where there is a similar mechanism of uptake. Just as reactive bone formation or turnover often accounts for more bone tracer localization than uptake by viable tumor, it is predicted that ^{18}F-PET would be similarly unsuccessful (64).

There are more studies of ^{18}F-PET for metastatic surveys. Although these have again been mostly adult patients with unselected cancers, many of the observations should be relevant here. Conventional bone scans have a lower resolution, and almost all are planar images, with single photon emission computed tomography (SPECT) limited to a localized region of the body. The higher resolution and whole-body tomography intrinsic to ^{18}F-PET predicts superior diagnostic performance. Schirrmeister et al. (65–67) found this to be the case in series of patients with breast, lung, prostate, and thyroid cancer. Supe-rior resolution in the spine allowed more specific diagnosis over con-ventional planar bone scans (67). This observation was taken a step further with the more recent study of ^{18}F-PET-CT vs. ^{18}F-PET from Even-Sapir et al. (68). One would expect that the improved lesion localization from PET/CT would improve diagnostic accuracy, and this was the case. Their study population ranged in age from 15 to 81 years old. There were three cases of ES, one chondrosarcoma, and one giant cell tumor. In a patient-based analysis for the detection of metastatic disease, ^{18}F-PET-CT was superior to ^{18}F-PET alone in sensi-tivity (100% vs. 88%, $p < .05$) and specificity (88% vs. 56%, not signifi-cant). Therefore, this is the most promising area for ^{18}F-PET; more studies of specific tumor types, including pediatric primary bone tumors, are awaited. The feasibility of acquiring ^{18}F-PET and ^{18}F-FDG-

PET scans at one clinic attendance is another interesting area for study.

^{18}F-α-Methyltyrosine

After promising initial studies with iodine-123–labeled methyltyrosine (69), fluorine-18 α-methyltyrosine (^{18}FMT) was developed for PET imaging (70). It is a tracer for the increased amino acid utilization by tumors, as is carbon-11 (^{11}C) methionine (see below), but it has a significant advantage by virtue of its tumor-specific transport. Watanabe et al. (71) reported a comparison between ^{18}FMT and ^{18}F-FDG in baseline pretreatment musculoskeletal tumors. The study group comprised 75 patients with benign and malignant tumors and included three patients (ages 14 to 34 years) with OS, a 12-year-old patient with ES, and adult patients with chondrosarcoma and giant cell tumor. All malignant bone tumors showed ^{18}FMT uptake. Of note, there was also uptake within a pulmonary metastasis from OS. There was higher uptake in malignant lesions than benign, and there was good correlation with ^{18}F-FDG uptake. Using ^{18}FMT mean SUV cutoff of 1.2 to differentiate benign vs. malignant lesions, the diagnostic accuracy was 81.3%, which was higher than the respective analysis for ^{18}F-FDG. Thirteen of 18 lesions that were false positive on ^{18}F-FDG were found to have an ^{18}FMT mean SUV lower than the cutoff and would have been correctly classified as benign. However, ^{18}FMT was found to be inferior for grading of malignancy. It was suggested that the lower absolute values and ranges of its mean SUV were responsible. In summary, another promising alternative to ^{18}F-FDG and more studies are awaited.

Fluorine-18 fluoro-3′-deoxy-3′-L-fluorothymidine

Fluorine-18 fluoro-3′-deoxy-3′-L-fluorothymidine (FLT) has been developed as a proliferative tracer to provide a noninvasive staging tool and to measure response to anticancer therapy (72). Proliferating cells synthesize DNA during the S phase of the cell cycle. FLT is a pyrimidine analogue and uses the salvage pathway of DNA synthesis for imaging proliferation. The ability to image cell proliferation may offer the possibility to differentiate between benign and malignant disease. FLT is taken up by the cell via passive diffusion and facilitated transport by Na^+-dependent carriers. FLT is then phosphorylated by thymidine kinase (TK) into FLT monophosphate, after which it is trapped in the cell. Preliminary comparisons with FDG show that FLT can visualize malignant cancers but at a lower sensitivity than FDG. Some tumors metabolically rely on the de novo synthesis of DNA precursors, resulting in little or no uptake of thymidine and FLT. As a proliferative marker, because FLT is phosphorylated by TK, which has high activity in the S phase of cell synthesis. There are higher concentrations of FLT in malignant cells compared to normal cells. There have been several reports of strong correlation of FLT with other proliferative markers (Ki-67 index). As tumor mass heterogeneity is visualized, there is the potential for determining optimal biopsy sites (Fig. 15.8).

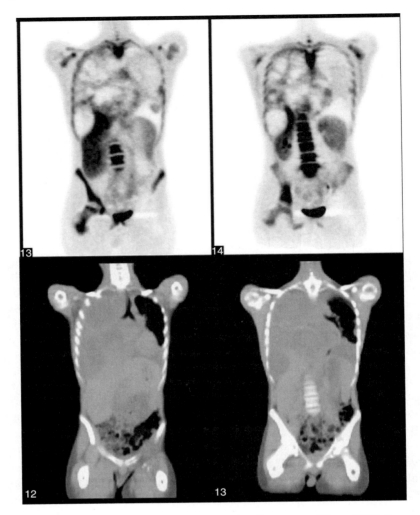

Figure 15.8. Fluorine-18 fluoro-3'-deoxy-3'-L-fluorothymidine (FLT) in sarcoma. Following radiotherapy for a synovial sarcoma of the left hip, this adolescent boy developed progressive right lung metastases and bilateral pleural effusions. ^{18}F-FLT-PET scanning demonstrates heterogeneous uptake in the opacified right hemithorax with very low uptake in the bilateral basal pleural effusions and in areas of necrotic tumor but relatively high uptake at the periphery of solid tumoral deposits indicating active proliferation. Note the high uptake in the bone marrow with the exception of the irradiated left hip, where there is no uptake consistent with local marrow ablation. High uptake in the kidneys and liver reflect normal excretion but limit detection of metastatic disease in these organs. The spleen is also visualized, displaced inferiorly and medially by the left basal pleural effusion. In our experience, the spleen is not normally visualized in adults except in cases of extramedullary hematopoiesis or malignant infiltration.

In the initial data on assessment of response to anticancer therapy, FLT uptake has been shown to decrease after some therapy but may increase after other types. This would most likely be due to the various metabolic actions of the different chemotherapeutic agents. Preliminary studies using FLT have been reported in various tumors, including soft tissue sarcoma. Cobben et al. (73) found correlations among SUV and T/NT and mitotic score, Ki-67, and the French and Japanese grading systems. Visualization of the tumors was good, and FLT was able to differentiate between low- and high-grade tumors. However, no differentiation could be made between benign and low-grade tumors. This agent appears promising and potentially may be useful in primary bone tumors. However, further research is needed to clarify the value of FLT in cancer management. High uptake of FLT in normal proliferating marrow may limit sensitivity for detection of bone metastases and for evaluating the extent of marrow spread in marrow-containing regions of the skeleton. This poses a potential limitation, particularly in pediatric patients, because of more extensive appendicular marrow than seen in adults (72,73).

Carbon-11–Based Tracers

Carbon-11–labeled methionine (^{11}C-Met) was developed as a tracer for the increased amino acid metabolism in tumors. There are few studies on extracranial tumors, in part because of its participation in too many metabolic pathways to allow kinetic modeling (74). Of the published studies of ^{11}C-Met, only a few relate to primary bone tumors. Inoue et al. (75) studied 24 adult patients with clinically suspected recurrent or residual tumors, using ^{11}C-Met and ^{18}F-FDG-PET. Their group included one case of proven recurrent pelvic ES where ^{11}C-Met was false negative but was detected by ^{18}F-FDG. Both PET agents were false negative in one case of recurrent pelvic chondrosarcoma, but both were true positive in two cases of recurrent giant cell tumor. Therefore, the early report card for ^{11}C-Met is mixed; it is not clearly superior to ^{18}F-FDG.

Methyl-C-11 choline (^{11}C-choline) takes advantage of increased tumor requirements for choline, which is phosphorylated, integrated within lecithin, and finally becomes a component of the phospholipid cell membrane (76). After injection, tumor uptake equilibrates at 5 minutes, allowing earlier image acquisition than is the case with ^{18}F-FDG. Another potential advantage of ^{11}C-choline is that it does not accumulate in the bladder compared with the usual urinary excretion of FDG, a consideration when evaluating pelvic lesions. The application to bone and soft tissue tumors has been published in two articles from the Gunma University group comparing ^{11}C-choline and ^{18}F-FDG-PET scans, with what appears to be some overlap of both study samples (77,78). Yanagawa et al. (77) reported only patients at pretreatment baseline. Their first group included 5 ranging in age from 11 to 20 years with OS. Zhang et al. (78) appear to have included some patients undergoing therapy, but the 2 scans were acquired within 2 weeks of each other with no change in therapy. This second group included 2 older patients with OS and 2 patients (17 and 24 years old) with ES. Both studies included other benign and malignant tumors. All malignant tumors showed ^{11}C-choline uptake, and their mean tumor SUV was higher than benign tumors. ^{11}C-choline uptake showed good correlation with ^{18}F-FDG uptake. However, significant ^{11}C-choline uptake was also seen in some benign tumors in both study groups, viz. giant cell tumor, desmoid tumor, fibroma, neurofibroma, inflammatory granulation tissue, and pigmented villonodular synovitis. When analyzing the ability of ^{11}C-choline to differentiate benign from malignant lesions, both groups used different mean SUV cutoff values—2.7 for a diagnostic accuracy of 90.9% (77) and 2.59 for a diagnostic accuracy of 75.6% (78). The differing result was attributed to the inclusion of more benign lesions in the latter analysis. However, when compared with the respective ^{18}F-FDG mean SUV cutoffs in a receiver operating characteristic analysis, both studies found that ^{11}C-choline had a higher diagnostic accuracy. In summary, if ^{11}C-choline becomes more widely available, it may be a useful alternative to ^{18}F-FDG. It may have a problem-solving role in tumors located near the urinary bladder and possibly in cases where there is uncertainty about benign vs. malignant pathology. Newer fluorinated choline analogues (79) are of interest and may be more practical for clinical use due to a longer physical half-life.

Technical Issues

In oncology, radiation dosimetry from diagnostic imaging tests is a more important consideration for pediatric than for adult patients because of a generally higher survival rate and a longer potential period of life to manifest adverse consequences of radiation exposure in children, as well as issues of differential susceptibility to the effects of radiation. Accordingly, minimization of radiation dose is an important consideration in the pediatric population. Although PET utilizes isotopes with relatively high gamma photon energy (511 keV) and with a particulate (positron) emission, the short half-life of ^{18}F and other PET tracers offer significant advantages compared to other competing tracers used for oncologic imaging, such as ^{201}Tl and [67]Ga. The high sensitivity of PET generally allows administration of relatively small doses of radiotracer to pediatric patients, particularly if three-dimensional (3D) imaging is performed. Although 3D body imaging using PET can be degraded by a significant scatter fraction in adults, this is seldom an issue in children. We believe that 3D acquisition is preferable, if available, for imaging children less than 60 kg in weight. Sensitive PET detectors like thick sodium iodide crystals used in the C-PET (Philips [Milpitas, California]) and various modified gamma cameras have particular appeal for pediatric patients, although their performance is somewhat compromised in larger patients compared to modern bismuth germanate oxide (BGO) and lutetium oxyorthosilicate (LSO) based PET scanners. The incremental benefits of PET-CT in terms of diagnostic confidence and localization ability also need to be balanced with the additional radiation burden of adding a helical CT acquisition to the PET procedure. Low-dose CT acquisitions yield very good quality CT for correlation and attenuation correction purposes in our opinion.

Conclusion

Positron emission tomography imaging with ^{18}F-FDG has been shown to significantly impact patient management in primary bone tumors by improving the initial diagnosis with more accurate staging, determining whether there is metastatic disease, providing an accurate indicator of response to treatment, detecting early recurrence, and finally by providing an accurate indicator for patient prognosis. The most efficient method is a combination of PET with other anatomic imaging modalities, that is, CT and MRI. Several other PET radiopharmaceuticals also show great promise. For the medical imaging evaluation of primary bone tumors in our young patients, the already essential role of PET is likely to expand further with newer developments and applications. Recognition that PET, as a molecular imaging technique, is more about lesion characterization than lesion counting will enable realistic expectations of how and when to use PET in the diagnostic process. With such a disparate range of diseases, outcomes, and therapeutic options, we believe that prognostic stratification may well be the most important function provided by PET.

References

1. Phan A, Patel S. Advances in neoadjuvant chemotherapy in soft tissue sarcomas. Curr Treat Options Oncol 2003;4(6):433–439.
2. Bacci G, Lari S. Current treatment of high grade osteosarcoma of the extremity: review. J Chemother 2001;13(3):235–243.
3. Ballo MT, Zagars GK. Radiation therapy for soft tissue sarcoma. Surg Oncol Clin North Am 2003;12:449–467.
4. Meyers PA, Gorlick R. Osteosarcoma. Pediatr Clin North Am 1997;4: 973–989.
5. Grier HE. The Ewing family of tumors. Pediatr Clin North Am 1997;4: 991–1104.
6. Mirra JM. Osteosarcoma: intramedullary variants. In: Mirra JM, ed. Bone Tumors. Philadelphia: Lea & Febiger, 1989:249–389.
7. Mirra JM, Picci P. Ewing's sarcoma. In: Mirra JM, ed. Bone Tumors. Philadelphia: Lea & Febiger, 1989:1087–1117.
8. Arndt CAS, Crist WM. Common musculoskeletal tumors of childhood and adolescence. N Engl J Med 1999;341(5):342–352.
9. Rodriguez-Galindo C, Spunt SL, Pappo AS. Treatment of Ewing sarcoma family of tumors: current status and outlook for the future. Med Pediatr Oncol 2003;40:276–287.
10. Bruland OS, Pihl A. On the current management of osteosarcoma: a critical evaluation and a proposal for a modified treatment strategy. Eur J Cancer 1997;33:1725–1731.
11. Raymond AK, Chawla SP, Carrasco CH, et al. Osteosarcoma chemotherapy effect: a prognostic factor. Semin Diagn Pathol 1987;4:212–236.

12. Eary JF, Conrad EU, Bruckner JD, et al. Quantitative [F-18] fluorodeoxyglucose positron emission tomography in pretreatment and grading of sarcoma. Clin Cancer Res 1998;4:1215–1220.
13. Brenner W, Bohuslavizki KH, Eary JF. PET imaging of osteosarcoma. J Nucl Med 2003;44(6):930–942.
14. Messa C, Landoni C, Pozzato C, Fazio F. Is there a role for FDG PET in the diagnosis of musculoskeletal neoplasms? J Nucl Med 2000;41(10): 1702–1703.
15. Oliveira AM, Nascimento AG. Grading in soft tissue tumors: principles and problems. Skeletal Radiol 2001;30:543–559.
16. Hicks RJ. Nuclear medicine techniques provide unique physiologic characterization of suspected and known soft tissue and bone sarcomas. Acta Orthop Scand 1997;273(suppl):25–36.
17. Hicks RJ. Functional imaging techniques for evaluation of sarcomas. Cancer Imaging 2005;5:58–65.
18. Hicks RJ, Toner G, Choong PFM. Clinical applications of molecular imaging in sarcoma evaluation. Cancer Imaging 2005;5:66–72.
19. Miller SL, Hoffer FA. Malignant and benign bone tumors. Radiol Clin North Am 2001;39:673.
20. Siegel MJ. Magnetic resonance imaging of musculoskeletal soft tissue masses. Radiol Clin North Am 2001;39:701–720.
21. Rosen G, Caparros B, Groshen S. Primary osteogenic sarcoma of the femur: a model for the use of preoperative chemotherapy in high risk malignant tumours. Cancer Invest 1984;2:181–192.
22. Picci P, Rougraff BT, Bacci G, et al. Prognostic significance of histopathologic response to chemotherapy in non metastatic Ewing sarcoma of the extremity. J Clin Oncol 1993;11:1763–1769.
23. San-Julian M, Dolz R, Garcia-Barrecheguren E, et al. Limb salvage in bone sarcomas in patients younger than age 10. J Pediatr Orthop 2003;23: 753–762.
24. Wodajo FM, Bickels J, Wittig J, Malawer M. Complex reconstruction in the management of extremity sarcomas. Curr Opinion Oncol 2003;15:304–312.
25. Picci P, Sangiorgi L, Rougraff BT, et al. Relationship of chemotherapy-induced necrosis and surgical margins to local recurrence in osteosarcoma. J Clin Oncol 1994;12:2699–2705.
26. Glasser D, Lane J, Huvos A, et al. Survival, prognosis and therapeutic response in osteogenic sarcoma: the Memorial Hospital experience. Cancer 1992;69:698–708.
27. Townsend DW, Beyer T, Blodgett TM. PET/CT scanners: a hardware approach to image fusion. Semin Nucl Med 2003;33:193–204.
28. Kern KA, Brunetti A, Norton JA, et al. Metabolic imaging of human extremity musculoskeletal tumors by PET. J Nucl Med 1988;29:181–186.
29. Adler LP, Blair HF, Makley JT, et al. Noninvasive grading of musculoskeletal tumors using PET. J Nucl Med 1991;32(8):1508–1512.
30. Hoh CK, Hawkins RA, Glaspy JA, et al. Cancer detection with whole-body PET using 2–[^{18}F]fluoro-2–deoxy-D-glucose. J Comput Assist Tomogr 1993;17:582–589.
31. Eary JF, O'Sullivan F, Powitan Y, et al. Sarcoma tumor FDG uptake measured by PET and patient outcome: a retrospective analysis. Eur J Nucl Med Mol Imaging 2002;29(9):1149–1154.
32. Folpe AL, Lyles RH, Sprouse JT, Conrad EU III, Eary JF. (F-18) fluorodeoxyglucose positron emission tomography as a predictor of pathologic grade and other prognostic variables in bone and soft tissue sarcoma. Clin Cancer Res 2000;6(4):1279–1287.

33. Schulte M, Brecht-Krauss D, Heymer B, et al. Grading of tumors and tumorlike lesions of bone: evaluation by FDG PET. J Nucl Med 2000; 41(10):1695–1701.
34. Feldman F, van Heertum R, Manos C. 18FDG PET scanning of benign and malignant musculoskeletal lesions. Skeletal Radiol 2003;32(4):201–208.
35. Dimitrakopoulou-Strauss A, Strauss LG, Heichel T, et al. The role of quantitative (18)F-FDG PET studies for the differentiation of malignant and benign bone lesions. J Nucl Med 2002;43(4):510–518.
36. Aoki J, Watanabe H, Shinozaki T, et al. FDG PET of primary benign and malignant bone tumors: standardized uptake value in 52 lesions. Radiology 2001;219(3):774–777.
37. Watanabe H, Shinozaki T, Yanagawa T, et al. Glucose metabolic analysis of musculoskeletal tumours using 18-fluorine-FDG PET as an aid to preoperative planning. J Bone Joint Surg [Br] 2000;82(5):760–767.
38. Kole AC, Nieweg OE, Hoekstra HJ, van Horn JR, Koops HS, Vaalburg W. Fluorine-18–fluorodeoxyglucose assessment of glucose metabolism in bone tumors. J Nucl Med 1998;39(5):810–815.
39. Franzius C, Bielack S, Flege S, Sciuk J, Jurgens H, Schober O. Prognostic significance of (18)F-FDG and (99m)Tc-methylene diphosphonate uptake in primary osteosarcoma. J Nucl Med 2002;43(8):1012–1017.
40. Jaramillo D, Laor T, Gebhardt MC. Pediatric musculoskeletal neoplasms: evaluation with MR imaging. MRI Clin North Am 1996;4(4):749–770.
41. Schulte M, Brecht-Krauss D, Werner M, et al. Evaluation of neoadjuvant therapy response of osteogenic sarcoma using FDG PET. J Nucl Med 1999;40(10):1637–1643.
42. Franzius C, Daldrup-Link HE, Sciuk J, et al. FDG-PET for detection of pulmonary metastases from malignant primary bone tumors: comparison with spiral CT. Ann Oncol 2001;12:479–486.
43. Lucas JD, O'Doherty MJ, Wong JC, et al. Evaluation of fluorodeoxyglucose positron emission tomography in the management of soft-tissue sarcomas. J Bone Joint Surg [Br] 1998;80:441–447.
44. Pitman AG, Hicks RJ, Binns DS, et al. Performance of sodium iodide based ^{18}F-fluorodeoxyglucose positron emission tomography in the characterisation of indeterminate pulmonary nodules or masses. Br J Radiol 2002;75:114–121.
45. Franzius C, Sciuk J, Daldrup-Link HE, Jurgens H, Schober O. FDG-PET for detection of osseous metastases from malignant primary bone tumours: comparison with bone scintigraphy. Eur J Nucl Med 2000;27(9):1305–1311.
46. Franzius C, Daldrup-Link HE, Wagner-Bohn A, et al. FDG-PET for detection of recurrences from malignant primary bone tumors: comparison with conventional imaging. Ann Oncol 2002;13:157–160.
47. Daldrup-Link HE, Franzius C, Link TM, et al. Whole-body MR imaging for detection of bone metastases in children and young adults: comparison with skeletal scintigraphy and FDG PET. AJR 2001;177(1):229–236.
48. Tacikowska M. Dynamic magnetic resonance imaging in soft tissue tumors—assessment of the diagnostic value of tumor enhancement rate indices. Med Sci Monitor 2002;8(4):MT53–MT57.
49. Negendank WG. MR spectroscopy of musculoskeletal soft-tissue tumors. MRI Clin North Am 1995;3:713–725.
50. Kostakoglu L, Panicek DM, Divgi CR, et al. Correlation of the findings of thallium-201 chloride scans with those of other imaging modalities and histology following therapy in patients with bone and soft tissue sarcomas [erratum in Eur J Nucl Med 1996;23(11):1558]. Eur J Nucl Med 1995;22(11): 1232–1237.

51. Jones DN, McCowage GB, Sostman HD, et al. Monitoring of neoadjuvant therapy response of soft-tissue and musculoskeletal sarcoma using fluorine-18–FDG PET. J Nucl Med 1996;37(9):1438–1444.

52. Franzius C, Sciuk J, Brinkschmidt C, Jurgens H, Schober O. Evaluation of chemotherapy response in primary bone tumors with F-18 FDG positron emission tomography compared with histologically assessed tumor necrosis. Clin Nucl Med 2000;25(11):874–881.

53. Hawkins DS, Rajendran JG, Conrad EU III, Bruckner JD, Eary JF. Evaluation of chemotherapy response in pediatric bone sarcomas by [F-18]-fluorodeoxy-D-glucose positron emission tomography [erratum appears in Cancer 2003;97(12):3130]. Cancer 2002;94(12):3277–3284.

54. Larson SM, Erdi Y, Akhurst T, et al. Tumor treatment response based on visual and quantitative changes in global tumor glycolysis using PET-FDG imaging: the Visual Response Score and the change in total lesion glycolysis. Clin Positron Imaging 1999;2(3):159–171.

55. Nair N, Ali A, Green AA, et al. Response of osteosarcoma to chemotherapy: evaluation with F-18 FDG-PET scans. Clin Positron Imaging 2000;3:79–83.

56. Ma LD, Frassica FJ, Scott WW, et al. Differentiation of benign and malignant musculoskeletal tumors: potential pitfalls with MR imaging. Radiographics 1995;15:349–366.

57. Garcia R, Kim EE, Wong FC, et al. Comparison of fluorine-18–FDG PET and technetium-99m-MIBI SPECT in evaluation of musculoskeletal sarcomas. J Nucl Med 1996;37(9):1476–1479.

58. el-Zeftawy H, Heiba SI, Jana S, et al. Role of repeated F-18 fluorodeoxyglucose imaging in management of patients with bone and soft tissue sarcoma. Cancer Biother Radiopharm 2001;16(1):37–46.

59. Fletcher BD. Imaging pediatric bone sarcomas: diagnosis and treatment related issues. Radiol Clin North Am 1997;35:1477–1494.

60. Hains SF, O'Doherty MJ, Lucas JD, Smith MA. Fluorodeoxyglucose PET in the evaluation of amputations for soft tissue sarcoma. Nucl Med Commun 1999;20(9):845–848.

61. Blau M, Nagler W, Bender MA. Fluorine-18: a new isotope for bone scanning. J Nucl Med 1962;3:332–334.

62. Schiepers C, Nuyts J, Bormans G, et al. Fluoride kinetics of the axial skeleton measured in vivo with fluorine-18–fluoride PET. J Nucl Med 1997;38(12):1970–1976.

63. Hoh CK, Hawkins RA, Dahlbom M, et al. Whole body skeletal imaging with [18F]fluoride ion and PET. J Comput Assist Tomogr 1993;17(1):34–41.

64. Cook GJ, Fogelman I. Detection of bone metastases in cancer patients by 18F-fluoride and 18F-fluorodeoxyglucose positron emission tomography. Q J Nucl Med 2001;45(1):47–52.

65. Schirrmeister H, Guhlmann A, Kotzerke J, et al. Early detection and accurate description of extent of metastatic bone disease in breast cancer with fluoride ion and positron emission tomography. J Clin Oncol 1999;17(8):2381–2389.

66. Schirrmeister H, Glatting G, Hetzel J, et al. Prospective evaluation of the clinical value of planar bone scans, SPECT, and (18)F-labeled NaF PET in newly diagnosed lung cancer. J Nucl Med 2001;42(12):1800–1804.

67. Schirrmeister H, Guhlmann A, Elsner K, et al. Sensitivity in detecting osseous lesions depends on anatomic localization: planar bone scintigraphy versus 18F PET. J Nucl Med 1999;40(10):1623–1629.

68. Even-Sapir E, Metser U, Flusser G, et al. Assessment of malignant skeletal disease: initial experience with 18F-fluoride PET/CT and comparison

between 18F-fluoride PET and 18F-fluoride PET/CT. J Nucl Med 2004; 45(2):272–278.

69. Jager PL, Franssen EJ, Kool W, et al. Feasibility of tumor imaging using L-3–[iodine-123]-iodo-alpha-methyl-tyrosine in extracranial tumors. J Nucl Med 1998;39(10):1736–1743.

70. Tomiyoshi K, Amed K, Muhammad S, et al. Synthesis of isomers of ^{18}F-labelled amino acid radiopharmaceutical: position 2- and 3-L-^{18}F-alpha-methyltyrosine using a separation and purification system. Nucl Med Commun 1997;18(169):175.

71. Watanabe H, Inoue T, Shinozaki T, et al. PET imaging of musculoskeletal tumours with fluorine-18 alpha-methyltyrosine: comparison with fluorine-18 fluorodeoxyglucose PET. Eur J Nucl Med 2000;27(10):1509–1517.

72. Been LB, Suurmeijer AJH, Cobben DCP, et al. [F18]FLT-PET in oncology: current status and opportunities. Eur J Nucl Med Mol Imaging 2004; 31:1659–1672.

73. Cobben DC, Elsinga PH, Suurmeijer AJH, et al. Detection and grading of soft tissue sarcomas of the extremities with (18)F-fluoro-3'-deoxy-L-thymidine. Clin Cancer Res 2004;10:1685–1690.

74. Ishiwata K, Enomoto K, Sasaki T, et al. A feasibility study on L-[1-carbon-11]tyrosine and L-[methyl-carbon-11]methionine to assess liver protein synthesis by PET. J Nucl Med 1996;37(2):279–285.

75. Inoue T, Kim EE, Wong FC, et al. Comparison of fluorine-18-fluorodeoxyglucose and carbon-11-methionine PET in detection of malignant tumors. J Nucl Med 1996;37(9):1472–1476.

76. Hara T, Yuasa M. Automated synthesis of [11C]choline, a positron-emitting tracer for tumor imaging. Appl Radiat Isotopes 1999;50(3):531–533.

77. Yanagawa T, Watanabe H, Inoue T, et al. Carbon-11 choline positron emission tomography in musculoskeletal tumors: comparison with fluorine-18 fluorodeoxyglucose positron emission tomography. J Comput Assist Tomogr 2003;27(2):175–182.

78. Zhang H, Tian M, Oriuchi N, et al. 11C-choline PET for the detection of bone and soft tissue tumours in comparison with FDG PET. Nucl Med Commun 2003;24(3):273–279.

79. De Grado TR, Coleman RE, Wang S, et al. Synthesis and evaluation of ^{18}F-labelled choline as an oncologic tracer for positron emission tomography: initial findings in prostate cancer. Cancer Res 2001;61:110–117.

16

Soft Tissue Sarcomas

Marc P. Hickeson

Soft tissue sarcomas are a heterogeneous group of malignant neo-plasms of mesenchymal origin. They account for approximately 1% of all cancer diagnoses and 7% of pediatric malignancies (1,2). Just over half of these patients eventually succumb as a result of the disease. Soft tissue sarcomas typically present as asymptomatic large masses within the retroperitoneum or the proximal lower limbs but can also affect other sites of the body. In adults, the most common histologic origins are liposarcomas (21%), malignant fibrous histiocytomas (MFHs) (20%), leiomyosarcomas (20%), fibrosarcomas (11%), and tendosyn-ovial sarcomas (10%) (3). In children, rhabdomyosarcoma comprise approximately 70% of the soft tissue sarcomas (3). Despite this highly variable histopathologic origin, the three negative predictive factors at the time of initial diagnosis for disease-free survival are primary site in the superficial trunk or in the limbs, high tumor grade, and large tumor size, rather than the histologic origin (4).

Roles of PET

For soft tissue sarcomas, positron emission tomography (PET) has been shown to be useful in the following capacities:

1. Evaluation of the primary lesion
2. Staging of the disease
3. Monitoring therapy and detection of recurrence
4. Prognostic information

Evaluation of the Primary Lesion

Correct diagnosis of the soft tissue sarcoma is important because treat-ment is effective for many if diagnosed early. However, benign soft tissue masses can appear very similar to soft tissue sarcoma on physi-cal examination and radiologic investigation. The most specific method to diagnose sarcoma is by biopsy. An alternative noninvasive method is PET with fluorine-18 (^{18}F)-fluorodeoxyglucose (FDG), which has been used for the initial diagnosis and grading of soft tissue sarcomas in several series (5–14). On a meta-analysis with a total of 441 lesions (15), the sensitivity and specificity were 92% and 73% by qualitative evaluation, 87% and 79% for a standard uptake value (SUV) of 2.0, and 70% and 87% for SUV 3.0 to diagnose malignant versus benign lesions. The sensitivity of FDG-PET is higher for high-grade malignant lesions than for low-grade lesions (5,16). All intermediate/high-grade sarcomas were detected with qualitative visualization as compared to 74% of low-grade sarcomas and 39% of benign lesions on a meta-analysis (15). Another meta-analysis including 341 patients with soft tissue sarcomas reported sensitivity and specificity of 88% and 86%, respectively, and showed that FDG-PET can discriminate low- and high-grade sarcomas based on the SUV (17). The most common cause for false-negative studies is low-grade sarcoma with low FDG uptake; the most common cause for false-positive studies is inflammation. Fluorodeoxyglucose-PET may also be useful as noninvasive screening modality for malignant transformation of premalignant lesions.

The kinetics of FDG uptake differ in benign and malignant tumors. Hamberg et al. (18) reported that malignant tumors reach maximal uptake of FDG approximately 5 hours after the time of injection. However, benign lesions reach a maximum much earlier, within 30 minutes after FDG injection (12). It is unclear why malignant and benign lesions demonstrate different uptake patterns over time. Although it is well known that an increased number of glucose transporters are present in tumor cells, this does not account for FDG trapping. Hexokinase and glucose-6-phosphatase mediate the phosphorylation and dephosphorylation, respectively, of FDG. It has been reported that the rate of dephosphorylation of FDG-6-phosphate is responsible for the difference in kinetics in malignant and benign lesions (19,20). Unless FDG-6-phosphate is dephosphorylated to FDG by glucose-6-phosphatase, it is unable to leave the cell. Lodge et al. (12) reported an improved differentiation of high-grade sarcomas from benign lesions using a SUV measured at 4 hours postinjection as compared to earlier after FDG injection.

Another approach is to obtain dual-time point imaging to differentiate benign from malignant lesions (21–24). This method has been particularly helpful for lesions associated with low-grade increased FDG activity. In this approach, the lesion's SUV is measured at two different time points after FDG injection. Malignant lesions tend to increase in intensity between the two scans, whereas benign lesions tend to remain stable or decrease slightly in intensity. This technique has been validated for the evaluation of solitary pulmonary nodules (22–24). This difference of kinetics of FDG uptake has also been observed for soft tissue sarcomas (12).

Computed tomography (CT) and magnetic resonance imaging (MRI) have an important role in determining the site of the disease and its local extent. The most specific method for the diagnosis and grading of the lesion is by biopsy of the mass. Although the site and extent of the lesion can be accurately delineated with anatomic imaging modalities, these tumors are sometimes highly heterogeneous. For this reason, the portion of the tumor with the highest grade may be missed on biopsy of only a small region. Hain et al. (25) have reported that in malignant masses the site that was the most likely to be malignant on FDG-PET was found to be representative of the most malignant site on the whole mass histology. Fluorodeoxyglucose-PET can be used to direct preoperative biopsy of soft tissue mass and to prevent the underestimation of the grade of the sarcoma that would result in suboptimal management of the disease (25,26). The availability of PET-CT imaging further enhances the usefulness of this application by providing the precise CT anatomic localization of the metabolic abnormalities on PET.

Staging for Metastases

Magnetic resonance imaging, CT scan, and FDG-PET imaging have complementary roles in staging soft tissue sarcomas (Table 16.1). Lucas et al. (11) reported sensitivity and specificity of 86.7% and 100%, respectively, with FDG-PET and sensitivity and specificity of 100% and 96.4%, respectively, with CT for the detection of pulmonary metastases. However, an additional 13 unsuspected sites of metastases were demonstrated on FDG-PET. One advantage of FDG-PET over other imaging modalities is that all organ systems can be visualized in a single examination. Johnson et al. (27) reported that FDG-PET correctly diagnosed or excluded local recurrence and distant metastases in 33 patients. In some cases, FDG-PET detected metastases before they were present on CT scan and MRI. These data suggest that FDG-PET is useful for staging for distant metastases and offers complementary information provided by anatomic imaging modalities.

Monitoring Therapy and Detection of Recurrence

Approximately 10% to 15% of patients develop local recurrence and 35% to 45% develop distant metastases despite adequate treatment.

Table 16.1. American Joint Committee on Cancer (AJCC) staging system for soft tissue sarcoma

Stage	Description
IA	Low-grade sarcoma; tumor ≤5 cm; no nodal or systemic metastases (G1T1N0M0)
IB	Low-grade sarcoma; tumor >5 cm; no nodal or systemic metastases (G1T2N0M0)
IIA	Moderate-grade sarcoma; tumor ≤5 cm; no nodal or systemic metastases (G2T1N0M0)
IIB	Moderate-grade sarcoma; tumor >5 cm; no nodal or systemic metastases (G2T2N0M0)
IIIA	High-grade sarcoma; tumor ≤5 cm; no nodal or systemic metastases (G3T1N0M0)
IIIB	High-grade sarcoma; tumor >5 cm; no nodal or systemic metastases (G3T2N0M0)
IVA	Any grade sarcoma; any tumor size; with regional node metastases; no systemic metastases (any G, any T, N1M0)
IV	Any grade sarcoma; any tumor size; any nodal status; with systemic metastases (any G, any T, any N, M1)

Early detection of recurrence allows a larger variety of treatment options and results in better prognosis than late detection of recurrence. Therefore, early detection of recurrence is important for the treatment of sarcomas.

There has been a significant evolution in the treatment of soft tissue sarcoma. For aggressive tumors, surgical resection is the method of choice of local control. For sarcomas involving the limbs, limb-sparing procedures can be appropriately performed by chemotherapy in the neoadjuvant (presurgical) setting. The primary objective is tumor eradication. However, the response to therapy varies considerably with different tumors. Identification of resistant or nonresponding tumors early or immediately after initiation of therapy would be most advantageous, so that an alternative, potentially more effective, treatment can be instituted in a timely manner. Toxicities from ineffective therapy can also be prevented. Unlike anatomic imaging modalities, which assess tumor response by size criteria, PET assesses the metabolic activity of tumors. Studies have shown that therapy-induced anatomic changes lag behind metabolic changes of the tumor (28).

One specific example that FDG-PET has demonstrated its utility for early prediction of response to therapy is with the treatment of gastrointestinal intestinal stromal tumors (GISTs), which are tumors of mesenchymal origin arising from the gastrointestinal tract. A significant percentage of these tumors have an exceptional response to the tyrosine kinase inhibitor, imatinib mesylate (Gleevec/Glivec). Fluorodeoxyglucose-PET has been shown to be an early indicator of tumor response to treatment (Figs. 16.1 to 16.3) (29). In all responders, a significant decrease of FDG uptake was observed as early as 24 hours after the administration of a single dose of Gleevec. Subsequent studies have indicated that FDG-PET is the imaging modality of choice for early

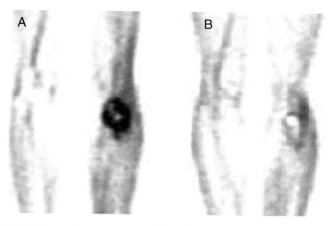

Figure 16.1. Patient has a tenosynovial cell sarcoma in the left knee, which is demonstrated on the baseline fluorodeoxyglucose–positron emission tomography (FDG-PET) scan (A). The posttherapy FDG-PET scan (B) demonstrated a complete metabolic response to therapy.

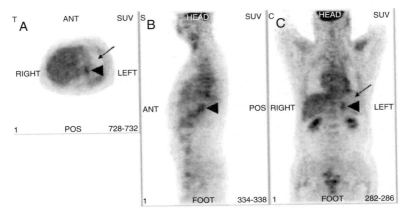

Figure 16.2. Patient with gastrointestinal stroma tumor of the stomach who had undergone FDG-PET study after chemotherapy. The transaxial (A), sagittal (B), and coronal images (C) are shown and demonstrate a large mass with no evidence of FDG metabolism (arrows) with the exception of a focus of hypermetabolism at its stalk (arrowheads), which was proven to be residual tumor.

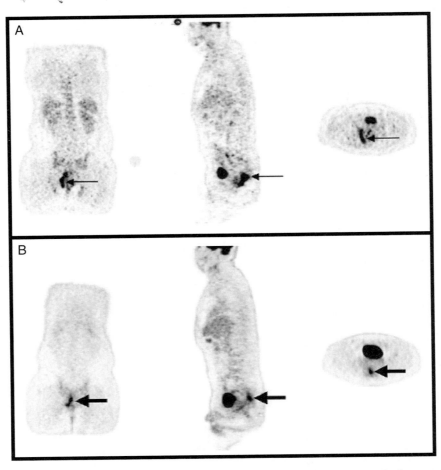

Figure 16.3. Partial metabolic response in this patient with history of gastrointestinal stromal tumor of the rectum who had undergone FDG-PET study prior to (A, narrow arrows) and 3 weeks after initiation of therapy (B, wide arrows).

Table 16.2. Tumor response using FDG-PET with the European Organization for Research and Treatment of Cancer (EORTC) criteria

Response	Definition
Progressive metabolic disease	Increase in FDG tumor SUV of equal or greater than 25% within the tumor region as compared to the baseline study or appearance of new FDG uptake in metastatic lesions
Stable disease	Increase in tumor FDG uptake of less than 25% or a decrease of less than 15% of FDG uptake within the tumor region as compared to the baseline study
Partial metabolic response	Reduction of at least 15% of FDG uptake within the tumor as compared to the baseline study
Complete metabolic response	Complete resolution of FDG uptake within the tumor

prediction of response to therapy for a patient with GIST treated with Gleevec (30–32).

The metabolic response of tumor from therapy can be defined using the European Organization for Research and Treatment of Cancer (EORTC) criteria (Table 16.2) (33).

Hain et al. (34) studied the findings of 16 patients with amputation in either the upper or lower limb on FDG-PET. Diffuse hypermetabolism at the amputation stump up to 18 months postsurgery is a common finding. However, focal hypermetabolism may be associated with a pressure area if there is clinical evidence of skin breakdown at that site. However, if there is no evidence of localized skin breakdown at the site of focal hypermetabolism, then the finding indicates a recurrence, and a skin biopsy is indicated. Kole et al. (35) have also reported a 93% sensitivity of FDG-PET for the detection of recurrence of soft tissue sarcomas in 14 patients.

Prognostic Information

A noninvasive method to determine tumor regional glucose metabolism is with FDG-PET. Eary et al. (36) reported that FDG-PET provides independent prognostic information in a retrospective analysis of 209 patients with sarcomas. They have shown that the risk of death increases by approximately 60% for each doubling of the maximal baseline lesion SUV. Schuetze et al. (37) have demonstrated that soft tissue sarcomas with a pretreatment SUV of greater than 6.0 are associated with a higher risk of recurrence and of mortality than those with SUV of less than 6.0. Another negative prognostic finding provided by FDG-PET is lack of reduction in SUV of the lesion with therapy (Fig. 16.4) (37). In general, FDG tumor activity is positively associated with the metabolic activity, and tumor metabolic activity is positively associated with aggressiveness. Aggressive tumors have a worse prognosis than those with less aggressive histology.

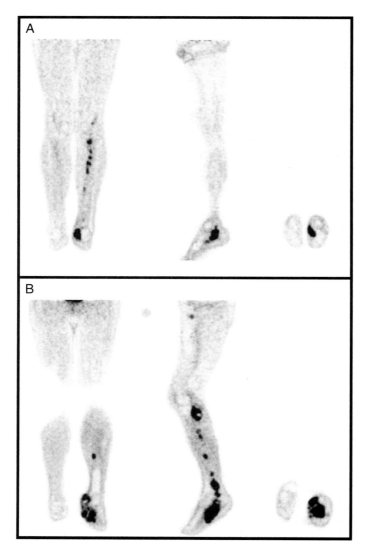

Figure 16.4. Evidence of progression in this patient with an aggressive metastatic sarcoma of the left foot who had undergone FDG-PET study prior to (A) and after completing chemotherapy (B). The baseline SUV was 13.9; this increased to 18.2 on the posttherapy scan, which indicates a poor prognosis.

Conclusion

Positron emission tomography with ^{18}F-fluorodeoxyglucose has been shown to have potential value in the evaluation of primary malignant lesions, for staging, for the response to treatment and detection of recurrence, and for prognostic information.

References

1. Landis SH, Murray T, Bolden S, Wingo PA. Cancer statistics, 1998. CA Cancer J Clin 1998;48(1):6–29.
2. Marina NM, Krance R, Ribeiro RC, Crist WM. Diagnosis and treatment of the most common solid tumors in childhood. Prim Care 1992;19(4): 871–889.
3. Nijhuis PH, Schaapveld M, Otter R, Molenaar WM, van der Graaf WT, Hoekstra HJ. Epidemiological aspects of soft tissue sarcomas (STS)—consequences for the design of clinical STS trials. Eur J Cancer 1999;35(12): 1705–1710.
4. Zagars GK, Ballo MT, Pisters PW, Pollock RE, Patel SR, Benjamin RS. Prognostic factors for disease-specific survival after first relapse of soft-tissue sarcoma: analysis of 402 patients with disease relapse after initial conservative surgery and radiotherapy. Int J Radiat Oncol Biol Phys 2003;57(3): 739–747.
5. Schwarzbach MH, Dimitrakopoulou-Strauss A, Willeke F, et al. Clinical value of [18–F] fluorodeoxyglucose positron emission tomography imaging in soft tissue sarcomas. Ann Surg 2000;231(3):380–386.
6. Watanabe H, Shinozaki T, Yanagawa T, et al. Glucose metabolic analysis of musculoskeletal tumours using 18-fluorine-FDG PET as an aid to preoperative planning. J Bone Joint Surg Br 2000;82(5):760–767.
7. Griffeth LK, Dehdashti F, McGuire AH, et al. PET evaluation of soft-tissue masses with fluorine-18 fluoro-2-deoxy-D-glucose. Radiology 1992;182(1): 185–194.
8. Schulte M, Brecht-Krauss D, Heymer B, et al. Fluorodeoxyglucose positron emission tomography of soft tissue tumours: is a non-invasive determination of biological activity possible? Eur J Nucl Med 1999;26(6):599–605.
9. Lucas JD, O'Doherty MJ, Cronin BF, et al. Prospective evaluation of soft tissue masses and sarcomas using fluorodeoxyglucose positron emission tomography. Br J Surg 1999;86(4):550–556.
10. Kern KA, Brunetti A, Norton JA, et al. Metabolic imaging of human extremity musculoskeletal tumors by PET. J Nucl Med 1988;29(2):181–186.
11. Lucas JD, O'Doherty MJ, Wong JC, et al. Evaluation of fluorodeoxyglucose positron emission tomography in the management of soft-tissue sarcomas. J Bone Joint Surg Br 1998;80(3):441–447.
12. Lodge MA, Lucas JD, Marsden PK, Cronin BF, O'Doherty MJ, Smith MA. A PET study of 18FDG uptake in soft tissue masses. Eur J Nucl Med 1999; 26(1):22–30.
13. Ferner RE, Lucas JD, O'Doherty MJ, et al. Evaluation of (18)fluorodeoxyglucose positron emission tomography ((18)FDG PET) in the detection of malignant peripheral nerve sheath tumours arising from within plexiform neurofibromas in neurofibromatosis 1. J Neurol Neurosurg Psychiatry 2000;68(3):353–357.
14. Adler LP, Blair HF, Williams RP, et al. Grading liposarcomas with PET using [18F]FDG. J Comput Assist Tomogr 1990;14(6):960–962.
15. Ioannidis JP, Lau J. 18F-FDG PET for the diagnosis and grading of soft-tissue sarcoma: a meta-analysis. J Nucl Med 2003;44(5):717–724.
16. Nieweg OE, Pruim J, van Ginkel RJ, et al. Fluorine-18-fluorodeoxyglucose PET imaging of soft-tissue sarcoma. J Nucl Med 1996;37(2):257–261.
17. Bastiaannet E, Groen H, Jager PL, et al. The value of FDG-PET in the detection, grading and response to therapy of soft tissue and bone sarcomas; a systematic review and meta-analysis. Cancer Treat Rev 2004;30(1): 83–101.

18. Hamberg LM, Hunter GJ, Alpert NM, Choi NC, Babich JW, Fischman AJ. The dose uptake ratio as an index of glucose metabolism: useful parameter or oversimplification? J Nucl Med 1994;35(8):1308–1312.

19. Gallagher BM, Fowler JS, Gutterson NI, MacGregor RR, Wan CN, Wolf AP. Metabolic trapping as a principle of radiopharmaceutical design: some factors responsible for the biodistribution of [18F] 2-deoxy-2-fluoro-D-glucose. J Nucl Med 1978;19(10):1154–1161.

20. Nelson CA, Wang JQ, Leav I, Crane PD. The interaction among glucose transport, hexokinase, and glucose-6-phosphatase with respect to 3H-2-deoxyglucose retention in murine tumor models. Nucl Med Biol 1996; 23(4):533–541.

21. Hustinx R, Smith RJ, Benard F, et al. Dual time point fluorine-18 fluorodeoxyglucose positron emission tomography: a potential method to differentiate malignancy from inflammation and normal tissue in the head and neck. Eur J Nucl Med 1999;26(10):1345–1348.

22. Zhuang H, Pourdehnad M, Lambright ES, et al. Dual time point 18F-FDG PET imaging for differentiating malignant from inflammatory processes. J Nucl Med 2001;42(9):1412–1417.

23. Matthies A, Hickeson M, Cuchiara A, Alavi A. Dual time point 18F-FDG PET for the evaluation of pulmonary nodules. J Nucl Med 2002;43(7): 871–875.

24. Demura Y, Tsuchida T, Ishizaki T, et al. 18F-FDG accumulation with PET for differentiation between benign and malignant lesions in the thorax. J Nucl Med 2003;44(4):540–548.

25. Hain SF, O'Doherty MJ, Bingham J, Chinyama C, Smith MA. Can FDG PET be used to successfully direct preoperative biopsy of soft tissue tumours? Nucl Med Commun 2003;24(11):1139–1143.

26. Israel-Mardirosian N, Adler LP. Positron emission tomography of soft tissue sarcomas. Curr Opin Oncol 2003;15(4):327–330.

27. Johnson GR, Zhuang H, Khan J, Chiang SB, Alavi A. Roles of positron emission tomography with fluorine-18-deoxyglucose in the detection of local recurrent and distant metastatic sarcoma. Clin Nucl Med 2003;28(10): 815–820.

28. Jansson T, Westlin JE, Ahlstrom H, Lilja A, Langstrom B, Bergh J. Positron emission tomography studies in patients with locally advanced and/or metastatic breast cancer: a method for early therapy evaluation? J Clin Oncol 1995;13(6):1470–1477.

29. Demetri GD, von Mehren M, Blanke CD, et al. Efficacy and safety of imatinib mesylate in advanced gastrointestinal stromal tumors. N Engl J Med 2002;347(7):472–480.

30. Gayed I, Vu T, Iyer R, et al. The role of 18F-FDG PET in staging and early prediction of response to therapy of recurrent gastrointestinal stromal tumors. J Nucl Med 2004;45(1):17–21.

31. Goerres GW, Stupp R, Barghouth G, et al. The value of PET, CT and in-line PET/CT in patients with gastrointestinal stromal tumours: long-term outcome of treatment with imatinib mesylate. Eur J Nucl Med Mol Imaging 2005;32(2):153–162.

32. Antoch G, Kanja J, Bauer S, et al. Comparison of PET, CT, and dual-modality PET/CT imaging for monitoring of imatinib (STI571) therapy in patients with gastrointestinal stromal tumors. J Nucl Med 2004;45(3): 357–365.

33. Young H, Baum R, Cremerius U, et al. Measurement of clinical and subclinical tumour response using [18F]-fluorodeoxyglucose and positron

emission tomography: review and 1999 EORTC recommendations. European Organization for Research and Treatment of Cancer (EORTC) PET Study Group. Eur J Cancer 1999;35(13):1773–1782.

34. Hain SF, O'Doherty MJ, Lucas JD, Smith MA. Fluorodeoxyglucose PET in the evaluation of amputations for soft tissue sarcoma. Nucl Med Commun 1999;20(9):845–848.

35. Kole AC, Nieweg OE, van Ginkel RJ, et al. Detection of local recurrence of soft-tissue sarcoma with positron emission tomography using [18F]fluorodeoxyglucose. Ann Surg Oncol 1997;4(1):57–63.

36. Eary JF, O'Sullivan F, Powitan Y, et al. Sarcoma tumor FDG uptake measured by PET and patient outcome: a retrospective analysis. Eur J Nucl Med Mol Imaging 2002;29(9):1149–1154.

37. Schuetze SM, Rubin BP, Vernon C, et al. Use of positron emission tomography in localized extremity soft tissue sarcoma treated with neoadjuvant chemotherapy. Cancer 2005;103(2):339–348.

17

Other Tumors

Jian Qin Yu and Martin Charron

Positron emission tomography (PET) is a new and powerful imaging tool that has been successfully employed to diagnose many adult tumors. Incidental tumor detection by PET has been reported (1–5), as well as detection of chronic cholecystitis, aspiration pneumonia, and other benign conditions (6–8). The implementation of this new technology has been slower in the pediatric population than in the adult population.

PET has shown promise in a variety of pediatric tumors such as those of the central nervous system, lymphomas, neuroblastoma, bone, and soft tissue tumors; these are discussed in other chapters. Positron emission tomography evaluations for diagnosis and therapy in the pediatric population were reported in the early and mid-1980s (9–11). The early studies focused on brain tumors, metastatic tumors to the brain, and metabolic abnormalities such as Sturge-Weber syndrome (12). Many of the studies in the 1990s also focused on brain tumor. This chapter discusses other rare tumors not covered in other parts of this book.

Ewing's Sarcoma

There are few reports regarding PET with Ewing's sarcoma. One early scientific report in a pediatric population was by Shulkin et al. (13) from the University of Michigan Medical Center in the mid-1990s, in which the author showed that PET is superior to bone scan in detecting bone metastasis in a patient with Ewing's sarcoma. A case report later demonstrated that PET is superior to both bone scan and gallium, especially when the disease involves the bone marrow (14). Another study comparing PET and magnetic resonance imaging (MRI) for detection of Ewing's metastasis concluded that PET is more sensitive (15). The findings reinforced the uses of a functional imaging modality, such as PET, over anatomic imaging.

A large amount of clinical research has assessed the role of PET in evaluating the response to chemotherapy. Fluorodeoxyglucose (FDG)-PET standard uptake values (SUVs), or tumor-to-nontumor ratio

(T/NT) before and after chemotherapy, were analyzed and correlated with the chemotherapy response assessed by histopathology in surgically excised tumors. Good response correlated with relatively benign histology and had markedly decreased SUV or T/NT on posttherapy scans (16,17).

Two reviews by Franzius et al. (17,18) found that for the detection of osseous metastases of Ewing's sarcoma, therapy monitoring, and the diagnosis of recurrences, FDG-PET was useful. This conclusion is echoed by a recent paper by McCarville et al. (19) that stated that PET is useful in monitoring response to different therapies and aids the postoperative evaluation of tumor resection sites.

Neurofibromatosis Type 1

Neurofibromatosis type 1 (NF1) is an autosomal-dominant genetic disorder commonly associated with neuropsychological complications. Focal areas of high signal intensity on magnetic resonance imaging (MRI) scans occur commonly. However, there is inconsistent correlation with neuropsychological problems. Biopsy may be the gold standard for a definitive answer, but it is invasive, unpleasant, and prone to sampling errors. Kaplan et al. (20) reported the findings of PET scans utilizing FΔ6 and MRI studies on 10 children with NF1. This study focused on multiple focal areas of high signal intensity to evaluate the regional cerebral metabolic rate for glucose in these lesions and other central nervous system structures. Visual inspection and semiquantitative analysis of PET images demonstrated thalamic hypometabolism and varying degrees of cortical inhomogeneity in all cases of NF1 compared to normal controls. The metabolic abnormalities noted in this study suggest a potential relationship between these structures and the neuropsychological dysfunctions noted in NF1.

We recently reported our experience in 28 patients (16 males, 12 females) with an age range from 4 years to 35 years (21,22). Twenty-six were clinically stable, but were considered high risk for progression, based on the anatomic location or the change in the size of the lesion over time. All patients enrolled from Children's Hospital of Philadelphia (CHOP) had undergone MRI studies as part of standard patient care. FΔ6 PET scans were obtained for baseline assessment of the disease activity within 2 weeks of the first MRI study. Positron emission tomography images were performed with a dedicated PET camera following a standard protocol. The images were interpreted with and without attenuation correction. Correlation was made to MRI on a lesion-by-lesion basis whenever possible. Standard uptake value was determined for all identifiable lesions on PET scan. The common sites of involvement by plexiform neurofibromas were the face, neck, trunk, and extremities. Twenty-three of 28 patients (82%) showed various degrees of FDG uptake as focal abnormalities. The number of lesions ranged from one to over 10 per patient. The location of FDG-PET abnormalities in these patients corresponded to those noted on the MRI scans. The SUV was calculated for all identifiable lesions on PET, and their values ranged from 1.0 to 5.3. Most lesions had a low SUV, which further corroborates the benign nature of these lesions. Five of 28 patients (18%) did not show any identifiable abnormal focal uptake. Now MRI is used as the gold standard to determine progression of the lesions. Our findings agree with those of Ferner et al. (23,24), who reported an SUV range of 0.56 to 3.3 for benign plexiform neurofibromas

Pheochromocytoma

The first report evaluating PET in pheochromocytoma was by Shulkin's group (25) using C-11 hydroxyephedrine (HED); they reported excellent imaging quality superior to that obtained from planar and tomographic meta-iodobenzylguanidine (mIBG) studies. A recent study confirmed the accuracy of the C-11 HED (26). However, its clinical availability is limited by the tracer C-11, which needs an on-site cyclotron, which is not generally available for most daily clinical practice. Another early study suggested using iodine-124 mIBG probes (27), which also faces the problem of tracer availability.

Several later studies evaluated FDG-PET scanning for the detection of pheochromocytoma (28). Shulkin et al. (29) demonstrated that most pheochromocytomas accumulate FDG to a greater percentage in malignant versus benign pheochromocytoma. Fluorodeoxyglucose-PET is especially useful in defining the distribution of those pheochromocytoma that fail to concentrate mIBG (29). A PET scan with both FDG and rubidium 82 has been reported to be successful (30).

Carbon-11 metomidate (31) was evaluated for its ability to discriminate lesions of adrenal cortical origin from noncortical lesions. However, a favored tracer is 6-^{18}F-fluorodopamine, which has been shown to detect pheochromocytoma with high sensitivity in patients with known disease (32–34). In those reports PET is much more sensitive than iodine-131 mIBG (35). One German study reported results with ^{18}F-DOPA (36). To discriminate between benign and malignant lesions, FDG is the tracer of choice (37).

Because pheochromocytomas are potentially curable with surgery, the diagnosis and exact localization are very important. The recent imaging recommendations are anatomic imaging followed by mIBG scintigraphy. A negative mIBG study should be followed by an F-DOPA study, which is more specific (38–42).

Other Neuroendocrine Tumors

Neuroendocrine tumors were evaluated with FDG-PET with variable success. Scintigraphy with mIBG and octreotide are still the studies of choice. However, in our experience PET scan showed some potential clinical application. We evaluated whether FDG-PET can be successfully utilized in the evaluation of tumors that are commonly examined by Octreoscan; we retrospectively reviewed 34 FDG-PET scans performed from 1998 to 2002 to evaluate recurrent or metastatic tumors that were considered optimal candidates for Octreoscan (43). Among these, 25 patients were noted to have complete follow-up and therefore were included for final analysis; five had carcinoid, seven had islet cell tumors, five had pheochromocytoma, seven had medullary carcinoma of the thyroid, and one had Cushing's syndrome. Thirteen of these patients also had concurrent ostreoscan. Final diagnosis was made based on surgical findings, clinical follow-up, and results of other imaging modalities. Fluorodeoxyglucose-PET detected 16 of 17 patients who were proven to have recurrent or metastatic disease, with a sensitivity of 94.1%. It excluded seven of eight patients proven not to have recurrent or metastatic disease—a specificity of 87.5%. Among 13 patients with both FDG-PET and Octreoscan in whom eight patients were proven to have disease, FDG-PET correctly detected seven whereas Octreoscan detected five. On the other hand, five patients with negative results on both tests proved to be disease-free. One patient had islet cell tumor that was detected by neither FDG-PET nor Octreoscan. Fluorodeoxyglucose-PET excluded four of five patients with one false-positive result (inflammation), whereas Octreoscan excluded five of five patients. Thus our data indicate that FDG-PET and Octreoscan provide comparable results in patients who are considered optimal candidates for Octreoscan, although FDG-PET is slightly more sensitive whereas Octreoscan appears to be slightly more specific. Considering the similar cost of these two examinations, FDG-PET may prove to be more efficient in this setting because of its substantially superior image quality (whole body vs. regional tomographic images) and convenience to the patient (2 hours vs. 24 hours for completion of the test).

There is little in the current literature to document the utility of PET in pediatric endocrine tumors (44,45). A recent article suggests that ^{18}F-fluoro-L-DOPA could be an accurate noninvasive technique to distinguish between focal and diffuse forms of hyperinsulinism (46).

Liver Tumors

Primary liver tumors' uptake of FDG showed good correlation with the patient's α-fetoprotein (AFP) (47). Another series from Germany demonstrates that PET is better than computed tomography (CT) and ultrasonography, but not MRI (48). The greatest value of PET scan appears to be in the detection of extrahepatic tumor, which is a very useful addition to the currently used anatomically based images in all cases of advanced tumor.

Germ Cell Tumors

Fluorodeoxyglucose-PET scan has been used in the detection and management of different germ cell tumors since 1995 (49–51). Post-therapy studies employed PET soon afterward (52–55). A pilot study in 2000 tested the utility of PDG-PET in the initial staging of the germ cell tumors (56). The sample size is small (31 patients), and a large prospective study is needed. A later study failed to find a benefit of FDG-PET over CT (57). However, it confirmed the value of PET in restaging patients. Positron emission tomography appears to be less sensitive to detect small retroperitoneal nodes (58). L-[1–11C] tyrosine was found to be insufficiently sensitive for clinical use (59).

Histiocytosis X

Studies evaluating histiocytosis were recent (8,60–67), and most of them were case reports (8,64–67). There are no large-scale studies with sufficient patient sample size. Anatomic imaging remains the favored modality. Positron emission tomography may provide additional information for evaluation of distant sites.

Retinoblastoma

Currently, there is only one report of FDG-PET being used to detect retinoblastoma (68). This study did not support the use of FDG-PET, as the PET findings did not correlate with clinical or histopathologic features. Further study with more patients will be of value.

Conclusion

Fluorodeoxyglucose remains the most frequently used tracer. New tracers for different conditions are currently being evaluated worldwide. Positron emission tomography remains poorly evaluated in the pediatric population (69). The recent merger of the Children's Cancer Group and the Pediatric Oncology Group to form the Children's Oncology Group creates an opportunity to examine the use of FDG-PET in the management of childhood tumors in multiinstitutional, cooperative efforts (70).

References

1. Ramos CD, Chisin R, Yeung HW, Larson SM, Macapinlac HA. Incidental focal thyroid uptake on FDG positron emission tomographic scans may represent a second primary tumor. Clin Nucl Med 2001;26:193–197.
2. Davis PW, Perrier ND, Adler L, Levine EA. Incidental thyroid carcinoma identified by positron emission tomography scanning obtained for metastatic evaluation. Am Surg 2001;67:582–584.
3. Tatlidil R, Jadvar H, Bading JR, Conti PS. Incidental colonic fluorodeoxyglucose uptake: correlation with colonoscopic and histopathologic findings. Radiology 2002;224:783–787.
4. Kamel EM, Thumshirn M, Truninger K, et al. Significance of incidental 18F-FDG accumulations in the gastrointestinal tract in PET/CT: correlation with endoscopic and histopathologic results. J Nucl Med 2004;45: 1804–1810.

5. Agress H Jr, Cooper BZ. Detection of clinically unexpected malignant and premalignant tumors with whole-body FDG PET: histopathologic comparison. Radiology 2004;230:417–422.

6. Yu JQ, Kumar R, Xiu Y, Alavi A, Zhuang H. Diffuse FDG uptake in the lungs in aspiration pneumonia on positron emission tomographic imaging. Clin Nucl Med 2004;29:567–568.

7. Yu JQ, Kung JW, Potenta S, Xiu Y, Alavi A, Zhuang H. Chronic cholecystitis detected by FDG-PET. Clin Nucl Med 2004;29:496–497.

8. Yu JQ, Zhuang H, Xiu Y, Talati E, Alavi A. Demonstration of increased FDG activity in Rosai-Dorfman disease on positron emission tomography. Clin Nucl Med 2004;29:209–210.

9. Reiman RE, Benua RS, Gelbard AS, Allen JC, Vomero JJ, Laughlin JS. Imaging of brain tumors after administration of L-(N-13)glutamate: concise communication. J Nucl Med 1982;23:682–687.

10. Mineura K, Yasuda T, Kowada M, et al. Positron emission tomographic evaluations in the diagnosis and therapy of multifocal glioblastoma. Report of a pediatric case. Pediatr Neurosci 1985;12:208–212.

11. Mineura K, Yasuda T, Suda Y, Kowada M, Shishido F, Uemura K. Ewing's sarcoma with intracranial metastasis presenting depressed cerebral blood flow and metabolism in the contralateral gray matter. Comput Med Imaging Graph 1989;13:185–190.

12. Chugani HT, Mazziotta JC, Phelps ME. Sturge-Weber syndrome: a study of cerebral glucose utilization with positron emission tomography. J Pediatr 1989;114:244–253.

13. Shulkin BL, Mitchell DS, Ungar DR, et al. Neoplasms in a pediatric population: 2–[F-18]-fluoro-2–deoxy-D-glucose PET studies. Radiology 1995;194:495–500.

14. Hung GU, Tan TS, Kao CH, Wang SJ. Multiple skeletal metastases of Ewing's sarcoma demonstrated on FDG-PET and compared with bone and gallium scans. Kaohsiung J Med Sci 2000;16:315–318.

15. Daldrup-Link HE, Franzius C, Link TM, et al. Whole-body MR imaging for detection of bone metastases in children and young adults: comparison with skeletal scintigraphy and FDG PET. AJR 2001;177:229–236.

16. Hawkins DS, Rajendran JG, Conrad EU 3rd, Bruckner JD, Eary JF. Evaluation of chemotherapy response in pediatric bone sarcomas by [F-18]-fluorodeoxy-D-glucose positron emission tomography. Cancer 2002;94:3277–3284.

17. Franzius C, Sciuk J, Brinkschmidt C, Jurgens H, Schober O. Evaluation of chemotherapy response in primary bone tumors with F-18 FDG positron emission tomography compared with histologically assessed tumor necrosis. Clin Nucl Med 2000;25:874–881.

18. Franzius C, Schulte M, Hillmann A, et al. [Clinical value of positron emission tomography (PET) in the diagnosis of bone and soft tissue tumors. 3rd Interdisciplinary Consensus Conference, "PET in Oncology": results of the Bone and Soft Tissue Study Group]. Chirurg 2001;72:1071–1077.

19. McCarville MB, Christie R, Daw NC, Spunt SL, Kaste SC. PET/CT in the evaluation of childhood sarcomas. AJR 2005;184:1293–1304.

20. Kaplan AM, Chen K, Lawson MA, Wodrich DL, Bonstelle CT, Reiman EM. Positron emission tomography in children with neurofibromatosis-1. J Child Neurol 1997;12:499–506.

21. Yu J, Shrikanthan S, Dontu V, et al. FDG-PET imaging in the assessment of disease activity in patients with plexiform neurofibromatosis. (abstr). J Nucl Med 2004;45:34.

22. Yu J, Shrikanthan S, Dontu V, et al. PET experience with plexiform neurofibromatosis: a preliminary data. Clin Nucl Med 2004;29:139.

23. Ferner RE, Gutmann DH. International consensus statement on malignant peripheral nerve sheath tumors in neurofibromatosis. Cancer Res 2002; 62:1573–1577.

24. Ferner RE, Lucas JD, O'Doherty MJ, et al. Evaluation of (18) fluorodeoxyglucose positron emission tomography ((18)FDG PET) in the detection of malignant peripheral nerve sheath tumours arising from within plexiform neurofibromas in neurofibromatosis 1. J Neurol Neurosurg Psychiatry 2000;68:353–357.

25. Shulkin BL, Wieland DM, Schwaiger M, et al. PET scanning with hydroxyephedrine: an approach to the localization of pheochromocytoma. J Nucl Med 1992;33:1125–1131.

26. Trampal C, Engler H, Juhlin C, Bergstrom M, Langstrom B. Pheochromocytomas: detection with 11C hydroxyephedrine PET. Radiology 2004;230: 423–428.

27. Ott RJ, Tait D, Flower MA, Babich JW, Lambrecht RM. Treatment planning for 131I-mIBG radiotherapy of neural crest tumours using 124I-mIBG positron emission tomography. Br J Radiol 1992;65:787–791.

28. Musholt TJ, Musholt PB, Dehdashti F, Moley JF. Evaluation of fluorodeoxyglucose-positron emission tomographic scanning and its association with glucose transporter expression in medullary thyroid carcinoma and pheochromocytoma: a clinical and molecular study. Surgery 1997; 122:1049–1060; discussion 1060–1061.

29. Shulkin BL, Koeppe RA, Francis IR, Deeb GM, Lloyd RV, Thompson NW. Pheochromocytomas that do not accumulate metaiodobenzylguanidine: localization with PET and administration of FDG. Radiology 1993;186: 711–715.

30. Neumann DR, Basile KE, Bravo EL, Chen EQ, Go RT. Malignant pheochromocytoma of the anterior mediastinum: PET findings with [18F]FDG and 82Rb. J Comput Assist Tomogr 1996;20:312–316.

31. Bergstrom M, Juhlin C, Bonasera TA, et al. PET imaging of adrenal cortical tumors with the 11beta-hydroxylase tracer 11C-metomidate. J Nucl Med 2000;41:275–282.

32. Pacak K, Linehan WM, Eisenhofer G, Walther MM, Goldstein DS. Recent advances in genetics, diagnosis, localization, and treatment of pheochromocytoma. Ann Intern Med 2001;134:315–329.

33. Pacak K, Goldstein DS, Doppman JL, Shulkin BL, Udelsman R, Eisenhofer G. A "pheo" lurks: novel approaches for locating occult pheochromocytoma. J Clin Endocrinol Metab 2001;86:3641–3646.

34. Pacak K, Ilias I, Adams KT, Eisenhofer G. Biochemical diagnosis, localization and management of pheochromocytoma: focus on multiple endocrine neoplasia type 2 in relation to other hereditary syndromes and sporadic forms of the tumour. J Intern Med 2005;257:60–68.

35. Ilias I, Yu J, Carrasquillo JA, et al. Superiority of 6–[18F]-fluorodopamine positron emission tomography versus [131I]-metaiodobenzylguanidine scintigraphy in the localization of metastatic pheochromocytoma. J Clin Endocrinol Metab 2003;88:4083–4087.

36. Hoegerle S, Nitzsche E, Altehoefer C, et al. Pheochromocytomas: detection with 18F DOPA whole body PET–initial results. Radiology 2002;222: 507–512.

37. Zettinig G, Mitterhauser M, Wadsak W, et al. Positron emission tomography imaging of adrenal masses: (18)F-fluorodeoxyglucose and the 11beta-

hydroxylase tracer (11)C-metomidate. Eur J Nucl Med Mol Imaging 2004; 31:1224–1230.

38. Lenz T, Gossmann J, Schulte KL, Salewski L, Geiger H. Diagnosis of pheochromocytoma. Clin Lab 2002;48:5–18.

39. Ilias I, Pacak K. Anatomical and functional imaging of metastatic pheochromocytoma. Ann N Y Acad Sci 2004;1018:495–504.

40. Maurea S, Caraco C, Klain M, Mainolfi C, Salvatore M. Imaging characterization of non-hypersecreting adrenal masses. Comparison between MR and radionuclide techniques. Q J Nucl Med Mol Imaging 2004;48: 188–197.

41. Brink I, Hoegerle S, Klisch J, Bley TA. Imaging of pheochromocytoma and paraganglioma. Fam Cancer 2005;4:61–68.

42. Minn H, Salonen A, Friberg J, et al. Imaging of adrenal incidentalomas with PET using (11)C-metomidate and (18)F-FDG. J Nucl Med 2004;45: 972–979.

43. Zhuang H, Yu J, Dadparvar S, et al. Accuracy of FDG-PET in the evaluation of metastatic or recurrent tumors which are candidates for Octreoscan (abstract). J Nucl Med 2003;44:73.

44. Sasi OA, Sathiapalan R, Rifai A, et al. Colonic neuroendocrine carcinoma in a child. Pediatr Radiol 2005;35:339–343.

45. Scanga DR, Martin WH, Delbeke D. Value of FDG PET imaging in the management of patients with thyroid, neuroendocrine, and neural crest tumors. Clin Nucl Med 2004;29:86–90.

46. Ribeiro MJ, De Lonlay P, Delzescaux T, et al. Characterization of hyperinsulinism in infancy assessed with PET and 18F-fluoro-L-DOPA. J Nucl Med 2005;46:560–566.

47. Shang JB, Li YH, Liu FY, et al. [18F-Fluorodeoxyglucose uptake in hepatocellular carcinoma on positron emission tomography correlates with alphafetoprotein]. Di Yi Jun Yi Da Xue Xue Bao 2004;24:697–699.

48. Bohm B, Voth M, Geoghegan J, et al. Impact of positron emission tomography on strategy in liver resection for primary and secondary liver tumors. J Cancer Res Clin Oncol 2004;130:266–272.

49. Wilson CB, Young HE, Ott RJ, et al. Imaging metastatic testicular germ cell tumours with 18FDG positron emission tomography: prospects for detection and management. Eur J Nucl Med 1995;22:508–513.

50. Okamura T, Kawabe J, Kobashi T, et al. [A case of peritoneal metastasis from retroperitoneal yolk sac tumor diagnosed by 67Ga-scan and 18F-FDG-PET]. Kaku Igaku 1995;32:495–499.

51. Bachor R, Kocher F, Gropengiesser F, Reske SN, Hautmann RE. [Positron emission tomography. Introduction of a new procedure in diagnosis of urologic tumors and initial clinical results]. Urologe A 1995;34:138–142.

52. Cremerius U, Effert PJ, Adam G, et al. FDG PET for detection and therapy control of metastatic germ cell tumor. J Nucl Med 1998;39:815–822.

53. Nuutinen JM, Leskinen S, Elomaa I, et al. Detection of residual tumours in postchemotherapy testicular cancer by FDG-PET. Eur J Cancer 1997;33: 1234–1241.

54. Hartmann JT, Schmoll HJ, Kuczyk MA, Candelaria M, Bokemeyer C. Postchemotherapy resections of residual masses from metastatic nonseminomatous testicular germ cell tumors. Ann Oncol 1997;8:531–538.

55. Stephens AW, Gonin R, Hutchins GD, Einhorn LH. Positron emission tomography evaluation of residual radiographic abnormalities in postchemotherapy germ cell tumor patients. J Clin Oncol 1996;14: 1637–1641.

56. Hain SF, O'Doherty MJ, Timothy AR, Leslie MD, Partridge SE, Huddart RA. Fluorodeoxyglucose PET in the initial staging of germ cell tumours. Eur J Nucl Med 2000;27:590–594.

57. Spermon JR, De Geus-Oei LF, Kiemeney LA, Witjes JA, Oyen WJ. The role of (18)fluoro-2–deoxyglucose positron emission tomography in initial staging and re-staging after chemotherapy for testicular germ cell tumours. BJU Int 2002;89:549–556.

58. Cremerius U, Wildberger JE, Borchers H, et al. Does positron emission tomography using 18–fluoro-2–deoxyglucose improve clinical staging of testicular cancer?—results of a study in 50 patients. Urology 1999;54: 900–904.

59. Kole AC, Hoekstra HJ, Sleijfer DT, Nieweg OE, Schraffordt Koops H, Vaalburg W. L-[1–carbon-11]tyrosine imaging of metastatic testicular non-seminoma germ-cell tumors. J Nucl Med 1998;39:1027–1029.

60. Steiner M, Prayer D, Asenbaum S, et al. Modern imaging methods for the assessment of Langerhans' cell histiocytosis-associated neurodegenerative syndrome: case report. J Child Neurol 2005;20:253–257.

61. Buchler T, Cervinek L, Belohlavek O, et al. Langerhans cell histiocytosis with central nervous system involvement: follow-up by FDG-PET during treatment with cladribine. Pediatr Blood Cancer 2005;44:286–288.

62. Hoshino A, Kawada E, Ukita T, et al. Usefulness of FDG-PET to diagnose intravascular lymphomatosis presenting as fever of unknown origin. Am J Hematol 2004;76:236–239.

63. Binkovitz LA, Olshefski RS, Adler BH. Coincidence FDG-PET in the evaluation of Langerhans' cell histiocytosis: preliminary findings. Pediatr Radiol 2003;33:598–602.

64. Blum R, Seymour JF, Hicks RJ. Role of 18FDG-positron emission tomography scanning in the management of histiocytosis. Leuk Lymphoma 2002;43:2155–2157.

65. Menzel C, Hamscho N, Dobert N, et al. PET imaging of Rosai-Dorfman disease: correlation with histopathology and ex-vivo beta-imaging. Arch Dermatol Res 2003;295:280–283.

66. Lim R, Wittram C, Ferry JA, Shepard JA. FDG PET of Rosai-Dorfman disease of the thymus. AJR 2004;182:514.

67. Pereira Neto CC, Roman C, Johnson M, Jagasia M, Martin WH, Delbeke D. Positron emission tomography/computed tomography of a rare xanthogranulomatous process: Erdheim-Chester disease. Mol Imaging Biol 2004;6:63–67.

68. Moll AC, Hoekstra OS, Imhof SM, et al. Fluorine-18 fluorodeoxyglucose positron emission tomography (PET) to detect vital retinoblastoma in the eye: preliminary experience. Ophthalmic Genet 2004;25:31–35.

69. Connolly LP, Drubach LA, Ted Treves S. Applications of nuclear medicine in pediatric oncology. Clin Nucl Med 2002;27:117–125.

70. Jadvar H, Alavi A, Mavi A, Shulkin BL. PET in pediatric diseases. Radiol Clin North Am 2005;43:135–152.

Section 3

Neurology and Psychiatry

18

The Developing Brain

Lorcan A. O'Tuama and Paul R. Jolles

This chapter reviews the development of the normal brain primarily as studied with nuclear imaging methods, with an emphasis on radio-pharmaceutical-based methods [positron emission tomography (PET), single photon emission computed tomography (SPECT), and PET—computed tomography (PET-CT)]. These methods retain unchallenged specificity and sensitivity for certain important neurochemical events. We will also cover advances in allied techniques, including magnetic resonance imaging (MRI)-based and electrophysiologic methods. The functional modalities of PET and SPECT are best studied concurrently with structural modalities, including MRI and CT. In selected cases, both functional MRI (fMRI) and nonimaging modalities such as magnetic resonance spectroscopy (MRS) allow for in vivo molecular speciation, and can be brought to bear as well as magnetoencephalography (MEG). The recent introduction of hybrid PET-CT methods introduces a further dimension by allowing direct comparison of functional and structural features in a fused data set. By including these intermodality comparisons we hope to provide a more integrated and mutually explanatory exposition of the imaging of normal brain development.

Brain Imaging Studies

Anatomic Studies of Normal Brain Development

It is essential to discuss the basic structural framework before going on to the more functional insights of MRI. In an early study, Barkovich et al. (1) used 1.5-tesla MRI with the classic spin-echo sequences (T1, T2) to examine 82 neurologically normal-appearing infants, and gave a useful review of the time course of attainment of the major structural developmental milestones. The authors found by these imaging criteria that brain maturation commenced in the brainstem and spread centrifugally to the cerebellum and supratentorial levels. T1-weighted images were most sensitive for assessment of normal brain development in the first 6 to 8 months of life, and T2-weighted images were most sensitive thereafter.

Radiopharmaceutical-Based Studies of Normal Brain Development

Advances in radiolabeling have resulted in the development of a large number of radiopharmaceuticals utilized to evaluate metabolism, blood flow and perfusion, neuroreceptor occupancy, genetic targets, and a host of other biochemical processes. These include both gamma-emitting and positron-emitting tracers. As applied to brain imaging, markers of cerebral glucose and amino acid metabolism [in particular, fluorine-18 (^{18}F)-2-fluorodeoxyglucose (FDG) and carbon-11 (^{11}C)-L-methionine, respectively] and cerebral blood flow/perfusion [oxygen-15 (^{15}O)-CO_2, ^{15}O-water, xenon 133 (^{133}Xe), iodine-123 (^{123}I)-iodoamphetamine, technetium-99m (^{99m}Tc)-bicisate and ^{99m}Tc-exametazime] have been employed most often.

SPECT Study of Normal Developmental Changes in Cerebral Blood Flow

Rubinstein et al. (2), using ^{123}I-iodomethylamphetamine (^{123}I-IMP) SPECT, assessed normal evolution of regional cerebral blood flow (rCBF) as a function of age. Thirty babies with normal clinical examination were retrospectively studied. Perfusion in thalamic structures exceeded that of the cortex until the end of the second month. Within the supratentorial brain, the parietal and occipital areas initially visualized about the 40th week and rose rapidly in the postnatal period. Frontal activity was clearly detectable only by the second month and rose markedly to reach adult levels by the second year. The authors felt rCBF changes paralleled achievement of early behavioral milestones. Thus the early emphasis on brainstem perfusion partly paralleled the morphologic developmental sequence reported by Barkovich et al. (1).

Chiron et al. (3) examined rCBF with ^{133}Xe-SPECT in 42 infants and children (ages 2 days to 19 years) considered developmentally normal. Regions of interest (ROIs) were placed to depict the cortical regions, cerebellum, and thalamus. At birth, cortical rCBFs were lower than those for adults; after birth they increased up to 6 years of age to values 50% to 85% higher than in adults and thereafter decreased, reaching adult levels at between 15 and 19 years of age. Neonatal values of rCBF in cerebellum and thalamus were slightly higher than adult levels, but not significantly; after age 1, they followed the common pattern for cortical curves. The time needed to reach normal adult values differed for each cortical region. The shortest time was found for the primary sensorimotor cortex and the longest for the visual associative cortex.

This work provided an important clinical rationale for pursuing brain perfusion SPECT studies in that cognitive development of the child seemed to be related to changes in blood flow of the corresponding brain regions. The study hinted at another interesting aspect of brain development, suggesting an initial period of "overperfusion" or "luxury" perfusion. These changes somewhat paralleled PET studies, as discussed below, which also provide evidence for an initial hypermetabolic period in the immature brain, with overperfusion followed by a drop to typical adult values.

PET Studies of Metabolic Brain Development

Positron emission tomography has become an indispensable imaging tool in clinical nuclear medicine (4). Especially in combination with CT (now optimized by the direct simultaneous acquisition feasible with PET-CT) and MRI, PET is an established method with wide application in neurology, cardiology, infectiology, and oncology. Compared with its widespread application in adults, however, clinical use of PET in pediatrics is still relatively limited. Possible reasons include the small number of clinical and prospective studies of PET obtained for pediatric as compared with adult imaging indications. Furthermore, only a limited number of PET scanners are available for pediatric imaging. Generally recognized current important indications for pediatric PET include diagnosis and follow-up assessment of Hodgkin's and non-Hodgkin's lymphoma and primary brain tumors, and in defining the seizure focus site for epileptic seizures.

Positron emission tomography study of normal brain development has been less emphasized but is of potentially far-reaching importance. Studies using functional imaging techniques such as PET scans have shown a pattern of metabolic activity that varies in different regions of the brain at different ages.

Fluorodeoxyglucose Studies

Unless under conditions of starvation (in which ketones are available), the brain utilizes glucose as an energy substrate (5). The most commonly utilized marker of glucose metabolism is FDG, a tracer method that evolved from Sokoloff et al.'s (6) original work involving autoradiography and the localization of ^{14}C-2-deoxyglucose in the rat substrate. Although earlier investigations of cerebral circulation and metabolism in children were also conducted (7), the ability to image and quantify vivo metabolic processes was significantly advanced after the development and evolution of modern PET instrumentation (8).

In a classic study, Chugani et al. (9) studied 29 infants and children (ages 5 days to 15.1 years) who had suffered transient neurologic events not significantly affecting normal neurodevelopment. In infants less than 5 weeks old, the local cerebral metabolic rate of glucose (lCMRGl) utilization, a PET parameter, was highest in sensorimotor cortex, thalamus, brainstem, and cerebellar vermis. In cortex, lCMRGl increased first in divisions of occipital cortex and by 2 years had reached essentially adult values in all or most regions. Between 6 months and a year, metabolic activity was marked in the frontal cortex, paralleling development clinically of higher cortical functions, including individual interpersonal interactions, stranger anxiety, and other behaviors. Rates of up to 65 mmol/min/100 g were reached in most regions and persisted until about 9 years. Thereafter, a progressive decline set in, with adult values being reached around 20 years of age. The time course of this metabolic time profile paralleled the phases of production and regression of neurons, synapses, and dendritic spines, as established from morphologic studies. The detailing of this sequence was reasonably postulated as a prerequisite to study of the brain metabolic response in diverse encephalopathies. This sequence of imaging-defined functional events may underlie and provide the biologic basis for the clinically observed critical period of learning and emotional development.

More recently, the effect of brain development on cerebral glucose metabolism was evaluated in 20 neurodevelopmentally normal infants (postconceptional age: 32.7 to 60.3 weeks) (10). It was reported that the lCMRGl in various cortical regions and in the basal ganglia was low at birth (from 4 to 16 μmol/min/100 g). Infants 2 months of age and younger showed the highest lCMRGl in the sensorimotor cortex, thalamus, and brainstem. At 5 months, there was an increase in the lCMRGl in the frontal, parietal, temporal, occipital, and cerebellar cortical regions. Generally, the whole brain lCMRGl correlated with postconceptional age, and the change in the glucose metabolic pattern reflected functional maturation of these regions. Based on these data, it seems that regional glucose metabolism is a credible marker of brain maturation.

The effect of neonatal hypoglycemia on cerebral glucose metabolism was studied in a small group of eight infants (11). The infants were studied with FDG-PET at ages 5.3 ± 6.2 days during normoglycemia and compared to the age-adjusted lCMRGl of eight infants with suspected hypoxic-ischemic brain injury but with normal neurologic development. After neonatal hypoglycemia, the whole brain age-adjusted lCMRGl was not lower than that of the control group and seemed to be normal.

Although the ability to quantify regional cerebral metabolic rates is highly desirable, techniques less invasive than arterial blood sampling have been proposed for early infancy (12). Using a Patlak analysis, the input function was derived by using a combined time-activity curve (derived from left ventricular activity and venous whole blood activity concentration) and by using the activity concentration in whole blood venous samples. These methods showed good correlation, as did an alternative method using standard uptake values (SUV) correlated to lCMRGl values. It appears that reasonable estimations of lCMRGl can be obtained with techniques other than arterial sampling.

Labeled Amino Acid PET Studies

O'Tuama used a dual-probe positron detection system and also retrospective data fit on normal-appearing brain regions of ^{11}C-L-methionine PET to study age-associated changes in amino acid transport from blood to normal frontal cortex (13). Seventeen patients, 1.8 to 71 years of age, were studied. Each patient received two scans in an attempt to assess competitive inhibition of ^{11}C-L-methionine uptake. The first study was performed using tracer doses of the radiopharmaceutical only. One hour before a second PET study, each subject received either oral L-phenylalanine or an intravenous infusion of amino acids, as competing substrates for the neutral amino acid transport system. Uptake of ^{11}C-L-methionine by frontal cortex decreased sevenfold between 1.8 and 71 years of age ($r = -0.71$; $p < .05$). Concomitantly measured blood-to-brain transfer of ^{11}C-L-methionine, at 4.5 years, exceeded mean adult values by more than fivefold. Competitive inhibition reduced L-methionine uptake in all patients older than 4.6 years. These developmental changes parallel findings in animals.

The results of Chugani et al. (9) and O'Tuama, as pointed out by Robinson et al. (14), suggest a significant age-dependence for two different neurometabolic systems—the overall rate of glycolysis and glucose cell membrane transport (FDG), versus amino acid transport and protein synthesis (methionine).

PET Radiation Exposure

A concern intrinsic to the medical and research use of PET radiopharmaceuticals is whether the radiation dose to the newborn or young child is acceptable. Based on the medical internal radiation dose (MIRD) model, the radiation dose to newborn children from FDG has been estimated and has been found to differ from that noted in adults. The radioactivity concentration in the brain and urinary bladder was measured to determine accumulated activity in 21 infant FDG studies. A greater proportion of the tracer was noted to accumulate in the brain of infants than in adults (9% versus 7%, respectively, perhaps partly due to relatively greater brain mass), and less was excreted into the urine (7% versus 20%, respectively). However, there was a large individual variation in the latter. Overall, the dose to the bladder wall was less than for adults, and the greater amount of radioactivity remaining in the body of infants may increase the dose to other organs. Although the calculations were based on upper estimates, the estimated radiation dose from FDG studies was lower in infants compared to adults. Infant FDG studies also had a lower calculated radiation dose compared to conventional nuclear medicine studies such as ^{99m}Tc-methylene diphosphonate bone scintigraphy.

Correlation of SPECT with Other Modalities: MR Imaging and MRS

Tokumaru et al. (15) noted that the precise relationship between function and anatomic brain maturation remains unclear. They studied the changes of rCBF in 42 infants and children, ages 2 days to 19 years, using ^{123}I-IMP-SPECT correlated with MR findings and known developmental changes. The subjects suffered transient neonatal neurologic events, without an overt effect on subsequent neurodevelopment. Beginning at the 34th postconceptional week, there was predominant uptake in the thalami, brainstem, and paleocerebellum, with less cortical activity. Subsequent evolution of rCBF showed a similar regional pattern to the studies of Rubinstein et al. (2) and Chiron et al. (3), and a general parallel to the values for lCMRGl as established by Chugani et al. (9). Also, these changes paralleled T1 and T2 standard spin-echo MRI, and were consequently attributed presumptively to the major neurodevelopmental event of myelination. Minor limitations in the study include lack of specific inversion recovery MR pulse sequences for characterization of myelin development, and the spatial limitations of region definition with ^{123}I-IMP-SPECT. Interesting speculations from these results included the idea that metabolic demands associated with myelination may "drive" the rCBF pattern in the developing brain. At the practical level, it was pointed out that awareness of evolving normal MRI and PET or SPECT patterns during development is crucial

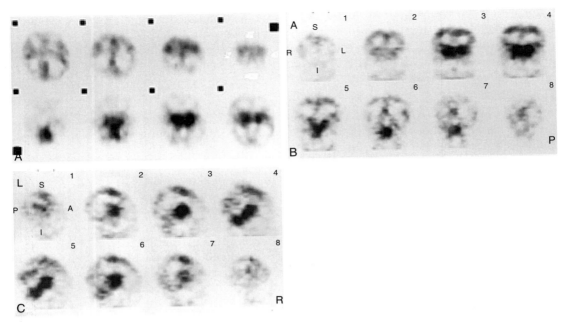

Figure 18.1. Patient at about 34 weeks' gestational age. Axial (A), coronal (B), and sagittal (C) SPECT scans show prominent cerebral perfusion in thalami, brainstem, and cerebellum. There was low activity in the paracentral gyri area.

for interpretation of pediatric studies. Thus the time course of the changes in ^{123}I-IMP uptake in the developing brain as detected by SPECT is similar to that of myelination and most likely reflects an overall topologic maturational pattern of the brain (Fig. 18.1). Ogawa et al. (16) obtained similar results.

Subsequently, newer imaging methods and pulse sequences have been applied to extend our knowledge of the physiology of the developing brain. Zhang et al. (17) used diffusion-weighted sequences, with fitting of data to a triple-gaussian model, to show that brain diffusion decreases and brain volume increases during maturation. They focused on regions showing a range of gray and white matter composition.

Filippi et al. (18) showed changes in diffusion constant and anisotropy in infants with developmental delay despite a normal appearance with conventional MRI techniques. These results further illustrate the potential importance of techniques beyond conventional structural MRI for objective assessment of neurodevelopment.

Other parameters of normal brain development that can be approached by imaging methods include changes in brain water diffusion as studied by diffusion-tensor MRI (18). This study had 167 participants, ages 31 gestational weeks to 11 postnatal years. An isotropic diffusion model was applied to the gray matter of the basal ganglia and thalamus. Maturational decreases of the diffusion tensor eigenvalues were consistent with models reflecting influence of brain water content and myelination.

Magnetic resonance spectroscopy represents another noninvasive method for the study of normal brain development (19). In a review article, Hedlund (20) illustrated how normal white matter spectra with identification of critical neurometabolites can be achieved in children as young as 2 years. These neurometabolites include compounds such as N-acetylaspartate (NAA), a primarily neuronal marker as well as choline, a marker of turnover of myelin and other important cell membranes. Abnormal metabolites such as lactate are undetectable in the normal spectra and are readily revealed in encephalopathies. The studies have relatively short acquisition times, are noninvasive, and thus are feasible even in young sedated patients.

More recently, the technique of dynamic susceptibility contrast-enhanced (DSCE) MRI technique has been used to measure rCBF in newborns (21). This method requires a first-pass contrast bolus, which presents a formidable limitation in neonates and infants, as does the problem of artifacts resulting from bulkhead motion. However, images of perfusion were calculated in 12 of 27 subjects. Major vascular structures such as the circle of Willis could be identified. Values of rCBF were generally larger in gray matter than in white matter.

Attempts have been made to obtain three-dimensional (3D) MRS to study the anatomic distributions of choline, creatine, and NAA in a small group of premature and term infants (22). The basic feasibility of such studies was demonstrated. The results showed topologic and age-dependent variations in the white matter regions of the premature infants. However, there is concern about small sample size and lower signal-to-noise ratio. There is need for substantial further effort to establish an adequate normal database for this age group.

The notion of human brain plasticity is an important concept developed in part from developmental imaging studies of the kind just reviewed. For example, Chugani (23) discussed correlations between lCMRGl and synaptogenesis and has advocated that the PET findings have important implications with respect to potential recovery of regional brain functions following injury and for the concept of "critical periods" for learning capacity. Indirect support for the existence of normal brain functional plasticity has been inferred from studies of abnormal conditions. Thus Helmstaedter and Elger (24), studying patients undergoing left anterior temporal lobectomy, showed varying regional effects on parenchymal plasticity depending on extent of damage and the specific neocortical function involved.

Pediatric PET-CT Brain Imaging

The advent of PET-CT offers further opportunity to delineate these events with increased spatial accuracy with the use of both intermodality fused data sets, as well as high-resolution positron imaging. In normal subjects, uniformly high metabolic uptake in the brain, particularly in brain parenchymal gray matter (GM) structures such as basal ganglia, thalamus, and cerebellum, has limited its use for lesion detection, as discussed elsewhere. However, this feature is a boon for evaluation of normal metabolic variants. The technique involves coupling of PET and CT scanning into a hybrid system. This allows both studies to be done together in what is now known as a PET-CT scanner. The CT acquisition, designed (in many centers) so as not to be diagnostic, but rather to provide adequate attenuation correction and resolution for co-registration, is performed with approximately 2 to 4.25 mm thick contiguous slices, 100 mAs, 140 kVp.

The PET phase of the study is performed with 5- to 10-minute acquisition per imaging level. These systems have the outstanding advantage for pediatric sets of minimizing study times. One platform combines a high resolution and ultrafast multislice CT system with PET optimized for routine 2D and 3D acquisitions. The attached software facilitates postprocessing stages and allows interactive analysis of both data sets. Ionic oral contrast (often administered 1 hour prior to imaging to opacify the bowel for whole-body applications) is omitted. A dose of ^{18}F-FDG, titrated by weight and standard conversion factor, is given intravenously 1 hour prior to imaging, and the patient voids prior to imaging to decrease bladder activity (25). The older, cooperative child is positioned supine on the imaging table, with the head comfortably positioned in a cushioned head holder and arms at the patient's side. Following tracer injection, it is useful to have the patient rest in a quiet environment, instructed to limit verbal and physical activity during the major tracer uptake phase (about 20 minutes).

A qualitative analysis is the most common method for pediatric brain PET-CT and, with an experienced observer, is usually adequate. Typically, a workstation review is made of all orthogonal images with varying gray scale and color image presentation, rotating views, and maximum intensity projection images (Fig. 18.2).

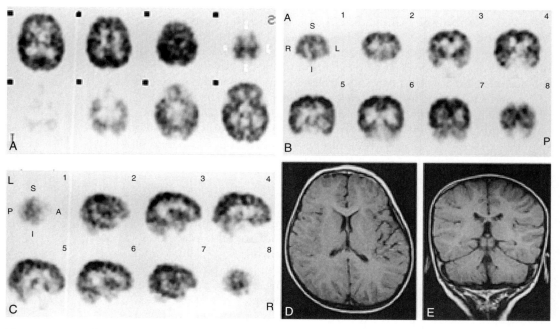

Figure 18.2. A–C: SPECT scans show almost similar appearance to adult pattern. D,E: Axial spin echo (600/15) MR images show myelination in frontal and temporal areas. [*Source:* Tokumaru et al., (14) with permission.]

Conclusion

Techniques used for mapping of brain function are usefully reviewed by Santosh (26). Brain morphology and tissue composition will continue to be elucidated mainly with MRI and CT. Information on neuronal activity and communication will continue to be provided at the electromagnetic (EEG, MEG) level. Biochemical aspects of neurotransmission will be studied by general mapping of blood flow and tissue metabolism with standard PET and SPECT methods, supplemented by tissue typing using MRS. Energy-dependent metabolic processes will be assessed most specifically with selective PET ligand and metabolite radiopharmaceuticals. Clinically relevant neurotransmitters and receptors include D_1 antagonists in prefrontal cortex, hippocampus, and amygdala; D_2 receptor agonist, which localizes mainly in the striatum; and 5-hydroxytryptamine $(5HT)_{1A}$, $5HT_{2A}$, and $5HT_{\alpha 2}$ receptor ligands. Also, ligands that help quantify receptors such as N-methyl-D-aspartate (NMDA), α-amino-3-hydroxy-5-methyl-4-isoxazolepropionate (AMPA), etc., will help understanding both of normal function of these systems, and of their specific abnormalities in the neurodevelopmental disorders. Functional MRI will assist these efforts, mainly by measuring activation-associated changes in brain perfusion.

Advances in MR technique will contribute significantly. These will include rapid MR scanning (gradient echo, fast spin echo, and planar sequences), contrast-based fMRI techniques, diffusion MRI, arterial spine labeling (ASL), and dynamic susceptibility MR perfusion imaging of the brain. Other important anticipated improvements in technology will relate to reduction of movement artifacts, imaging data reduction, and postimaging data processing.

Among these exciting future developments, nuclear medicine technology is likely to continue to play a unique and unchallenged role. Radiopharmaceutically based imaging technology retains the highest sensitivity of available modalities (including MRI, fMRI, MRS, EEG, and MEG) for depiction of biochemical processes occurring in the picomolar to nanomolar range. This specificity extends to presynaptic neurotransmitter molecules, which can be separated from receptor systems that are mainly postsynaptic, only 20 to 50 nM apart. Therefore, nuclear techniques will play an increasingly important and visible role as developmental mapping of neurotransmitters and synaptic systems comes to the fore. Correlation with the more spatially detailed modalities reviewed here will be important in gleaning the ultimate information from such studies. In this regard, ultimately the use of combined functional and structural data sets as pioneered with PET-CT systems will provide the method of choice. Studies on normal children, within ethical limits, will continue to give important and critical new insights into the neurofunctional underpinnings of normal childhood cognitive and emotional processes.

References

1. Barkovich AJ, Kjos BO, Jackson DE Jr, Norman D. Normal maturation of the neonatal and infant brain: MR imaging at 1.5 T. Radiology 1988; 166(1 pt 1):173–180.
2. Rubinstein M, Denays R, Ham HR, et al. Functional imaging of brain maturation in humans using iodine-123 iodoamphetamine and SPECT. J Nucl Med 1989;30(12):1982–1985.
3. Chiron C, Raynaud C, Maziere B, et al. Changes in regional cerebral blood flow during brain maturation in children and adolescents. J Nucl Med 1992;33(5):696–703.
4. Hahn K, Pflunger T. Has PET become an important clinical tool in the paediatric imaging? Eur J Nucl Med Mol Imaging 2004;31(5):615–621.
5. Sokoloff L, Relationships among local functional activity, energy metabolism, and blood flow in the central nervous system. Fed Proc 1981;40(8): 2311–2316.
6. Sokoloff L, Revich M, Kennedy C, et al. The [14C]deoxyglucose method for the measurement of local cerebral glucose utilization: theory, procedure, and normal values in the conscious and anesthetized albino rat. J Neurochem 1977;28:897–916.
7. Kennedy C, Sokoloff L, Anderson W, Duffy P. Studies in cerebral circulation and metabolism in children. Trans Am Neurol Assoc 1954;13:196–198.
8. Phelps ME, Huang SC, Hoffman EJ, Selin C, Sokoloff L, Kuhl DE. Tomographic measurement of local cerebral glucose metabolic rate in humans with (F-18)2–fluoro-2–deoxy-D-glucose: validation of method. Ann Neurol 1979;6:371–388.
9. Chugani HT, Phelps ME, Mazziotta JC. Positron emission tomography study of human brain functional development. Ann Neurol 1987;22(4): 487–497.
10. Kinnala A, Suhonen-Polvi H, Aarimaa T, et al. Cerebral metabolic rate for glucose during the first six months of life: an FDG positron emission tomography study. Arch Dis Child (Fetal Neonatal Ed) 1996;74:F153–157.
11. Kinnala A, Nuutila P, Ruotsalainen U, et al. Cerebral metabolic rate for glucose after neonatal hypoglycaemia. Early Human Dev 1997;24:63–72.
12. Suhonen-Polvi H, Ruotsalainen U, Kinnala A, et al. FDG-PET in early infancy: simplified quantification methods to measure cerebral glucose utilization. J Nucl Med 1995;36:1249–1254.
13. O'Tuama LA, Guilarte TR, Douglass KN, et al. Assessment of ll-C-L-methionine transport into the human brain. J Cereb Blood Flow Metab. 1998;8:341–345.
14. Robinson RO, Ferrie CD, Capra M, Maisey MN. Positron emission tomography and the central nervous system. Arch Dis Child 1999;81(3):263–270.
15. Tokumaru AM, Barkovicha AJ, O'uchia T, Massuo T, Kusano S. The evolution of cerebral blood flow in the developing brain: evaluation with iodine-123 iodoamphetamine SPECT and correlation with MR imaging. AJNR 1999;20(5):845–852.
16. Ogawa A, Sakurai Y, Kayama T, Yoshimoto T. Regional cerebral blood flow with age: changes in rCBF in childhood. Neurol Res 1989;11(3):173–176.
17. Zhang L, Thomas KM, Davidson MC, Casey BJ, Heier LA, Ulug AM. MR quantitation of volume and diffusion changes in the developing brain. AJNR 2005;26(1):45–49.
18. Filippi CG, Lin DD, Tsiouris AJ, et al. Diffusion-tensor MR imaging in children with developmental delay: preliminary findings. Radiology 2003; 229(1):44–50.

19. Mukherjee P, Miller JH, Shimony JS, et al. Diffusion-tensor MR imaging of gray and white matter development during normal human brain maturation. AJNR 2002;23(9):1445–1456.

20. Hedlund GL. Neuroradiology of the central nervous system in childhood. Neurol Clin 2002;20(4):965–981.

21. Tanner SF, Cornette L, Ramenghi LA, et al. Cerebral perfusion in infants and neonates: preliminary results obtained using dynamic susceptibility contrast enhanced magnetic resonance imaging. Arch Dis Child (Fetal Neonatal Ed) 2003;88(6):F525–530.

22. Vigneron DB, Barkovich AJ, Noworolski SM, et al. Three-dimensional proton MR spectroscopic imaging of premature and term neonates. AJNR 2001;22(7):1424–1433.

23. Chugani HT. PET scanning Studies of human brain development and plasticity. Dev Neuropsychol 1999;16(3):379–381.

24. Helmstaedter C, Elger CE. Functional plasticity after left anterior temporal lobectomy: reconstitution and compensation of verbal memory functions. Epilepsia 1998;39(4):399–406.

25. Stabin MG, Gelfand MJ. Dosimetry of pediatric nuclear medicine procedures. Q J Nucl Med 1998;42(2):93–112.

26. Santosh P. Neuroimaging in child and adolescent psychiatric disorders. Arch Dis Child 2000;82(5):412–419.

19

Neurodevelopmental and Neuropsychiatric Disorders

Marianne Glanzman and Josephine Elia

Positron emission tomography (PET) and single photon emission computed tomography (SPECT) scans offer great promise in helping to unravel the scientific basis for neurodevelopmental and neuropsychiatric disorders. To date, results have been somewhat limited by the difficulty in obtaining adequate control groups, technical difficulties in studying children, small numbers of subjects, variable analytic methods, and the inability to repeat scans in order to understand the effects of development and intervention due to concerns about exposure to radiopharmaceuticals. Nonetheless, some consistent findings have emerged, and intriguing new results point toward future directions of study.

Attention-Deficit/Hyperactivity Disorder

Background

Attention-deficit/hyperactivity disorder (ADHD) is one of the most common neurodevelopmental/neuropsychiatric disorders of childhood, with a prevalence of between 5% and 12% in school-aged children, and persistence into adulthood in 50% to 75% of cases (1,2). It is characterized by age-inappropriate difficulty in sustaining mental effort, excessive distractibility, restlessness or overactivity, and impulsivity that is chronic, present across settings, functionally impairing, and not due primarily to another diagnosis such as cognitive or language impairment, autism, mood or anxiety disorders, or medical or other neurologic disorders. Its symptoms have important functional implications for learning, socializing, self-esteem, educational and occupational achievement, driving safety, risk for depression, and the stability of employment and significant relationships. Though "invisible," it typically has tremendous impact on the lives of the affected individual and family members; thus, improvement in our understanding of its nature and treatment is critical.

Neuropsychological testing of individuals who demonstrate the behavioral criteria for ADHD typically reveals evidence of executive dysfunction. Executive functions are prefrontal cortical functions including sustaining and shifting attention, vigilance, organization, planning, self-monitoring, conception of time, and the ability to inhibit behavior as well as modify it based on past experience and future expectations. Attention-deficit/hyperactivity disorder is highly heritable, and there are probably several genes that confer susceptibility. The most important ones are likely yet to be discovered, though specific alleles at the loci for the dopamine transporter (DAT), dopamine type 4 receptor, and dopamine type 5 receptor appear to be associated (3). Converging evidence from neuropsychological, neurochemical, electrophysiologic, and neuroimaging studies indicate that ADHD is most likely the result of altered dopamine (DA) and norepinephrine neurotransmission in the prefrontal cortex and its targets, particularly the basal ganglia (2,4).

Structural imaging studies done for clinical purposes, such as computed axial tomography (CAT) or magnetic resonance imaging (MRI) scans, are not typically revealing in children with ADHD. However, volumetric MRI scans document alterations in the size of various brain regions in subjects compared with controls. Consistent findings include smaller frontal lobes (most notable on the right), globus pallidus, corpus callosum (most often anteriorly), and the posterior inferior cerebellar vermis. The caudate nucleus in subjects with ADHD is also consistently different from that in controls, but the findings between studies are more complex and variable, with some authors reporting a smaller caudate on one side or the other or an absence or reversal of the typical "left greater-than right" asymmetry (5,6). The most recent studies show that, although frontostriatal regions continue to be most markedly implicated, there is a widespread volume loss of approximately 5% to 9% involving both gray and white matter, consistent with involvement of widespread attention and cognitive processing networks (5,7). A developmental study comparing volumetric analysis from children with ADHD and controls across the age span of 5 to 18 indicates that cerebellar, cerebellar vermis, caudate, and gray and white matter from all four cerebral lobes are smaller in subjects from the youngest ages. With correction for total cerebral volume, the cerebellar vermis remained smaller in subjects. The differences remained throughout childhood, with the exception that caudate volumes were similar by 18 due to the lack of the "normal" decline in size in subjects (7). In individual studies, the degree of volume reduction in one or more regions may correlate with specific symptoms or severity, but across studies, findings are somewhat inconsistent (5). This highlights the need for a functional imaging approach.

Many functional imaging studies support the role of the prefrontal cortex in working memory, one of the executive functions that is often impaired in individuals with ADHD (4,8). In general, subjects with ADHD are found to activate frontal areas to a lesser degree than controls when performing a memory/attention demanding task, but may activate a wider, more posterior (and behaviorally less effective) set of neural networks to accomplish the task (4,5).

Three studies using functional MRI (fMRI) in children with ADHD have been reported. These lend support to the role of frontostriatal differences in ADHD, though these studies employed behavioral inhibition rather than working memory tasks during scanning. Rubia et al. (9) studied seven adolescent boys with ADHD and matched controls during two different motor tasks involving pushing a button in response to a target on a screen—one demanding motor inhibition and one stressing motor timing. On the response inhibition task, subjects demonstrated increased right inferior and mid-prefrontal and left caudate activation compared with controls. On the motor timing task, subjects demonstrated decreased right mid-prefrontal activation compared with controls. Vaidya et al. (10) used a "go/no go" task in which subjects responded by pressing a button either to all letters presented on a screen (go task) or all letters except X (no go task). Two different formats were used for the "go" task involving different rates of presentation. This was used as the "control" condition from which to compare activation during the "no go" condition. Different results were obtained with the two different formats, highlighting the importance of slight differences in the behavior portion of the experimental protocol in fMRI results. In the stimulus-controlled, more demanding presentation rate, striatal activation was greater in controls than subjects, and medication typically used to treat ADHD (methylphenidate, MPH) given prior to the task, increased activation in subjects and decreased it in controls. Methylphenidate increased frontal activation in both groups. In the response-controlled, less demanding presentation rate, subjects had more frontal activation than controls and there were no effects of MPH (4). Durston et al. (5) studied the effects of increasing the number of "go" trials that preceded a "no go" trial on the likelihood of making a "no go error" in adults, in typically developing children, and in children with ADHD. In normally developing children, increasing the number of "go" trials before a "no go" trial increased the likelihood of a "no go" error; this effect of interference improved with maturity. In adults, the maintenance of accurate performance with increasing interference resulted in increased activation of the ventral prefrontal cortex, but in children any level of interference results in maximal increases in activation of this area. Seven school-aged, right-handed children with ADHD were compared with matched controls and were found to have similar accuracy and reaction times on the "go" trials. However, though accuracy on the "no go" trials decreased with increasing preceding "go" trials in controls, in subjects even one preceding "go" trial significantly decreased accuracy on a subsequent "no go" trial. When compared with controls, subjects showed less activation in ventral prefrontal cortex, anterior cingulate gyrus, and basal ganglia, and increased activation in posterior parietal and occipital cortices (5).

PET/SPECT Imaging in ADHD

The first SPECT studies of ADHD were performed in children with ADHD by Lou and colleagues (11) from 1984 to 1990. These studies employed xenon-133 (^{133}Xe) inhalation to reflect regional perfusion in children with ADHD; however, these studies were initially criticized because many of the children had coexisting disorders such as language delays. Initial results indicated bilateral central frontal hypoperfusion and occipital hyperperfusion, and MPH treatment was found to increase perfusion in the frontal regions, basal ganglia, and mesencephalon while decreasing it in cortical sensorimotor regions. In later studies, this group employed controls and evaluated subjects with pure ADHD separately from those with language disorders, though the pure ADHD group still may have had more generalized neurologic dysfunction than children typically referred to as having pure ADHD today (12,13). The results were similar with the additional finding in ADHD of decreased perfusion in the striatum (more so on the right). Once again, scans taken after acute MPH treatment tended to show normalization of both under- and overperfusion.

In 1990 Zametkin and colleagues (14) undertook a series of PET studies initiated by landmark research often used to the present to prove the biologic basis of ADHD. They used fluorine-18 (^{18}F)-fluoro-2-deoxy-D-glucose (^{18}F-FDG) to measure regional cerebral glucose metabolism (rCGM) in 25 adult subjects carefully diagnosed as having persistent ADHD from childhood and 50 matched controls during performance of an auditory continuous performance task that taxed attention, persistence of mental effort, and working memory (though there may have been ceiling effects in terms of its clinical difficulty). Adults with ADHD had an overall 8% decrease in global CGM and 30 of 60 measured regions were lower in subjects, with the largest reductions in the superior prefrontal and premotor cortices. This study was repeated in a smaller number of adolescents, with the expectation that even greater differences from controls would be found in the more clinically symptomatic adolescents, but this was not the case. Left anterior frontal perfusion was found to correlate inversely with symptom severity, however (15).

Subsequent studies by this group suggested that females with ADHD might have more pronounced PET findings than males, though findings were not consistent (16–18). During this time frame, other researchers using methods to evaluate regional perfusion or glucose metabolism also found decreased prefrontal cortical perfusion in subjects with ADHD compared with controls (19,20). Sieg et al. (19) also found decreased temporal perfusion using N-isopropyl-123p-iodoamphetamine (^{123}I-IMP) SPECT in children with normal structural MRIs, some of whom had learning differences. Amen and Carmichael (20) found that subjects actually showed a decrease in prefrontal perfusion (the opposite of what was expected from studies of controls) during an attention-demanding task. More recent studies employing ligands related to general perfusion continue to show decreases in frontal or frontotemporal perfusion in children with ADHD compared with controls, but the laterality of findings differs between studies, perhaps related to differences in learning profiles or coexisting conditions among subject groups (21–24). Even within a study, perfusion abnormalities differ among subjects (21). Decreases in temporal lobe perfusion may be related to the presence of coexisting conditions. Lorberboym and colleagues (23) studied young adolescent boys with "pure" ADHD, ADHD plus oppositional, conduct, learning, or mood disorders, and controls during a computerized continuous performance task using technetium-99m ethylcysteinate dimer (^{99m}Tc-ECD) SPECT. Although there were differences among subjects, all subjects with an additional diagnosis had decreased perfusion in one or both temporal lobes.

Several studies have also been done using ligands related to specific neurotransmitters rather than glucose utilization or perfusion. Ernst and colleagues (25,26) used ^{18}F-fluorodopa (^{18}F-FD) to assess the integrity of DA uptake processes in the midbrain, striatum, and prefrontal cortex of adults and children with ADHD compared with controls. Adults showed more than a 50% decrease in uptake in medial and lateral prefrontal cortex (25), whereas children showed an almost 50% increase in the right midbrain (26). The most common neurotransmitter component studied in ADHD is DAT. Methylphenidate, the most commonly prescribed medication for treating ADHD, blocks dopamine reuptake at the transporter (27). Many types of studies implicate the DA system in ADHD symptoms (28,29), and genetic studies implicate DAT polymorphisms in ADHD (30). Several studies (31–33), though not all (34), have found elevated levels of DAT binding in adults with ADHD; one study in children (35) showed that medication-naive children with ADHD have 14% to 70% increases in DAT binding in the striatum compared with controls.

In summary, decreased perfusion in the frontal lobes and basal ganglia are typically found in subjects with ADHD compared with controls. Subjects tend to activate more widespread neural networks in response to attention-demanding tasks. Findings between studies differ with respect to laterality (5,21–24). Findings in children and adults show both similarities and differences, but developmental changes over the course of childhood have not been well studied. Gender differences are likely to be important but require further study. Finally, the small numbers of subjects has limited the ability of researchers to separate the findings specifically related to ADHD from those related to commonly coexisting conditions, but work is beginning in this direction.

PET/SPECT Imaging and Medications for ADHD

Stimulants have been used for decades and are the treatment of choice for ADHD. There are two categories of stimulants, MPH and amphetamine (AMPH), with a variety of products available in each category with different durations of action and release properties. Functional imaging studies investigating medication effects have typically been performed with short-acting (3 to 4 hours) MPH or dextroamphetamine (d-AMPH) even though most children actually take longer-acting formulations. Strattera, a selective norepinephrine reuptake inhibitor, was recently approved for the treatment of ADHD (36). To date, there are no functional imaging studies of its effects in children with ADHD.

Approximately 30% of students with ADHD do not respond to or do not tolerate stimulants due to side effects (27). The presence of comorbidities related to mood and anxiety, and repetitive behaviors such as tics or compulsions may increase the risk for medication side effects or limit stimulant effectiveness (37). Alternative medications, including antidepressants, antihypertensives, atypical antipsychotics, and modafinil (a medication approved for narcolepsy) are sometimes used in these children but have not been studied with functional imaging in children with ADHD.

Matochik et al. (38,39) evaluated the effects of acute and subchronic (6 week) MPH and d-AMPH on rCGM in adults with ADHD using ^{18}F-FDG. There was no change in global metabolism in any condition, and very few changes at all were noted with subchronic administration. With acute administration, some regions increased and others decreased, not necessarily in the pattern that would have been expected based on previous studies reported herein. The findings with MPH and d-AMPH differed, even though behavioral improvements were similar. Schweitzer et al. (40) compared rCBF using oxygen-15 (^{15}O)-H$_2$O in adults with ADHD before and after 3 weeks of optimally dosed MPH. In conjunction with improved behavioral measures, post-treatment scans showed higher rCBF in the posterior cerebellum and decreased rCBF in the bilateral precentral gyrus, left caudate, and right claustrum. Volkow et al. (41) also noted differences between acute and chronic administration. They also showed that, in healthy adults, the regions activated by MPH administration, as demonstrated by ^{18}F-FDG uptake, differed between subjects with high and low DA type 2 (D2) receptor binding assessed concomitantly with ^{11}C-raclopride (42). Mattay et al. (43) administered d-AMPH during neuropsychological tasks that taxed different brain regions and measured rCBF with ^{15}O-H$_2$O. d-AMPH was found to increase rCBF in a task-dependent manner. Thus, characteristics of the subjects or the brain activity during scanning may influence results.

Two studies have investigated the effects of MPH in children and adolescents with ADHD using PET/SPECT scanning. Szobot et al. (44) measured blood flow with ^{99m}Tc-ECD before and after 4 days of MPH or placebo treatment in 36 boys with ADHD without severe comorbidities (but boys with oppositional defiant disorder and learning disorders were not excluded). Statistical parametric mapping showed a decrease in the left parietal region in the treated group compared with the placebo group, suggesting that the posterior attentional system may also be involved in the behavioral effects of MPH. Langleben et al. (45) studied the effects on rCBF of discontinuing MPH in boys with ADHD and controls with ^{99m}Tc-ECD SPECT and found increased rCBF in the motor, premotor, and anterior cingulated cortices, but this study was not designed in such a way as to determine whether ADHD treatment lowers rCBF in these areas, or whether the increase was a specific response to withdrawal of subchronic treatment.

Several researchers have evaluated the effects of MPH on the DAT and other specific measures of DA function using PET/SPECT scans.

Volkow and colleagues (46) have shown that (1) oral MPH reaches peak concentrations in the brain at 60 to 90 minutes, (2) therapeutic doses block about 50% of striatal DATs, (3) MPH's relatively slow uptake and egress from the brain is most likely responsible for its lack of euphorogenic properties in contrast to cocaine, and (4) it is the d-isomer of MPH that effectively blocks the DAT. Furthermore, they have shown that DAT blockade leads to increased extracellular DA in the striatum and that variability in response to MPH is more likely due to variability between individuals in their dopaminergic neuronal activity, which modulates the degree of extracellular DA increase in response to DAT blockade rather than differences in the degree of MPH-induced DAT blockade itself (46).

Researchers have also begun to think about how to use PET/SPECT to assess the long-term effects of medication on the dopamine system. Vles et al. (47) studied six, non-comorbid, medication-naive boys with ADHD at baseline and after 3 to 4 months of clinically optimized MPH treatment. Behavior and neuropsychological test performance improved. They used ^{123}I-loflupane (FP-CIT) to label DAT and ^{123}I-benzamide (IBZM) to label postsynaptic D2 receptors in the caudate and putamen. Due to the small number of subjects, only descriptive statistics are used. At baseline, D2 receptor binding was similar in the left and right caudate and putamen. After 3 months of treatment, five of the six subjects showed a decrease (average of 14%) in D2 receptor binding in the striatum. One subject was re-scanned after 1 month off medication, and his D2 receptor binding returned to pretreatment levels. Baseline DAT binding was less in the left compared to right caudate in all six subjects. Whether this reflects normal development or is characteristic of ADHD is still unclear. Binding differences in the left and right putamen varied among subjects. After treatment, binding decreased in both the caudate and putamen by an average of 58% and the left < right asymmetry disappeared. In the subject who was scanned after a month off medication, binding in the right caudate and putamen returned to pretreatment levels, but binding in the left caudate and putamen was increased by 30% and 50%, respectively. This study suggests that further study is warranted regarding the possibility of long-term alterations in DAT function as a result of MPH treatment. Ilgin et al. (48) evaluated D2 receptor availability in the caudate and putamen of medication-naive children with ADHD before and after 3 months of MPH treatment. At baseline, subjects demonstrated normal to increased D2 receptor binding compared to published values for healthy young adults. It is known that D2 receptor binding decreases with age, but even taking this into account, these values were higher than anticipated. However, the lack of age-matched controls in the same study makes any conclusions about higher D2 receptor binding in children with ADHD preliminary. No right/left asymmetry in binding was detected in either region. Chronic medication effect studies are critical but are complicated by the need for controls for normal developmental changes and potential differences in effects of long- and short-acting medications.

Tourette Syndrome

Background

Tourette syndrome (TS) is the most complex form of tic disorder and occurs in approximately 0.1% to 1% of children. Tics are brief, repetitive, staccato, involuntary movements or vocalizations that tend to occur in clusters, and typically fluctuate in type, frequency, and severity over time. It is diagnosed when an individual displays multiple motor tics and at least one vocal tic that fluctuate in character and severity over time, have persisted for more than a year, and have not occurred solely during the course of treatment with a medication that is known to induce or exacerbate tics (e.g., stimulants for ADHD). Other tic disorders, which occur more commonly than full TS, include chronic single tic disorder (1% to 2% of children) and transient tic disorder (approximately 5% of children) (49,50). Chronic tic disorders of any variety, however, appear to be genetically related (51,52). Although most cases of TS are mild in terms of tic severity and tic-related functional impairment, it is common for individuals with TS to have comorbidities that are far more functionally impairing including ADHD, obsessive-compulsive disorder (OCD), other forms of anxiety, aggression, and learning disabilities (LDs) (49). Not only do tic disorders of varying severity probably have a common genetic etiology, but there appear to be genetic relationships among tics, ADHD, and OCD as well (53). The search for the genetic etiology of TS has been ongoing for over 20 years, and, as with the genetics of other complex behavioral disorders, progress has been slow. Recently, linkages have been identified on chromosomes 2, 4, 5, 8, 11, and 19, but specific genes in these areas remain to be identified (51). Immune reactions to streptococcal bacteria and other agents that produce antibodies that cross-react with basal ganglia neurons may be etiologic in some cases, and this phenomenon may have genetic underpinnings. Nongenetic factors including uterine and hormonal milieu, and maternal stress during pregnancy may also play a role (49,54).

Multiple lines of evidence, including various neuroimaging modalities, support the involvement of the basal ganglia in movement disorders, including TS. However, dyscontrol of movement can occur at any level in cortical–basal ganglia–thalamocortical circuitry. Multiple lines of evidence also indicate a role for the dopamine system in TS, including the effects of medications (dopaminergic medications can exacerbate tics, whereas dopamine-blocking agents are used to treat tics), studies of dopamine metabolites, and functional imaging studies involving dopamine-related ligands.

PET/SPECT Imaging in TS

Imaging studies of tic disorders have focused on TS; however, the high rate of multiple comorbid conditions in individuals with TS has complicated the interpretation of results. Volumetric MRI studies in adults with TS show decreased size of the prefrontal cortex and left caudate and putamen, whereas children with TS show larger prefrontal volumes and left caudate reductions (55). A recent study that used parcellation into more specific subregions of the frontal lobes and distinguished white and gray matter found that boys with TS had decreased volume of the left deep white matter, suggesting abnormalities of association and projection bundles, in contrast to boys with ADHD who were found to have reduced volumes of gray and white matter within the prefrontal cortex (56).

Positron emission tomography/SPECT studies assessing regional metabolism or blood flow in TS have been performed in adults, primarily, and have confirmed decreased activity in the striatum in comparison with controls, though specific locations have differed between studies and have included ventral striatum, ventral globus pallidus, and basal ganglia in general. Some, but not all, studies suggest a greater decrease in left-sided structures (55). Other researchers have also found decreases in the midbrain (57), thalamus (58), cingulate, and prefrontal cortex (59) and one group found an increase in frontal CBF (60). Limitations in anatomic resolution may contribute to discrepancies in these studies. In addition, the role of tics themselves and tic suppression during scanning may complicate findings. A study of blood flow in conjunction with tic frequency during scanning indicates that multiple brain areas associated with motor activity as well as several not generally associated with motor activity show increased flow in association with tics (61). Studies under the identical conditions assessing similar voluntary motor behaviors would need to be done to identify the regions associated specifically with tic generation as opposed to the motor activity itself. Finally, areas activated or deactivated by the acute or chronic process of suppressing tics are largely unknown and may be relevant to studies of both etiology and changes in findings over the life span. An fMRI study of tic suppression showed that it was associated with increases and decreases in signal in a variety of regions, some unilateral and some bilateral. In particular, prefrontal and right caudate showed increased signal, associated with decreased signal in the rest of the basal ganglia (62).

Positron emission tomography/SPECT studies assessing striatal dopaminergic innervation using ^{18}F-FD, ^{123}I-2β-carbomethoxy-3β-(4-iodophenyl)tropane (β-CIT), and IBZM have been done primarily in adults and have shown conflicting results, initially thought to be due to potential effects of prior or current medication exposure (55). Initial studies showed increased binding to DAT sites in adults with TS compared with controls (63–65), and a study in children without current medication showed increased ^{18}F-FD activity in the left caudate and right midbrain (66). Later studies controlled for this variable but still showed conflicting results. For example, a study by Stamenkovic et al. (67) evaluated medication-naive and actively medicated subjects (adolescents and primarily young adults) separately and found no increase in DAT binding in either group but more variability among the medicated group.

Serra-Mestres et al. (68) found higher 2β-carbomethoxy-3β-(4-iodophenyl)-N-(3-fluoropropyl)nortropane (^{123}I-FP-CIT) binding in both caudate and putamen in 10 neuroleptic naive/free adults compared with controls, but the binding did not correlate with any of the measured indices of TS severity. Other important variables may include past history of medication use and coexisting disorders. In a study that looked more specifically at different anatomic regions within the striatum, Albin et al. (69) studied 19 adults with TS and various medication histories and comorbidities with ^{11}C-dihydrotetrabenazene (^{11}C-DTBZ), a ligand for the type 2 vesicular monoamine transporter. They found no difference compared with controls in the dorsal striatum but an increase in binding in the right ventral striatum. Finally, Cheon et al. (35) studied nine drug-naive children aged 6 to 12 with TS (excluding those with comorbid OCD, ADHD, anxiety, and depression) and matched controls with ^{123}I-N-(3-iodoproprn-2-yl)-2β-carbomethoxy-3β-(4-clorophenyl)tropane (^{123}I-IPT) SPECT and found subjects to have an increase in specific to nonspecific (measured in cerebellum) binding in the basal ganglia, though this did not correlate with tic severity. D2 receptor density has been studied with PET/SPECT in adult subjects with TS and generally found not to differ from controls (55), though one study suggests that a subgroup of adults with TS may have an increased binding capacity (70). One study comparing five sets of adult monozygotic twins found a 17% increase in D2 binding capacity in the more severely affected twin (71), and one study found a decrease in D2 binding capacity in subjects affected for more than 15 years and in subjects on neuroleptic medication. Because both of these conditions are associated with a lessening of tic severity, it may be hypothesized that a decline in D2 binding may be associated with symptom improvement (64).

Dyslexia

Background

Learning disability can be described (as proposed by the National Joint Committee on Learning Disabilities) as a generic term that refers to a heterogeneous group of disorders manifested by significant difficulties in the acquisition and use of listening, speaking, reading, writing, spelling, reasoning, or mathematical abilities. It is intrinsic to the individual and presumed due to dysfunction of the central nervous system and not due to cognitive impairment, sensory dysfunction, inadequate educational exposure, social/emotional disturbance, or environmental disadvantage (72). A learning disability in reading, or dyslexia, is the most common form of learning disability, affecting approximately 10% of children. Many children with dyslexia have associated language, spelling, writing, attention, and fine motor deficits (73).

Multiple lines of evidence indicate that three types of underlying processing deficits occur in dyslexia: phonologic, visual, and temporal. The best studied, and most central, is phonologic; children with dyslexia are impaired in their ability to segment words verbally as well as graphically into their component phonemes (sound segments), and, in the reverse, to combine phonemes accurately into words. Visual processing deficits are inferred from the types of reading errors children make (substitutions of visually similar letters, words, etc.) as well as studies that show slower visual processing. Temporal processing deficits were identified most recently. Alterations have been found in the magnocellular component of the auditory and visual pathway, known to be relevant for the rapid detection of changes in and sequences of stimuli, and it has been hypothesized that the left hemisphere in particular is involved in the processing of transient sensory events. Studies of event-related potentials suggest that dyslexics are impaired in the distinction between speech sounds in the preattentive phase, as measured by mismatch negativity, and have lower or later P300 waves reflecting inefficient processing of target stimuli (73). Classic studies of language-impaired and dyslexic children by Tallal et al. (74) indicate that they are impaired in distinguishing phonemes that differ by rapid or subtle frequency differences but not those that differ by slower or more prolonged frequency characteristics. This may be true for other sensory modalities as well. Electrophysiologic evidence supports both slower auditory and visual processing in dyslexics (75). It is likely that children with dyslexia differ from each other with respect to the degree of each different type of impairment they manifest. Some may be more phonologically dyslexic, whereas others are more visually dyslexic, though the ultimate clinical impairment is the same.

Dyslexia is commonly genetic, but the specific inheritance pattern is unknown. It appears that genes on a variety of different chromosomes may be related to different neuropsychological processes that are weak in dyslexics. For example, a gene on chromosome 15 appears related to rapid single word reading, whereas one on chromosome 6 appears related to a phonologic awareness task (73). A twin study indicates that the phonologic component of dyslexia is more strongly heritable than the visual component (76), supporting a role for the prenatal environment in the latter as has previously been proposed (77,78).

Anatomic studies of the brains of dyslexic individuals show two types of consistent abnormalities: ectopias in the bilateral frontal and left temporal and parietal cortices with associated adjacent dysplasia, and loss of the normal left > right size of the planum temporale. These findings indicate that dyslexia is associated with altered mid-gestation brain development. Less frequent findings include vascular micromalformations and microgyria (73).

Functional MRI studies of the brain during reading by Shaywitz (79) and others showed that women activate both the left and right inferior frontal gyrus (Broca's area) while reading, whereas men activate only the left. This part of the brain appears to be specifically involved in sounding out words, as it is activated by the reading of nonsense words. An occipitotemporal region is important in storing information about word form, which allows automatic recognition of words previously accurately analyzed, and a parietotemporal area is important in slowly analyzing words. As readers become more skilled, they activate the occipitotemporal area (automatic word recognition) more and the parietotemporal and frontal areas (word analysis) less. Dyslexic readers have less posterior activation but also show a change in activation pattern over the course of development, unlike skilled readers who show more posterior than anterior activation at all ages. Dyslexics increasingly activate the front of the brain as well as right-sided auxiliary pathways as they become adolescents, suggesting that they increasingly compensate for poor word recognition by the slower process of word analysis. These findings are present in dyslexics in all languages and at all ages (79,80). Functional MRI has been used to demonstrate that dyslexics do not activate motion-sensitive regions of the magnocellular system located in the posterior part of the inferior temporal sulcus, which supports the temporal processing theory of dyslexia (81). Functional MRI has also been used to show that effective reading intervention leads to "brain repair" in that in response to the specific type of instruction known to improve reading in dyslexics, and with confirmation of improved skills, dyslexic children show increased activation of the left posterior region similar to that of controls (82,83).

PET/SPECT Imaging in Dyslexia

Oxygen-15 (^{15}O)-H$_2$O, ^{18}F-FDG, and ^{133}Xe inhalation have been used to study reading and its subprocesses in dyslexics and controls. To date, there have been no studies in children. The vast majority of studies find differences between dyslexics and controls in one or more regions of the brain known to be involved in language or reading, but specific findings cannot be compared across studies because different tasks are used and the coexistence of ADHD has not typically been considered. Different patterns of abnormal left hemisphere blood flow have been found in several studies (84). For example, Flowers et al. (85) found that although language tasks activated the expected supratemporal area (Wernicke's area) in controls, it activated a slightly posterior temporoparietal area in adults who were poor readers in childhood, perhaps related to additional effort required.

In a series of studies by Rumsey and colleagues (86), different types of reading tasks were performed by controls and adult dyslexics. Dyslexics showed reduced activation of the left parietal region at rest, and bilateral reduced activation of the mid-to-posterior temporal cortices and left inferior parietal cortex during phonologic processing tasks. During tasks requiring syntactical (word meaning) processing, dyslexics showed similar activation to controls in the left mid-to-anterior temporal lobe and inferior frontal cortex. Gross-Glenn et al. (87) showed symmetry rather than the asymmetry seen in controls in metabolic activity in the prefrontal cortex and lingual area of the occipital lobes during oral reading in adult dyslexic men. Hagman et al. (88) found higher metabolic rates in the medial temporal cortices bilaterally in adults who had been diagnosed with dyslexia in childhood compared with controls during a task taxing attention and speech discrimination. This study and others reviewed by Frank and Pavlakis (84) and McCandiss and Noble (83) suggest that dyslexia may be related to a disconnection between anterior and posterior language areas. In general, adults with dyslexia show underactivation of left temporoparietal language processing areas, and in some cases, more symmetry of activation and increased anterior activation. A similar constellation of findings was shown in two proton MRI studies in children with dyslexia. Both showed differences from controls, but one showed a decreased ratio of choline to *N*-acetylaspartate in the left temporoparietal region (89), whereas the other showed a larger anterior number of voxels with elevated lactate during phonologic tasks (90), again suggesting increased compensatory anterior activity. In addition to differences in age and task requirements, future studies should take into account the remediation history, current types and severity of reading difficulty, and related conditions, especially ADHD and language impairment.

Autism

Background

Autism, a developmental disorder first described by Kanner in 1943, is characterized by impairment in social reciprocity, language impairment, restricted interests, and repetitive behaviors (91–93). The etiology remain unknown; however, there is some support for genetic, environmental, neurologic, and immunologic factors in its development (93–96). Autistic features can also present in some neurologic disorders such as tuberous sclerosis, neurofibromatosis, fragile X, Rett syndrome, and phenylketonuria (97). Mental retardation co-occurs in 70% of cases and seizures in 33% (97). Epidemiologic studies are suggesting an increase in prevalence of 1 in 250 to 500 children, which is thought to be due to improved and expanded diagnostic criteria (98,99).

Abnormalities in cerebral cortex (100), cerebral asymmetry (101), ventricles (97,102,103) and cerebellum (104–107) have been reported in computed tomography (CT) and MRI scans. Clinical manifestations usually emerge between ages 2 and 4 and may reflect abnormal brain development (108). As reviewed by Courchesne et al. (108,109), accelerated head circumference from birth to age 2 in autistic children may reflect rapid brain overgrowth. Brain volumes in autistic children ages 2 to 3, measured by MRI, show an enlargement in the frontal, parietal white matter volumes, and frontal and temporal gray matter. This is in contrast to the cerebellar hypoplasia (primarily posterior vermis) noted in autistic children and adolescents. Between ages 5 and 12, brain volumes in autistic children compare to those of normal children, suggesting an abnormally decelerated growth pattern.

PET/SPECT Imaging in Autism

A review by Boddaert and Zilbovicius (110) of PET/SPECT studies conducted at rest in autistic subjects show mixed results including increased global metabolism (111–113), bitemporal hypoperfusion (114,115) and temporofrontal hypoperfusion (116,117), whereas others found no localized abnormalities (118–120). Autistic children were the focus of several of these studies (112,114,116,119,120) with one including autistic subjects with seizures (116). Zilbovicius et al. (121) conducted the first longitudinal study, measuring rCBF twice during development (age 2 to 4 and then at ages 6 to 7) in the same group of five autistic children matched to five nonautistic children with normal development. Frontal hypoperfusion was found in the autistic group at ages 3 to 4 that normalized by the time these children reached 6 to 7 years of age.

Functional brain imaging has also been conducted during various tasks aimed at elucidating cortical activation patterns involved in language, cognitive, and emotional functions. A well-controlled PET study using ^{15}O-H$_2$O found differences in thalamic blood flow and the dentate-thalamocortical pathway in four autistic men compared with five healthy controls performing an expressive language task (122). Another study in seven autistic patients and seven sex- and age-matched controls evaluated with both PET and MRI while performing a serial verbal learning task, showed decreased glucose metabolism in the right anterior cingulate cortex (specifically in Brodmann's area 24′, which is thought to be involved in executive functions and information processing) (123,124). These investigators increased their study sample to 10 individuals with autism and seven individuals with Asperger's syndrome—an autistic spectrum disorder in which there is normal language development but abnormalities in pragmatic language, impairment in nonverbal communication and social interaction, and restricted interests or activities. Patients were compared to 15 men and two women controls, using ^{18}F-FDG uptake, and smaller volumes for right anterior cingulate gyrus were identified. The authors divided the anterior cingulate gyrus into three segments (Brodmann's areas 25, 24, and 24′), and Brodmann's area 24′ was found to be significantly smaller in patients with autism. No volume differences were noted for the left anterior and posterior cingulate gyri. No significant differences were found in glucose metabolic rate of the amygdala or hippocampus. Significantly lower glucose metabolism was found in both the anterior and posterior cingulate gyri in the autistic group. Patients with Asperger's syndrome had bilateral glucose hypometabolism in the anterior cingulate cortex compared to controls, whereas the autistic patients differed only in the right anterior cingulate gyrus. Within the autistic and Asperger groups, hypometabolism was found in the right posterior cingulate gyrus in autistic patients, whereas hypometabolism was bilateral in Asperger patients (125).

Garreau et al. (126) performed the first activated SPECT study in autistic children and found activation in the right posterior associative cortex in contrast to the control group in which left-sided activation was seen. Studies of auditory cortical processing using ^{15}O-H$_2$O PET in five autistic adults and eight controls at rest and while listening to speech-like sounds found bilateral activation of the superior temporal gyrus in both groups. However, in the autistic group there was significantly greater activation in the right middle frontal gyrus and less activation in the left temporal area, suggesting a dysfunction of temporal regions specializing in perception and integration of complex sounds (127). The same investigators (Zilbovicius et al.), using the same PET technique, reported essentially similar results in a group of 11 autistic children. They found that although significant activation of the auditory cortex in the bilateral superior temporal gyrus (Brodmann's area 22) occurred in both groups while subjects were listening to speech-like stimuli, control children activated the superior temporal cortex bilaterally with left-biased asymmetry. This left dominance, not observed in the autistic groups, suggests abnormal auditory cortical processing (128). In another PET study of 33 autistic children compared to 10 nonautistic children with idiopathic mental retardation, the same group of investigators found significant hypoperfusion of both temporal lobes (114). Using SPECT, Ohnishi et al. (115) reported hypoperfusion bilaterally in the superior temporal gyrus and in the left frontal region in 23 autistic children compared with 26 control children.

Muller et al. (129) scanned five autistic individuals and five normal controls, using ^{15}O-H$_2$O at rest, while the subjects were listening to tones and listening, repeating, and generating sentences. The autistic group had reversed hemispheric dominance during verbal auditory stimulation, a trend toward reduced activation of auditory cortex during acoustic stimulation, and reduced cerebellar activation during nonverbal auditory perception. A reanalysis of these studies focusing on brain regions identified in previous studies [left thalamus, dorsolateral prefrontal cortex, dentate nucleus (130)] showed reduced activation in the right dentate nucleus and left frontal area 46 during a verbal auditory and expressive language task that increased during motor speech (122).

Patterns of brain activity measured in normal volunteers while reading stories involving complex mental states, nonmental stories, and unconnected sentences showed the left medial prefrontal cortex (on the border between Brodmann areas 8 and 9) as the brain area specifically associated with "mentalizing" story comprehension (131). Autistic individuals may do well on cognitive tasks but lack the ability to attribute mental states to themselves or others (explain and predict the behavior of others in terms of their beliefs or desires) (132). Five adult men with Asperger's syndrome and normal volunteers were scanned using a CTI model 953B PET scanner (CTI, Knoxville, USA) after receiving a bolus of ^{15}O-H$_2$O. Results showed that individuals with Asperger's syndrome performed as well as controls with unlinked sentences but performed worse on the story conditions. The PET scans showed activation in most of the same brain areas [temporal pole (left), temporal pole (right) and angular gyrus (left)] with one exception—the medial frontal cortex (133).

Serotonin abnormalities reported in autism include increased blood serotonin (134), symptom exacerbation with tryptophan depletion (135), and improvement with serotonin reuptake inhibitors (136–138). Positron emission tomography studies using α-^{11}C-methyl-L-tryptophan that allows direct in vivo measurement of serotonin synthesis in humans have shown an asymmetry of serotonin synthesis in the frontal cortex, thalamus, and cerebellum in autistic boys compared with normal controls (130). Using the same method, these investigators measured serotonin synthesis capacity in 24 boys and six girls with autism and eight of their siblings as well as 16 children with epilepsy. In the nonautistic children, serotonin synthesis capacity was more than 200% of adult values until age 5 and then declined toward adult levels, with the decline occurring earlier in girls than in boys. In autistic children, serotonin synthesis capacity increased gradually between the ages of 2 and 15 to values one and a half times adult values; no gender differences were noted (139). Using a cluster analysis of autism subscales, significant differences in α-^{11}C-methyl-L-tryptophan uptake was noted between the two clusters (stereotyped behavior and social isolation subscales) in the right cerebellar cortex, cerebellar vermis, dentate nucleus, and pineal gland (140). This may be of significance given that areas of the dentate-thalamocortical pathway in the dorsolateral prefrontal lobe are thought to be involved in language processing (141).

In summary, findings from earlier functional brain imaging studies in autism did not detect consistent abnormalities, but none had used both PET and MRI to localize precise anatomic differences in metabolic activity patterns that distinguished autistics from controls. More recent, well-controlled studies have shown bilateral hypoperfusion of the temporal lobes and abnormal patterns of thalamocortical activation. These brain areas, thought to be involved in language and emotional function, may be sites of pathologic processes in autism. The lack of age normative data and the frequent occurrence of other conditions also affecting brain function (different levels of mental retardation, seizures) have also impeded interpretation of PET data.

Anxiety and Mood Disorders

Anxiety disorders occur in 5% to 15% of children and can be classified as one or more of several types including separation anxiety, overanxious disorder, panic disorder, specific phobias, and OCD (142). There are no PET studies in children with anxiety disorders.

In adult studies, anxiety symptoms provoked in healthy controls result in increased regional cerebral metabolic rate (rCMR) (measured as glucose uptake) in the orbitofrontal, temporal, and cuneus gyri, left anterior cingulate and inferior frontal gyri, and left insula. Also the rCMR for glucose (rCMRGlu) is decreased in the right posterior temporoparietal, superior frontal, and medial frontal cortices (143,144). A review by Osuch et al. (145) of functional brain imaging in adults with anxiety disorders indicates involvement of several brain areas including increased cerebral blood flow and metabolism in the right compared to the left parahippocampal gyrus (146–148).

A comparison of patients with anxiety disorders and healthy volunteers found flumazenil volume distribution lower in anxiety patients in all areas sampled (149). A 20% decrease in benzodiazepine binding was reported in patients with panic disorder using ^{11}C-flumazenil localized primarily to the orbitofrontal, anterior insula, and anterior temporal cortices, brain areas thought to play role in anxiety (150). A PET study investigating serotonin type 1A receptor [5-hydroxytryptamine type 1A receptor (5HT$_{1A}$R)] binding in patients with panic disorder shows marked reduction in the anterior and posterior cingulate cortices (151).

Symptom provocation studies in OCD, simple phobia, and post-traumatic stress disorder (PTSD) showed increased cerebral metabolism in the insular cortex, right frontal and posterior medial orbitofrontal cortices, and lenticular nucleus (152). Decreased cerebral blood flow was reported in superior frontal cortices and right caudate in OCD and PTSD (153).

Studies with medications and behavioral therapy used to treat some of the anxiety disorders also give us some insight. In patients with OCD, chronic administration of fluoxetine or clomipramine improved OCD symptoms and normalized abnormally elevated rCMRGlu in the right head of the caudate and orbitofrontal regions (areas thought to be involved in OCD symptomatology). Behavioral therapy produced similar results as medications (154–156). Eighteen adults with childhood-onset OCD were studied using ^{18}F-FDG. Increased glucose metabolism was found in the OCD group in left orbital frontal, right sensorimotor, and bilateral prefrontal and anterior cingulate cortices compared to controls. There was a significant relationship between metabolic activity, state and trait measurements of OCD and anxiety, and response to clomipramine (157).

There are no PET studies of children with mood disorders; however, in studies of adults PET scans are proving to be useful in exploring these conditions. As reviewed by Videbech (158), although PET studies in adult patients with major depression have many limitations, some consistent results include reduced blood flow and glucose metabolism in the prefrontal cortex (159–162), anterior cingulate cortex (163), and caudate nucleus (159,164) during rest as well as during cognitive tasks. Increased blood flow and metabolism was reported in the amygdalae of depressed patients (164–166). Recovery has been associated with normalization of reduced glucose metabolism of the prefrontal cortex (160,161,167), cingulated cortex (168), and caudate nucleus (159). Increased blood flow in the amygdala may be a trait marker because it persists after recovery (164). Decreased blood flow and metabolic rate has been reported in depressed patients with bipolar disorder (159,161) and not in unipolar depression (169,170). A PET study of patients with depression and anxiety showed that comorbid anxiety was associated with specific metabolic findings that differ from those found in patients with depression alone (145). Successful psychotherapy has also been shown to result in adaptive regional brain metabolic changes (171,172). Because depression commonly develops in adolescents and young adults, it would be useful to use PET technology to identify trait or predictive findings in those at risk, as well as those that signal active depression, treatment response, and recovery.

References

1. American Psychiatric Association. Diagnostic and statistical manual of mental disorders, 4th ed. (DSM-IV). Washington, DC: APA, 1994.
2. Spencer TJ, Biederman J, Wilens TE, Faraone SV. Overview and neurobiology of attention-deficit/hyperactivity disorder. J Clin Psychiatry 2002; 63(suppl 12):3–9.
3. Glanzman M. Genetics, imaging, and neurochemistry in attention deficit and hyperactivity in children and adults. In: Accardo P, Blondis T, Whitman B, Stein M, eds. Baltimore: Paul H, Brookes, in press, 2006.
4. Durston S. A review of the biological bases of ADHD: what have we learned from imaging studies? Ment Retard Dev Disabil Res Rev 2003;9(3): 184–195.
5. Durston S, Tottenham NT, Thomas KM, et al. Differential patterns of striatal activation in young children with and without ADHD. Biol Psychiatry 2003;53(10):871–878.
6. Giedd JN, Blumenthal J, Molloy E, Castellanos FX. Brain imaging of attention deficit/hyperactivity disorder. Ann N Y Acad Sci 2001;931:33–49.
7. Castellanos FX, Lee PP, Sharp W, et al. Developmental trajectories of brain volume abnormalities in children and adolescents with attention-deficit/hyperactivity disorder. JAMA 2002;288(14):1740–1748.
8. Schweitzer JB, Faber TL, Grafton ST, Tune LE, Hoffman JM, Kilts CD. Alterations in the functional anatomy of working memory in adult attention deficit hyperactivity disorder. Am J Psychiatry 2000;157(2):278–280.
9. Rubia K, Overmeyer S, Taylor E, et al. Hypofrontality in attention deficit hyperactivity disorder during higher-order motor control: a study with functional MRI. Am J Psychiatry 1999;156(6):891–896.
10. Vaidya CJ, Austin G, Kirkorian G, et al. Selective effects of methylphenidate in attention deficit hyperactivity disorder: a functional magnetic resonance study. Proc Natl Acad Sci U S A 1998;95(24):14494–14499.
11. Lou HC, Henriksen L, Bruhn P. Focal cerebral hypoperfusion in children with dysphasia and/or attention deficit disorder. Arch Neurol 1984;41(8): 825–829.
12. Lou HC, Henriksen L, Bruhn P, Borner H, Nielsen JB. Striatal dysfunction in attention deficit and hyperkinetic disorder. Arch Neurol 1989;46(1): 48–52.
13. Lou HC, Henriksen L, Bruhn P. Focal cerebral dysfunction in developmental learning disabilities. Lancet 1990;335(8680):8–11.
14. Zametkin AJ, Nordahl TE, Gross M, et al. Cerebral glucose metabolism in adults with hyperactivity of childhood onset. N Engl J Med 1990;323(20): 1361–1366.
15. Zametkin AJ, Liebenauer LL, Fitzgerald GA, et al. Brain metabolism in teenagers with attention-deficit hyperactivity disorder. Arch Gen Psychiatry 1993;50(5):333–340.
16. Ernst M, Liebenauer LL, King AC, Fitzgerald GA, Cohen RM, Zametkin AJ. Reduced brain metabolism in hyperactive girls. J Am Acad Child Adolesc Psychiatry 1994;33(6):858–868.
17. Ernst M, Cohen RM, Liebenauer LL, Jons PH, Zametkin AJ. Cerebral glucose metabolism in adolescent girls with attention-deficit/hyperactivity disorder. J Am Acad Child Adolesc Psychiatry 1997;36(10):1399–1406.
18. Ernst M, Zametkin AJ, Phillips RL, Cohen RM. Age-related changes in brain glucose metabolism in adults with attention-deficit/hyperactivity disorder and control subjects. J Neuropsychiatry Clin Neurosci 1998; 10(2):168–177.

19. Sieg KG, Gaffney GR, Preston DF, Hellings JA. SPECT brain imaging abnormalities in attention deficit hyperactivity disorder. Clin Nucl Med 1995;20(1):55–60.

20. Amen DG, Carmichael BD. High-resolution brain SPECT imaging in ADHD. Ann Clin Psychiatry 1997;9(2):81–86.

21. Kaya GC, Pekcanlar A, Bekis R, et al. Technetium-99m HMPAO brain SPECT in children with attention deficit hyperactivity disorder. Ann Nucl Med 2002;16(8):527–531.

22. Kim BN, Lee JS, Shin MS, Cho SC, Lee DS. Regional cerebral perfusion abnormalities in attention deficit/hyperactivity disorder. Statistical parametric mapping analysis. Eur Arch Psychiatry Clin Neurosci 2002;252(5):219–225.

23. Lorberboym M, Watemberg N, Nissenkorn A, Nir B, Lerman-Sagie T. Technetium 99m ethylcysteinate dimer single-photon emission computed tomography (SPECT) during intellectual stress test in children and adolescents with pure versus comorbid attention-deficit hyperactivity disorder (ADHD). J Child Neurol 2004;19(2):91–96.

24. Spalletta G, Pasini A, Pau F, Guido G, Menghini L, Caltagirone C. Prefrontal blood flow dysregulation in drug naive ADHD children without structural abnormalities. J Neural Transm 2001;108(10):1203–1216.

25. Ernst M, Zametkin AJ, Matochik JA, Jons PH, Cohen RM. DOPA decarboxylase activity in attention deficit hyperactivity disorder adults. A (fluorine-18) fluorodopa positron emission tomographic study. J Neurosci 1998;18(15):5901–5907.

26. Ernst M, Zametkin AJ, Matochik JA, Pascualvaca D, Jons PH, Cohen RM. High midbrain (18F)DOPA accumulation in children with attention deficit hyperactivity disorder. Am J Psychiatry 1999;156(8):1209–1215.

27. Solanto MV. Neuropsychopharmacological mechanisms of stimulant drug action in attention-deficit hyperactivity disorder: a review and integration. Behav Brain Res 1998;94(1):127–152.

28. Ohno M. The dopaminergic system in attention deficit/hyperactivity disorder. Congenit Anom (Kyoto) 2003;43(2):114–122.

29. Solanto MV. Dopamine dysfunction in AD/HD: integrating clinical and basic neuroscience research. Behav Brain Res 2002;130(1–2):65–71.

30. DiMaio S, Grizenko N, Joober R. Dopamine genes and attention-deficit hyperactivity disorder: a review. J Psychiatry Neurosci 2002;29:27–38.

31. Dougherty DD, Bonab AA, Spencer TJ, Rauch SL, Madras BK, Fischman AJ. Dopamine transporter density in patients with attention deficit hyperactivity disorder. Lancet 1999;354(9196):2132–2133.

32. Dresel S, Krause J, Krause KH, et al. Attention deficit hyperactivity disorder: binding of (99mTc)TRODAT-1 to the dopamine transporter before and after methylphenidate treatment. Eur J Nucl Med 2000;27(10):1518–1524.

33. Krause KH, Dresel SH, Krause J, Kung HF, Tatsch K. Increased striatal dopamine transporter in adult patients with attention deficit hyperactivity disorder: effects of methylphenidate as measured by single photon emission computed tomography. Neurosci Lett 2000;285(2):107–110.

34. van Dyck CH, Quinlan DM, Cretella LM, et al. Unaltered dopamine transporter availability in adult attention deficit hyperactivity disorder. Am J Psychiatry 2002;159(2):309–312.

35. Cheon KA, Ryu YH, Kim YK, Namkoong K, Kim CH, Lee JD. Dopamine transporter density in the basal ganglia assessed with (123I)IPT SPET in children with attention deficit hyperactivity disorder. Eur J Nucl Med Mol Imaging 2003;30(2):306–311.

36. Simpson D, Plosker GL. Atomoxetine: a review of its use in adults with attention deficit hyperactivity disorder. Drugs 2004;64(2):205–222.

37. Hunt RD, Paguin A, Payton K. An update on assessment and treatment of complex attention-deficit hyperactivity disorder. Pediatr Ann 2001; 30(3):162–172.

38. Matochik JA, Nordahl TE, Gross M, et al. Effects of acute stimulant medication on cerebral metabolism in adults with hyperactivity. Neuropsychopharmacology 1993;8(4):377–386.

39. Matochik JA, Liebenauer LL, King AC, Szymanski HV, Cohen RM, Zametkin AJ. Cerebral glucose metabolism in adults with attention deficit hyperactivity disorder after chronic stimulant treatment. Am J Psychiatry 1994;151(5):658–664.

40. Schweitzer JB, Lee DO, Hanford RB, et al. A positron emission tomography study of methylphenidate in adults with ADHD: alterations in resting blood flow and predicting treatment response. Neuropsychopharmacology 2003;28(5):967–973.

41. Volkow ND, Wang GJ, Fowler JS, et al. Differences in regional brain metabolic responses between single and repeated doses of methylphenidate. Psychiatry Res 1998;83(1):29–36.

42. Volkow ND, Wang GJ, Fowler JS, et al. Effects of methylphenidate on regional brain glucose metabolism in humans: relationship to dopamine D2 receptors. Am J Psychiatry 1997;154(1):50–55.

43. Mattay VS, Berman KF, Ostrem JL, et al. Dextroamphetamine enhances "neural network-specific" physiological signals: a positron-emission tomography rCBF study. J Neurosci 1996;16(15):4816–4822.

44. Szobot CM, Ketzer C, Cunha RD, et al. The acute effect of methylphenidate on cerebral blood flow in boys with attention-deficit/hyperactivity disorder. Eur J Nucl Med Mol Imaging 2003;30(3):423–426.

45. Langleben DD, Acton PD, Austin G, et al. Effects of methylphenidate discontinuation on cerebral blood flow in prepubescent boys with attention deficit hyperactivity disorder. J Nucl Med 2002;43(12):1624–1629.

46. Volkow ND, Fowler JS, Wang G, Ding Y, Gatley SJ. Mechanism of action of methylphenidate: insights from PET imaging studies. J Atten Disord 2002;6(suppl 1):S31–43.

47. Vles JS, Feron FJ, Hendriksen JG, Jolles J, van Kroonenburgh MJ, Weber WE. Methylphenidate down-regulates the dopamine receptor and transporter system in children with attention deficit hyperkinetic disorder (ADHD). Neuropediatrics 2003;34(2):77–80.

48. Ilgin N, Senol S, Gucuyener K, Gokcora N, Sener S. Is increased D2 receptor availability associated with response to stimulant medication in ADHD. Dev Med Child Neurol 2001;43(11):755–760.

49. Leckman JF. Tourette's syndrome. Lancet 2002;360(9345):1577–1586.

50. Robertson MM. Diagnosing Tourette syndrome: is it a common disorder? J Psychosom Res 2003;55(1):3–6.

51. Pauls DL. An update on the genetics of Gilles de la Tourette syndrome. J Psychosom Res 2003;55(1):7–12.

52. Comings DE. Clinical and molecular genetics of ADHD and Tourette syndrome. Two related polygenic disorders. Ann N Y Acad Sci 2001; 931:50–83.

53. Comings D. Tourette Syndrome and Human Behavior. Duarte, CA: Hope Press, 1990.

54. Power T, Glanzman M. Tic disorders in children's needs. III: Development, problems and alternatives. In: Bear G, Mike K, Thomas A, eds. Bethesda, MD: National Association of Psychologists, in press, 2006.

55. Gerard E, Peterson BS. Developmental processes and brain imaging studies in Tourette syndrome. J Psychosom Res 2003;55(1):13–22.
56. Kates WR, Frederikse M, Mostofsky SH, et al. MRI parcellation of the frontal lobe in boys with attention deficit hyperactivity disorder or Tourette syndrome. Psychiatry Res 2002;116(1–2):63–81.
57. Braun A, Randolph C, Stoetter B, et al. The functional neuroanatomy of Tourette's syndrome: an FDG-PET Study. II: relationships between regional cerebral metabolism and associated behavioral and cognitive features of the illness. Neuropsychopharmacology 1995;13:151–168.
58. Eidelberg D, Moeller J, Antonini A, et al. The metabolic anatomy of Tourette's syndrome. Neurology 1997;48:927–934.
59. Moriarty J, Costa D, Schmitz B, Trimble M, Ell P, Robertson MM. Brain perfusion abnormalities in Gilles de la Tourette's syndrome. Br J Psychiatry 1995;167:249–254.
60. George M, Trimble M, Costa DC, Robertson MM, Ring H, Ell PJ. Elevated frontal cerebral blood flow in Gilles de la Tourette syndrome: a 99 Tcm-HMPAO SPECT study. Psychiatry Res Neuroimaging 1992;45: 143–151.
61. Stern E, Silbersweig D, Chee K, et al. A functional neuroanatomy of tics in Tourette syndrome. Arch Gen Psychiatry 2000;57:741–748.
62. Peterson BS, Skudlarski P, Anderson AW, et al. A functional magnetic resonance imaging study of tic suppression in Tourette syndrome. Arch Gen Psychiatry 1998;55(4):326–333.
63. Malison RT, McDougle CJ, van Dyck CH, et al. 123I B-CIT SPECT imaging of striatal dopamine transporter binding in Tourette's disorder. Am J Psychiatry 1995;152:1359–1361.
64. Muller-Vahl K, Berding G, Brucke T, et al. Dopamine transporter binding in Gilles de la Tourette syndrome. J Neurol 2000;247:514–520.
65. Wong D, Singer HS, Marenco S, et al. Dopamine transporter reuptake sites measured by (11C)WIN 35,428 PET imaging are elevated in Tourette syndrome (abstract). J Nucl Med 1994;35:130.
66. Ernst M, Zametkin A, Jons PH, Matochik JA, Pascualvaca D, Cohen RM. High presynaptic dopaminergic activity in children with Tourette's disorder. J Am Acad Child Adolesc Psychiatry 1999;38:86–94.
67. Stamenkovic M, Schindler S, Asenbaum S, et al. No change in striatal dopamine re-uptake site density in psychotropic drug naive and in currently treated Tourette's disorder patients: a(123)-beta-CIT SPECT study. Eur Neuropsychopharmacol 2001;11:69–74.
68. Serra-Mestres J, Ring H, Costa D, et al. Dopamine transporter binding in Gilles de la Tourette syndrome: a (123I)FP-CIT/SPECT study. Acta Psychiatr Scand 2004;109:140–146.
69. Albin RL, Koeppe RA, Bohnen NI, et al. Increased ventral striatal monoaminergic innervation in Tourette syndrome. Neurology 2003;61(3): 310–315.
70. Wong D, Singer HS, Brandt J, et al. D2–like dopamine receptor density in Tourette's syndrome measured by PET. J Nucl Med 1997;38:1243–1247.
71. Wolf S, Jones D, Knable M, et al. Tourette syndrome prediction of phenotypic variation in monozygotic twins by caudate nucleus D2 receptor binding. Science 1996;273:1225–1227.
72. Hammill D. On defining learning disabilities: an emerging consensus. J Learning Disabil 1990;23:74–84.
73. Habib M. The neurological basis of developmental dyslexia. An overview and working hypothesis. Brain 2000;123:2373–2399.
74. Tallal P, Miller S, Fitch R. Neurobiological basis of speech: a case for the preeminence of temporal processing. Irish J Psychol 1995;16:194–219.

75. Breznitz Z, Meyler A. Speed of lower-level auditory and visual processing as a basic factor in dyslexia: electrophysiological evidence. Brain Language 2003;16:785–803.
76. Castles A, Datta H, Gayan J, Olson R. Varieties of developmental reading disorders: genetic and environmental influences. J Exp Child Psychol 1999;72:73–94.
77. Geschwind N, Behan P. Left-handedness: association with immune disease, migraine and developmental disorder. Proc Natl Acad Sci U S A 1982;79:5097–5100.
78. Bryden M, McManus I, Bulman-Fleming M. Evaluating the empirical support for the Geschwind-Behan-Galaburda model of cerebral lateralization. Brain Cog 1994;266:276–279.
79. Shaywitz S. Overcoming Dyslexia. New York: Alfred A. Knopf, 2003.
80. Paulesu E, Desmond J-F, Fazio F, et al. Dyslexia: cultural diversity and biological unity. Science 2001;291:2165–2167.
81. Eden GF, VanMeter JW, Rumsey JM, Maisog JM, Woods RP, Zeffiro TA. Abnormal processing of visual motion in dyslexia revealed by functional brain imaging. Nature 1996;382(6586):66–69.
82. Simos P, Fletcher J. Dyslexia-specific brain activation profile becomes normal following successful remedial training. Neurology 2002;58:1203–1213.
83. McCandiss B, Noble K. The development of reading impairment: a cognitive neuroscience model. MRDD Res Rev 2003;9:196–205.
84. Frank Y, Pavlakis S. Brain imaging in neurobehavioral disorders. Pediatr Neurol 2001;25:278–287.
85. Flowers D, Wood F, Naylor C. Regional cerebral blood flow correlates of language processes in reading disability. Arch Neurol 1991;48:637–643.
86. Rumsey J, Nace K, Donohue B, Wise D, Maisog J, Andreason P. A positron emission tomographic study of impaired word recognition and phonological processing in dyslexic men. Arch Neurol 1997;54:562–573.
87. Gross-Glenn K, Duara R, Barker W, et al. Positron emission tomographic studies during serial word reading by normal and dyslexic adults. J Clin Exp Neuropsychol 1999;13:531–544.
88. Hagman J, Wood F, Buchsbaum M, Tallal P, Flowers L, Katz W. Cerebral brain metabolism in adult dyslexic subjects assessed with positron emission tomography during performance of an auditory task. Arch Neurol 1992;49:734–739.
89. Rae C, Lee M, Dixon R. Metabolic abnormalities in developmental dyslexia detected by 1H magnetic resonance spectroscopy. Lancet 1998;351:1849–1852.
90. Richards T, Dager S, Corina D, et al. Dyslexia children have abnormal brain lactate response to reading related language tasks. AJNR 1999;20:1393–1398.
91. Rapin I. Autism. N Engl J Med 1997;337(2):97–104.
92. Kanner L. Autistic disturbances of affective contact. Nerv Child 1943;2:217–250.
93. Rapin I, Katzman R. Neurobiology of autism. Ann Neurol 1998;43(1):7–14.
94. Folstein SE, Rosen-Sheidley B. Genetics of autism: complex aetiology for a heterogeneous disorder. Nat Rev Genet 2001;2(12):943–955.
95. Korvatska E, Van de Water J, Anders TF, Gershwin ME. Genetic and immunologic considerations in autism. Neurobiol Dis 2002;9(2):107–125.
96. Vargas DL, Nascimbene C, Krishnan C, Zimmerman AW, Pardo CA. Neuroglial activation and neuroinflammation in the brain of patients with autism. Ann Neurol 2005;57(1):67–81.

97. Gilberg C, Coleman M. The Biology of Autistic Syndromes. London: MacKeith Press, 1992.

98. Fombonne E. Epidemiological surveys of autism and other pervasive developmental disorders: an update. J Autism Dev Disord 2003;33(4):365–382.

99. Yeargin-Allsopp M, Rice C, Karapurkar T, Doernberg N, Boyle C, Murphy C. Prevalence of autism in a US metropolitan area. JAMA 2003;289(1):49–55.

100. Piven J, Berthier ML, Starkstein SE, Nehme E, Pearlson G, Folstein S. Magnetic resonance imaging evidence for a defect of cerebral cortical development in autism. Am J Psychiatry 1990;147(6):734–739.

101. Hier DB, LeMay M, Rosenberger PB. Autism and unfavorable left-right asymmetries of the brain. J Autism Dev Disord 1979;9(2):153–159.

102. Campbell M, Rosenbloom S, Perry R, et al. Computerized axial tomography in young autistic children. Am J Psychiatry 1982;139(4):510–512.

103. Damasio H, Maurer RG, Damasio AR, Chui HC. Computerized tomographic scan findings in patients with autistic behavior. Arch Neurol 1980;37(8):504–510.

104. Courchesne E, Yeung-Courchesne R, Press GA, Hesselink JR, Jernigan TL. Hypoplasia of cerebellar vermal lobules VI and VII in autism. N Engl J Med 1988;318(21):1349–1354.

105. Courchesne E, Townsend J, Saitoh O. The brain in infantile autism: posterior fossa structures are abnormal. Neurology 1994;44(2):214–223.

106. Piven J, Nehme E, Simon J, Barta P, Pearlson G, Folstein SE. Magnetic resonance imaging in autism: measurement of the cerebellum, pons, and fourth ventricle. Biol Psychiatry 1992;31(5):491–504.

107. Filipek PA. Quantitative magnetic resonance imaging in autism: the cerebellar vermis. Curr Opin Neurol 1995;8(2):134–138.

108. Courchesne E. Brain development in autism: early overgrowth followed by premature arrest of growth. Ment Retard Dev Disabil Res Rev 2004;10(2):106–111.

109. Courchesne E, Redcay E, Kennedy DP. The autistic brain: birth through adulthood. Curr Opin Neurol 2004;17(4):489–496.

110. Boddaert N, Zilbovicius M. Functional neuroimaging and childhood autism. Pediatr Radiol 2002;32(1):1–7.

111. Rumsey JM, Duara R, Grady C, et al. Brain metabolism in autism. Resting cerebral glucose utilization rates as measured with positron emission tomography. Arch Gen Psychiatry 1985;42(5):448–455.

112. De Volder A, Bol A, Michel C, Congneau M, Goffinet AM. Brain glucose metabolism in children with the autistic syndrome: positron tomography analysis. Brain Dev 1987;9(6):581–587.

113. Horwitz B, Rumsey JM, Grady CL, Rapoport SI. The cerebral metabolic landscape in autism. Intercorrelations of regional glucose utilization. Arch Neurol 1988;45(7):749–755.

114. Zilbovicius M, Boddaert N, Belin P, et al. Temporal lobe dysfunction in childhood autism: a PET study. Positron emission tomography. Am J Psychiatry 2000;157(12):1988–1993.

115. Ohnishi T, Matsuda H, Hashimoto T, et al. Abnormal regional cerebral blood flow in childhood autism. Brain 2000;123(pt 9):1838–1844.

116. Mountz JM, Tolbert LC, Lill DW, Katholi CR, Liu HG. Functional deficits in autistic disorder: characterization by technetium-99m-HMPAO and SPECT. J Nucl Med 1995;36(7):1156–1162.

117. Gillberg C, Bjure J, Vestergen E. SPECT in 31 children and adolescents with autism and autistic-like conditions. Eur Child Adolesc Psychiatry 1993;2:50–59.

118. Herold S, Frackowiak RS, Le Couteur A, Rutter M, Howlin P. Cerebral blood flow and metabolism of oxygen and glucose in young autistic adults. Psychol Med 1988;18(4):823–831.

119. Zilbovicius M, Garreau B, Tzourio N, et al. Regional cerebral blood flow in childhood autism: a SPECT study. Am J Psychiatry 1992;149(7): 924–930.

120. Chiron C, Leboyer M, Leon F, Jambaque I, Nuttin C, Syrota A. SPECT of the brain in childhood autism: evidence for a lack of normal hemispheric asymmetry. Dev Med Child Neurol 1995;37(10):849–860.

121. Zilbovicius M, Garreau B, Samson Y, et al. Delayed maturation of the frontal cortex in childhood autism. Am J Psychiatry 1995;152(2):248–252.

122. Muller RA, Chugani DC, Behen ME, et al. Impairment of dentato-thalamo-cortical pathway in autistic men: language activation data from positron emission tomography. Neurosci Lett 1998;245(1):1–4.

123. Devinsky O, Morrell MJ, Vogt BA. Contributions of anterior cingulate cortex to behaviour. Brain 1995;118(pt 1):279–306.

124. Haznedar MM, Buchsbaum MS, Metzger M, Solimando A, Spiegel-Cohen J, Hollander E. Anterior cingulate gyrus volume and glucose metabolism in autistic disorder. Am J Psychiatry 1997;154(8):1047–1050.

125. Haznedar MM, Buchsbaum MS, Wei TC, et al. Limbic circuitry in patients with autism spectrum disorders studied with positron emission tomography and magnetic resonance imaging. Am J Psychiatry 2000;157(12): 1994–2001.

126. Garreau B, Zilbovicius M, Guerin P. Effects of auditory stimulation on regional cerebral blood flow in autistic children. Dev Brain Dysfunction 1994;7:119–128.

127. Boddaert N, Belin P, Chabane N, et al. Perception of complex sounds: abnormal pattern of cortical activation in autism. Am J Psychiatry 2003;160(11):2057–2060.

128. Boddaert N, Chabane N, Belin P, et al. Perception of complex sounds in autism: abnormal auditory cortical processing in children. Am J Psychiatry 2004;161(11):2117–2120.

129. Muller RA, Behen ME, Rothermel RD, et al. Brain mapping of language and auditory perception in high-functioning autistic adults: a PET study. J Autism Dev Disord 1999;29(1):19–31.

130. Chugani DC, Muzik O, Rothermel R, et al. Altered serotonin synthesis in the dentatothalamocortical pathway in autistic boys. Ann Neurol 1997; 42(4):666–669.

131. Fletcher PC, Happe F, Frith U, et al. Other minds in the brain: a functional imaging study of "theory of mind" in story comprehension. Cognition 1995;57(2):109–128.

132. Baron-Cohen S, Leslie AM, Frith U. Does the autistic child have a "theory of mind"? Cognition 1985;21(1):37–46.

133. Happe F, Ehlers S, Fletcher P, et al. "Theory of mind" in the brain. Evidence from a PET scan study of Asperger syndrome. Neuroreport 1996;8(1):197–201.

134. Schain RJ, Freedman DX. Studies on 5–hydroxyindole metabolism in autistic and other mentally retarded children. J Pediatr 1961;58:315–320.

135. McDougle CJ, Naylor ST, Cohen DJ, Aghajanian GK, Heninger GR, Price LH. Effects of tryptophan depletion in drug-free adults with autistic disorder. Arch Gen Psychiatry 1996;53(11):993–1000.

136. Gordon CT, State RC, Nelson JE, Hamburger SD, Rapoport JL. A double-blind comparison of clomipramine, desipramine, and placebo in the treatment of autistic disorder. Arch Gen Psychiatry 1993;50(6):441–447.

137. Cook EH Jr, Rowlett R, Jaselskis C, Leventhal BL. Fluoxetine treatment of children and adults with autistic disorder and mental retardation. J Am Acad Child Adolesc Psychiatry 1992;31(4):739–745.

138. McDougle CJ, Naylor ST, Cohen DJ, Volkmar FR, Heninger GR, Price LH. A double-blind, placebo-controlled study of fluvoxamine in adults with autistic disorder. Arch Gen Psychiatry 1996;53(11):1001–1008.

139. Chugani DC, Muzik O, Behen M, et al. Developmental changes in brain serotonin synthesis capacity in autistic and nonautistic children. Ann Neurol 1999;45(3):287–295.

140. Chugani DC, Behen M, Asano E, et al. Behavioral subtypes of autistic children show differences in regional brain serotonin synthesis. Soc Neurosci Abstracts 2000;26(1–2).

141. Dow RS. Cerebellar cognition. Neurology 1995;45(9):1785–1786.

142. Cohen P, Cohen J, Kasen S, et al. An epidemiological study of disorders in late childhood and adolescence—I. Age- and gender-specific prevalence. J Child Psychol Psychiatry 1993;34(6):851–867.

143. Kimbrell TA, George MS, Parekh PI, et al. Regional brain activity during transient self-induced anxiety and anger in healthy adults. Biol Psychiatry 1999;46(4):454–465.

144. Chua P, Krams M, Toni I, Passingham R, Dolan R. A functional anatomy of anticipatory anxiety. Neuroimage 1999;9(6 pt 1):563–571.

145. Osuch EA, Ketter TA, Kimbrell TA, et al. Regional cerebral metabolism associated with anxiety symptoms in affective disorder patients. Biol Psychiatry 2000;48(10):1020–1023.

146. Nordahl TE, Semple WE, Gross M, et al. Cerebral glucose metabolic differences in patients with panic disorder. Neuropsychopharmacology 1990;3(4):261–272.

147. Reiman EM, Raichle ME, Butler FK, Herscovitch P, Robins E. A focal brain abnormality in panic disorder, a severe form of anxiety. Nature 1984; 310(5979):683–685.

148. Reiman EM, Raichle ME, Robins E, et al. The application of positron emission tomography to the study of panic disorder. Am J Psychiatry 1986;143(4):469–477.

149. Abadie P, Boulenger JP, Benali K, Barre L, Zarifian E, Baron JC. Relationships between trait and state anxiety and the central benzodiazepine receptor: a PET study. Eur J Neurosci 1999;11(4):1470–1478.

150. Malizia AL, Cunningham VJ, Bell CJ, Liddle PF, Jones T, Nutt DJ. Decreased brain GABA(A)-benzodiazepine receptor binding in panic disorder: preliminary results from a quantitative PET study. Arch Gen Psychiatry 1998;55(8):715–720.

151. Neumeister A, Bain E, Nugent AC, et al. Reduced serotonin type 1A receptor binding in panic disorder. J Neurosci 2004;24(3):589–591.

152. Rauch SL, Savage CR, Alpert NM, Fischman AJ, Jenike MA. The functional neuroanatomy of anxiety: a study of three disorders using positron emission tomography and symptom provocation. Biol Psychiatry 1997;42(6):446–452.

153. Lucey JV, Costa DC, Adshead G, et al. Brain blood flow in anxiety disorders. OCD, panic disorder with agoraphobia, and post-traumatic stress disorder on 99mTcHMPAO single photon emission tomography (SPET). Br J Psychiatry 1997;171:346–350.

154. Baxter LR Jr, Schwartz JM, Bergman KS, et al. Caudate glucose metabolic rate changes with both drug and behavior therapy for obsessive-compulsive disorder. Arch Gen Psychiatry 1992;49(9):681–689.

155. Schwartz JM, Stoessel PW, Baxter LR Jr, Martin KM, Phelps ME. Systematic changes in cerebral glucose metabolic rate after successful behavior modification treatment of obsessive-compulsive disorder. Arch Gen Psychiatry 1996;53(2):109–113.

156. Swedo SE, Pietrini P, Leonard HL, et al. Cerebral glucose metabolism in childhood-onset obsessive-compulsive disorder. Revisualization during pharmacotherapy. Arch Gen Psychiatry 1992;49(9):690–694.

157. Swedo SE, Schapiro MB, Grady CL, et al. Cerebral glucose metabolism in childhood-onset obsessive-compulsive disorder. Arch Gen Psychiatry 1989;46(6):518–523.

158. Videbech P. PET measurements of brain glucose metabolism and blood flow in major depressive disorder: a critical review. Acta Psychiatr Scand 2000;101(1):11–20.

159. Baxter LR Jr, Phelps ME, Mazziotta JC, et al. Cerebral metabolic rates for glucose in mood disorders. Studies with positron emission tomography and fluorodeoxyglucose F 18. Arch Gen Psychiatry 1985;42(5): 441–447.

160. Baxter LR Jr, Schwartz JM, Phelps ME, et al. Reduction of prefrontal cortex glucose metabolism common to three types of depression. Arch Gen Psychiatry 1989;46(3):243–250.

161. Martinot JL, Hardy P, Feline A, et al. Left prefrontal glucose hypometabolism in the depressed state: a confirmation. Am J Psychiatry 1990;147(10): 1313–1317.

162. Hurwitz TA, Clark C, Murphy E, Klonoff H, Martin WR, Pate BD. Regional cerebral glucose metabolism in major depressive disorder. Can J Psychiatry 1990;35(8):684–688.

163. Mayberg HS, Brannan SK, Mahurin RK, et al. Cingulate function in depression: a potential predictor of treatment response. Neuroreport 1997;8(4):1057–1061.

164. Drevets WC, Videen TO, Price JL, Preskorn SH, Carmichael ST, Raichle ME. A functional anatomical study of unipolar depression. J Neurosci 1992;12(9):3628–3641.

165. Abercrombie HC, Schaefer SM, Larson CL, et al. Metabolic rate in the right amygdala predicts negative affect in depressed patients. Neuroreport 1998;9(14):3301–3307.

166. Drevets WC, Price JL, Bardgett ME, Reich T, Todd RD, Raichle ME. Glucose metabolism in the amygdala in depression: relationship to diagnostic subtype and plasma cortisol levels. Pharmacol Biochem Behav 2002;71(3):431–447.

167. Smith GS, Reynolds CF 3rd, Pollock B, et al. Cerebral glucose metabolic response to combined total sleep deprivation and antidepressant treatment in geriatric depression. Am J Psychiatry 1999;156(5): 683–689.

168. Wu JC, Gillin JC, Buchsbaum MS, Hershey T, Johnson JC, Bunney WE Jr. Effect of sleep deprivation on brain metabolism of depressed patients. Am J Psychiatry 1992;149(4):538–543.

169. Biver F, Goldman S, Delvenne V, et al. Frontal and parietal metabolic disturbances in unipolar depression. Biol Psychiatry 1994;36(6):381–388.

170. Bench CJ, Friston KJ, Brown RG, Frackowiak RS, Dolan RJ. Regional cerebral blood flow in depression measured by positron emission tomography: the relationship with clinical dimensions. Psychol Med 1993;23(3): 579–590.

171. Brody AL, Saxena S, Stoessel P, et al. Regional brain metabolic changes in patients with major depression treated with either paroxetine or interpersonal therapy: preliminary findings. Arch Gen Psychiatry 2001; 58(7):631–640.
172. Martin SD, Martin E, Rai SS, Richardson MA, Royall R. Brain blood flow changes in depressed patients treated with interpersonal psychotherapy or venlafaxine hydrochloride: preliminary findings. Arch Gen Psychiatry 2001;58(7):641–648.

20

Epilepsy

Nicolaas I. Bohnen and James M. Mountz

PET for Functional and Neurochemical Imaging

Positron emission tomography (PET) can be used to perform neuro-chemical and functional brain imaging studies. First, neurochemical imaging studies allow assessment of the regional distribution and quantitative measurement of neurotransmitters, enzymes, or receptors in the living brain. Benzodiazepine receptor binding scans are an example of neurochemical receptor studies that are used in the evaluation of children with epilepsy. Second, functional brain imaging studies can measure regional cerebral blood flow (rCBF) or glucose metabolism. These studies may be performed in the resting state when the child is not having seizures (interictal) or at the time of a seizure (ictal study). Seizure activation of the brain is accompanied by increases in rCBF and glucose consumption. Interictal fluorodeoxyglucose (FDG)-PET studies are most commonly performed in the clinical PET imaging evaluation of children with epilepsy at the present time. Although technically more challenging, ictal FDG- or rCBF-PET studies may be performed when children have frequent or predictable seizures.

Imaging for Presurgical Workup

Epileptic syndromes are classified as generalized and partial types of seizures. Primary generalized epilepsy is associated with diffuse and bilateral epileptiform discharges on an electroencephalogram (EEG) without evidence of focal brain lesions. In contrast, partial epilepsy is thought to arise from a focal gray matter lesion (localization-related epilepsy). Partial-onset seizures may remain partial or may secondarily generalize. Medically refractory epilepsy is defined by seizure syndromes that are not effectively controlled by antiepileptic drugs. The management of medically refractory partial epilepsy has been revolutionized by neurosurgical techniques aimed at the resection of the epileptogenic brain focus. Therefore, precise seizure localization is the primary objective of the presurgical workup. Electroencephalogram monitoring and structural brain imaging using magnetic resonance imaging (MRI) are part of the standard workup of epilepsy patients undergoing presurgical evaluation. Functional imaging studies, such as FDG-PET, can provide additional localizing information in patients with nonlocalizing surface ictal EEG and can reduce the number of patients requiring intracranial EEG studies (1). Even when intracranial EEG is required, FDG-PET can be helpful in guiding placement of subdural grids or depth electrodes prior to surgical ablative therapy. Obtaining a FDG-PET scan is strongly recommended before performing intracranial EEG because prior depth electrode insertion can cause small hypometabolic regions that may lead to false-positive PET interpretations (2). The FDG-PET scan in the routine clinical setting is usually interpreted in a qualitative analysis by physicians experienced in the normal cerebral distribution of the tracer in the brain.

Figure 20.1 shows a normal FDG-PET brain scan of a 16-year-old girl. It was performed on the Siemens (CTI PET Systems, Knoxville, TN)

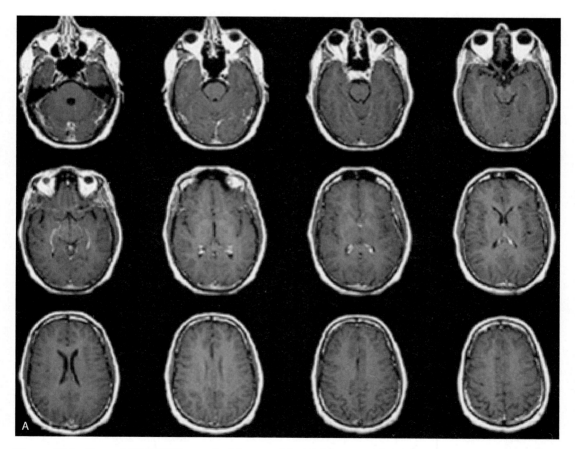

Figure 20.1. Normal FDG-PET scan in 16–year-old girl. The normal mild asymmetry in metabolism typically seen in the temporal lobe is illustrated, as well as the normal degree of apparent reduction in metabolism in the anterior and mesial temporal lobe regions. A: Normal MRI scan. B: Normal FDG-PET scan.

HR+ dedicated brain PET scanner. After the intravenous injection of 7.2 mCi of fluorine-18 (^{18}F)-FDG, the patient waited on a comfortable recliner in a dimly lit, quiet room for approximately 30 minutes to allow for tracer incorporation into the brain. The figure illustrates the typical pattern of FDG uptake in the brain of a child. It has been previously reported that there is increased metabolic activity in the anterior cingulate cortex and thalamus in children (3). Figure 20.1 also illustrates the importance of using symmetry or other semiqualitative methods to establish the presence of abnormally reduced metabolism in the temporal lobes, because there is a variability of symmetrical uptake of approximately 15% in this location (4). The PET scan should be interpreted as being abnormal if there is a definite focal area of reduced FDG uptake identified during the interictal state. It is also highly recommended that the FDG-PET scan be reviewed with full information available including the current MRI scan, clinical history, neurologic examination, seizure semiology, and EEG results.

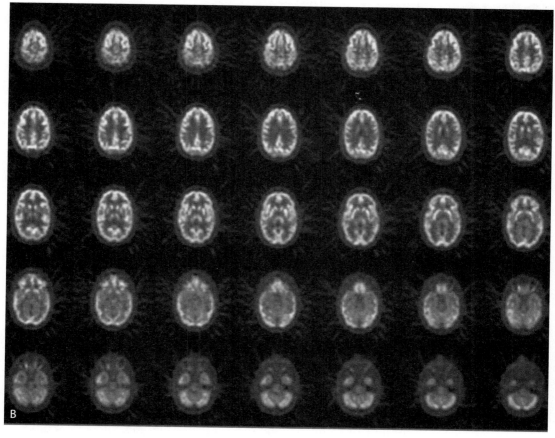

Figure 20.1. *Continued.*

Regional Glucose Hypometabolism and Epileptogenic Focus

The use of FDG-PET in clinical epilepsy emerged from early observations of regionally reduced cortical glucose metabolism at the site of the epileptogenic focus (5). It should be noted that FDG-PET may show more widespread hypometabolism than suspected on the basis of the scalp-recorded EEG (1). The pathophysiology of interictal cortical hypometabolism in partial epilepsy is incompletely understood. Areas of interictal hypometabolism in epileptogenic cortex appear to be partially uncoupled from blood flow with metabolic reductions being greater relative to flow (6). Although there are significant correlations between hippocampal volume and inferior mesial and lateral temporal lobe cerebral metabolic rates in patients with temporal lobe epilepsy (7), hippocampal neuronal loss cannot fully account for the regional interictal hypometabolism of temporal lobe epilepsy (8). Children with new onset of seizures are less likely to have hypometabolism (9). Therefore, it is uncertain whether hypometabolism reflects the effects of repeated seizures on the brain, the underlying pathologic process, or an initial insult such as early status epilepticus (9). It is possible that synaptic mechanisms rather than cell loss may contribute to the observed hypometabolism (10).

Ictal SPECT Combined with Interictal FDG

Single photon emission computed tomography (SPECT) is a nuclear medicine imaging method that facilitates the measurement of rCBF (11). Its utility is based on the fact that partial seizures are associated with an increase in rCBF (12). In ictal SPECT, a photon-emitting radiotracer [usually technetium-99m (^{99m}Tc)-hexamethylproleneamineoxime (HMPAO) or ^{99m}Tc-ethylcysteinate dimer (ECD)] is injected intravenously at the onset of a seizure and the subject is scanned when stable using a rotating gamma camera to obtain SPECT images. This provides a three-dimensional image of the distribution of the radiotracer during the seizure, for the radiotracer accumulates and remains "fixed" in different areas of the brain proportional to the cerebral perfusion to those regions at the time of injection. In partial seizures, the increased blood flow closely corresponds with the site of seizure origin. The interpretation of ictal rCBF-SPECT has several potential limitations. Extratemporal seizures are often associated with multiple areas of increased rCBF that may be due to seizure propagation or to individual variability in the baseline rCBF patterns of tracer uptake (13–15). Also, if the epileptogenic zone is hypoperfused at baseline (interictal), the ictal increase in tracer uptake may be obscured despite relative hyperperfusion (15,16). These factors have led to the widespread but not universal practice of combining an ictal with an interictal study (13,15,16). Typically, qualitative comparison of the ictal and interictal studies is undertaken when both are available; otherwise, qualitative or semi-

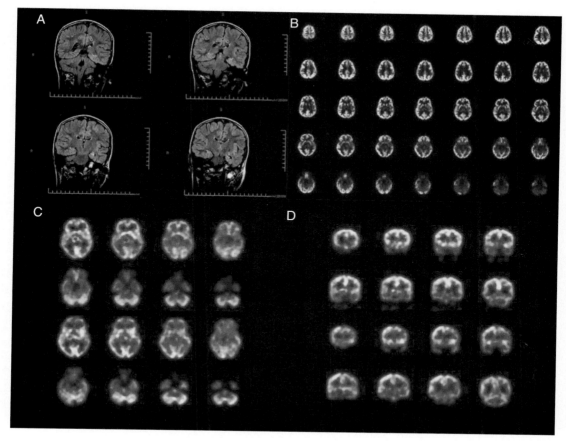

Figure 20.2. A 9–year-old, right-handed boy with history of intractable partial epilepsy. A: MRI coronal sections through the mesial temporal lobe region show left mesial temporal lobe sclerosis with villous atrophy. B: Transverse sections from a FDG-PET scan show left temporal lobe hypometabolism with greatest reduction in the left mesial temporal lobe. C: Transverse interictal regional cerebral blood flow (rCBF)-SPECT (top two rows) compared with ictal rCBF-SPECT (bottom two rows) shows increased blood flow to the lateral temporal lobe region during ictus. D: Coronal interictal rCBF-SPECT of the same scan as shown in C (top two rows) compared with ictal rCBF-SPECT (bottom two rows) shows increased blood flow to the lateral temporal lobe region during ictus.

quantitative side-to-side comparison of the ictal study alone is performed. More recently it has been shown that the accuracy of this method may be enhanced by subtraction of the interictal from the ictal SPECT and then co-registration of the resulting images onto MRI (15).

Ictal SPECT can corroborate the findings on interictal FDG, as shown in Figure 20.2. However, due to late propagation and cross-hemispheric electrocortical activation, the findings on ictal SPECT must be carefully interpreted. This difficulty with ictal SPECT is illustrated in a 9-year-old, right-handed boy with history of intractable partial epilepsy. Seizure onset was in the first few months of life. The EEG showed left temporal slowing as well as left sharp waves. An MRI scan showed left medial temporal sclerosis with villous atrophy. The FDG-PET scan showed left medial temporal hypometabolism. However, the ictal SPECT showed an increase in left lateral temporal lobe perfusion. Thus, although ictal SPECT correctly lateralized the epileptogenic focus to the correct lobe of the brain, only interictal FDG-PET localized the true epileptogenic focus to the left mesial temporal lobe.

Interictal FDG-PET Studies in Temporal Lobe Epilepsy (TLE)

Mesial temporal lobe epilepsy is commonly associated with hippocampal sclerosis. Fluorodeoxyglucose-PET has high sensitivity in detecting temporal hypometabolic foci and can be visualized as a region of reduced metabolism that, when compared to the normal temporal lobe, may show a significant asymmetry in FDG uptake (4). Figure 20.3 illustrates concordance between abnormalities on MRI and FDG-PET in a 16-year-old boy with temporal lobe epilepsy. The MRI shows abnormal high signal intensity in the right hippocampal region. The FDG-PET shows a corresponding area of focal reduction of FDG uptake in the right hippocampal region.

Fluorodeoxyglucose-PET is most useful for those patients with TLE who have equivocal or no structural MRI abnormalities to provide the necessary lateralization information (7,17). Although most patients with TLE will have the findings of hippocampal sclerosis on a high resolution MRI, a significant minority of patients with electroclinically well-lateralized temporal lobe seizures have no evidence of sclerosis on

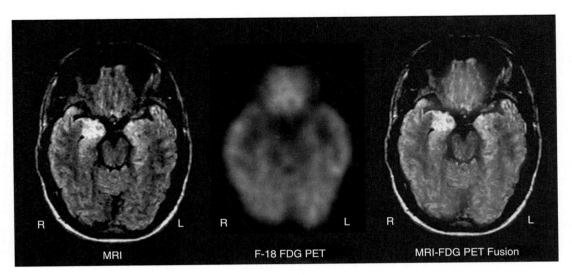

Figure 20.3. Right mesial temporal lobe sclerosis in a 16–year-old boy. The MRI-PET fusion image illustrates that the reduction in FDG corresponds to the region of MRI increase in signal intensity in the right mesial temporal lobe (hippocampal region).

MRI (18). Figure 20.4 illustrates a normal MRI scan and an abnormal FDG-PET scan in a 15-year-old boy with intractable complex partial seizures. He averaged about one to two complex partial seizures a month and two to three simple partial seizures per day. His surface EEG showed ictal discharges from the right frontotemporal region. The MRI and interictal rCBF-SPECT studies were normal. An interictal FDG-PET showed right temporal hypometabolism involving medial and anterior aspects of the right temporal lobe.

It should be noted that false lateralization is rare but may occur in FDG-PET studies of temporal lobe epilepsy. For example, unrecognized epileptic activity can make the contralateral temporal lobe appear spuriously depressed (2). Furthermore, normal right-to-left asymmetry between temporal lobes should not be interpreted as pathologic hypometabolism. Although FDG-PET images can be analyzed visually, additional information can be obtained by semiquantitative analysis, such as left-to-right asymmetry indices. Semiquantitative analysis using the asymmetry index is generally considered significant when a difference of 15% or greater exists between the affected and contralateral sides (19). Quantitative asymmetry indices should reduce potential error due to misinterpreting these normal left-to-right variations (20). Registration programs can be used to align structural MRI and PET for more precise anatomic localization of the hypometabolic area. Although regional hypometabolism is typically present in the temporal lobe ipsilateral to EEG seizure onset, other brain regions may also show patterns of glucose hypometabolism. For example, an FDG-PET study of patients with temporal lobe epilepsy demonstrated hypometabolic regions ipsilateral to seizure onset that included lateral temporal (in 78% of patients), mesial temporal (70%), thalamic (63%), basal ganglia (41%), frontal (30%), parietal (26%), and occipital (4%) regions (21). In pure TLE, however, the extratemporal hypometabolic regions rarely show epileptiform activity on EEG but may be affected by rapid seizure propagation (21).

Cerebellar hypometabolism may be ipsilateral, contralateral, or bilateral, depending on the distribution and spread of ictal activity and possible effects of phenytoin therapy (2,22). Bilateral cerebellar hypometabolism, which often is present, cannot be fully explained by the effects of phenytoin (22). Unilateral temporal hypometabolism predicts good surgical outcome from temporal lobectomy. The greater the metabolic asymmetry, the greater the chance of becoming seizure-free (2). Bilateral temporal hypometabolism may represent a relative contraindication for surgery (2). Similarly, thalamic asymmetry on FDG-PET is a strong predictor of surgical outcome; hypometabolism in the thalamus contralateral to the presumed EEG focus almost invariably predicts poor surgical outcome (23).

FDG-PET Imaging in Extratemporal Epilepsy

The localization of epileptic foci in patients who have intractable extratemporal epilepsy remains a major diagnostic challenge in the

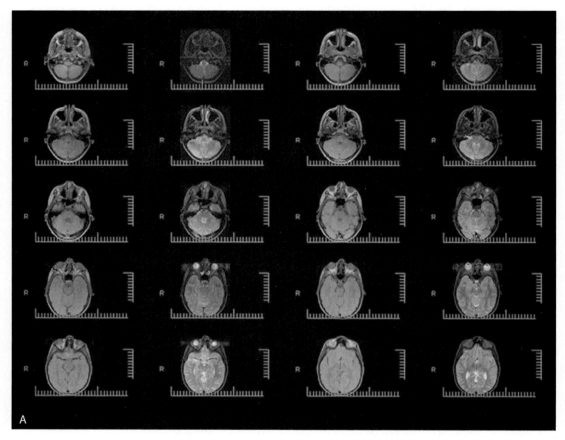

Figure 20.4. A 15–year-old boy with intractable complex partial seizures. A: Normal MRI scan. B: Inter-ictal FDG-PET shows right temporal hypometabolism in the hippocampal region.

presurgical evaluation of children with epilepsy. The most common underlying pathology in extratemporal neocortical epilepsy is micro-scopic focal cortical dysplasia, which cannot be readily detected by current MRI techniques (24). Fluorodeoxyglucose-PET may not be as valuable in the evaluation of patients with extratemporal seizures, such as frontal lobe epilepsy, because of limited sensitivity (20,25). Areas of hypometabolism in frontal lobe epilepsy have been found to be focal, regional, or hemispheric (26). Interictal hypometabolism may be uncom-mon in the absence of co-localized structural imaging abnormality in frontal lobe epilepsy (27). Furthermore, large zones of extrafrontal, par-ticularly temporal, hypometabolism are commonly observed ipsilateral to frontal hypometabolism in frontal lobe epilepsies (27). Figure 20.5 illustrates this limitation on the localization capability of interictal FDG-PET in extratemporal lobe epilepsy in a 14-year-old girl with intractable epilepsy. The patient had one to two brief seizures per day. Video-EEG monitoring was nonlocalizing. The MRI scan was normal. Ictal ^{99m}Tc-HMPAO showed focal intense right frontal lobe hyperperfusion. Inter-ictal FDG-PET was nonlocalizing, but in retrospect, after review of the

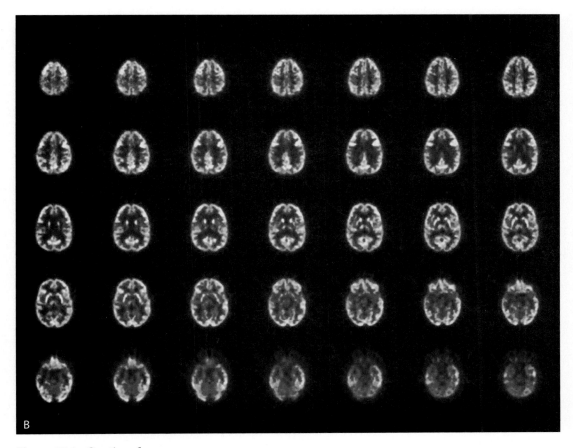

Figure 20.4. *Continued.*

ictal rCBF study, showed subtle right frontal hypometabolism. In this case interictal FDG was confirmatory but by itself was not localizing.

Recent data show that observer-independent automatic statistical brain mapping techniques may increase the usefulness of FDG-PET in patients with extratemporal lobe epilepsy (28). For example, a study using an automated brain mapping method found significantly higher sensitivity in detecting the epileptogenic focus (67%) than visual analysis (19% to 38%) in patients with extratemporal epilepsy (29). Hypometabolic regions in partial epilepsies of neocortical origin have been usually associated with structural imaging abnormalities (25). Therefore, PET data should always be interpreted in the context of high-quality anatomic MRI, providing a structural-functional correlation. The importance of precise localization using an an automated registration mapping method is illustrated in Figure 20.6,

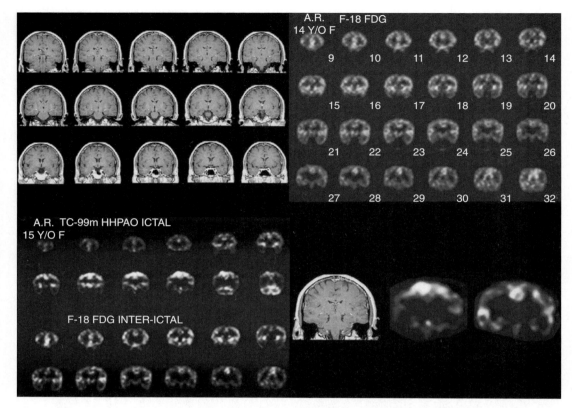

Figure 20.5. A 14–year-old girl with a history of intractable epilepsy with seizure frequency as one to two seizures per day. MRI coronal sections are normal (left upper quadrant). FDG-PET shows normal variability in metabolic uptake with no convincing areas of metabolic reduction that are diagnostic for the epileptogenic focus (right upper quadrant). Ictal technetium-99m (^{99m}Tc)-hexamethylproleneamine-oxime (HMPAO) SPECT in coronal section (top) demonstrates a region of focal intense blood flow in the right medial frontal lobe compared with co-registered coronal sections from the interictal FDG-PET scan. In retrospect, a region of hypometabolism is detectable (left lower quadrant). Co-registered MRI, ictal SPECT, and FDG-PET images show the MRI is normal in the location of intense hyperemia on ictal SPECT, in the same area retrospectively showing hypometabolism on PET (right upper quadrant).

Figure 20.6. A 15–year-old boy with generalized tonic-clonic seizures from a right parieto-occipital cavernous venous angioma. A: MRI shows right parieto-occipital cavernous venous angioma. B: FDG-PET scan shows reduced metabolism in the area of the cavernous venous angioma. C: Ictal SPECT transverse section (bottom) shows increased blood flow to the right parietal lobe in the location of the angioma. Interictal SPECT (top) shows reduced blood flow corresponding to the location of the angioma. D: Ictal SPECT sagittal section (bottom) shows increased blood flow to the right parietal lobe in the location anterior to the angioma. Interictal SPECT (top) shows reduced blood flow corresponding to the location of the angioma. E: Statistical pixel analysis map in transverse section of significant ictal rCBF greater than interictal rCBF (yellow) or less that interictal rCBF (blue). Map shows significant ictal associated hyperemia in the region of the angioma. F: Statistical pixel analysis map in sagittal section of significant ictal rCBF greater than interictal rCBF (yellow) or less that interictal rCBF (blue). Map shows significant ictal associate hyperemia anterior to the angioma. (See color insert, parts E and F only.)

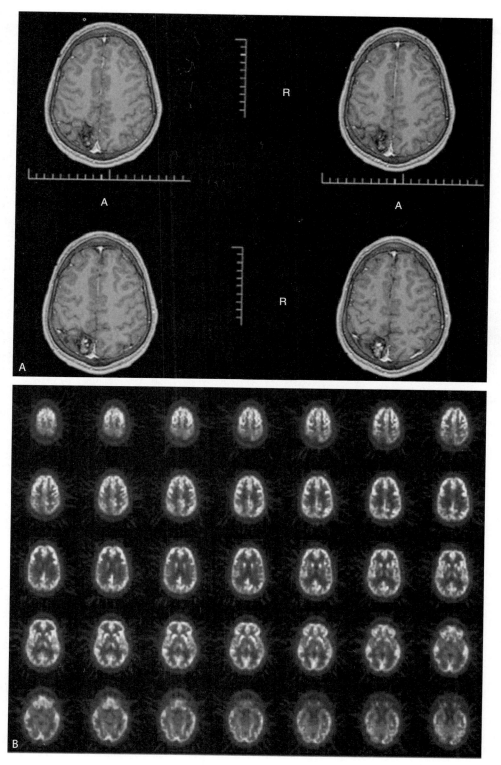

(Continued)

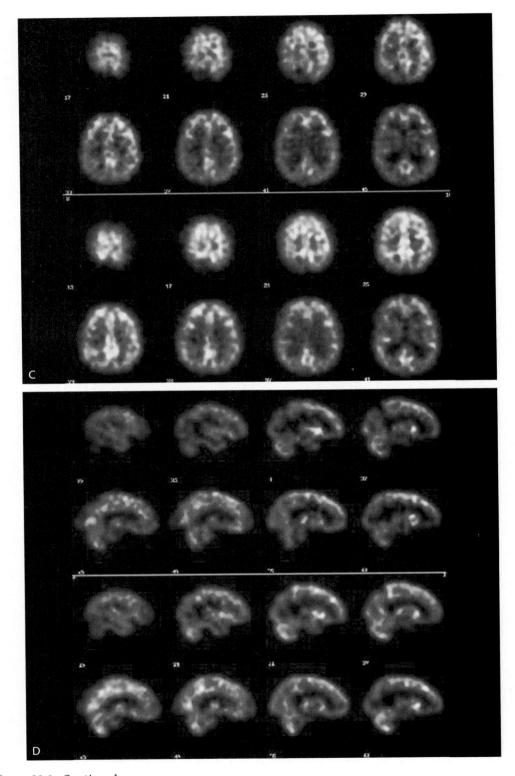

Figure 20.6. *Continued.*

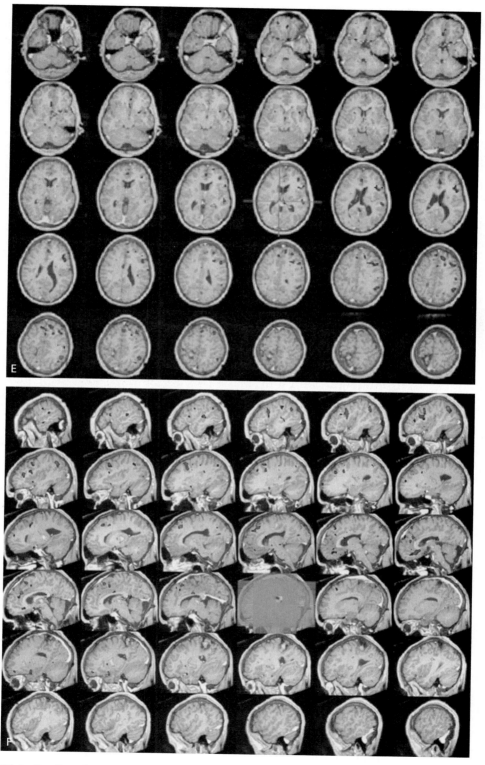

Figure 20.6. *Continued.*

see color insert, by the example of a 15-year-old, right-handed boy undergoing evaluation for a generalized tonic-clonic seizure disorder caused by a right parietooccipital cavernous venous angioma. The EEG showed right parieto-occipital focal slow and sharp waves. The MRI showed right parieto-occipital cavernous venous angioma with evidence of bleeding. The FDG-PET scan showed reduced metabolism in the area of the cavernous venous angioma. An ictal SPECT showed increased uptake in the right parietal lobe, anterior and medial to the area of reduction of blood flow in right parietal lobe caused by the angioma. The patient underwent electrocorticography and mapping of the lesion for subsequent resection of the lesion and surrounding epileptogenic area. On electrocorticography and intraoperative mapping, the area of increased epileptogenesis was found to correlate with the findings of ictal SPECT.

Interictal FDG-PET studies have limited usefulness in the presence of multiple hypometabolic regions in patients with multifocal brain syndromes, such as in children with tuberous sclerosis. Such children with multifocal lesions represent a special challenge during presurgical evaluation. The goal of functional imaging in these cases is to identify the epileptogenic lesions and differentiate them from nonepileptogenic ones. In this context, ictal rCBF-SPECT may have useful clinical applications but may be technically challenging when seizures are short, as is particularly common in frontal lobe epilepsy and in children who have infantile spasms that are associated with multifocal cortical dysplasia (30). Figure 20.7 shows such a case in a 1-year-old boy with tuberous sclerosis. Several lesions appeared anatomically abnormal on the CT portion of the PET-CT scan. These areas also showed reduced FDG uptake on PET. Ictal SPECT was able to identify the dominant area of presumed epileptogenesis associated with a large tuber in the right frontal lobe.

Figure 20.7. A 1–year-old boy with tuberous sclerosis underwent a PET–computed tomography (CT) scan as well as ictal and interictal rCBF-SPECT. A: CT portion of PET-CT scan showing the tubers. B: FDG-PET portion of PET-CT scan showing reduced metabolism in the multiple areas of the tubers. C: PET-CT fusion image showing that the areas of decreased metabolism correspond to the numerous tuber abnormalities identified on the CT scan. D: FDG-PET scan coronal sections showing reduced metabolism in multiple areas of the tubers. E: Ictal rCBF-SPECT coronal section (bottom) showing intense hyperemia corresponding to the large tuber in the right frontal lobe. Interictal rCBF-SPECT does not show blood flow reduction to the degree of metabolic reduction identified on interictal PET.

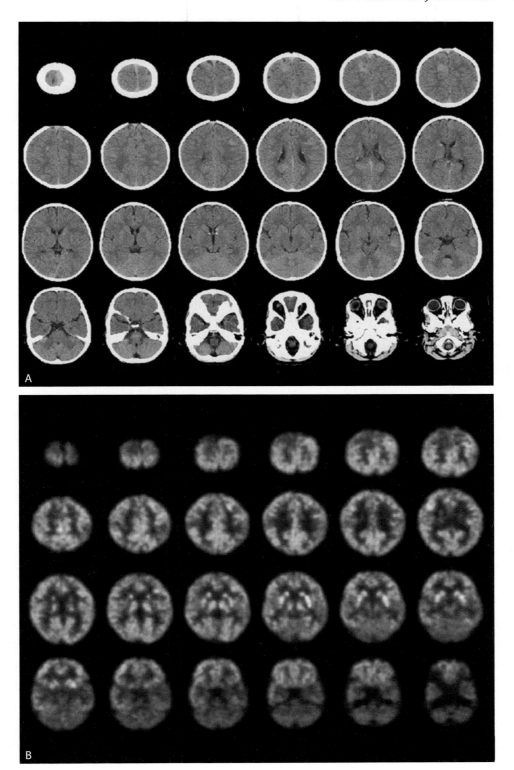

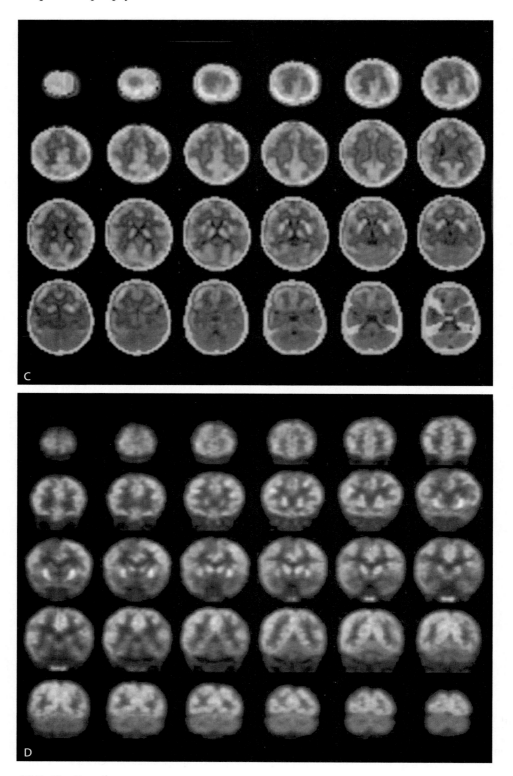

Figure 20.7. *Continued.*

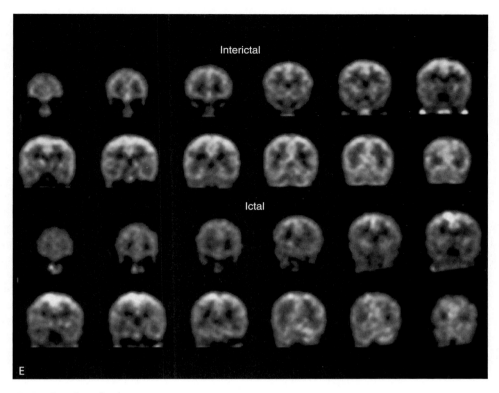

Figure 20.7. *Continued.*

FDG-PET Studies of Children with Infantile Spasms (West Syndrome)

An infantile spasm is an epileptic syndrome that begins in early infancy in which children have tonic and myoclonic seizures, arrhythmia on EEG, and development arrest. Among patients with infantile spasms, FDG-PET studies suggest that the spasms are the result of secondary generalization from cortical foci and that maturational factors result in the recruitment of basal ganglia and brainstem serotonin mechanisms that lead to secondary generalization and the unique semiology of the spasms (31,32). Most infants who are diagnosed with "cryptogenic" spasms have focal or multifocal cortical regions of decreased (or occasionally increased) glucose metabolic activity on PET that are often consistent with areas of cortical dysplasia missed by MRI (31,33). When a single region of abnormal glucose hypometabolism is apparent on PET and corresponds to the EEG focus, and the seizures are intractable, surgical removal of the PET focus results in seizure control and in complete or partial reversal of the associated developmental delay (30). When the pattern of glucose hypometabolism is generalized and symmetric, a lesional cause is not likely, and neurometabolic or neurogenetic disorders should be considered when further evaluating the child

(30). Results of serial FDG-PET imaging have shown that when PET after the initial treatment shows no abnormalities, even though the first PET shows hypometabolism, infants with cryptogenic West syndrome may have a favorable developmental or seizure outcome (34).

FDG-PET Studies in Lennox-Gastaut Syndrome

Lennox-Gastaut syndrome is a childhood epileptic encephalopathy characterized by an electroclinical triad of generalized slow spike wave activity in the EEG, multiple types of epileptic seizures, and slow mental development. It is usually subdivided into symptomatic and crypto-genic types, the latter accounting for at least one fourth of all patients. Symptomatic cases are due to diverse cerebral conditions, which are usually bilateral, diffuse, or multifocal, involving cerebral gray matter (35). Fluorodeoxyglucose-PET studies have shown that Lennox-Gastaut syndrome can be classified into four predominant subtypes, each with a distinct metabolic pattern: unilateral focal hypometabolism, unilateral diffuse hypometabolism, bilateral diffuse hypometabolism, and normal (36). Patients who have the unilateral focal and unilateral diffuse patterns may be considered for cortical resection provided that there is concordance between FDG-PET and ictal EEG findings (30).

Interictal and Ictal PET Studies

Interictal ^{15}O-H$_2$O rCBF-PET Studies

It should be noted that interictal oxygen-15 (^{15}O)-H$_2$O rCBF-PET studies, when compared to FDG-PET studies, have reduced sensitivity in localizing epileptogenic zones and sometimes may be false lateralizing (37). Furthermore, rCBF-PET scans are noisier than FDG-PET, which may increase partial volume effects and make detection of a hypoperfused area more difficult. Therefore, interictal rCBF-PET studies are unreliable markers for epileptic foci and should not be used in the presurgical evaluation of patients with epilepsy (6).

Ictal PET

Although not always practical, FDG-PET can also be used for ictal studies in patients who have frequent seizures (38). It should be noted that FDG-PET may be less accurate for ictal compared to interictal glucose metabolic measurements because seizures may alter the "lumped constant," which describes the relationship between FDG and its physiologic substrate glucose (2). Furthermore, a typical seizure is much shorter than the average 30-minute FDG uptake period. Therefore, an "ictal" scan may include interictal, ictal, and postictal metabolic changes with combinations of hypermetabolic and hypometabolic regions (2). ^{15}O-H$_2$O PET imaging has been used to study quantitative alterations in rCBF accompanying seizures induced by pentylenetetrazole (39). Patients with generalized tonic-clonic seizures demonstrated asymmetric flow increases. One patient with a complex partial seizure demonstrated 70% to 80% increases in bitemporal flow. Thalamic flow increased during both complex partial and generalized seizures, indicating the importance of this subcortical structure during ictal activation (39).

Factors That May Affect Interpretation of Interictal and Ictal FDG-PET Studies

A number of other factors need to be considered when interpreting brain PET images of children with epilepsy. It should be realized that brain glucose metabolic or blood flow PET images are functional in nature. For example, when a child is moving or talking around the time of injection, increased activity in specific brain regions, like the basal ganglia, motor cortex, or language centers, may be present. Metabolic activity in the visual cortex was increased in subjects studied with their eyes open when compared to a baseline of subjects studied with their eyes closed (40). Therefore, knowledge of the clinical or behavioral state of the patient at the time of the injection and study is critical for proper image interpretation.

Positron emission tomography in children often requires sedation. An FDG-PET study of propofol sedation in children found significant hypometabolism in the medial parieto-occipital cortex bilaterally, including the lingual gyrus, cuneus, and middle occipital gyrus (41). The bilateral parieto-occipital hypometabolism is likely to be a sedation-specific effect and should be taken into account when evaluating cerebral FDG-PET scans in sedated children. Diazepam sedation has been found to reduce cerebral glucose metabolism globally by about 20% (42). A study by Wang et al. (43) found that lorazepam significantly decreased whole-brain metabolism over 10%. However, regional effects of lorazepam were largest in the thalamus and occipital cortex (about 20% reduction). Similarly, antiepileptic drugs have been found to reduce glucose metabolism and rCBF. Studies on valproate have shown global FDG (about 9% to 10%) and global CBF (about 15%) reductions with greatest regional reductions in the thalamus (44). Phenytoin has been found to cause an average reduction of cerebral glucose metabolism by 13% (45). Cerebellar metabolism may also be reduced by phenytoin, although the effect of the drug is probably less than that due to early onset of uncontrolled epilepsy (22,46). Studies on the barbiturate phenobarbital and cerebral glucose metabolism have shown very prominent global reductions of about 37% (47).

Emerging Clinical Applications of Neurochemical PET Imaging

The inhibitory neurotransmitter γ-aminobutyric acid (GABA) has anticonvulsant properties. Benzodiazepine receptor ligands, such as carbon-11 (^{11}C)-flumazenil (FMZ), have been used to study the regional cerebral distribution of benzodiazepine receptor binding sites that are related to GABA$_A$ receptors. The high density of GABA$_A$ receptors in the normal hippocampus accounts for the high sensitivity of FMZ-PET to detect even mild decreases in binding that are consistent with hippocampal sclerosis in TLE. Where available, FMZ-PET provides a useful alternative for FDG-PET in the evaluation of children with epilepsy. A regional decrease in benzodiazepine receptor binding has been associated with the presence of a possible epileptogenic focus. Unilaterally decreased temporal FMZ binding can also help to lateralize the epileptic focus in patients who have TLE that is associated with bilateral temporal hypometabolism on FDG-PET (30). When compared to FDG studies, FMZ-PET studies have been reported to demonstrate less extensive cortical involvement. For example, a study comparing FDG and FMZ-PET imaging in patients with temporal lobe epilepsy found a wide range of mesial temporal, lateral temporal, and thalamic glucose hypometabolism ipsilateral to ictal EEG changes as well as extratemporal hypometabolism. In contrast, each patient demonstrated decreased benzodiazepine-receptor binding in the ipsilateral anterior mesial temporal region, without neocortical changes. Thus, interictal metabolic dysfunction can be variable and usually is extensive in temporal lobe epilepsy, whereas decreased central benzodiazepine-receptor density appears to be more restricted to mesial temporal areas (48). Similar benzodiazepine receptor findings have been reported for patients with extratemporal lobe seizures caused by focal cortical dysplasia (49). Unlike the more widespread glucose hypometabolic patterns, benzodiazepine receptor changes may reflect localized neuronal loss that is more specific to the epileptogenic zone (48). Therefore, FMZ imaging may be useful in the presurgical evaluation of children with epilepsy. However, focal increases of benzodiazepine receptor binding have also been reported in the temporal lobe as well as extratemporal sites in patients with temporal lobe epilepsy when statistical brain mapping analysis is performed (50). This may lead to false-localizing information when attention is paid only to areas of decreased uptake.

The development of radioligands that are specific for excitatory amino acid and selected opioid receptor subtypes, such as ^{11}C-carfentanil for mu-opiate receptors, may help to better explore the pathophysiology of epileptic syndromes. Another promising direction in the development of new PET tracers for epilepsy is to target serotonergic neurotransmission. A novel tracer, α-^{11}C-methyl-L-tryptophan (AMT), which accumulates in epileptic foci in the interictal state, can be a useful approach to identify epileptogenic sites in children with multifocal brain lesions (30,51). This radiotracer may also be useful in identifying nonresected epileptic cortex in young patients with a previously failed neocortical epilepsy surgery (52).

Conclusion

The use of FDG-PET in clinical epilepsy emerged from early observations of regionally reduced cortical glucose metabolism at the site of the epileptogenic focus. Fluorodeoxyglucose is the most commonly used PET radiotracer in the diagnostic and presurgical evaluation of children with epilepsy at the present time. Measurement of receptors or neurotransmitter metabolism is a unique ability of PET that has not achieved its full potential in the study of pediatric epilepsy. For example, PET measures of central benzodiazepine receptor binding and serotonin synthesis may have increasing clinical applications in the presurgical evaluation of children with localization-related epilepsy. It is anticipated that the use of such tracers will further enhance the clinical yield of PET in the diagnostic workup and presurgical evaluation of children with medically intractable epilepsy and will further improve our understanding of the pathophysiology of pediatric epilepsy.

References

1. Theodore WH, Newmark ME, Sato S, et al. [^{18}F]fluorodeoxyglucose positron emission tomography in refractory complex partial seizures. Ann Neurol 1983;14:429–437.
2. Theodore WH. Positron emission tomography in the evaluation of seizure disorders. Neurosci News 1998;1:18–22.
3. Van Bogaert P, Wikler D, Damhaut P, Szliwowski HB, Goldman S. Regional changes in glucose metabolism during brain development from the age of 6 years. Neuroimage 1998;8:62–68.
4. Henry TR, Van Heertum RL. Positron emission tomography and single photon emission computed tomography in epilepsy care. Semin Nucl Med 2003;33:88–104.
5. Kuhl DE, Engel J, Phelps ME, Selin C. Epileptic patterns of local cerebral metabolism and perfusion in humans determined by emission computed tomography of ^{18}FDG and ^{13}NH3. Ann Neurol 1980;8:348–360.
6. Gaillard WD, Fazilat S, White S, et al. Interictal metabolism and blood flow are uncoupled in temporal lobe cortex of patients with complex partial epilepsy. Neurology 1995;45:1841–1847.
7. Gaillard WD, Bhatia S, Bookheimer SY, Fazilat S, Sato S, Theodore WH. FDG-PET and volumetric MRI in the evaluation of patients with partial epilepsy. Neurology 1995;45:123–126.
8. Henry TR, Babb TL, Engel J Jr, Mazziotta JC, Phelps ME, Crandall PH. Hippocampal neuronal loss and regional hypometabolism in temporal lobe epilepsy. Ann Neurol 1994;36:925–927.
9. Theodore WH. Cerebral blood flow and glucose metabolism in human epilepsy. In: Advances in Neurology, vol. 79. Philadelphia: Lippincott Williams & Wilkins, 1999:873–881.
10. Hajek M, Wieser HG, Khan N, et al. Preoperative and postoperative glucose consumption in mesiobasal and lateral temporal lobe epilepsy. Neurology 1994;44:2125–2132.
11. Mountz JM, Deutsch G, Kuzniecky R, Rosenfeld SS. Brain SPECT: 1994 Update. In: Freeman LM, ed. Nuclear Medicine Annual 1994. New York: Raven Press, 1994:1–54.
12. Horsely V. An address on the origin and seat of epileptic disturbance. Br Med J 1892;1:693–696.
13. Marks DA, Katz A, Hoffer P, Spencer SS. Localization of extratemporal epileptic foci during ictal single photon emission computed tomography. Ann Neurol 1992;31:250–255.

14. Ho SS, Berkovic SF, Newton MR, Austin MC, McKay WJ, Bladin PF. Parietal lobe epilepsy: clinical features and seizure localization by ictal SPECT. Neurology 1994;44:2277–2284.

15. O'Brien TJ, So EL, Mullan BP, et al. Subtraction ictal SPECT co-registered to MRI improves clinical usefulness of SPECT in localizing the surgical seizure focus. Neurology 1998;50:445–454.

16. Spanaki MV, Spencer SS, Corsi M, MacMullan J, Seibyl J, Zubal IG. Sensitivity and specificity of quantitative difference SPECT analysis in seizure localization. J Nucl Med 1999;40:730–736.

17. Lamusuo S, Jutila L, Ylinen A, et al. [^{18}F]FDG-PET reveals temporal hypometabolism in patients with temporal lobe epilepsy even when quantitative MRI and histopathological analysis show only mild hippocampal damage. Arch Neurol 2001;58:933–939.

18. Carne RP, O'Brien TJ, Kilpatrick CJ, et al. MRI-negative PET-positive temporal lobe epilepsy: a distinct surgically remediable syndrome. Brain 2004;127:2276–2285.

19. Delbeke D, Lawrence SK, Abou-Khalil BW, Blumenkopf B, Kessler RM. Postsurgical outcome of patients with uncontrolled complex partial seizures and temporal lobe hypometabolism on ^{18}FDG-positron emission tomography. Invest Radiol 1996;31:261–266.

20. Theodore WH, Sato S, Kufta CV, Gaillard WD, Kelley K. FDG-positron emission tomography and invasive EEG: seizure focus detection and surgical outcome. Epilepsia 1997;38:81–86.

21. Henry TR, Mazziotta JC, Engel J. Interictal metabolic anatomy of mesial temporal lobe epilepsy. Arch Neurol 1993;50:582–589.

22. Theodore WH, Fishbein D, Dietz M, Baldwin P. Complex partial seizures: cerebellar metabolism. Epilepsia 1987;28:319–323.

23. Newberg AB, Alavi A, Berlin J, Mozley PD, O'Connor M, Sperling M. Ipsilateral and contralateral thalamic hypometabolism as a predictor of outcome after temporal lobectomy for seizures. J Nucl Med 2000;41:1964–1968.

24. Crino PB, Eberwine J. Cellular and molecular basis of cerebral dysgenesis. J Neurosci Res 1987;50:907–916.

25. Henry TR, Sutherling WW, Engel J, et al. Interictal cerebral metabolism in partial epilepsies of neocortical origin. Epilepsy Res 1991;10:174–182.

26. Swartz BE, Halgren E, Delgado-Escueta AV, et al. Neuroimaging in patients with seizures of probable frontal lobe origin. Epilepsia 1989;30:547–558.

27. Henry TR, Mazziotta JC, Engel JJ. The functional anatomy of frontal lobe epilepsy studied with PET. Adv Neurol 1992;57:449–463.

28. Knowlton RC, Lawn ND, Mountz JM, Kuzniecky RI. Ictal SPECT analysis in epilepsy: subtraction and statistical parametric mapping techniques. Neurology 2004;63:10–15.

29. Drzezga A, Arnold S, Minoshima S, et al. ^{18}F-FDG PET studies in patients with extratemporal and temporal epilepsy: evaluation of an observer-independent analysis. J Nucl Med 1999;40:737–746.

30. Juhasz C, Chugani HT. Imaging the epileptic brain with positron emission tomography. Neuroimag Clin North Am 2003;13:705–716.

31. Chugani HT, Shields WD, Shewmon DA, Olson DM, Phelps ME, Peacock WJ. Infantile spasms: I. PET identifies focal cortical dysgenesis in cryptogenic cases for surgical treatment. Ann Neurol 1990;27:406–413.

32. Chugani HT, Chugani DC. Basic mechanisms of childhood epilepsies: studies with positron emission tomography. Adv Neurol 1999;79:883–891.

33. Chugani HT, Shewmon DA, Shields WD, et al. Surgery for intractable infantile spasms: neuroimaging perspectives. Epilepsia 1993;34:764–771.

34. Itomi K, Okumura A, Negoro T, et al. Prognostic value of positron emission tomography in cryptogenic West syndrome. Dev Med Child Neurol 2002;44:107–111.

35. Markand ON. Lennox-Gastaut syndrome (childhood epileptic encephalopathy). J Clin Neurophysiol 2003;20:426–441.

36. Chugani HT, Mazziotta JC, Engel JJ, Phelps ME. The Lennox-Gastaut syndrome: metabolic subtypes determined by 2–deoxy-2[^{18}F]fluoro-D-glucose positron emission tomography. Ann Neurol 1987;21:4–13.

37. Leiderman DB, Balish M, Sato S, et al. Comparison of PET measurements of cerebral blood flow and glucose metabolism for the localization of human epileptic foci. Epilepsy Res 1992;13:153–157.

38. Meltzer CC, Adelson PD, Brenner RP, et al. Planned ictal FDG PET imaging for localization of extratemporal epileptic foci. Epilepsia 2000;41: 193–200.

39. Theodore WH, Balish M, Leiderman D, Bromfield E, Sato S, Herscovitch P. Effect of seizures on cerebral blood flow measured with ^{15}O-H2O and positron emission tomography. Epilepsia 1996;37:796–802.

40. Mazziotta JC, Phelps ME, Carson RE, Kuhl DE. Tomographic mapping of human cerebral metabolism: sensory deprivation. Ann Neurol 1982;12: 435–444.

41. Juengling FD, Kassubek J, Martens-Le Bouar H, et al. Cerebral regional hypometabolism caused by propofol-induced sedation in children with severe myoclonic epilepsy: a study using fluorodeoxyglucose positron emission tomography and statistical parametric mapping. Neurosci Lett 2002;335:79–82.

42. Foster NL, VanDerSpek AF, Aldrich MS, et al. The effect of diazepam sedation on cerebral glucose metabolism in Alzheimer's disease as measured using positron emission tomography. J Cereb Blood Flow Metab 1987;7:415–420.

43. Wang GJ, Volkow ND, Overall J, et al. Reproducibility of regional brain metabolic responses to lorazepam. J Nucl Med 1996;37:1609–1613.

44. Gaillard WD, Zeffiro T, Fazilat S, DeCarli C, Theodore WH. Effect of valproate on cerebral metabolism and blood flow: an ^{18}F-2–deoxyglucose and ^{15}O water positron emission tomography study. Epilepsia 1996;37: 515–521.

45. Theodore WH, Bairamian D, Newmark ME, et al. Effect of phenytoin on human cerebral glucose metabolism. J Cereb Blood Flow Metab 1986;6: 315–320.

46. Seitz RJ, Piel S, Arnold S, et al. Cerebellar hypometabolism in focal epilepsy is related to age of onset and drug intoxication. Epilepsia 1996;37:1194–1199.

47. Theodore WH. Antiepileptic drugs and cerebral glucose metabolism. Epilepsia 1988;29(suppl 2):S48–S55.

48. Henry TR, Frey KA, Sackellares JC, et al. In vivo cerebral metabolism and central benzodiazepine-receptor binding in temporal lobe epilepsy. Neurology 1993;43:1998–2006.

49. Arnold S, Berthele A, Drzezga A, et al. Reduction of benzodiazepine receptor binding is related to the seizure onset zone in extratemporal focal cortical dysplasia. Epilepsia 2000;41:818–824.

50. Koepp MJ, Hammers A, Labbe C, Woermann FG, Brooks DJ, Duncan JS. ^{11}C-flumazenil PET in patients with refractory temporal lobe epilepsy and normal MRI. Neurology 2000;54:332–339.

51. Juhasz C, Chugani DC, Muzik O, et al. Alpha-methyl-L-tryptophan PET detects epileptogenic cortex in children with intractable epilepsy. Neurology 2003;60:960–968.
52. Juhasz C, Chugani DC, Padhye UN, et al. Evaluation with alpha-[^{11}C]methyl-L-tryptophan positron emission tomography for reoperation after failed epilepsy surgery. Epilepsia 2004;45:124–130.

21

Neurotransmitter Imaging

Alan J. Fischman and Rajendra D. Badgaiyan

In recent years, investigators have used a variety of techniques to study human neurotransmission in health and disease. One of the most promising of these techniques is molecular or neurotransmitter imaging, which, despite being an emerging technique, has made significant contribution to our understanding of human neurotransmission (1,2). Molecular imaging has been used by numerous investigators to establish maps of the functional anatomy of neuroreceptor-radioligand interaction (3,4). Recently, it has been applied to the detection of dynamic changes in neurotransmitter activity induced by behavioral, cognitive, or pharmacologic interventions (5–12). This chapter includes a brief outline of the basic concepts of neurotransmitter imaging, important information acquired using this technique, and a discussion of dynamic receptor imaging.

Basic Concepts

Neurotransmitter imaging techniques exploit the competition between an endogenous neurotransmitter and a radiolabeled ligand (usually an agonist or antagonist of the neurotransmitter) that binds to the target receptor. With this technique, the concentration of the radiolabeled ligand (administered intravenously or orally) is measured at different brain regions, using positron emission tomography (PET) or single photon emission computed tomography (SPECT). These measurements provide information concerning active receptors and facilitate estimation of changes induced by a challenge (13). Because the reliability and accuracy of the estimation depend on the kinetics of receptor-ligand interaction, selection of an appropriate ligand is critical for success (14).

An ideal ligand has high affinity and selectivity for the target receptor, is permeable across the blood–brain barrier, has low nonspecific binding, and is not metabolized in brain tissue (15). Another factor that affects the accuracy of measurement is the proportion of administered ligand that actually binds to the target receptor (specific binding).

Tomographic methods measure the concentration of ligand in areas of interest; this concentration includes ligand that is bound to the receptor, that is present in the extracellular fluid, or that is bound to the tissue or plasma proteins (nonspecific binding). Because only specific binding provides information concerning neurotransmission, nonspecific binding must be estimated and excluded from the ligand concentration detected by the camera. The exclusion of nonspecific binding is done by applying a correction to the total concentration. Because this correction is calculated using models that provide only an approximate estimation of the amount of nonspecifically bound ligand, measurements of specific binding are more accurate if nonspecific binding is low (16–18).

A number of models have been developed for the estimation of specific binding. The most commonly used model (three-compartment model) assumes that in the brain, a ligand is distributed in three compartments (Fig. 21.1): the plasma compartment, the nondisplaceable compartment (free and nonspecifically bound ligand), and the receptor compartment (3,4). The concentration of ligand in these compartments changes if there is a positive gradient between the blood and tissue concentration. It eventually approaches equilibrium, and a steady-state volume of distribution is achieved. In this state, the ligand concentration in different compartments remains constant (17). In this model, the relationship between the concentration of specifically bound ligand at steady state (B), the maximum number of receptors (B_{max}), the concentration of free ligand (F), and the dissociation rate constant of the ligand (K_D) can be defined using the Michaelis-Menton equation (19):

$$B = \frac{B_{max} \cdot F}{K_D + F}$$

If a tracer dose of ligand is administered (as is the usual practice), the value of F is very small (as compared to that of K_D) and can be disregarded in the denominator of this formula. Thus the specific binding of a tracer can be expressed as

$$B = \frac{B_{max} \cdot F}{K_D}$$

Conventionally, the specific binding is expressed in terms of binding potential (BP), which indicates the capacity of a brain region for specific binding. Most investigators define BP as the steady state ratio

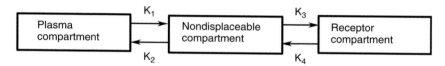

Figure 21.1. Schematic diagram of the compartmental model used to analyze PET and SPECT data in receptor imaging studies. K_1, k_2, k_3, and k_4 represent the rate constants of the ligand movement between compartments.

of the specifically bound (*B*) to free ligand (*F*). It is clear from the above equation that this ratio is equal to the ratio of B_{max} and K_D for tracers:

$$BP = \frac{B}{F} = \frac{B_{max}}{K_D}$$

Specific binding in a brain area can be measured by calculating the difference between ligand concentration in the area of interest and that in another area that is devoid of target receptor (or has a negligible number of receptors, e.g., cerebellum for dopamine receptor studies). The other variable, *F*, the free concentration of ligand in the brain cannot be measured directly. However, because ligands diffuse through the blood–brain barrier by passive diffusion, it can be assumed that, at equilibrium, the brain concentration equals the plasma concentration (20). This measurement of *F*, however, is not required if the objective of the study is to compare the *BP* in two groups of subjects. If the free ligand concentration is the same in the two groups, changes in specific binding will be proportional to the changes in *BP*. Further, by assuming that the free ligand concentration in the target and reference regions is the same at equilibrium, *BP* can be calculated by estimating the ratio of ligand concentration (*C*) in the target and reference region (*BP* = C_{TARG}/C_{REF} − 1). Theoretically, the ratio of ligand that enters the receptor compartment (k_3) to that which leaves (k_4) this compartment (*BP* = k_3/k_4) provides the best estimate of *BP* (3).

If an intervention induces release of an endogenous neurotransmitter, the number of receptors occupied by the neurotransmitter will increase. Consequently, smaller number of receptors will be available for the radioligand, and *BP* will be reduced. The reduction, however, may not occur if the neurotransmitter modifies the behavior of ligand-receptor complex. Thus the *BP* of some ligands (e.g., ^{3}H-spiperone) show a paradoxical increase after endogenous release of the neurotransmitter (21). This paradoxical behavior is caused by the neurotransmitter-promoted receptor internalization that results in trapping of the ligand in the cell (22).

Neurotransmitter imaging has been used to study a variety of psychiatric and neurologic disorders to understand the nature of impairments of neurotransmission. Because dopaminergic and serotonergic ligands are most appropriate for molecular imaging, many studies have examined these systems. The following section provides a brief survey of the findings of these investigations.

Dopaminergic System

Dopamine has been the most extensively studied neurotransmitter. The reason for the focus on dopaminergic transmission is its involvement in the pathogenesis of psychiatric and neurologic conditions. Availability of a number of dopamine ligands that are suitable for molecular imaging also contributed to the interest of investigators. Dopamine ligands have been developed from a host of agonists and antagonists of dopamine D_1 and D_2 receptors. Each of these ligands has different binding properties, and is therefore suitable for specific kinds of study. For example, the D_2 receptor antagonist raclopride is the preferred ligand for studying striatal dopamine (Fig. 21.2), but it cannot be used to examine dopamine transmission in the extrastriatal brain areas because of its extremely low binding in areas where D_2 receptor concentration are low (10,23). Newer D_2 receptor ligands, ^{18}F-fallypride, ^{11}C-FLB 457, and ^{11}C-nemonapride have high affinity for extrastriatal D_2 receptors, but their utility in detection of striatal dopamine has not yet been established (24–27).

Most of the studies on dopamine neurotransmission have been conducted to understand the pathogenesis of psychiatric disorders. Schizophrenia has attracted many investigators because of the uncertainty concerning the role of the dopamine system in its pathogenesis (28). The findings of receptor imaging studies, however, are equivocal. Based on the ligand used, these studies have found either increased (29,30) or normal (31) density of D_2 receptors in schizophrenia. Experiments that have used dopamine D_1 receptor ligands have also reported contradictory findings. These studies have found normal, increased, or decreased density in the prefrontal cortex (32). Both increased and reduced densities are correlated with the degree of impairment in prefrontal functions (measured by tests of working memory and by Wisconsin card sorting tasks). The contradictory findings of these studies are possibly due to the diversity of ligands used. It is known that each ligand has different vulnerability to competition by endogenous dopamine (33,34). The most significant increase in D_2 receptor density has been observed in studies that have used raclopride. The studies that have found decreased D_1 receptor density have used the ligand SCH 23390, whereas increased D_1 receptor density has been reported with ^{11}C-NNC (4). Apparent contradictory findings, however, may be consistent with a single pathologic process—dopamine depletion. In rats chronic dopamine depletion is known to cause decreased binding of SCH 23390 (32,35) and increased binding of ^{11}C-NNC (32).

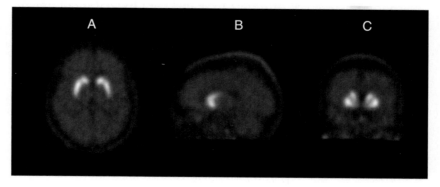

Figure 21.2. Binding potential map of ^{11}C-raclopride in a healthy volunteer showing ligand binding in the striatum (A, transaxial; B, sagittal; and C, axial view).

In receptor imaging experiments, the activity of a neurotransmitter can be evaluated by either inducing or inhibiting its release, using a pharmacologic agent. The inducers reduce the *BP* of the ligand, and inhibitors have an opposite effect. It has been shown that the *BP* of raclopride is reduced after administration of amphetamine, which induces dopamine release (36). This reduction is exaggerated in schizophrenic patients (37–39), even if they are drug naive (40). The altered response to amphetamine in schizophrenia has been shown to be proportional to the severity of symptoms and therefore is observed only in the patients who have active symptoms (37). Depletion studies have also been conducted on schizophrenic patients, using a tyrosin analogue α-methyl-para-tyrosin (AMPT), which inhibits dopamine release. These studies have found that a higher proportion of D_2 receptors are occupied by dopamine at basal level in schizophrenic patients as compared to healthy controls (41).

All of these studies examined dopaminergic activity of postsynaptic neurons. Neurotransmitter imaging can also be used to evaluate presynaptic dopaminergic activity. Presynaptic dopamine activity can be evaluated by measuring DOPA decarboxylase activity, using the ligand ^{18}F-DOPA, or by studying dopamine transporter (DAT) activity. Imaging with ^{18}F-DOPA has been used extensively to study Parkinson's disease in which dopamine synthesis is reduced (42). It has also been used to study enhanced synthesis in schizophrenia (43). Presynaptic activity has however been studied mostly by imaging the DAT, which is involved in a number of neurologic and psychiatric disorders.

Dopamine Transporter (DAT)

The DAT is a plasma membrane protein, expressed exclusively by dopamine synthesizing neurons. By removing dopamine released into the extracellular space, it regulates the amplitude and duration of dopaminergic signals (44). Molecular imaging has played a major role in our understanding of the functions of DAT, and its involvement in disorders like Parkinson's disease, attention-deficit hyperactivity disorder (ADHD), and drug abuse. The DAT has been imaged (Fig. 21.3) using a variety of cocaine (a DAT inhibitor) analogues [e.g., ^{11}C-altropane, ^{123}I-β-CIT, ^{18}F-CFT and ^{123}I-FP-CIT]. Because DAT density changes with the density of dopaminergic neurons, DAT ligands have been used to estimate neuronal loss in Parkinson's disease. Reduction in *BP* of DAT ligands such as ^{123}I-altropane (45) and ^{11}C-methylphenidate (46) has been documented in Parkinson's disease (Fig. 21.4). Because Parkinsonian symptoms appear only after destruction of >85% of dopamine innervations, and because DAT tracers can detect a loss of as low as 50% of innervations, these tracers are useful for the diagnosis of early Parkinson's disease in asymptomatic individuals (42,45,47).

In addition to Parkinson's disease, DAT imaging has been used extensively to study pathogenesis of ADHD (48,49). Though DAT binding is significantly elevated (20% to 70%) in adults (50) and children (51) with ADHD (Fig. 21.5), it is not clear whether its depletion is

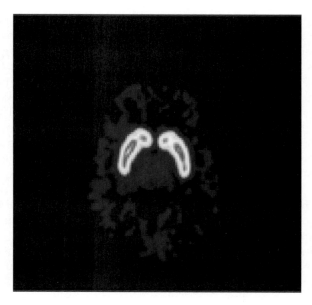

Figure 21.3. Binding potential map of ^{11}C-altropane in a healthy volunteer.

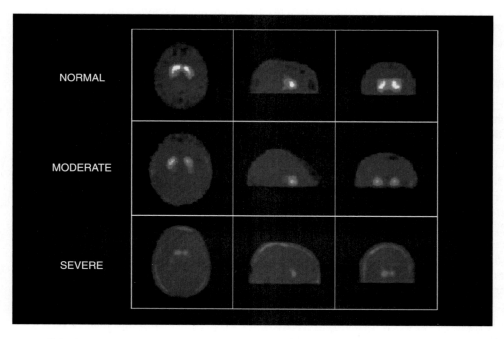

Figure 21.4. ^{11}C-altropane binding in a healthy volunteer (normal) and in patients with moderate and severe Parkinson's disease.

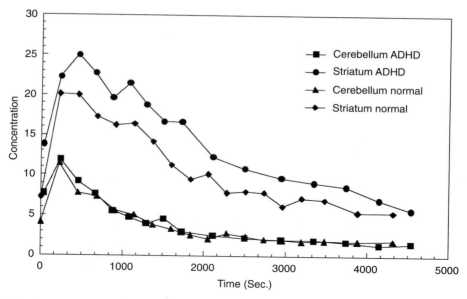

Figure 21.5. Concentration of ^{11}C-altropane in the striatum, and in the reference region (cerebellum) in a healthy volunteer and in an attention-deficit/hyperactivity disorder (ADHD) patient. There is increased striatal binding in ADHD.

the cause of the disorder or is a reflective compensatory mechanism (49). It has been shown, however, that methylphenidate treatment downregulates the elevated DAT density in these patients (52,53).

The DAT has also been associated with substance abuse (54). It has been shown that the degree of DAT blockade correlates positively with self-reported "high" following intravenous administration of cocaine or methylphenidate. Further, the abuse potential and dependency on these substances depends on the rate of DAT blockade. The incidence of dependency is greater if the blockade is faster. This is the reason why oral methylphenidate has lower abuse potential than cocaine administered parentally (55).

Changes in DAT expression have been reported in a number of other disorders including dementia with Lewy bodies, Wilson's disease, Tourette's syndrome, and Lesch-Nyhan disease (44). The role of DAT in pathogenesis of these diseases, however, is uncertain because of a limited number of studies.

Molecular imaging of the DAT has been used to elucidate the mechanism of actions of drugs that alter dopaminergic transmission. These studies have indicated that amphetamine promotes reverse transport of dopamine by internalizing DAT and making it available to intracellular dopamine, which is transported to the extracellular space. The internalization causes decrease in DAT activity (B_{max}) on the cell surface. Cocaine, on the other hand, blocks the amphetamine-induced internalization and increases DAT expression, but it also attenuates DAT activity (56,57). Further, it has been shown that methamphetamine causes degeneration of dopamine nerve terminals, resulting in the loss of DAT binding in multiple brain regions (58–60).

Serotonergic System

A number of radioligands have been developed to study serotonin [5-hydroxytryptamine ($5HT_{2A}$ and $5HT_{1A}$)] and serotonin transporter (SERT) activities. Commonly used ligands for serotonin receptors include ^{11}C-WAY 100635, ^{18}F-seroperone, and SERT ligands including ^{11}C-McN5652, ^{123}I-ADAM, and ^{11}C-DASB.

Abnormal serotonin transmission has been implicated in a number of disorders, including major depression, epilepsy, and schizophrenia (61). Serotonergic receptors have been studied extensively to understand epileptic processes because they are believed to mediate antiepileptic and anticonvulsive effects through $5HT_{1A}$ receptors located in the limbic area (62,63). Antiepileptic effect of serotonin is supported by studies that have found reduced binding of serotonin ligands (^{18}F-MPPF and ^{18}F-WAY) in epileptic zones of patients, as compared to the binding in the same areas of healthy controls. Further, the reduction is strongly correlated with the degree of epileptic activity (62,63). These results, however, are different from studies that have used a tryptophan (a serotonin precursor) derivative AMT, as ligand. These studies have found higher binding in the hippocampus of temporal lobe epilepsy (TLE) patients (64). Because AMT binding is positively correlated with the number of serotonergic neurons, it appears that receptor availability is reduced in epilepsy, even though there is an increase in serotonergic neurons.

Another disorder that has been studied using serotonergic receptor imaging is major depression in which reduced uptake of the ligand ^{11}C-WAY 100635 is found in the cingulate, hippocampus, and midbrain of depressed patients (65).

Studies that have used specific SERT ligands have not yielded definitive results because of their high nonspecific binding and slow clearance. These studies, however, have found lower binding of ^{11}C-McN5652, and ^{11}C-DASB in multiple brain regions, most significantly in the striatal and limbic regions of depressed patients (61). Many investigators have studied the SERT using nonspecific transporter ligands. These studies have reported reduced binding of ^{123}I-β-CIT in mood disorders (66).

Other Neurotransmitter Systems

γ-Aminobutyric Acid

γ-Aminobutyric acid (GABA) is the most abundant inhibitory transmitter in the central nervous system and is distributed throughout the brain (2). A benzodiazepine derivative ^{11}C-flumazenil (FMZ) has been used as a ligand to study GABA receptor activity in a variety of disorders that are associated with changes in GABAergic transmission. These disorders include schizophrenia, Huntington's disease, Alzheimer's disease, and epilepsy (67–75). Because GABA receptors are considered markers of neuronal loss (76), ^{11}C-FMZ has been used to evaluate hippocampal atrophy in TLE by a number of investigators (77–79). These investigators have found that FMZ binding is a sensitive localizer of the regions of epileptic foci in intractable TLE. The localization of epileptic zones is more precise with FMZ than with FDG (80). Because resection of the areas of FMZ abnormalities is associated with excellent outcome, it is recommended that imaging studies using ^{11}C-FMZ-PET be performed as a part of the routine surgical evaluation of TLE. In epileptic patients, the extent of FMZ-PET abnormalities correlates positively with the seizure frequency and duration of interictal period. Further, these abnormalities are corrected after surgery (81,82).

Opiate Receptors

The three types of opiate receptors (μ, κ, and δ) are widely distributed in human brain. These receptors are involved in many pathologic conditions, including, addiction, Alzheimer's disease, and epilepsy (83). A number of ligands are available for studying these receptors in humans (e.g., ^{11}C-carfentanil, ^{11}C-diprenorphine, ^{11}C-buprenorphine, ^{18}F-cyclofoxy, ^{11}C-naltrindole, and ^{11}C-GR103545). Receptor imaging studies have shown that opiate receptors mediate addictive behavior by either stimulating (μ receptors) or inhibiting (κ receptors) the striatal dopamine system. Thus, high density of μ receptors in the striatum is associated with alcohol dependence and craving (84). In Alzheimer's disease, the binding of both μ and κ receptors is decreased (85). Binding studies in epileptic patients have yielded variable results. Although no change in opiate receptor density is found, if a nonspecific opiate receptor ligand ^{11}C-diprenorphine is used, studies with the specific μ-receptor ligand ^{11}C-carfentanil are associated with increased binding at epileptic foci (86). It has also been shown that, after surgical removal of epileptic foci, the opiate receptors downregulate (87).

Norepinephrine

Alterations in the noradrenergic system have been reported in a number psychiatric disorders including depression and posttraumatic stress disorder. This system is also altered in Parkinson's and Alzheimer's disease (88). Most studies of norepinephrine neurotransmission have used ligands that bind to the norepinephrine transporter (NET), which is located on presynaptic noradrenergic neurons. Because of their location in presynaptic neurons, NET activity is considered an indicator of the density of norepinephrinergic neurons. A number of ligands have been developed to study the NET. These ligands include ^{11}C-talopram and ^{11}C-talsupram. Because the NET represents an important target for a number of psychoactive compounds including some antidepressants and drugs of abuse, NET ligands may play an important role in the study of pathophysiology and pharmacotherapy of neuropsychiatric disorders. Alterations of the noradrenergic system have been reported in depressed patients and in postmortem brain tissue obtained from these patients (89). Further, decreased NET density is observed in the locus ceruleus of depressed individuals who committed suicide (90). Although the involvement of the noradrenergic system in mood disorders is well established, a unifying theory regarding the role of this system in depression has remained elusive. Imaging agents that evaluate NET activity can be a useful tool for clarifying the role of noradrenergic system in major depression. However, because the brain uptake of current NET ligands is very low, their application in neurotransmitter imaging is limited.

Acetylcholine

Cholinergic ligands are selective for either muscarinic or nicotinic receptors. Nicotinic receptors have been studied using ^{11}C-nicotine and its derivatives. These studies have reported significant reduction (up to 50%) in the binding of these ligands in Alzheimer's patients (67). The degree of reduction corresponds to the severity of cognitive impairment (68,69). Further, it has been shown that increase in receptor density (following treatment) correlates well with improvement in cognitive abilities of these patients (70). Because cholinergic receptor density parallels cognitive abilities, tracers that bind either to nicotinic or muscarinic receptors can be used to detect early Alzheimer's disease. This condition can also be detected using tracers (e.g., ^{11}C-MP4A-PET) that image acetylcholinesterase activity (71).

Dynamic Receptor Imaging

The models used in conventional receptor imaging assume a steady state in which there is no change in synaptic concentration of endogenous neurotransmitter during the study. Therefore, these models cannot be used to detect acute changes in the amount of neurotransmitter released in response to a challenge, unless two separate scans (before and after the challenge) are performed. Separate scans, however, significantly reduce sensitivity and do not measure the gradient of change in neurotransmitter release. The conventional models, therefore, have been modified to allow detection of acute changes in neurotransmitter release. The modified models are particularly useful for the study of neurotransmission associated with a cognitive or behavioral task because these studies require comparison of the activated and control states and assume a change in the state during task performance.

A number of simulation studies have been performed to evaluate the ability of these models to detect task-induced dynamic changes in synaptic concentration of neurotransmitters (91,92). These models prompted Koepp and colleagues to conduct an experiment and demonstrate that the BP of a dopamine ligand, raclopride, decreases significantly during performance of a goal-directed activity (11). The model used in this study, however, assumed a steady state. Consequently, the experiment was performed in two separate scan sessions. In one session, *BP* was measured while the volunteers were in the activated state (playing a video game). In the other, it was measured during a "no-activation" control condition. A comparison of *BP* measured in the two sessions indicated that dopamine is released during the task performance and that the release can induce measurable displacement of the ligand from receptor sites (93,94). However, because this method required two separate scan sessions, it is not considered sensitive enough to isolate changes induced by finer cognitive activities like memory and attention (5). Cognitive and behavioral studies are considered more sensitive if the two measurements are made in the same session. This issue was addressed to some extent by the development of a method for assessment of time-dependent changes in ligand displacement (95). This method allowed detection of ligand displacement in a single scan session. Using this approach, striatal dopamine release was detected during reward processing in healthy volunteers (12). In this experiment the rate of ligand displacement was increased relative to the rate observed in a control (no activation) task performed by a different group of volunteers. Moreover, the pattern of ligand displacement during activation was modeled using simulations. Because the control data were not specific to the subjects studied and the rate of ligand displacement was not derived from real data, the approach of this study was not ideal.

This approach was modified by designing a method based on the simplified reference region model (96). In the modified method, an activation parameter was included in the model to quantify change in the rate of ligand displacement during task performance (5,9). By not assuming a steady state, this model allowed for fluctuations in synaptic concentration of endogenous transmitter. Using the data from a reference region (cerebellum) to estimate the effect of arterial input function (96), we explicitly modeled the kinetics of ligand delivery, receptor binding and dissociation, and the competition of ligand and endogenous neurotransmitter for the receptor. The solution of the differential equation of the model for the instantaneous concentration history of the tracer has the following form:

$$PET(t) = R \cdot C_R(t) + k_2 \int_0^t C_R(u)du - k_{2a} \int_0^t PET(u)du$$
$$- \gamma \int_0^t v(u-T)e^{-\tau(u-T)} PET(u)du$$

where C_R is the concentration of radioligand in a region devoid of specific binding (reference region), *PET* is the concentration of radioligand in a region with specific binding, *R* is the ratio of transport rates for the binding and reference regions, k_2 describes the clearance of nonspecifically bound tracer, k_{2a} includes the information about dissociation from the receptor, γ represents the amplitude of transient effects, *t* denotes the measurement time, *T* is the task initiation time, and

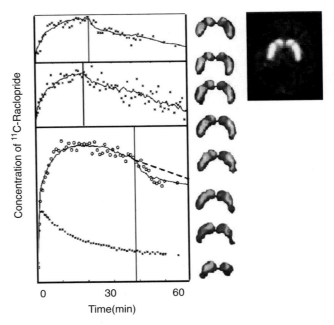

Figure 21.6. Changes in the rate of displacement of ^{11}C-raclopride in the left putamen during a motor planning task in healthy volunteers. The vertical lines indicate the time of task initiation, and the lowest line depicts displacement in a reference region (cerebellum). The figure also shows horizontal sections of the striatum from dorsal to ventral aspect in 2.4-mm steps (left striatum on the right). The *t*-map showing areas of significant changes ($t > 3.0$) in the rate of displacement is superimposed on the binding potential map (inset).

$v(u - T)$ is the unit step function. Positive values of γ represent task-related ligand displacement. Using this model we demonstrated the release of striatal dopamine during the performance of a variety of behavioral and cognitive tasks (Fig. 21.6). These tasks included motor planning, implicit motor memory, explicit motor memory and explicit cued recall (5–10).

The dynamic receptor imaging method, at its current stage of development, has a number of limitations. It is not able to detect dopamine if the task induces release of a relatively small amount of neurotransmitter. Simulation experiments suggest that the method can detect dopamine release only if the change is >30% of baseline. The sensitivity of the method, however, can be enhanced by optimization of the signal-to-noise ratio (using advanced signal processing techniques). It can be further enhanced by averaging the data acquired from a cohort of subjects. Another limitation of the method is its inability to detect dopamine released in extrastriatal regions of the brain. Two newer ligands have kinetic properties that should favor detection of dopamine in the extrastriatal areas. These ligands are ^{18}F-fallypride and ^{11}C-FLB 457 (isoremoxipride). Experiments conducted on human volunteers and laboratory animals suggest that both of these ligands have high affinity for extrastriatal receptors and are displaced from the receptor sites by amphetamine-induced dopamine release (27,97,98).

Even though dynamic receptor imaging has so far been used only for detection of striatal dopamine, it is theoretically possible to develop ligands that can detect release of other neurotransmitters in other brain areas. Such developments will go a long way in enhancing our understanding of human cognitive control.

Conclusion

Neurotransmitter imaging has resulted in a considerable amount of new information concerning the pathogenesis of a number of neurologic and psychiatric conditions that include schizophrenia, addiction, Parkinson's disease, Alzheimer's disease, ADHD, epilepsy, anxiety, and affective disorders. Further, the use of these techniques in the diagnoses of subclinical Alzheimer's and Parkinson's disease in asymptomatic patients can help in early diagnosis and intervention. In addition, localization of epileptic foci by GABA receptor imaging has been shown to improve postsurgical clinical outcome. Neurotransmitter imaging for drug evaluation has aided in the development of new compounds that target specific receptors that are dysregulated in various disorders. Evolving molecular imaging techniques, like dynamic receptor imaging, offer even more exciting possibilities. These techniques can identify and localize areas of the brain where specific neurotransmitters are released during a task performance or symptom provocation. It will greatly expand our understanding of the fundamental alterations in neurochemistry in psychiatric and neurologic disorders. In addition, these methods will provide empirical data that can be used to formulate novel therapeutic strategies for treatment and prevention of the disorders that are associated with altered neurotransmission.

References

1. Jacobs AH, Li H, Winkeler A, et al. PET-based molecular imaging in neuroscience. Eur J Nucl Med Mol Imaging 2003;30:1051–1065.
2. Blankenberg FG. Molecular imaging: the latest generation of contrast agents and tissue characterization techniques. J Cell Biochem 2003;90: 443–453.
3. Gjedde A, Wong DF, Rosa-Neto P, Cumming P. Mapping neuroreceptors at work: on the definition and interpretation of binding potentials after 20 years of progress. Int Rev Neurobiol 2005;63:1–20.
4. Laruelle M. Imaging synaptic neurotransmission with in vivo binding competition techniques: a critical review. J Cereb Blood Flow Metab 2000; 20:423–451.
5. Alpert NM, Badgaiyan RD, Livini E, Fischman AJ. A novel method for noninvasive detection of neuromodulatory changes in specific neurotransmitter systems. NeuroImage 2003;19:1049–1060.

6. Badgaiyan RD, Alpert NM, Fischman AJ. Detection of striatal dopamine release during an implicit motor memory task. Annual meeting of the Society of Nuclear Medicine, Philadelphia, 2004.

7. Badgaiyan RD, Alpert NM, Fischman AJ. Detection of striatal dopamine released during an explicit motor memory task. Annual meeting of the Society of Nuclear Medicine, Toronto, 2005.

8. Badgaiyan RD, Alpert NM, Fischman AJ. Detection of striatal dopamine release during a motor planning task in human volunteers. Brain'03, XXIst International Symposium on Cerebral Blood Flow, Metabolism and Function (abstract 706). Calgarg, 2003.

9. Badgaiyan RD, Fischman AJ, Alpert NM. Striatal dopamine release during unrewarded motor task in human volunteers. NeuroReport 2003;14:1421–1424.

10. Badgaiyan RD, Fischman AJ, Alpert NM. Striatal dopamine release during unrewarded motor task in human volunteers. Neuroreport 2003;14:1421–1424.

11. Koepp MJ, Gunn RN, Lawrence AD, et al. Evidence for striatal dopamine release during a video game. Nature 1998;393:266–268.

12. Pappata S, Dehaene S, Poline JB, et al. In vivo detection of striatal dopamine release during reward: a PET study with ((11)C)raclopride and a single dynamic scan approach. NeuroImage 2002;16:1015–1027.

13. Morris ED, Alpert NM, Fischman AJ. Comparison of two compartmental models for describing receptor ligand kinetics and receptor availability in multiple injection PET studies. J Cereb Blood Flow Metab 1996;16:841–853.

14. Choy G, Choyke P, Libutti SK. Current advances in molecular imaging: noninvasive in vivo bioluminescent and fluorescent optical imaging in cancer research. Mol Imaging 2003;2:303–312.

15. Maria Moresco R, Messa C, Lucignani G, et al. PET in psychopharmacology. Pharmacol Res 2001;44:151–159.

16. Wagner HNJ, Dannals RF, Frost JJ, et al. Imaging neuroreceptors in the human brain in health and disease. Radioisotopes 1985;34:103–107.

17. Wong DF, Gjedde A, Wagner HNJ. Quantification of neuroreceptors in the living human brain. I. Irreversible binding of ligands. J Cereb Blood Flow Metab 1986;6:137–146.

18. Wong DF, Young D, Wilson PD, Meltzer CC, Gjedde A. Quantification of neuroreceptors in the living human brain: III. D2–like dopamine receptors: theory, validation, and changes during normal aging. J Cereb Blood Flow Metab 1997;17:316–330.

19. Mintun MA, Raichle ME, Kilbourn MR, Wooten GF, Welch MJ. A quantitative model for the in vivo assessment of drug binding sites with positron emission tomography. Ann Neurol 1984;15:217–227.

20. Laruelle M, al-Tikriti MS, Zea-Ponce Y, et al. In vivo quantification of dopamine D2 receptor parameters in nonhuman primates with (123I)iodobenzofuran and single photon emission computerized tomography. Eur J Pharmacol 1994;263:39–51.

21. Saelens JK, Simke JP, Neale SE, Weeks BJ, Selwyn M. Effects of haloperidol and d-amphetamine on in vivo 3H-spiroperiodol binding in the rat forebrain (1). Arch Int Pharmacodyn Ther 1980;246:98–107.

22. Chugani DC, Ackermann RF, Phelps ME. In vivo (3H)spiperone binding: evidence for accumulation in corpus striatum by agonist-mediated receptor internalization. J Cereb Blood Flow Metab 1988;8:291–303.

23. Laruelle M, Huang Y. Vulnerability of positron emission tomography radiotracers to endogenous competition. New insights. Q J Nucl Med 2001;45:124–138.

24. Christian BT, Narayanan TK, Shi B, Mukherjee J. Quantitation of striatal and extrastriatal D-2 dopamine receptors using PET imaging of ((18)F) fallypride in nonhuman primates. Synapse 2000;38:71–79.
25. de Paulis T. The discovery of epidepride and its analogs as high-affinity radioligands for imaging extrastriatal dopamine D(2) receptors in human brain. Curr Pharm Des 2003;9:673–696.
26. Mukherjee J, Christian BT, Dunigan KA, et al. Brain imaging of 18F-fallypride in normal volunteers: Blood analysis, distribution, test-retest studies, and preliminary assessment of sensitivity to aging effects on dopamine D-2/D-3 receptors. Synapse 2002;46:170–188.
27. Mukherjee J, Christian BT, Narayanan TK, Shi B, Collins D. Measurement of d-amphetamine-induced effects on the binding of dopamine D-2/D-3 receptor radioligand, 18F-fallypride in extrastriatal brain regions in nonhuman primates using PET. Brain Res 2005;1032:77–84.
28. Abi-Dargham A. Do we still believe in the dopamine hypothesis? New data bring new evidence. Int J Neuropsychopharmacol 2004;7(suppl 1):S1–5.
29. Wong DF, Wagner HNJ, Tune LE, et al. Positron emission tomography reveals elevated D2 dopamine receptors in drug-naive schizophrenics. Science 1986;234:1558–1563.
30. Marzella PL, Hill C, Keks N, Singh B, Copolov D. The binding of both (3H)nemonapride and (3H)raclopride is increased in schizophrenia. Biol Psychiatry 1997;42:648–654.
31. Farde L, Wiesel FA, Stone-Elander S, et al. D2 dopamine receptors in neuroleptic-naive schizophrenic patients. A positron emission tomography study with (11C)raclopride. Arch Gen Psychiatry 1990;47:213–219.
32. Guo N, Hwang DR, Lo ES, Huang YY, Laruelle M, Abi-Dargham A. Dopamine depletion and in vivo binding of PET D1 receptor radioligands: implications for imaging studies in schizophrenia. Neuropsychopharmacology 2003;28:1703–1711.
33. Seeman P. Brain dopamine receptors in schizophrenia: PET problems. Arch Gen Psychiatry 1988;45(6):598–600.
34. Seeman P, Guan HC, Niznik HB. Endogenous dopamine lowers the dopamine D2 receptor density as measured by (3H)raclopride: implications for positron emission tomography of the human brain. Synapse 1989;3:96–97.
35. Xu ZC, Ling G, Sahr RN, Neal-Beliveau BS. Asymmetrical changes of dopamine receptors in the striatum after unilateral dopamine depletion. Brain Res 2005;1038:163–170.
36. Laruelle M. The role of endogenous sensitization in the pathophysiology of schizophrenia: implications from recent brain imaging studies. Brain Res Brain Res Rev 2000;31:371–384.
37. Breier A, Su TP, Saunders R, et al. Schizophrenia is associated with elevated amphetamine-induced synaptic dopamine concentrations: evidence from a novel positron emission tomography method. Proc Natl Acad Sci U S A 1997;94:2569–2574.
38. Laruelle M, Abi-Dargham A, van Dyck CH, et al. Single photon emission computerized tomography imaging of amphetamine-induced dopamine release in drug-free schizophrenic subjects. Proc Natl Acad Sci U S A 1996;93:9235–9240.
39. Abi-Dargham A, Gil R, Krystal J, et al. Increased striatal dopamine transmission in schizophrenia: confirmation in a second cohort. Am J Psychiatry 1998;155:761–767.
40. Laruelle M, Abi-Dargham A, Gil R, Kegeles L, Innis R. Increased dopamine transmission in schizophrenia: relationship to illness phases. Biol Psychiatry 1999;46:56–72.

41. Voruganti L, Slomka P, Zabel P, et al. Subjective effects of AMPT-induced dopamine depletion in schizophrenia: correlation between dysphoric responses and striatal D(2) binding ratios on SPECT imaging. Neuropsychopharmacology 2001;25:642–650.

42. Fischman AJ. Role of (18F)-dopa-PET imaging in assessing movement disorders. Radiol Clin North Am 2005;43:93–106.

43. McGowan S, Lawrence AD, Sales T, Quested D, Grasby P. Presynaptic dopaminergic dysfunction in schizophrenia: a positron emission tomographic (18F)fluorodopa study. Arch Gen Psychiatry 2004;61:134–142.

44. Bannon MJ. The dopamine transporter: role in neurotoxicity and human disease. Toxicol Appl Pharmacol 2005;204:355–360.

45. Fischman AJ, Bonab AA, Babich JW, et al. Rapid detection of Parkinson's disease by SPECT with altropane: a selective ligand for dopamine transporters. Synapse 1998;29:128–141.

46. Lee CS, Samii A, Sossi V, et al. In vivo positron emission tomographic evidence for compensatory changes in presynaptic dopaminergic nerve terminals in Parkinson's disease. Ann Neurol 2000;47:493–503.

47. Marshall V, Grosset D. Role of dopamine transporter imaging in routine clinical practice. Mov Disord 2003;18:1415–1423.

48. DiMaio S, Grizenko N, Joober R. Dopamine genes and attention-deficit hyperactivity disorder: a review. J Psychiatry Neurosci 2003;28:27–38.

49. Madras BK, Miller GM, Fischman AJ. The dopamine transporter: relevance to attention deficit hyperactivity disorder (ADHD). Behav Brain Res 2002;130:57–63.

50. Dougherty DD, Bonab AA, Spencer TJ, Rauch SL, Madras BK, Fischman AJ. Dopamine transporter density in patients with attention deficit hyperactivity disorder. Lancet 1999;354(9196):2132–2133.

51. Cheon KA, Ryu YH, Kim YK, Namkoong K, Kim CH, Lee JD. Dopamine transporter density in the basal ganglia assessed with (123I)IPT SPET in children with attention deficit hyperactivity disorder. Eur J Nucl Med Mol Imaging 2003;30:306–311.

52. Dresel S, Krause J, Krause KH, et al. Attention deficit hyperactivity disorder: binding of (99mTc)TRODAT-1 to the dopamine transporter before and after methylphenidate treatment. Eur J Nucl Med 2000;27:1518–1524.

53. Vles JS, Feron FJ, Hendriksen JG, Jolles J, van Kroonenburgh MJ, Weber WE. Methylphenidate down-regulates the dopamine receptor and transporter system in children with attention deficit hyperkinetic disorder (ADHD). Neuropediatrics 2003;34:77–80.

54. Volkow ND, Wang GJ, Fowler JS, et al. Cardiovascular effects of methylphenidate in humans are associated with increases of dopamine in brain and of epinephrine in plasma. Psychopharmacology (Berl) 2003; 166:264–270.

55. Volkow ND, Fowler JS, Wang GJ, Goldstein RZ. Role of dopamine, the frontal cortex and memory circuits in drug addiction: insight from imaging studies. Neurobiol Learn Mem 2002;78:610–624.

56. Daws LC, Callaghan PD, Moron JA, et al. Cocaine increases dopamine uptake and cell surface expression of dopamine transporters. Biochem Biophys Res Commun 2002;290:1545–1550.

57. Kahlig KM, Binda F, Khoshbouei H, et al. Amphetamine induces dopamine efflux through a dopamine transporter channel. Proc Natl Acad Sci U S A 2005;102:3495–3500.

58. Volkow ND, Chang L, Wang GJ, et al. Loss of dopamine transporters in methamphetamine abusers recovers with protracted abstinence. J Neurosci 2001;21:9414–9418.

59. McCann UD, Wong DF, Yokoi F, Villemagne V, Dannals RF, Ricaurte GA. Reduced striatal dopamine transporter density in abstinent methamphetamine and methcathinone users: evidence from positron emission tomography studies with (11C)WIN-35,428. J Neurosci 1998;18:8417–8422.

60. Wilson JM, Kalasinsky KS, Levey AI, et al. Striatal dopamine nerve terminal markers in human, chronic methamphetamine users. Nat Med 1996;2: 699–703.

61. Parsey RV, Mann JJ. Applications of positron emission tomography in psychiatry. Semin Nucl Med 2003;33:129–135.

62. Merlet I, Ostrowsky K, Costes N, et al. 5–HT1A receptor binding and intracerebral activity in temporal lobe epilepsy: an (18F)MPPF-PET study. Brain 2004;127:900–913.

63. Toczek MT, Carson RE, Lang L, et al. PET imaging of 5–HT1A receptor binding in patients with temporal lobe epilepsy. Neurology 2003;60: 749–756.

64. Juhasz C, Chugani DC, Muzik O, et al. Alpha-methyl-L-tryptophan PET detects epileptogenic cortex in children with intractable epilepsy. Neurology 2003;60:960–968.

65. Farde L, Ginovart N, Ito H, et al. PET-characterization of (carbonyl-11C)WAY-100635 binding to 5–HT1A receptors in the primate brain. Psychopharmacology (Berl) 1997;133:196–202.

66. Parsey RV, Mann JJ. Applications of positron emission tomography in psychiatry. Semin Nucl Med 2003;33:129–135.

67. Sihver W, Langstrom B, Nordberg A. Ligands for in vivo imaging of nicotinic receptor subtypes in Alzheimer brain. Acta Neurol Scand Suppl 2000;176:27–33.

68. Nordberg A, Hartvig P, Lilja A, et al. Decreased uptake and binding of 11C-nicotine in brain of Alzheimer patients as visualized by positron emission tomography. J Neural Transm Park Dis Dement Sect 1990;2:215–224.

69. Nordberg A, Lundqvist H, Hartvig P, Lilja A, Langstrom B. Kinetic analysis of regional (S)(-)11C-nicotine binding in normal and Alzheimer brains— in vivo assessment using positron emission tomography. Alzheimer Dis Assoc Disord 1995;9:21–27.

70. Nordberg A, Amberla K, Shigeta M, et al. Long-term tacrine treatment in three mild Alzheimer patients: effects on nicotinic receptors, cerebral blood flow, glucose metabolism, EEG, and cognitive abilities. Alzheimer Dis Assoc Disord 1998;12:228–237.

71. Yoshida T, Kuwabara Y, Ichiya Y, et al. Cerebral muscarinic acetylcholinergic receptor measurement in Alzheimer's disease patients on 11C-N-methyl-4—piperidyl benzilate—comparison with cerebral blood flow and cerebral glucose metabolism. Ann Nucl Med 1998;12:35–42.

72. Maziere M, Hantraye P, Prenant C, Sastre J, Comar D. Synthesis of ethyl 8–fluoro-5,6–dihydro-5–(11C)methyl-6-oxo-4H-imidazo (1,5–a) (1,4)benzodiazepine-3-carboxylate (RO 15.1788–11C): a specific radioligand for the in vivo study of central benzodiazepine receptors by positron emission tomography. Int J Appl Radiat Isot 1984;35:973–976.

73. Hammers A. Flumazenil positron emission tomography and other ligands for functional imaging. Neuroimaging Clin North Am 2004;14:537–551.

74. Matheja P, Ludemann P, Kuwert T, et al. Disturbed benzodiazepine receptor function at the onset of temporal lobe epilepsy—lomanzenil-binding in de-novo TLE. J Neurol 2001;248:585–591.

75. Mitterhauser M, Wadsak W, Wabnegger L, et al. Biological evaluation of 2'-(18F)fluoroflumazenil ((18F)FFMZ), a potential GABA receptor ligand for PET. Nucl Med Biol 2004;31:291–295.

76. Heiss WD, Graf R, Fujita T, Ohta K, Bauer B, Lottgen J, Wienhard K. Early detection of irreversibly damaged ischemic tissue by flumazenil positron emission tomography in cats. Stroke 1997;28:2045–2051; discussion 2051–2052.

77. Savic I, Pauli S, Thorell JO, Blomqvist G. In vivo demonstration of altered benzodiazepine receptor density in patients with generalised epilepsy. J Neurol Neurosurg Psychiatry 1994;57:797–804.

78. Koepp MJ, Richardson MP, Brooks DJ, et al. Cerebral benzodiazepine receptors in hippocampal sclerosis. An objective in vivo analysis. Brain 1996;119:1677–1687.

79. Debets RM, Sadzot B, van Isselt JW, et al. Is 11C-flumazenil PET superior to 18FDG PET and 123I-iomazenil SPECT in presurgical evaluation of temporal lobe epilepsy? J Neurol Neurosurg Psychiatry 1997;62:141–150.

80. Juhasz C, Chugani DC, Muzik O, et al. Relationship of flumazenil and glucose PET abnormalities to neocortical epilepsy surgery outcome. Neurology 2001;56:1650–1658.

81. Bouvard S, Costes N, Bonnefoi F, et al. Seizure-related short-term plasticity of benzodiazepine receptors in partial epilepsy: a (11C)flumazenil-PET study. Brain 2005;128:1330–1343.

82. Savic I, Svanborg E, Thorell JO. Cortical benzodiazepine receptor changes are related to frequency of partial seizures: a positron emission tomography study. Epilepsia 1996;37:236–244.

83. Machulla HJ, Heinz A. Radioligands for brain imaging of the kappa-opioid system. J Nucl Med 2005;46:386–387.

84. Bencherif B, Wand GS, McCaul ME, et al. Mu-opioid receptor binding measured by (11C)carfentanil positron emission tomography is related to craving and mood in alcohol dependence. Biol Psychiatry 2004;55:255–262.

85. Cohen RM, Andreason PJ, Doudet DJ, Carson RE, Sunderland T. Opiate receptor avidity and cerebral blood flow in Alzheimer's disease. J Neurol Sci 1997;148:171–180.

86. Prevett MC, Cunningham VJ, Brooks DJ, Fish DR, Duncan JS. Opiate receptors in idiopathic generalised epilepsy measured with (11C)diprenorphine and positron emission tomography. Epilepsy Res 1994;19:71–77.

87. Bartenstein PA, Prevett MC, Duncan JS, Hajek M, Wieser HG. Quantification of opiate receptors in two patients with mesiobasal temporal lobe epilepsy, before and after selective amygdalohippocampectomy, using positron emission tomography. Epilepsy Res 1994;18:119–125.

88. McConathy J, Owens MJ, Kilts CD, et al. Synthesis and biological evaluation of (11C)talopram and (11C)talsupram: candidate PET ligands for the norepinephrine transporter. Nucl Med Biol 2004;31:705–718.

89. Ressler KJ, Nemeroff CB. Role of norepinephrine in the pathophysiology of neuropsychiatric disorders. CNS Spectr 2001;6:663–666, 670.

90. Klimek V, Stockmeier C, Overholser J, et al. Reduced levels of norepinephrine transporters in the locus coeruleus in major depression. J Neurosci 1997;17:8451–8458.

91. Morris ED, Fisher RE, Alpert NM, Rauch SL, Fischman AJ. In vivo imaging of neuromodulation using positron emission tomography: optimal ligand characteristics and task length for detection of activation. Hum Brain Map 1995;3:35–55.

92. Fisher RE, Morris ED, Alpert NM, Fischman AJ. In vivo imaging of neuromodulatory synaptic transmission using PET: A review of relevant neurophysiology. Hum Brain Map 1995;3:24–34.

93. Dewey SL, MacGregor RR, Brodie JD, et al. Mapping muscarinic receptors in human and baboon brain using (N-11C- methyl)-benztropine. Synapse 1990;5:213–223.

94. Seeman P, Guan HC, Niznik HB. Endogenous dopamine lowers the dopamine D2 receptor density as measured by (3H)raclopride: implications for positron emission tomography of the human brain. Synapse 1989;3:96–97.

95. Friston KJ, Malizia AL, Wilson S, Cunningham VJ, Jones T, Nutt DJ. Analysis of dynamic radioligand displacement or "activation" studies. J Cereb Blood Flow Metab 1997;17:80–93.

96. Gunn RN, Lammertsma AA, Hume SP, Cunningham VJ. Parametric imaging of ligand-receptor binding in PET using a simplified reference region model. Neuroimage 1997;6:279–287.

97. Mukherjee J, Yang ZY, Lew R, et al. Evaluation of d-amphetamine effects on the binding of dopamine D-2 receptor radioligand, 18F-fallypride in nonhuman primates using positron emission tomography. Synapse 1997; 27:1–13.

98. Chou YH, Halldin C, Farde L. Effect of amphetamine on extrastriatal D2 dopamine receptor binding in the primate brain: a PET study. Synapse 2000;38:138–143.

Section 4

Other Applications

22

Cardiovascular Applications

Miguel Hernandez-Pampaloni

An improved understanding of the pathophysiology of myocardial ischemia combined with the development of new diagnostic modalities has substantially modified the concepts of myocardial blood flow (MBF) and left ventricular function in coronary artery disease (CAD). Positron emission tomography (PET) has emerged as a unique tool to characterize physiologic and pathologic processes, and it already plays a significant role in different areas of clinical medicine, including cardiology. Cardiac PET is based on the properties of positron emitters and radiation detection to provide a noninvasive and in vivo assessment of regional myocardial perfusion and metabolism. Different study protocols have been largely used in the adult population to detect and grade the severity of coronary artery disease during the last two decades using cardiac PET technology. Further, cardiac PET using fluorine-18 (^{18}F) 2-fluoro-2-deoxyglucose (FDG) is considered the gold standard imaging modality for the assessment of myocardial viability (1) and is well recognized as providing accurate information on the long-term prognosis of the patients with chronic coronary ischemic disease (2).

Positron emission tomography offers unique capabilities for noninvasive assessment of regional myocardial function and can disclose information of utmost importance for the more accurate understanding of pathophysiologic processes and for the optimal management of the diseased patient. By detecting the very early functional regional abnormalities before the development of more severe structural changes, PET imaging can be useful in providing improved and preventive care to the patient. Thus, cardiac PET imaging can offer a more comprehensive understanding of the normal myocardial physiology and early recognition of functional abnormalities. This is even more important in pediatric cardiology where the early detection of myocardial dysfunction may be helpful in choosing the appropriate management for the prevention of long-term consequences. Recent surgical and technical advances in pediatric cardiology make even more important an accurate detection of potentially treatable coronary abnormalities. Positron emission tomography imaging's high spatial and temporal resolution provides better image quality, especially important in small pediatric hearts, and it allows the quantification in absolute terms of the MBF and regional myocardial metabolism. Single photon emission computed tomography (SPECT) imaging quality is usually limited by poor resolution and the low usable activity of thallium 201 (^{201}Tl), whereas images obtained after the administration of technetium-labeled compounds are compromised by the high liver activity in close proximity to the small heart.

This chapter describes the basic principles of PET applied to the study of the heart, and presents the current and potential future clinical applications of cardiac PET in pediatric patients.

Principles of Emission Tomography Applied to the Cardiovascular System

Positron emission tomography imaging features are based on the physical properties of the positron decay. A positron has the same characteristics as an electron, except for its positive charge. Positrons are emitted from unstable nuclei (that have an excess of protons) that dispose of their excess charge by emitting a positron. At the end of the positron range, after losing its kinetic energy, a positron combines with an electron and the two particles annihilate. The annihilation coincidence detection of the two colinear 511-keV gamma rays photons, emitted in diametrically opposite directions by opposing scintillator detectors, is the essence of the PET imaging formation (3). To detect the location of the annihilation event, detectors are placed on opposite sides of the source and are connected in a coincidence detection circuit. When a given event is recorded simultaneously, positron annihilation is assumed to have taken place on the line between the detectors, and hence the location can be accurately determined.

Radiopharmaceuticals

Cardiac PET studies are performed with radiopharmaceuticals specifically synthesized to assess determined cardiac functions or biochemical processes and with radiopharmaceuticals that have applications in other disciplines. The radiolabeled positron-emitting tracers used in cardiac PET studies are produced by a cyclotron or by a generator system. Currently, different processes of the heart have been studied using different radiopharmaceuticals (Table 22.1). The radiation exposure to PET radiotracers is lower compared to other radionuclides used for nuclear cardiology studies (Table 22.2).

Evaluation of Myocardial Blood Flow

The development of suitable radiotracers and appropriate mathematical models applied to PET imaging has been shown to allow for the noninvasive and accurate quantification of regional MBF. Different radiotracers have been used for measuring MBF, including nitrogen-13–labeled ammonia (^{13}NH$_3$) (4–6), oxygen-15 (^{15}O)-labeled water (^{15}O-

Table 22.1. Principal PET tracers for cardiac imaging

Radionuclide	Radiopharmaceutical	Physical half-life	Mean positron range	Production	Cardiac application
^{13}N	Ammonia	10.0 min	0.7 mm	Cyclotron	Blood flow
^{82}Rb	Rubidium chloride	78 s	2.6 mm	Generator	Blood flow
^{15}O	Water	2.0 min	1.1 mm	Cyclotron	Blood flow, perfusable tissue index
^{18}F	Deoxyglucose	110 min	0.2 mm	Cyclotron	Glucose metabolism
^{11}C	Acetate palmitate	20 min	0.28 mm	Cyclotron	Blood flow, oxygen consumption fatty acid metabolism

H_2O) (7–9), the potassium analogue rubidium-82 (^{82}Rb) (10), copper-62 (^{62}Cu)-pyruvaldehyde bis(N4-methylthio-semicarbazone (^{62}Cu-PTSM) (11,12), gallium-68 (^{68}Ga)-labeled albumin microspheres (13), and potassium 38 (^{38}K) (14). The choice of a specific radiotracer is finally frequently determined by different factors besides their physical properties, such as an individual institution's preference, experience, or accessibility. Currently, ^{13}NH$_3$, ^{15}O-H$_2$O, and ^{82}Rb are the most widely used PET perfusion tracers. Generator-produced ^{82}Rb has the advantages of not requiring a cyclotron and having a very short half-life (78 seconds), making it attractive for one-session rest/stress imaging. ^{82}Rb has a low first-pass myocardial extraction fraction (50% to 60%) that results in a nonlinear uptake in relation to blood flow, particularly at high flow rates (15). As a potassium analogue, ^{82}Rb is retained in the myocardium and equilibrates with the cellular potassium pool. Because of the dependence on the flow rate and the metabolic state,

Table 22.2. Dosimetry in cardiac pediatric nuclear medicine

	^{99m}Tc-sestamibi	^{201}Tl	^{13}N-ammonia	^{18}F-FDG
	Effective dose equivalent (mSv/MBq)			
Newborn (3.5 kg)	0.120	11.00	0.0320	0.310
1-yr-old (10 kg)	0.058	6.90	0.0130	0.100
5-yr-old (18 kg)	0.041	4.90	0.0067	0.077
10-yr-old (31 kg)	0.027	4.10	0.0043	0.050
15-yr-old (56 kg)	0.019	0.68	0.0028	0.038
Adult (70 kg)	0.015	0.34	0.0022	0.030
Critical organ	Kidney	Kidney	Bladder wall	Bladder wall
	Dose equivalent per body weight			
Newborn (3.5 kg)	0.89	12.22	0.34	1.64
1-yr-old (10 kg)	0.43	7.67	0.14	0.69
5-yr-old (18 kg)	0.30	5.44	0.07	0.41
10-yr-old (31 kg)	0.20	4.56	0.05	0.26
15-yr-old (56 kg)	0.14	0.76	0.03	0.20
Adult (70 kg)	0.11	0.38	0.02	0.16

Source: Modified from Radiopharmaceutical Internal Dose Information Center, Oak Ridge Associated Universities, Oak Ridge, Tennessee.

situations of hyperemia or metabolically impaired myocardium may limit the accuracy for quantifying MBF. $^{13}NH_3$ is a cyclotron-generated myocardial perfusion tracer with a high first-pass extraction fraction, a high tissue-to-blood contrast ratio within minutes following the radiotracer administration, and a relatively short half-life (9.8 minutes) that makes it also suitable for one-session studies. $^{13}NH_3$ is metabolically trapped in the myocardium based on the glutamine synthetase action. Under physiologic resting blood flow, the rate of metabolic conversion of $^{13}NH_3$ to glutamine inside the myocytes is sufficiently elevated to convert and retain a major fraction of $^{13}NH_3$ delivered to the myocardial tissue. However, in conditions of high flow, the amount of $^{13}NH_3$ delivered to the myocardial tissue exceeds the rate of conversion to glutamine, and therefore a significant amount of $^{13}NH_3$ is returned to the capillary blood and removed from the tissue. To overcome this nonlinear response to conditions of high flow rate, different kinetic modeling approaches have been developed (16,17). To minimize the limited spatial resolution of PET systems and the intrinsic motion of the heart, additional corrections have been included to account for the impact of the partial volume effect and spillover fraction (18,19).

^{15}O-H_2O has several attractive properties as a myocardial perfusion tracer including a high first-pass extraction fraction (nearly 100%), a freely diffusible uptake and washout mechanism limited only by myocardial perfusion, a much reduced accumulation of the tracer in background organs, and finally a short half-life (122 seconds) that permits repeated and sequential blood flow measurements. However, the rapid washout of ^{15}O-H_2O requires corrections to achieve a good tissue–blood contrast, necessary for an accurate MBF quantification. To correct for the high activity of ^{15}O-H_2O in the blood pool, an additional ^{15}O–carbon monoxide blood pool scanning, which binds hemoglobin in the red blood cells, was required to define regions of interest and delineate the vascular space. These correction techniques have recently been optimized by the generation of myocardial images directly from dynamic ^{15}O-H_2O scans, not requiring the ^{15}O-carbon monoxide blood pool scan (20,21).

Evaluation of Fatty Acid Metabolism and Oxygen Consumption

Cardiomyocytes metabolize various substrates as source of energy. Under fasting conditions, free fatty acids are the primary source of energy. Free fatty acids are extracted by the myocardium and, after the formation of long-chain acyl–coenzyme A (CoA), predominantly enter the mitochondria to suffer β-oxidation prior to going into the tricarboxylic acid cycle. The rate of fatty acid oxidation is controlled by the rate of transfer into the mitochondria. ^{11}C-palmitate, a 16-carbon, long-chain fatty acid, was the first PET radiotracer used to assess regional cardiac metabolism. Clearance of ^{11}C-palmitate follows a bioexponential kinetic model. The initial rapid-phase clearance reflects the immediate oxidation and the elimination of carbon dioxide. The second phase is believed to represent the incorporation of the radiotracer into

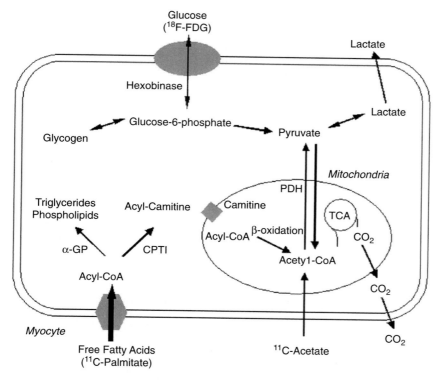

Figure 22.1. Radiotracers that can be used by PET to investigate different myocardial metabolic pathways.

the lipid metabolism as triglycerides and its final oxidation (22). The kinetics of ^{11}C-palmitate may theoretically be useful to evaluate cardiac metabolism in situations of ischemic compromise. During ischemia, the rate of elimination of ^{11}C-palmitate is decreased with a reduced oxidation of fatty acids. On the other hand, the increased cardiac work would produce an accelerated clearance of the radiotracer as the oxidative metabolism would be increased. However, the main disadvantage of this compound is the complexity of its kinetics because a very rapid clearance from the blood pool and β-oxidation allows only a very short time of analysis (Fig. 22.1).

To overcome the limitations presented by ^{11}C-palmitate, ^{11}C-acetate has been proposed as an alternative to evaluate oxidative cardiac metabolism (23,24). ^{11}C-palmitate is extracted proportionally to MBF with a first-pass extraction fraction of approximately 50% under resting conditions. Once inside the myocyte, ^{11}C-palmitate is converted to ^{11}C-acetyl-CoA, which enters the tricarboxylic acid cycle in the mitochondria (21,22). Clearance of ^{11}C activity in the form of ^{11}C-CO_2 does not occur for 4 to 5 minutes after tracer delivery, reflecting MBF except in conditions of high oxygen demand. Kinetics of ^{11}C-palmitate has allowed the quantification of oxygen consumption from the myocardial clearance rate as a parameter of the oxidative metabolism and MBF and its correlation with the presence of ischemia when this oxygen consumption diminishes (25–27).

Evaluation of Glucose Metabolism

In contrast to fasting conditions where free fatty acids predominate as a source of myocardial energy, after an ingestion of carbohydrates plasma glucose and insulin levels increase and levels of free fatty acids decline. In response, oxidation of free fatty acids decreases and utilization and oxidation of glucose increases. When myocardial ischemia ensues, contractile function declines, oxidation of free fatty acids decreases, and uptake and metabolism of glucose increase. Then glucose transport and metabolism are upregulated during ischemic conditions and after the complete resolution of these episodes, most likely due to an upregulation of the glucose transporter GLUT-1 (28,29). Regional cardiac glucose metabolic activity can be assessed with ^{18}F-FDG. The positron emitter [18]F (with a half-life of 109 minutes) linked to the glucose analogue FDG, passes the cellular membrane through facilitated diffusion, mostly mediated by the insulin-sensitive protein carrier GLUT-4 (30). Inside the myocyte the radiotracer is subjected to the first step of glycolysis by a hexokinase-mediated phosphorylation to FDG-6-phosphate. The phosphorylated glucose analogue becomes metabolically trapped in the myocardium so that the regional tracer activity concentrations reflect regional rates of exogenous glucose utilization. A more favorable standardized assessment of myocardial glucose utilization has been achieved assuming the conditions would have remained the same under physiologic and pathophysiologic conditions, by applying the so-called lumped constant, which corrects for the different kinetics affinities between ^{18}F-FDG and glucose itself (31).

Noninvasive approaches that assess exogenous glucose utilization, therefore, play an important role in the evaluation of myocardial viability in patients with coronary ischemic disease and left ventricular dysfunction. Because dysfunctional myocardium that can recover function after revascularization must retain sufficient blood flow and metabolic activity to sustain myocytes, the combined assessment of regional MBF and glucose metabolism provides additional and invaluable information.

Interpretation of PET Data

The acquisition of cardiac PET data can be achieved in either the static or dynamic mode. For static acquisitions prior to imaging, time is allowed after the injection of the radiotracer for adequate clearance from the bloodstream and uptake from the myocardium to obtain adequate myocardial-to-background activity ratios. Static imaging depicts the relative distribution of the radiotracers in the myocardium and is used for a semiquantitative or qualitative analysis of the distribution of the radiotracers within different regions of the myocardium. This approach, however, does not allow accurate quantifying functional myocardial processes. Imaging cardiac PET data are routinely acquired in transaxial slices with a field of view of approximately 10 to 15 cm. Reconstruction of the attenuation-corrected projection data is usually performed by filtered backprojection. Specific software is used to realign the image information perpendicular to the long axis of the left ventricle. This allows the visualization of the radiotracer distribution along the short and long axes of the left ventricle. The interpretation of the images is based on the visualization of the short, vertical, and horizontal long axes based on the relative regional distribution of the tracer (32). Further, the evaluation of circumferential profile analysis provides a more objective way to measure regional tracer differences and is based on specific analysis software packages, similar to that introduced for SPECT analysis (5,6). For the objective assessment of myocardial perfusion defects, individual patient data are compared with a database of normal controls. The assessment of regional myocardial defects is expressed as a percentage of pixels below two standard deviations of the control population for the corresponding area of myocardium.

Detailed knowledge of the myocardial biochemical processes is required to accurately analyze different patterns of the uptake of myocardial blood flow (^{13}N-ammonia, ^{15}O-H$_2$O, ^{82}Rb) and myocardial metabolism radiotracers (^{18}F-FDG). Three patterns of blood flow–metabolism uptake have been described in adults and largely used to analyze severe dysfunctional myocardium for assessing the presence of recoverable and, hence, viable myocardium (4). A normal distribution of the flow radiotracer regardless of the uptake of ^{18}F-FDG is seen in normal myocardium. On the other hand, absent or severely reduced regional blood flow and glucose metabolism is observed in akinetic and dyskinetic myocardium and represents myocardial necrosis. This pattern is described as a "match defect." Finally, the maintained reduced blood flow to the myocardium produces an adaptation with a normal or slightly reduced uptake of ^{18}F-FDG. This reduced or absent MBF with normal or slightly reduced glucose metabolism within the myocytes indicates myocardial hibernation and therefore viability. This pattern, described as a "mismatch pattern," characterizes severe dysfunctional myocardium supplied by a stenotic or almost totally occluded coronary artery (Fig. 22.2). The restoration of blood flow to these myocardial regions results in recovery of contractile function and normalization of the glucose metabolism (33,34). This more probably occurs after a period of time, described as stunned myocardium, where glucose metabolism may remain elevated with a normalized blood flow and a not entirely recovered contractile function.

Positron emission tomography cardiac radiotracers and physical properties of the PET system enable the absolute quantification of myocardial biochemical processes, such as myocardial blood flow and glucose metabolism. This is based on the short half-life and high energy of the radiotracers and the high temporal and spatial resolution of the current PET systems that provides the ground to accurately measure rapid changes in tissue tracer concentrations. Quantification of myocardial processes requires dynamic acquisition and the application of

NH$_3$

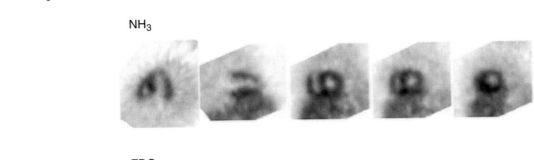

FDG

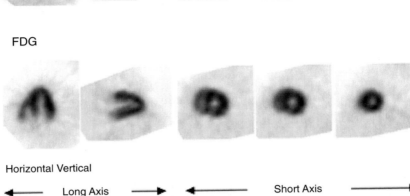

Horizontal Vertical

◄——— Long Axis ——► ◄——— Short Axis ———►

Figure 22.2. Reoriented images of the myocardial ^{13}N-ammonia (upper panel) and ^{18}F-FDG uptake (lower panel) in a patient with transposition of the great arteries after the arterial switch operation. Note the impaired perfusion in the anterolateral wall (arrows), evidenced by the decreased uptake of ^{13}N-ammonia, whereas the myocyte metabolism of ^{18}F-FDG is preserved, indicating viable myocardium. (Courtesy of Dr. Heinrich Schelbert, David Geffen School of Medicine, Los Angeles.)

tracer kinetic models (5,35). This means that the images are acquired by the system from the time of the tracer injection through a point of steady-state flux. Sampling with high temporal resolution is required to define the changes in radioactivity in the blood and the myocardial region of interest. The rapid sequential sampling and imaging enables the determination of the tracer delivery via the arterial plasma to the region of interest to define the arterial input function and the consequent tissue response to this input function. Arterial input function is generally defined by regions of interest placed over the left atrium or left ventricle to obtain temporal changes in radioactivity concentration in the different heart chambers. The rapid dynamic acquisition along with a late time frame enables the derivation of a myocardial tissue time-activity curve (19).

Dynamic acquisition, with its high volume of data, requires specific interactive software for image reconstruction, quantitative analysis, and visual presentation. The obtained regional MBF is expressed in milliliters per minute per 100 g of tissue, glucose utilization in micromoles per minute per gram of tissue, oxygen consumption in micromoles per minute per 100 g of tissue, and coronary flow reserve as the ratio of stress and resting myocardial perfusion.

Cardiac PET Protocols

Positron emission tomography studies in the pediatric population require special considerations for patient preparation and the data acquisition process. Experience in performing pediatric studies and expertise in dealing with pediatric patients will optimize the outcome of the entire study procedure minimizing the discomfort to the patients. A cardiac PET study requires the patient to remain still for the entire duration of the study. A routine myocardial blood flow–metabolism study may last up to 2 hours, and a rest/stress myocardial perfusion study may last up to 90 minutes. Thus, unlike adults, most pediatric patients would require sedation before the study is performed. This is especially necessary for infants and young children. Several intravenous premedication protocols have been used, mostly including chloral hydrate or midazolam (36,37). Due to the length of the study, further intravenous sedation may be necessary. Baseline vital signs (electrocardiogram, blood pressure, and heart rate) along with transcutaneous pulse oximetry should be recorded and monitored throughout the study.

Myocardial perfusion imaging and coronary reserve studies consist of a resting and stress examination using either pharmacologic stress (dipyridamole or adenosine) or exercise (ergometric bicycle). Patients should refrain from eating or drinking anything except water for 4 hours before the procedure, and they should abstain from caffeine-containing drinks or medications containing theophylline for 8 hours before. Adolescents should avoid cigarettes for at least 8 hours as well. Studies involving metabolic imaging with ^{18}F-FDG require a standardization of the substrate availability that optimizes myocardial glucose uptake. Older children and adolescents are routinely fasted overnight, and an oral glucose load dose is given 1 hour prior to the ^{18}F-FDG injection to facilitate glucose uptake in the myocardium. It is important to ascertain any history of diabetes or intolerance to glucose to ensure that proper steps are taken to optimize myocardial glucose uptake. Blood glucose monitoring during the study should be performed routinely to ensure that metabolic conditions are maintained along the entire acquisition process.

Clinical Applications

Coronary abnormalities, with impairments of regional myocardial perfusion, are a relevant cause of morbidity and mortality in the pediatric population. Although the experience of cardiovascular PET in pediatrics remains somewhat limited, this technique has been applied in several congenital and acquired heart diseases, providing new insights into the diseased pediatric heart and optimizing the clinical management of these patients. Recent surgical and technical advances have provided better treatment and long-term prognosis for many complex pediatric heart diseases, making the accurate diagnosis of ischemic but potentially recoverable myocardium even more important.

Transposition of the Great Arteries

In infants with transposition of the great arteries (TGA), correct cardiac anatomy is surgically restored by the arterial switch operation (ASO) of aorta and pulmonary artery. As the coronary arteries need to be excised and reinserted in the neo-aorta during the procedure, the long-term success of this operation is based on the continued patency and adequate functioning of the coronary arteries. The findings that post-surgical coronary occlusions have been described angiographically (38) and that acute myocardial infarctions and sudden deaths have been reported (39) in up to 10% of this patient population emphasize the prognostic implications of this issue. Regional reversible perfusion abnormalities were initially described by using exercise technetium-99m-sestamibi SPECT in patients following ASO (40). In contrast to SPECT imaging, higher spatial resolution of PET systems have allowed for the absolute quantification of MBF. Bengel et al. (41) were the first to report regional perfusion abnormalities with adenosine ^{13}N-ammonia PET in patients with no ischemic symptoms late after the ASO, with no correlation with any echocardiographic contractile dysfunction. They found a lower incidence of reversible perfusion defects when compared to the previous SPECT imaging studies, but quantitative hyperemic MBF and coronary flow reserve in response to adenosine were significantly lower in the patients after ASO, when compared to young healthy individuals. Similar results were described by others, which suggests that the global impairment of maximal MBF may represent alterations in the myocardial normal vasoreactivity as the early manifestation of changes in the coronary microcirculation (42). However, the procedure of coronary reimplantation alone seems to be not the only factor responsible for the myocardial perfusion abnormalities. By comparing two groups of patients with transposition of the great arteries, one after the ASO and the second after the Ross procedure to treat aortic valve disease with ^{13}N-ammonia adenosine PET, Hauser et al. (43) reported that in contrast to the patients who underwent the Ross operation, stress-induced perfusion defects and a diminished coronary flow reserve were documented in the patients after the ASO. Further follow-up and more extensive investigations are necessary to fully understand the etiology of these findings and to determine whether the reported myocardial perfusion abnormalities have significant long-term prognostic implications in these patients.

Metabolic ^{18}F-FDG imaging, along with myocardial perfusion assessment can provide useful information to identify viable but dysfunctional myocardium in patients who develop an acute cardiac event after the ASO or as a result of other coronary abnormalities. Rickers et al. (44) stated that ^{18}F-FDG–gated PET demonstrated viable myocardium in akinetic or hypokinetic regions subtended by stenotic coronary arteries after the ASO. Based on their findings, they treated patients surgically with coronary revascularization if viable myocardium was identified, whereas the patients with impaired glucose uptake, indicating myocardial scarring, were treated medically. To establish the accuracy of metabolic and perfusion PET imaging in

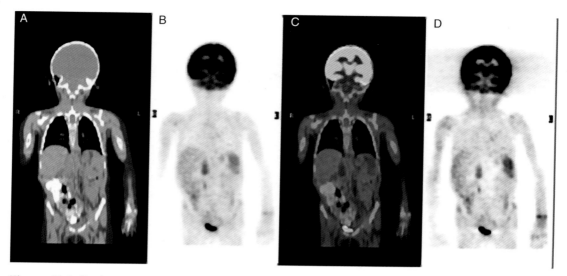

Figure 13.3. Positron emission tomography–computed tomography (PET-CT) coronal images of a 4-year-old girl with refractory neuroblastoma following bone marrow transplantation. A: CT scan. B: FDG-PET scan with attenuation correction. C: Fusion image of CT scan and FDG-PET scan with attenuation correction. D: FDG-PET scan without attenuation correction. Abnormal uptake of FDG in the abdomen is seen to the right of the midline medial to the liver, representing residual neuroblastoma.

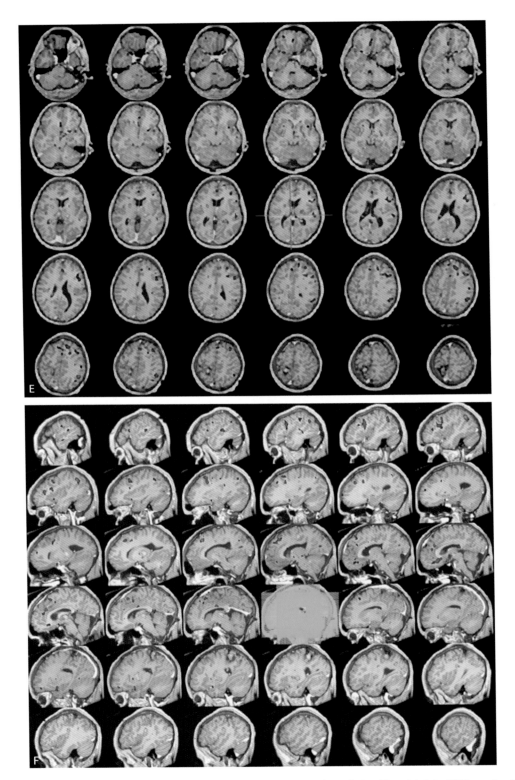

Figure 20.6. E: Statistical pixel analysis map in transverse section of significant ictal rCBF greater than interictal rCBF (yellow) or less that interictal rCBF (blue). Map shows significant ictal associated hyperemia in the region of the angioma. F: Statistical pixel analysis map in sagittal section of significant ictal rCBF greater than interictal rCBF (yellow) or less that interictal rCBF (blue). Map shows significant ictal associate hyperemia anterior to the angioma.

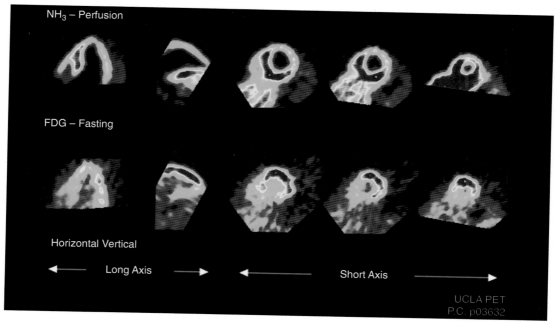

Figure 22.3. Reoriented images of the myocardial ^{13}N-ammonia (upper panel) and fasting ^{18}F-FDG uptake (lower panel) in a patient with transposition of the great arteries who had an acute episode of chest pain late after the arterial switch operation. Note the impaired perfusion in the anterolateral wall evidenced by the decreased uptake of ^{13}N-ammonia, whereas the myocyte metabolism of ^{18}F-FDG is preserved, indicating viable myocardium in that myocardial regions. (Courtesy of Dr. Heinrich Schelbert, David Geffen School of Medicine, Los Angeles.)

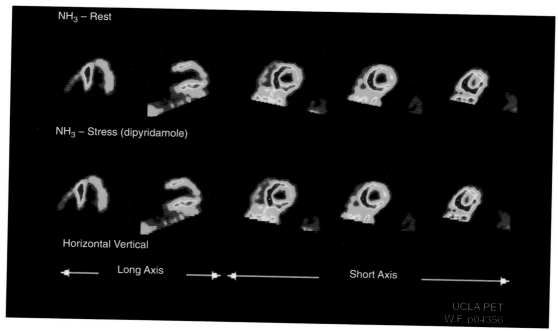

Figure 22.4. Reoriented images of the myocardial resting ^{13}N-ammonia (upper panel) and after dipyridamole-induced stress ^{13}N-ammonia (lower panel) PET study in a patient with anomalous origin of the left coronary artery arising from the pulmonary artery (ALCAPA). Note the fixed defect in the anterolateral wall that corresponds to an acute myocardial infarction in that region. (Courtesy of Dr. Heinrich Schelbert, David Geffen School of Medicine, Los Angeles.)

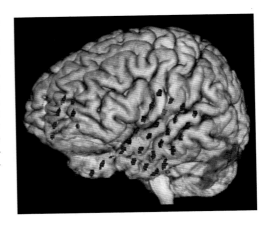

Figure 27.2. Three-dimensional (3D) reconstruction of a registered image data set. The cortical surface was rendered from MRI and red dots represent subdural EEG electrodes that were imaged with CT. The functional epileptogenic focus (orange) was defined by interictal fluorodeoxyglucose (FDG)-PET and ictal ECD–single photon emission computed tomography (SPECT).

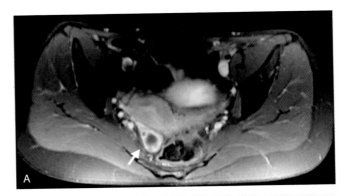

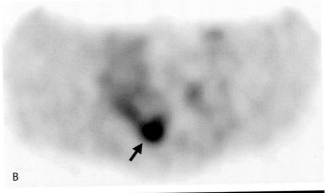

Figure 27.3. Histologically proven nonaffected cystic ovary in a patient with a recurrent yolk sack tumor: T1-weighted, fat-suppressed MR sequence after application of gadolinium–diethylenetriamine pentaacetic acid (Gd-DTPA) (A) depicts a physiologic-appearing cystic ovary (arrow). Corresponding PET (B) revealed a false-positive finding with an increased glucose uptake (arrow) suspect of a recurrent disease. Multimodality display of registered images (C) shows exact spatial correlation between the cystic ovary in MRI and increased glucose uptake in PET.

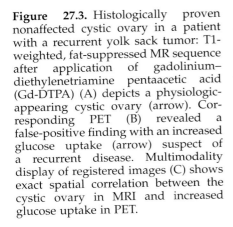

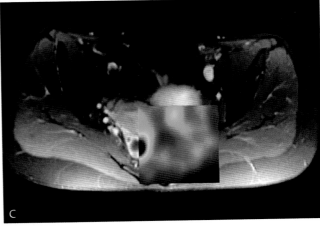

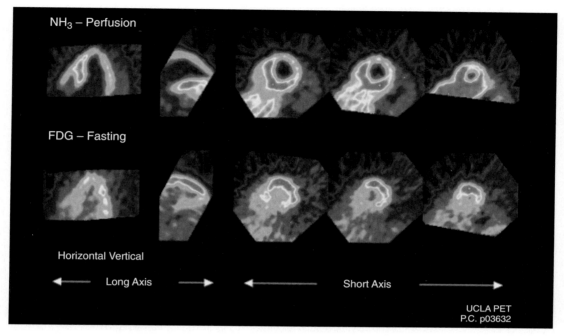

Figure 22.3. Reoriented images of the myocardial ^{13}N-ammonia (upper panel) and fasting ^{18}F-FDG uptake (lower panel) in a patient with transposition of the great arteries who had an acute episode of chest pain late after the arterial switch operation. Note the impaired perfusion in the anterolateral wall evidenced by the decreased uptake of ^{13}N-ammonia, whereas the myocyte metabolism of ^{18}F-FDG is preserved, indicating viable myocardium in that myocardial regions. (Courtesy of Dr. Heinrich Schelbert, David Geffen School of Medicine, Los Angeles.) (See color insert.)

detecting myocardial viability in children with myocardial dysfunction and its correlation with histopathological changes, Hernandez-Pampaloni et al. (45) studied a group of patients with different suspected coronary abnormalities after an acute cardiac event (Fig. 22.3, see color insert). They reported good agreement between the findings on myocardial perfusion PET and metabolic imaging with those on coronary angiography, echocardiography, and histopathology.

Anomalous Origin of the Left Coronary Artery Arising from the Pulmonary Artery

Anomalous origin of the left coronary artery arising from the pulmonary artery (ALCAPA) is a rare but serious congenital anomaly. It does not present prenatally because of the favorable fetal physiology that includes (1) equivalent pressure in the main pulmonary artery and aorta secondary to a nonrestrictive patent ductus arteriosus, and (2) relatively equivalent oxygen concentrations due to parallel circulations. As a result, myocardial perfusion is normal, and there is no stimulus for collateral formation between the right and left coronary artery

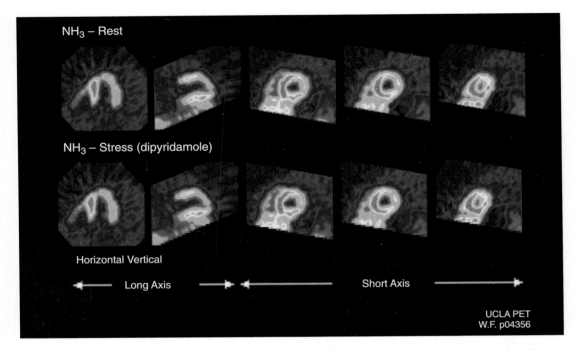

Figure 22.4. Reoriented images of the myocardial resting ¹³N-ammonia (upper panel) and after dipyridamole-induced stress ¹³N-ammonia (lower panel) PET study in a patient with anomalous origin of the left coronary artery arising from the pulmonary artery (ALCAPA). Note the fixed defect in the anterolateral wall that corresponds to an acute myocardial infarction in that region. (Courtesy of Dr. Heinrich Schelbert, David Geffen School of Medicine, Los Angeles.) (See color insert.)

systems. In the few weeks after birth, pulmonary artery pressure and resistance progressively decrease with a simultaneous decrease in oxygen content of pulmonary blood flow as the circulation becomes one in series. This results in the left ventricular myocardium being perfused by relatively desaturated blood under low pressure, leading to myocardial ischemia. Initially, myocardial ischemia is transient, occurring during periods of increased myocardial demands, such as when the infant is feeding and crying. Further increases in myocardial oxygen consumption lead to infarction of the anterolateral left ventricular free wall (Fig. 22.4, see color insert). This may lead to possible mitral valve papillary muscle dysfunction and variable degrees of insufficiency. Following surgical repair to establish blood flow to the left coronary arteries from the aorta, left ventricle (LV) function recovers and usually normalizes within 2 to 3 years. Perfusion abnormalities, however, are not uncommon in long-term survivors. Long-term survivors of ALCAPA repair demonstrate regional impairment of myocardial flow reserve. This may contribute to impaired exercise performance by limiting cardiac output reserve (46). Patients with severely reduced regional coronary flow reserve may be at risk of exercise-induced ischemic events. Thus, accurate identification of these patients by PET imaging can be of help regarding physical activity, antiischemic measures, and revascularization.

Kawasaki Disease

Kawasaki disease, also known as mucocutaneous lymph node syndrome, is an acute vasculitis that mostly affects infants and children under 5 years of age. It causes an acute vasculitis, particularly affecting medium-sized arteries such as the coronary arteries (47). The etiology and pathogenesis of Kawasaki disease remains unknown, although clinical and epidemiologic data support an infectious cause. The clinical features of Kawasaki disease can be divided into three phases. The first, or acute, phase lasts about 10 days and is marked by a temperature as high as 40°C accompanied by a polymorphous exanthem. Cardiac manifestations during this phase may include tachycardia, gallop rhythm, congestive heart failure, pericardial effusion, and arrhythmias. Arthritis and arthralgia occur during the second, or subacute, phase, which is characterized by gradual subsiding of fever, thrombocytosis, and desquamation of the palms and soles. Third is a convalescent phase where children continue to recover and all laboratory studies normalize but aneurysms of the coronary arteries may continue to enlarge (48).

Although this disease appears to be benign and self-limiting in most instances, coronary artery aneurysms or vascular ectasia develop in 20% to 25% of untreated Kawasaki patients and can lead to serious morbidity and even death (48,49). The cardiac lesions in Kawasaki disease occur in different stages, developing from an acute perivasculitis and vasculitis of the microvessels and small arteries to a panvasculitis of the coronary arteries with aneurysms and thrombosis. The late phase of development is characterized by myocardial scarring with severe stenosis in the major coronary arteries (47).

A specific diagnostic test, however, does not exit. Thus, the diagnosis of Kawasaki disease is based on the presence of a fever for at least 5 days as well as the presence at least four of the five classic clinical features: (1) bilateral nonexudative bulbar conjunctival injection, (2) unilateral nonsuppurative cervical adenopathy, (3) oral or lip erythema, (4) edema or erythema of hands and feet, and (5) a polymorphous erythematous rash.

Echocardiography is useful during the acute and subacute phase of the disease for the assessment of ventricular function and to delineate coronary aneurysms or ectasia. Up to 40% of untreated patients with Kawasaki disease have echocardiographically documented coronary artery dilatation and aneurysms in the third or convalescence phase of their disease (50). Cardiac involvement may cause different cardiac events, from silent chest pain to acute myocardial ischemia or sudden death due to myocardial infarction from occlusive coronary artery disease. Incidence, onset, and the time course of stenosis formation in the aneurysm are affected by various factors, such as the diameter of the aneurysm and the location and type of coronary arteries involved.

It is therefore critical to recognize aneurysms in Kawasaki disease to determine effective early therapy and to improve prognosis.

Two-dimensional echocardiography can detect coronary aneurysms. However, this method is not as effective for detecting coronary stenosis. Coronary angiography is an accurate method for assessing large and medium-sized coronary arteries but has little value in detecting microangiopathy (51). Furthermore, angiography is an invasive and potentially harmful procedure, with a nontrivial amount of radiation exposure that cannot be repeated often, especially in the pediatric population. Information about myocardial perfusion and regions of ischemia is necessary to make clinical decisions and to evaluate the prognosis.

In the past, children with a previous history of Kawasaki disease but no detectable angiographic coronary lesions during the acute and subacute phase were thought not to be at risk for myocardial ischemia. More recent studies have demonstrated the presence of reversible myocardial perfusion defects in children with angiographically normal coronary arteries. The clinical significance of these findings remains to be fully addressed (52). An alteration of the coronary microcirculation, possibly the result of a previous inflammatory process, has been suggested as a cause of the abnormalities in myocardial perfusion. Different authors have reported an abnormal hyperemic MBF and an impaired coronary flow reserve in patients with a previous history of Kawasaki disease but normal epicardial coronary arteries, after an adenosine-induced hyperemia PET study (53,54). These microcirculatory abnormalities, which could represent a risk factor for the development of atherosclerosis in adulthood, may correspond to an endothelium-dependent dysfunction. Furuyama et al. (55) described an impaired MBF response to the cold-pressor testing using ^{15}O-H$_2$O PET in patients with Kawasaki disease, when compared to normal controls, suggesting an intimal hypertrophy in these patients (55). An abnormal endothelium-dependent vasodilation in the brachial artery of patients with a previous history of Kawasaki disease seems to confirm that endothelial dysfunction may at least contribute to the microcirculatory changes responsible for myocardial perfusion alterations.

Positron emission tomography has been used in patients with Kawasaki and demonstrable coronary aneurysms as well to demonstrate an impaired hyperemic and coronary flow reserve, as reported by Ohmochi et al. (56). Interestingly, Yoshibayashi et al. (57) have correlated the presence of ischemic myocardial injury with the appearance of abnormal Q waves in the electrocardiogram (ECG) when compared to a ^{13}N-ammonia and ^{18}F-FDG PET. They reported that the presence of abnormal Q waves is a reliable clue to the presence of ischemic myocardial injury, whereas metabolic PET imaging showed viable myocardial tissue in those areas with an abnormal Q wave (57).

Monitoring the response to different therapies is another area of application of PET imaging. Hwang et al. (58) reported that the incidence of perfusion and metabolic PET abnormalities was reduced in patients in the convalescent stage of Kawasaki disease when they were treated with a 5-day dose of intravenous (IV) immunoglobulin, compared to those who received only a single dose of IV immunoglobulin.

Coronary arteries that have been previously aneurysmal have an abnormal response to vasodilators in Kawasaki patients. Intravascular ultrasound imaging of the coronary arteries demonstrated increased intimal thickening in many regions of resolved aneurysms but normal intimal thickness in those patients with Kawasaki disease and no previous history of a coronary artery lesion (59). These findings support the continuous surveillance of all children with a history of Kawasaki disease regardless of coronary artery status. Approximately 50% of patients who had coronary aneurysms show regression on follow-up coronary angiography (60). However, these angiographically normal vessels showed intimal thickening and endothelial dysfunction similar to that observed in early atherosclerotic lesions. Because these patients should be followed carefully to monitor potential late effects of Kawasaki disease in the coronary circulation, periodical PET measurement of MBF seems very appropriate in this particular setting. It has been reported that abnormal myocardial perfusion is present long-term after the resolution of complicated Kawasaki disease, and that unfavorable perfusion response to pharmacologic stress was coupled with an abnormal regional contractility. On the other hand, however, enhanced perfusion correlated poorly with segmental contractility response (52). Therefore, even if these abnormalities are modest and do not seem to diminish exercise performance in these patients, these findings may have implications later in life when other coronary risk factors may potentiate the development of coronary artery disease during adulthood.

Cardiac Transplant Vasculopathy

Allograft vasculopathy has emerged as the most important limiting factor for long-term survival and is the leading cause of death 1 year after transplantation. At 10 years after transplantation, as many as 20% of recipients have developed significant allograft vasculopathy. Because the donor heart is denervated, children with graft vasculopathy rarely present with angina. They may have atypical angina such as shoulder or back pain or, more frequently, abdominal pain. They may also present with syncope or sudden death. Several studies have demonstrated the diffuse nature of cardiac allograft vasculopathy, which affects the major epicardial vessels along their entire length from the base of the heart to the apex and the epicardial and intramyocardial branches (61). Available studies suggest that graft vasculopathy has a mixed etiology, based on the varied patterns of vascular disease seen by coronary angiography, that is, either diffuse and circumferential narrowing in the distal parts of the coronary arteries or focal segmental disorder in the middle and proximal branches similar to atherosclerosis. Major histologic findings include intact internal elastic lamina; rarely, calcification; occasionally, a low grade of vasculitis; and a tendency for the disease to progress rapidly (62). Although treatment of transplant vasculopathy is complex, several studies have showed that focal lesions have been treated successfully with percutaneous transluminal coronary angioplasty (63). On the other hand, the results of coronary artery bypass surgery have not been so successful, leaving only retransplantation as an alternative (64).

Annual coronary angiography and intravascular ultrasound have been used to detect coronary involvement and to assess the development and progression of this disease. These techniques are invasive and not event-free with a potential harmful effect, especially in the pediatric population. Therefore, it is paramount to introduce a noninvasive test to detect the progression of the disease and to predict future long-term outcome and cardiac events. Several studies have demonstrated in the adult population that technetium-based myocardial perfusion studies are useful to screen for significant coronary artery disease in the transplant vasculopathy (65). Additionally, they provide incremental data for the prediction of cardiac death in heart transplant patients, as described by Elhendy et al. (66).

Cardiac PET studies have shown a decreased coronary flow reserve in adult cardiac allografts after pharmacologically stress-induced hyperemia with dipyridamole (67,68). In addition to a decreased exercise capacity, PET imaging has described an incomplete reinnervation in the transplanted adult heart (69).

Cardiomyopathies of Diverse Origin

Cardiac PET has proven to be of utility in monitoring response to therapy and in predicting potential long-term outcome by measuring MBF after corrective surgery in specific cardiomyopathies. Donnelly et al. (70) reported on a small group of patients with a hypoplastic left heart syndrome assessed after corrective surgery, and found that coronary flow reserve was reduced due to a higher resting MBF. Also, long-term survivors of the Mustard operation have shown a high prevalence of right ventricular dysfunction. In these patients a decreased coronary flow reserve, as reported by Singh et al. (71), may help explain the systemic ventricular dysfunction they suffer. The long-term outcome of circulation driven by a single ventricular chamber remains a matter of concern as multiple sequelae, such as thromboembolic complications, ventricular dysfunction, arrhythmias, and reduced exercise capacity, can arise from subtle but continuous circulatory changes (72). Thus, coronary artery blood flow may be compromised if the ventricular mass increases significantly to reduce systolic and diastolic function. Hauser el al. (73) has reported an impaired stress MBF, impaired coronary flow reserve, and an elevated vascular resistance after vasodilation in patients with Fontan-like operations.

In the cardiomyopathy of Duchenne and Becker muscular dystrophies, studies at necropsy have shown that the posterolateral wall of the left ventricle is the first myocardial area suffering from dystrophy even in the absence of small vessel coronary artery disease in these regions. Perloff et al. (74) have reported areas of myocardial hibernation, identified by perfusion and metabolic PET imaging, in the lateral and posterolateral wall in a group of patients with Duchenne dystrophy.

Very low coronary flow reserve values measured with PET are reported in neonates with surgically treated congenital heart disease (75). Because the chronically dilated extramural coronary arteries in cyanotic congenital heart disease have a limited capacity to dilate further and because myocardial oxygen extraction is inherently maximal, the potential oxygen debt incurred by systemic arterial hypoxemia may be inadequately met. Basal coronary flow as determined by ^{13}N-ammonia PET was increased to the same degree in the right ventricular and left ventricular free walls and in the ventricular septum, but hyperemic perfusion, coronary vascular resistance, and flow reserve were normal in each of the three regions of interest. Although these studies were not designed to determine the mechanism(s) by which flow reserve is preserved in the face of increased basal coronary flow, the results may suggest remodeling of the intramyocardial coronary microcirculation and vasculogenesis in response to hypoxemic stimulation as potential causes for explaining the neonatal myocardial adaptation to different conditions.

Future Directions

Although current cardiac PET clinical applications in pediatrics are still limited, the greater availability of PET systems and infrastructure along with greater knowledge of its capabilities by the pediatric medical community are allowing PET imaging to become more than a tool for the noninvasive assessment of myocardial perfusion and glucose metabolism. It promises to have great potential for applications such as in vivo assessment of cardiac cellular metabolism and receptor function and gene expression. Finally, the potential of combined multimodality imaging, represented by PET–computed tomography (CT) imaging, may provide in the near future real-time assessment of function and structure of the diseased pediatric heart.

References

1. Bax JJ, et al. Metabolic imaging using F18-fluorodeoxyglucose to assess myocardial viability. Int J Card Imaging 1997;13(2):145–155; discussion 157–160.
2. Di Carli MF. Predicting improved function after myocardial revascularization. Curr Opin Cardiol 1998;13(6):415–424.
3. Hubbell JH. Review of photon interaction cross section data in the medical and biological context. Phys Med Biol 1999;44(1):R1–22.
4. Muzik O, et al. Validation of nitrogen-13-ammonia tracer kinetic model for quantification of myocardial blood flow using PET. J Nucl Med 1993; 34(1):83–91.
5. Hutchins GD, et al. Noninvasive quantification of regional blood flow in the human heart using N-13 ammonia and dynamic positron emission tomographic imaging. J Am Coll Cardiol 1990;15(5):1032–1042.

6. Schelbert HR, et al. Regional myocardial perfusion assessed with N-13 labeled ammonia and positron emission computerized axial tomography. Am J Cardiol 1979;43(2):209–218.

7. Bergmann SR, et al. Noninvasive quantitation of myocardial blood flow in human subjects with oxygen-15-labeled water and positron emission tomography. J Am Coll Cardiol 1989;14(3):639–652.

8. Araujo LI, et al. Noninvasive quantification of regional myocardial blood flow in coronary artery disease with oxygen-15-labeled carbon dioxide inhalation and positron emission tomography. Circulation 1991;83(3):875–885.

9. Kaufmann PA, et al. Assessment of the reproducibility of baseline and hyperemic myocardial blood flow measurements with 15O-labeled water and PET. J Nucl Med 1999;40(11):1848–1856.

10. Herrero P, et al. Noninvasive quantification of regional myocardial perfusion with rubidium-82 and positron emission tomography. Exploration of a mathematical model. Circulation 1990;82(4):1377–1386.

11. Tadamura E, et al. Generator-produced copper-62-PTSM as a myocardial PET perfusion tracer compared with nitrogen-13–ammonia. J Nucl Med 1996;37(5):729–735.

12. Beanlands RS, et al. The kinetics of copper-62-PTSM in the normal human heart. J Nucl Med 1992;33(5):684–690.

13. Beller GA, et al. Assessment of regional myocardial perfusion by positron emission tomography after intracoronary administration of gallium-68 labeled albumin microspheres. J Comput Assist Tomogr 1979;3(4):447–452.

14. Melon PG, et al. Myocardial kinetics of potassium-38 in humans and comparison with copper-62–PTSM. J Nucl Med 1994;35(7):1116–1122.

15. Mullani NA, et al. Myocardial perfusion with rubidium-82. I. Measurement of extraction fraction and flow with external detectors. J Nucl Med 1983;24(10):898–906.

16. Choi Y, et al. Quantification of myocardial blood flow using 13N-ammonia and PET: comparison of tracer models. J Nucl Med 1999;40(6):1045–1055.

17. Glatting G, Reske SN. Treatment of radioactive decay in pharmacokinetic modeling: influence on parameter estimation in cardiac 13N-PET. Med Phys 1999;26(4):616–621.

18. Hove JD, et al. Dual spillover problem in the myocardial septum with nitrogen-13–ammonia flow quantitation. J Nucl Med 1998;39(4):591–598.

19. Hutchins GD, Caraher JM, Raylman RR. A region of interest strategy for minimizing resolution distortions in quantitative myocardial PET studies. J Nucl Med 1992;33(6):1243–1250.

20. Hermansen F, et al. Generation of myocardial factor images directly from the dynamic oxygen-15-water scan without use of an oxygen-15-carbon monoxide blood-pool scan. J Nucl Med 1998;39(10):1696–1702.

21. Wyss CA, et al. Bicycle exercise stress in PET for assessment of coronary flow reserve: repeatability and comparison with adenosine stress. J Nucl Med 2003;44(2):146–154.

22. Schelbert HR, et al. Effects of substrate availability on myocardial C-11 palmitate kinetics by positron emission tomography in normal subjects and patients with ventricular dysfunction. Am Heart J 1986;111(6):1055–1064.

23. Brown M, et al. Delineation of myocardial oxygen utilization with carbon-11-labeled acetate. Circulation 1987;76(3):687–696.

24. Brown MA, Myears DW, Bergmann SR. Noninvasive assessment of canine myocardial oxidative metabolism with carbon-11 acetate and positron emission tomography. J Am Coll Cardiol 1988;12(4):1054–1063.

25. Buck A, et al. Effect of carbon-11–acetate recirculation on estimates of myocardial oxygen consumption by PET. J Nucl Med 1991;32(10):1950–1957.

26. Wolpers HG, et al. Assessment of myocardial viability by use of 11C-acetate and positron emission tomography. Threshold criteria of reversible dysfunction. Circulation 1997;95(6):1417–1424.

27. Armbrecht JJ, et al. Regional myocardial oxygen consumption determined noninvasively in humans with (1–11C)acetate and dynamic positron tomography. Circulation 1989;80(4):863–872.

28. Opie LH. Effects of regional ischemia on metabolism of glucose and fatty acids. Relative rates of aerobic and anaerobic energy production during myocardial infarction and comparison with effects of anoxia. Circ Res 1976;38(5 Suppl 1):I52–74.

29. Brosius FC 3rd, et al. Persistent myocardial ischemia increases GLUT1 glucose transporter expression in both ischemic and non-ischemic heart regions. J Mol Cell Cardiol 1997;29(6):1675–1685.

30. Sivitz WI, et al. Pretranslational regulation of two cardiac glucose transporters in rats exposed to hypobaric hypoxia. Am J Physiol 1992;263(3 pt 1): E562–569.

31. Krivokapich J, et al. Fluorodeoxyglucose rate constants, lumped constant, and glucose metabolic rate in rabbit heart. Am J Physiol 1987;252(4 pt 2): H777–787.

32. Laubenbacher C, et al. An automated analysis program for the evaluation of cardiac PET studies: initial results in the detection and localization of coronary artery disease using nitrogen-13–ammonia. J Nucl Med 1993;34(6): 968–978.

33. Tillisch J, et al. Reversibility of cardiac wall-motion abnormalities predicted by positron tomography. N Engl J Med 1986;314(14):884–888.

34. Knuuti MJ, et al. Myocardial viability: fluorine-18-deoxyglucose positron emission tomography in prediction of wall motion recovery after revascularization. Am Heart J 1994;127(4 Pt 1):785–796.

35. Kuhle WG, et al. Quantification of regional myocardial blood flow using 13N-ammonia and reoriented dynamic positron emission tomographic imaging. Circulation 1992;86(3):1004–1017.

36. American Academy of Pediatrics Committee on Drugs: Guidelines for monitoring and management of pediatric patients during and after sedation for diagnostic and therapeutic procedures. Pediatrics 1992;89(6 pt 1): 1110–1115.

37. Practice guidelines for sedation and analgesia by non-anesthesiologists. Anesthesiology 2002;96(4):1004–1017.

38. Tanel RE, et al. Coronary artery abnormalities detected at cardiac catheterization following the arterial switch operation for transposition of the great arteries. Am J Cardiol 1995;76(3):153–157.

39. Wernovsky G, et al. Factors influencing early and late outcome of the arterial switch operation for transposition of the great arteries. J Thorac Cardiovasc Surg 1995;109(2):289–301; discussion 301–302.

40. Weindling SN, et al. Myocardial perfusion, function and exercise tolerance after the arterial switch operation. J Am Coll Cardiol 1994;23(2):424–433.

41. Bengel FM, et al. Myocardial blood flow and coronary flow reserve late after anatomical correction of transposition of the great arteries. J Am Coll Cardiol 1998;32(7):1955–1961.

42. Yates RW, et al. Evaluation of myocardial perfusion using positron emission tomography in infants following a neonatal arterial switch operation. Pediatr Cardiol 2000;21(2):111–118.

43. Hauser M, et al. Myocardial blood flow and flow reserve after coronary reimplantation in patients after arterial switch and Ross operation. Circulation 2001;103(14):1875–1880.

44. Rickers C, et al. Myocardial viability assessed by positron emission tomography in infants and children after the arterial switch operation and suspected infarction. J Am Coll Cardiol 2000;36(5):1676–1683.

45. Hernandez-Pampaloni M, et al. Myocardial perfusion and viability by positron emission tomography in infants and children with coronary abnormalities: correlation with echocardiography, coronary angiography, and histopathology. J Am Coll Cardiol 2003;41(4):618–626.

46. Singh TP, et al. Myocardial flow reserve in long-term survivors of repair of anomalous left coronary artery from pulmonary artery. J Am Coll Cardiol 1998;31(2):437–443.

47. Shulman ST, Rowley AH. Advances in Kawasaki disease. Eur J Pediatr 2004;163(6):285–291.

48. Dajani AS, et al. Diagnosis and therapy of Kawasaki disease in children. Circulation 1993;87(5):1776–1780.

49. Dajani AS, et al. Guidelines for long-term management of patients with Kawasaki disease. Report from the Committee on Rheumatic Fever, Endocarditis, and Kawasaki Disease, Council on Cardiovascular Disease in the Young, American Heart Association. Circulation 1994;89(2):916–922.

50. Kondo C, et al. Detection of coronary artery stenosis in children with Kawasaki disease. Usefulness of pharmacologic stress 201Tl myocardial tomography. Circulation 1989;80(3):615–624.

51. Schillaci O, et al. Technetium-99m sestamibi single-photon emission tomography detects subclinical myocardial perfusion abnormalities in patients with systemic lupus erythematosus. Eur J Nucl Med 1999;26(7):713–717.

52. Iemura M, et al. Long term consequences of regressed coronary aneurysms after Kawasaki disease: vascular wall morphology and function. Heart 2000;83(3):307–311.

53. Muzik O, et al. Quantification of myocardial blood flow and flow reserve in children with a history of Kawasaki disease and normal coronary arteries using positron emission tomography. J Am Coll Cardiol 1996;28(3):757–762.

54. Hauser M, et al. Myocardial blood flow and coronary flow reserve in children with "normal" epicardial coronary arteries after the onset of Kawasaki disease assessed by positron emission tomography. Pediatr Cardiol 2004;25(2):108–112.

55. Furuyama H, et al. Altered myocardial flow reserve and endothelial function late after Kawasaki disease. J Pediatr 2003;142(2):149–154.

56. Ohmochi Y, et al. Assessment of effects of intravenous dipyridamole on regional myocardial perfusion in children with Kawasaki disease without angiographic evidence of coronary stenosis using positron emission tomography and H2(15)O. Coronary Artery Dis 1995;6(7):555–559.

57. Yoshibayashi M, et al. Regional myocardial perfusion and metabolism assessed by positron emission tomography in children with Kawasaki disease and significance of abnormal Q waves and their disappearance. Am J Cardiol 1991;68(17):1638–1645.

58. Hwang B, et al. Positron emission tomography for the assessment of myocardial viability in Kawasaki disease using different therapies. Nucl Med Commun 2000;21(7):631–636.

59. Dahdah NS, et al. Segmental myocardial contractility versus perfusion in Kawasaki disease with coronary arterial aneurysm. Am J Cardiol 1999; 83(1):48–51.

60. Kato H, et al. Long-term consequences of Kawasaki disease. A 10- to 21-year follow-up study of 594 patients. Circulation 1996;94(6):1379–1385.

61. Billingham ME. Histopathology of graft coronary disease. J Heart Lung Transplant 1992;11(3 pt 2):S38–44.

62. Grant SC, Brooks NH, Levy RD. Routine coronary angiography after heart transplantation. Heart 1997;78(2):101–102.

63. Wong PM, et al. Efficacy of coronary stenting in the management of cardiac allograft vasculopathy. Am J Cardiol 1998;82(2):239–241.

64. Halle AA 3rd, et al. Coronary angioplasty, atherectomy and bypass surgery in cardiac transplant recipients. J Am Coll Cardiol 1995;26(1):120–128.

65. Carlsen J, et al. Myocardial perfusion scintigraphy as a screening method for significant coronary artery stenosis in cardiac transplant recipients. J Heart Lung Transplant 2000;19(9):873–878.

66. Elhendy A, et al. Prediction of mortality in heart transplant recipients by stress technetium-99m tetrofosmin myocardial perfusion imaging. Am J Cardiol 2002;89(8):964–968.

67. Zhao XM, et al. Nitrogen-13–ammonia and PET to detect allograft coronary artery disease after heart transplantation: comparison with coronary angiography. J Nucl Med 1995;36(6):982–987.

68. Preumont N, et al. Early alterations of myocardial blood flow reserve in heart transplant recipients with angiographically normal coronary arteries. J Heart Lung Transplant 2000;19(6):538–545.

69. Uberfuhr P, et al. Incomplete sympathic reinnervation of the orthotopically transplanted human heart: observation up to 13 years after heart transplantation. Eur J Cardiothorac Surg 2000;17(2):161–168.

70. Donnelly JP, et al. Resting coronary flow and coronary flow reserve in human infants after repair or palliation of congenital heart defects as measured by positron emission tomography. J Thorac Cardiovasc Surg 1998;115(1):103–110.

71. Singh TP, et al. Myocardial flow reserve in patients with a systemic right ventricle after atrial switch repair. J Am Coll Cardiol 2001;37(8):2120–2125.

72. Fishberger SB, et al. Factors that influence the development of atrial flutter after the Fontan operation. J Thorac Cardiovasc Surg 1997;113(1):80–86.

73. Hauser M, et al. Myocardial perfusion and coronary flow reserve assessed by positron emission tomography in patients after Fontan-like operations. Pediatr Cardiol 2003;24(4):386–392.

74. Perloff JK, Henze E, Schelbert HR. Alterations in regional myocardial metabolism, perfusion, and wall motion in Duchenne muscular dystrophy studied by radionuclide imaging. Circulation 1984;69(1):33–42.

75. Oskarsson G. Coronary flow and flow reserve in children. Acta Paediatr Suppl 2004;93(446):20–25.

23

Fever of Unknown Origin

Hongming Zhuang and Ghassan El-Haddad

Definition and Classification

General Criteria

The original criteria for fever of unknown origin (FUO) as set forth in 1961 by Petersdorf and Beeson were fever higher than 38.3°C on several occasions of at least 3 weeks' duration and uncertain diagnosis after 1 week of study in the hospital (1). This definition was later revised, and the criterion of 1 week of hospitalization has been replaced by 3 days of hospitalization or three outpatient visits (2,3). In addition to the previously described classic FUO, additional categories have been added: nosocomial, neutropenic, and HIV-associated FUO (3,4).

Nosocomial FUO refers to the hospitalized patient with a temperature of ≥38.3°C (≥101°F) on several occasions, who is receiving acute care, and in whom infection was not manifest or incubating on admission. The diagnosis of nosocomial FUO is made after 3 days of illness under investigation, including at least 2 days' incubation of cultures. Examples of diseases causing nosocomial FUO are septic thrombophlebitis, sinusitis, *Clostridium difficile* colitis, and drug fever.

Neutropenic FUO includes patients with fever of ≥38.3°C (≥101°F) on several occasions, a neutrophil count either <500 cells/μL or expected to reach that level in 1 to 2 days, in whom initial cultures are negative and the diagnosis remains unknown after 3 days of investigation. Frequent causes of neutropenic FUO are perianal infection, aspergillosis, and candidemia.

The HIV-associated FUO refers to HIV-positive patients with fever of ≥38.3°C (≥101°F) on several occasions for 4 weeks as an outpatient or 3 days of illness as an inpatient under investigation, including at least 2 days for cultures to incubate. *Mycobacterium avium intracellulare* (MAI) infection, tuberculosis, non-Hodgkin's lymphoma, and drug fever are common causes of HIV-associated FUO.

Pediatric FUO

Fever is a common presenting problem in children. Approximately 30% of pediatric outpatient visits in the United States are because of fever, which is brief and self-limited in the majority of cases (5). Fever of unknown origin in children is a great diagnostic challenge for pediatricians. Due to the paucity of data in children, the definition of FUO is slightly different from adults, and there is no one agreed-upon definition. Several studies defined fever in children as FUO when it lasted 1 to 3 weeks without diagnosis (6–10). The definition of FUO in children that is currently used by most authorities is fever of at least 8 days' duration, in which no diagnosis is apparent after initial workup either in the hospital or as an outpatient. Fever of unknown origin has to be differentiated from fever without localizing signs, which does not meet the criteria for FUO, and where the development of additional clinical manifestations over a shorter period of time leads to less extensive diagnostic testing before confirming the nature of the disease.

Epidemiology and Etiology

Several studies on FUO carried out since 1961 found that infections, malignancies, and noninfectious inflammatory diseases cause the majority of classic FUO (1,11–13). In the current series on adults with FUO, infections were the most frequent causes of FUO, followed by malignancies, and then noninfectious inflammatory diseases (13,14). However, in children, infection is a more common cause of FUO than in adults, accounting for 30% to 50% of the cases, followed by connective tissue diseases (CTDs) and then neoplasm (7% to 13%) (8,9). Most cases of FUO in children as well as in adults represent unusual manifestations of common diseases, rather than a common manifestation of a rare disease. The common etiologies that should be considered in children with FUO are presented in Table 23.1.

The most common systemic infections in the United States that are implicated in children with FUO are salmonellosis, tuberculosis, rickettsial infections, spirochetal infections, cat-scratch disease, infectious mononucleosis, cytomegalovirus (CMV) infection, and viral hepatitis.

Autoimmune diseases occur with equal frequency in adults and children (10% to 20% of cases), but certain diseases such as systemic lupus erythematosus (SLE), Wegener's granulomatosis, and polyarteritis nodosa are more common in adults, whereas juvenile rheumatoid arthritis (JRA, now called juvenile idiopathic arthritis, JIA) is particularly common in children (8,15,16). Juvenile rheumatoid arthritis accounts for >90% of connective tissue diseases that cause FUO, followed by SLE and other types of vasculitis (6,8,9,17). Some autoimmune diseases that occur exclusively in adults are adult Still's disease, giant cell arteritis, and polymyalgia rheumatica. Temporal arteritis, polymyalgia rheumatica, sarcoidosis, rheumatoid arthritis, and Wegener's granulomatosis account for 25% to 30% of all FUOs in patients over 65 years of age (15).

Lymphoma and leukemia are the two most common malignancies presenting as FUO in children. The frequency of neoplasms decreased

Table 23.1. Etiologies to be considered in children with fever of unknown origin (FUO)

Infections	Noninfectious inflammatory diseases	Miscellaneous causes
Generalized	JRA	Central nervous system
Hepatitis viruses	SLE	dysfunction
Cytomegalovirus	Crohn's disease	Diabetes Insipidus
HIV	Ulcerative colitis	Drug fever
EBV	Sarcoidosis	Familial dysautonomia
Cat-scratch disease	Kawasaki's disease	(Riley-Day syndrome)
Tuberculosis (TB)		Factitious fever
Brucellosis	Neoplasms	Thyroiditis
Leptospirosis		Periodic fevers (e.g.
Malaria	Non-Hodgkin's	familial
Salmomellosis	lymphoma	Mediterranean fever)
Toxoplasmosis	Hodgkin's disease	Infantile cortical
Tularemia	Leukemia	hyperostosis
	Renal cell carcinoma	Pancreatitis
Localized	Hepatoma,	Hypothalamic-central
Arthritis	Neuroblastoma	fever
Osteomyelitis	Wilms' tumor	Thrombophlebitis
Intraabdominal		Pulmonary embolism
abscesses		Serum sickness
Upper respiratory tract		Factitious fever-
infections (URI)		Ectodermal dysplasia
Urinary tract infection		
(UTI)		

in two series (12,18), which was attributed to improved diagnostic imaging techniques.

Despite extensive investigations, 10% to 20% of FUO cases in children remain undiagnosed.

Diagnosis

Despite the fact that most children with FUO have a self-limited disease, it is still a very serious clinical problem, with mortality reaching 6% to 9% in two series of children with FUO (8,9). The diagnostic approach in children with FUO starts with a thorough history and physical examination, supplemented by laboratory and radiographic tests. Repeated histories and physical examination are important to better elucidate the etiology of FUO. The age of the patient, history of exposure to wild or domestic animals, history of unusual dietary habits or travel, medication history, and ethnic background are very helpful in evaluating FUO. After the screening laboratory and radiographic tests, additional tests should be guided by the history and physical examination.

Radiographic Evaluation of Children with FUO

After obtaining a regular chest radiograph, further radiographic examination of specific areas such as the nasal sinuses, mastoids, and gastrointestinal (GI) tract should be performed following special indications. Inflammatory bowel disease should be excluded in children with abdominal complaints, persistent fever, elevated erythrocyte sedimentation rate (ESR), anorexia, and weight loss. Finding a cost-effective diagnostic imaging procedure is challenging for the clinicians.

Echocardiograms are useful to evaluate the heart when suspecting infective endocarditis (19). Ultrasonography (US) is often used to investigate fluid collections, abscesses (20,21), and thrombophlebitis (22). Computed tomography (CT) or magnetic resonance imaging (MRI) is helpful in the detection of neoplasms and abscesses in the abdomen and in the investigation of lesions in the head, neck, and chest (23–28), as well as for osteomyelitis (29). Magnetic resonance imaging is rarely used in the initial evaluation of FUO except in certain cases such as spinal epidural abscesses (30). Laparotomy has been nearly replaced by noninvasive imaging techniques, especially in the search for occult abscesses or hematomas in patients with FUO. However, laparotomy is very helpful when noninvasive imaging measures are nondiagnostic and CT- or ultrasound-guided aspiration or biopsy fails to make the diagnosis (31).

Radionuclide Scans

Gallium-67– and indium-111–labeled leukocytes have a higher overall yield than CT or US in diagnosing FUO because the images cover the whole body (32,33). In patients with FUO, gallium 67 is useful for the detection of malignancies and of granulomatous and inflammatory disorders (34), whereas indium-111–labeled leukocytes are more useful for detecting localized infectious and inflammatory processes (35). Different technetium-99m (^{99m}Tc)-labeled compounds are being studied for potential clinical use in patients with FUO, such as ^{99m}Tc-hexamethylpropylene-amine-oxime (HMPAO)-labeled leukocytes (36), ^{99m}Tc-ciprofloxacin (37), and ^{99m}Tc-labeled monoclonal antibodies (38,39).

FDG-PET Scan

Mechanisms of FDG Uptake by the Cells
Currently, 18-fluoro-2-deoxyglucose (FDG) is the most clinically used radiotracer in positron emission tomography (PET). It competes with glucose for transport into the cell and for enzymatic phosphorylation by hexokinase, which enables us to image glucose metabolism in the body. Once FDG enters the cell, it is phosphorylated by hexokinase and trapped inside, which leads to an increase in its concentration with time (40). The uptake of FDG by the malignant cells is directly proportional to glucose metabolism (41). There is enhanced glycolysis in malignant

cells, which is related to high intracellular enzyme levels of hexokinase (42) and increased expression of surface glucose transporter proteins (GLUT) (43).

Infectious, inflammatory, and granulomatous diseases have increased glycolysis, which makes them readily visualized by FDG-PET scanning (44). Glycolysis is enhanced in inflammatory cells when the latter are stimulated, and this includes neutrophils, monocyte-macrophages, and lymphocytes (45–48). This has been mainly attributed to a high concentration of GLUT and a high affinity of these transporters for FDG. Especially, many investigations have demonstrated that there are increased levels of GLUT on the inflammatory cells when they are activated by inflammatory signals (46,47,49). Intratumoral inflammatory reactions also have a high rate of glycolysis (50,51).

Rationale for the Use of FDG-PET in FUO

The fact that FDG is not a tumor-specific substance can be exploited in a positive matter in the setting of FUO because infections, inflammations, and malignancies account for the great majority of FUO cases.

Fluorodeoxyglucose-PET has proven to be a very accurate modality for the detection of a large number of malignancies (52). Conventional anatomic imaging modalities rely on size as a criterion to distinguish between malignant and benign diseases; FDG-PET reflects the biochemical alterations within tumors, facilitating a functional assessment of malignancies. This has proven to provide a very accurate assessment of solitary pulmonary nodules, lymphoma, non–small cell lung cancer, colorectal cancer, malignant melanoma, head and neck cancers, and breast cancers (52). The success of PET is not limited to the staging of malignancies but goes beyond that to the accurate assessment of restaging and evaluation of response to therapy. This has been particularly proven in lymphoma in the adult (53,54) and pediatric (55) populations, and it has a direct impact on the management of patients with FUO because lymphoma accounts for the majority of cancers causing FUO. Fluorodeoxyglucose-PET is able to differentiate necrotic tissue from viable tumor and has proven its superiority to other imaging techniques in the initial staging of lymphoma, in monitoring response to therapy, and in detecting residual tumor (53,54).

Many metabolically active infectious and inflammatory disorders can be readily visualized by FDG-PET scanning (56,57) (Table 23.2). Fluorodeoxyglucose-PET has a high accuracy in detecting chronic osteomyelitis (58), especially in the central skeleton, which was found to be superior to antigranulocyte antibody scintigraphy (59,60) and to indium-111–labeled leukocytes (61). Although CT and MRI provide excellent anatomic details, they have limited capacity to differentiate postsurgical changes from infection, and, in contrast to FDG-PET, they are hindered by metal implants (62,63). Fluorodeoxyglucose-PET can differentiate between normal bone

Table 23.2. Common causes of FUO reportedly detected by FDG-PET

Infections	Inflammatory/granulomatous	Neoplasms
Subphrenic abscess	Takayasu's arteritis	Hodgkin's disease
Pneumonia	Rheumatoid arthritis	Non-Hodgkin's lymphoma
Osteomyelitis	Wegener's granulomatosis	Colon carcinoma
Vascular graft infection	Sarcoidosis	Renal cell carcinoma
Tuberculosis	Thyroiditis	Sarcoma
Sinusitis	Enterocolitis	Pheochromocytoma
Mastoiditis	Myositis	
	Gastritis	
	Giant cell arteritis	

healing following a fracture or surgical intervention and osteomyelitis or malignancy (64,65). In patients with prostheses, FDG-PET can assess the presence of a superimposed infection, especially in hip prostheses and, to a lesser extent, in knee prostheses (66). Fluorodeoxyglucose-PET can be used to diagnose infections related to diabetes, especially in the evaluation of the diabetic foot (67). Human immunodeficiency virus (HIV)-positive patients constitute a special group of patients because they are prone to opportunistic infections and malignancies, especially lymphoma. In a report on HIV-positive patients with FUO, FDG-PET had a sensitivity of 92% and a specificity of 94% for localizing a focal pathology that needed treatment (68). Fluorodeoxyglucose-PET was able to differentiate lymphoma from nonmalignant lesions in the central nervous system in HIV-positive patients (69). Although FDG-PET cannot clearly distinguish between granulomatous diseases such as sarcoidosis and lymphoma, it can localize the active lesions (70,71), which can be biopsied for a timely and minimally invasive diagnosis. The early diagnosis of vasculitis, especially large-vessel vasculitis, prevents progression to the occlusive phase of the disease. In this regard, FDG-PET has demonstrated high specificity and high sensitivity to detect and assess the activity of large-vessel vasculitis (72,73). It can noninvasively detect and quantitatively assess the disease activity in inflammatory bowel disease (74,75). Fluorodeoxyglucose uptake in the synovium measured using the standard uptake values (SUVs) facilitates the quantitative assessment of synovial activity (76), which has been particularly helpful in assessing the disease activity in patients with rheumatoid arthritis (77). The increase in SUV and the number of PET-positive joints correlated with swelling and tenderness of the joints, ultrasonography, synovial thickness, and inflammatory serum markers (ESR and C-reactive protein). This facilitates the measurement of disease activity in the joints of patients with rheumatologic diseases. Other infectious or inflammatory process that can be visualized with FDG-PET are thrombophlebitis (78,79), infected implantable devices (80), and pleural diseases (81).

Advantages of FDG-PET over Other Nuclear Medicine Techniques
Currently, gallium-67 scanning is the most commonly used radiotracer for the evaluation of FUO (32). However, FDG-PET has many advantages over conventional nuclear medicine techniques. Fluorodeoxyglucose offers a better tracer kinetic, a favorable 110-minute half-life, better spatial resolution (±5 to 8 mm resolution for PET vs. 10 to 15 mm for single photon emission computed tomography, SPECT), better lesion-to-background ratio (82), low dose to the patient, and the possibility for quantification decreasing the variability between readers. To date there have been no reported side effects from the injection of FDG. Whole-body FDG-PET scanning is completed approximately 2 hours from the injection, which results in earlier reporting than with other radiotracers (83). An important safety factor is that, in contrast to labeled leukocytes, in FDG-PET there is no handling of blood products. Fluorodeoxyglucose-PET is more sensitive in chronic, low-grade infections, has high accuracy in the central skeleton, and a high interobserver agreement (59,84,85). Another major advantage of FDG-PET over gallium in the evaluation of FUO patients is the ability to visualize and assess the degree of activity in a variety of inflammatory vessel diseases (83). It has been reported that FDG-PET can clearly visualize sarcoid lesions in the lungs and brain when concurrent gallium scans are negative (86).

Advantages of FDG-PET Over Anatomic Imaging
Timely identification and localization of the source of FUO is critical for the management of patients. Therefore, FDG-PET scanning is very helpful in this regard because it can detect early changes at the molecular level before they become apparent on anatomic imaging. Fluorodeoxyglucose-PET images the whole body in one study. Post-therapy tissue changes such as scarring, edema, and necrosis may alter the identification of recurrent tumor with anatomic imaging. Regardless of anatomic changes after chemotherapy and radiation therapy, FDG-PET can detect residual disease and has a high negative predictive value for viable disease in a residual anatomic abnormality, reaching 97% in some cases (87). Therefore, equivocal radiographic findings can be accurately characterized with FDG-PET. There is also increasing concern about the risk of radiation (88), radiocontrast-induced nephropathy (89), and allergic reactions (90) to patients imaged with CT. Furthermore, FDG-PET is able to detect early inflammatory and infectious lesions when anatomic imaging modalities reveal no abnormalities (91).

FDG-PET and Biopsy
As opposed to the other noninvasive diagnostic approaches in FUO, biopsy is a directed invasive intervention, which is often required to make a diagnosis. The most common biopsies performed in an FUO scenario are bone marrow, liver, lymph node, temporal artery, pleura, and pericardium. However, biopsy has spatial limitations, and a negative biopsy result may well be a false-negative finding due to sampling

errors. The combination of anatomic imaging and FDG-PET either through a software fusion or a combined PET-CT scanne leads to better localization of functional abnormalities. The registration of anatomic and functional images can be used to guide biopsies to the metabolically active area (92), which can increase the yield of this approach and decrease the need for unnecessary procedures.

Considerations for Accurate Reading of FDG-PET

When searching for the source of FUO, certain areas of the body can sometimes be difficult to evaluate because of normally high FDG uptake. The kidneys excrete FDG; therefore, there is intense FDG activity in the renal collecting systems, ureters, and bladder. There is also high FDG uptake in the brain and myocardium. Fluorodeoxyglucose activity in the bowel can be variably intense in the adult population (Fig. 23.1), which can decrease the accuracy of FDG-PET in the evaluation of the abdomen. However, FDG-PET can play a major role in the pediatric population because there is usually low FDG activity in the bowel (Fig. 23.2) (57). There is also physiologic activity in the thymus of children and young adults, which usually looks like an inverted V

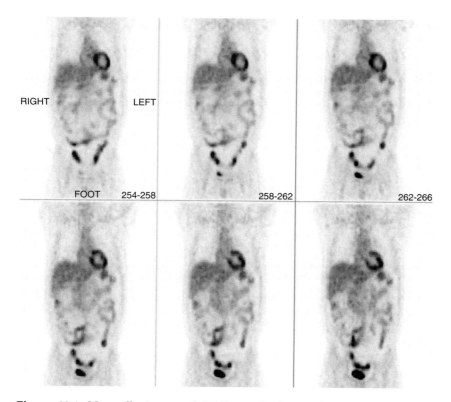

Figure 23.1. Normally increased FDG uptake is noted in the bowel of a 45–year-old patient with a history of tonsillar cancer.

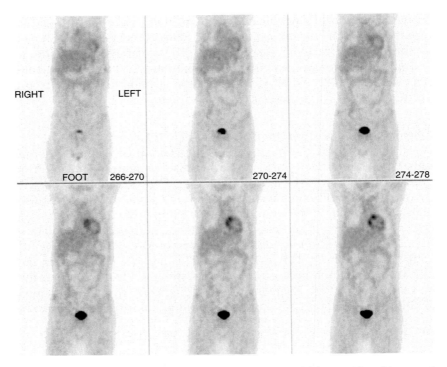

Figure 23.2. Normal FDG-PET scan of an 11–year-old boy with a history of Hodgkin's disease. There is a faint activity in the bowel.

(Fig. 23.3) (93). Therefore, accurate interpretation of FDG-PET images requires optimal knowledge of the normal distribution of FDG throughout the anatomic structures of the body and the variations that might occur with age (93).

Certain tumors cannot be easily detected with FDG-PET because of low FDG uptake, such as in hepatocellular carcinoma (94) or certain types of pancreatic tumors.(95) Because of the limited spatial resolution of PET (96), it is also difficult to detect low-grade tumors (e.g., cartilaginous tumors) (97), small lung nodules, and brain metastases (98). Although there has been a report of intra-vascular lymphomatosis presenting as fever of unknown origin (99), FDG-PET remains less effective in the detection of small-vessel disease.

Because FDG follows a similar pathway as glucose, a normalization of blood sugar level is a must in order not to miss any active malignant lesions because of suboptimal image quality (100). However, it is reported that the serum glucose levels do not necessarily affect the accuracy of FDG-PET when inflammatory and infectious lesion is evaluated (101).

Studies Regarding FDG-PET and FUO

There have been a limited number of prospective studies regarding FDG-PET scan and FUO. The percentage of FDG-PET scans helpful in the diagnosis of FUO as reported in the literature ranged from 37% to 69% (83,102–106). This variation is attributed to different factors, including a slightly different definition of FUO, a wide array of heterogeneous disorders, variable FDG-PET techniques, and no structured diagnostic protocol. However, the contributory effect of FDG-PET in the diagnosis of FUO was found to be higher than gallium scintigraphy (25%) (83). Fluorodeoxyglucose-PET was more helpful in the diagnostic process of patients with a suspected focal infection or localized inflammation than in FUO (104). Only one study found that indium-111–labeled granulocyte scintigraphy had a superior diagnostic performance compared to FDG-PET in the evaluation of FUO (106), but in the 19 patients studied, only one patient was diagnosed with malignancy (Hodgkin's disease).

Our Experience with FDG-PET

We retrospectively reviewed 30 FDG-PET scans of 30 patients (aged 13 to 73 years) who were evaluated at our institution for FUO during the period between 1999 and 2004. Clinical follow-up, which included subsequent conventional imaging studies and/or pathology results, was compared to the FDG-PET scan results. Fluorodeoxyglucose-PET contributed to the diagnosis of 71% of the cases. The causes of fever detected by FDG-PET included pneumonia, non-Hodgkin's lymphoma (Fig. 23.4), Hodgkin's disease (Fig. 23.5), Crohn's disease

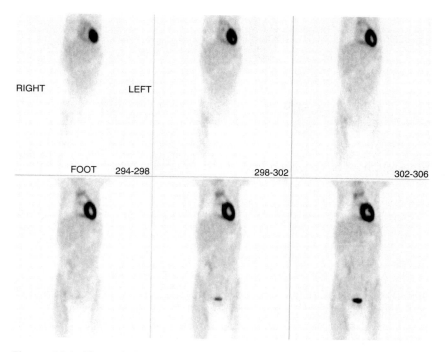

Figure 23.3. Normal FDG uptake is seen in the thymus of a 10–year-old patient.

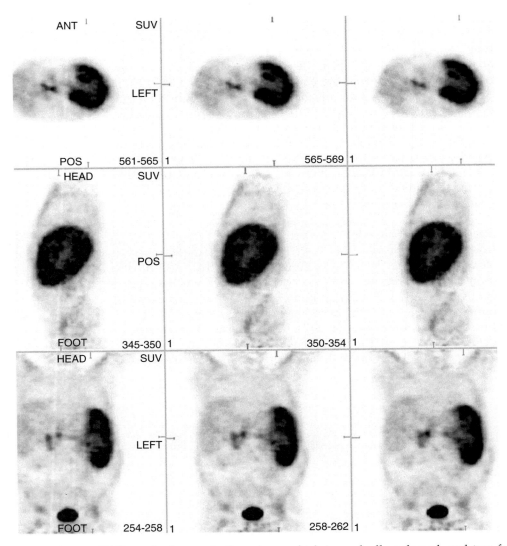

Figure 23.4. Intense FDG uptake is seen in the spleen, which is markedly enlarged, and two foci of abnormal uptake are visible in the upper abdomen, representing lymphadenopathy. The patient was diagnosed with non-Hodgkin's lymphoma.

(Fig. 23.6), surgical wound infection, infected liver cysts, leukemia, and metastatic renal cell carcinoma (Fig. 23.7). Fluorodeoxyglucose-PET was falsely negative in three cases of colitis, peritonitis (Fig. 23.8), and rejected renal transplant. Two FDG-PET scans were falsely positive in two patients with suspected abnormal activity in the abdomen; one of them had an eventual diagnosis of endocarditis.

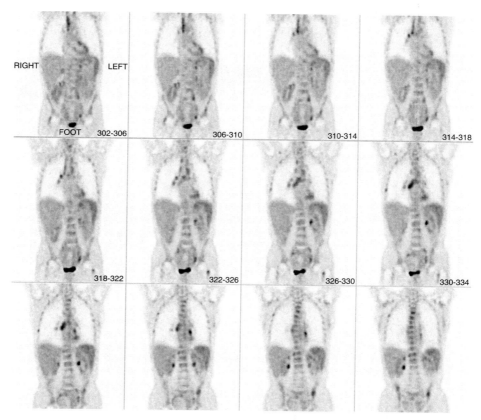

Figure 23.5. Abnormal FDG uptake is seen in the bone marrow, as well as in supraclavicular and mediastinal lymph nodes of a patient with FUO. The patient was diagnosed with Hodgkin's disease.

Figure 23.6. Diffuse FDG activity in the bowel. Although this pattern can be seen in normal adult patients, this finding was the only suspicious source of FUO in this patient, with a history of renal transplant. Subsequent colonoscopies and bone marrow biopsies were negative. The patient underwent a laparotomy; after segmental resection of the terminal ileum and cecum, he was diagnosed with Crohn's disease.

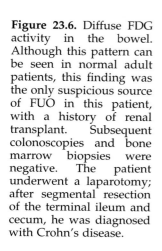

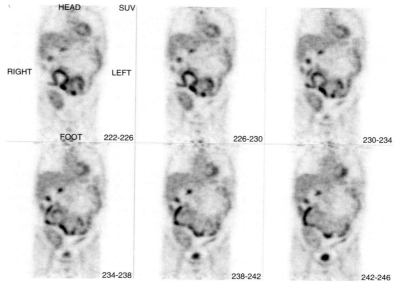

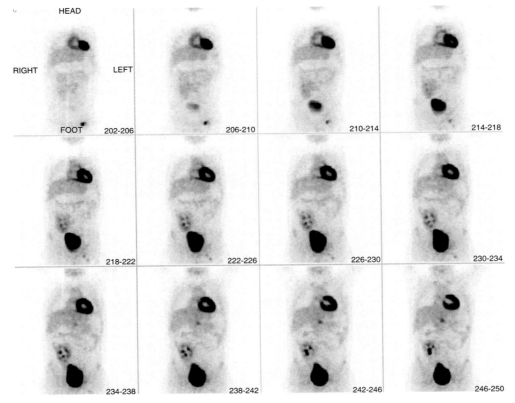

Figure 23.7. FDG-PET scan (coronal images) performed on a 13–year-old boy who underwent bilateral nephrectomies and renal transplant for polycystic kidney disease, after the patient developed a fever of unknown origin. Two foci of abnormal FDG uptake were noted in the left inguinal and in the portahepatic regions. There was no evidence of abnormal uptake in the transplanted kidney. Following biopsies, the patient was diagnosed with renal cell carcinoma in the transplanted kidney, which was removed.

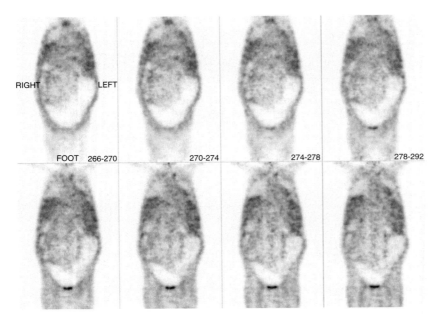

Figure 23.8. Coronal FDG-PET images of a 44–year-old patient who had a history of liver transplant, presenting with marked abdominal and pelvic ascites. There is a large photopenic area in the abdomen corresponding to the abdominal fluid but no definite evidence of a suspected source of FUO. The patient underwent a paracentesis and was diagnosed with peritonitis.

Conclusion

Fluorodeoxyglucose-PET is a valuable new imaging technique that has the potential for a major role in patients with FUO. It can detect malignancies as well as infectious and noninfectious inflammatory processes at an early stage of the disease. It has proven its superiority to other currently used conventional nuclear medicine imaging techniques. When ordered early in the diagnostic workup, FDG-PET has the potential to identify the area of abnormal activity where the cause of fever is likely to be found. This adds valuable information that can be used to focus the investigation and to eliminate unnecessary procedures, resulting in better management of the patients.

References

1. Petersdorf RG, Beeson PB. Fever of unexplained origin: report on 100 cases. Medicine (Baltimore) 1961;40:1–30.
2. Petersdorf RG. Fever of unknown origin. An old friend revisited. Arch Intern Med 1992;152:21–22.
3. Durack DT, Street AC. Fever of unknown origin—reexamined and redefined. Curr Clin Top Infect Dis 1991;11:35–51.
4. Konecny P, Davidson RN. Pyrexia of unknown origin in the 1990s: time to redefine. Br J Hosp Med 1996;56:21–24.
5. Finkelstein JA, Christiansen CL, Platt R. Fever in pediatric primary care: occurrence, management, and outcomes. Pediatrics 2000;105:260–266.
6. McClung HJ. Prolonged fever of unknown origin in children. Am J Dis Child 1972;124:544–550.
7. Dechovitz AB, Moffet HL. Classification of acute febrile illnesses in childhood. Clin Pediatr (Phila) 1968;7:649–653.
8. Pizzo PA, Lovejoy FH Jr, Smith DH. Prolonged fever in children: review of 100 cases. Pediatrics 1975;55:468–473.
9. Lohr JA, Hendley JO. Prolonged fever of unknown origin: a record of experiences with 54 childhood patients. Clin Pediatr (Phila) 1977;16:768–773.
10. Brewis EG. Child care in general practice. Undiagnosed fever. Br Med J 1965;5427:107–109.
11. Larson EB, Featherstone HJ, Petersdorf RG. Fever of undetermined origin: diagnosis and follow-up of 105 cases, 1970–1980. Medicine (Baltimore) 1982;61:269–292.
12. Knockaert DC, Vanneste LJ, Vanneste SB, et al. Fever of unknown origin in the 1980s. An update of the diagnostic spectrum. Arch Intern Med 1992;152:51–55.
13. de Kleijn EM, Vandenbroucke JP, van der Meer JW. Fever of unknown origin (FUO). I. A prospective multicenter study of 167 patients with FUO, using fixed epidemiologic entry criteria. The Netherlands FUO Study Group. Medicine (Baltimore) 1997;76:392–400.
14. Mourad O, Palda V, Detsky AS. A comprehensive evidence-based approach to fever of unknown origin. Arch Intern Med 2003;163:545–551.
15. Knockaert DC, Vanneste LJ, Bobbaers HJ. Fever of unknown origin in elderly patients. J Am Geriatr Soc 1993;41:1187–1192.

16. Cunha BA. Fever of unknown origin. Infect Dis Clin North Am 1996; 10:111–127.
17. Miller ML, Szer I, Yogev R, et al. Fever of unknown origin. Pediatr Clin North Am 1995;42:999–1015.
18. Iikuni Y, Okada J, Kondo H, et al. Current fever of unknown origin 1982–1992. Intern Med 1994;33:67–73.
19. Hoen B, Beguinot I, Rabaud C, et al. The Duke criteria for diagnosing infective endocarditis are specific: analysis of 100 patients with acute fever or fever of unknown origin. Clin Infect Dis 1996;23:298–302.
20. Carey BM, Williams CE, Arthur RJ. Ultrasound demonstration of pericardial empyema in an infant with pyrexia of undetermined origin. Pediatr Radiol 1988;18:349–350.
21. Picardi M, Morante R, Rotoli B. Ultrasound exploration in the work-up of unexplained fever in the immunocompromized host: preliminary observations. Haematologica 1997;82:455–457.
22. AbuRahma AF, Saiedy S, Robinson PA, et al. Role of venous duplex imaging of the lower extremities in patients with fever of unknown origin. Surgery 1997;121:366–371.
23. Gartner JC Jr. Fever of unknown origin. Adv Pediatr Infect Dis 1992;7: 1–24.
24. Cheng MF, Chiou CC, Hsieh KS. Mastoiditis: a disease often overlooked by pediatricians. J Microbiol Immunol Infect 2000;33:237–240.
25. Picus D, Siegel MJ, Balfe DM. Abdominal computed tomography in children with unexplained prolonged fever. J Comput Assist Tomogr 1984; 8:851–856.
26. de Leon DG, Shifteh S, Cunha BA. FUO due to sarcoidosis-lymphoma syndrome. Heart Lung 2004;33:124–129.
27. Gedalia A, Shetty AK, Ward KJ, et al. Role of MRI in diagnosis of childhood sarcoidosis with fever of unknown origin. J Pediatr Orthop 1997; 17:460–462.
28. Wagner AD, Andresen J, Raum E, et al. Standardised work-up programme for fever of unknown origin and contribution of magnetic resonance imaging for the diagnosis of hidden systemic vasculitis. Ann Rheum Dis 2005;64:105–110.
29. Berendt AR, Lipsky B. Is this bone infected or not? Differentiating neuro-osteoarthropathy from osteomyelitis in the diabetic foot. Curr Diab Rep 2004;4:424–429.
30. Bluman EM, Palumbo MA, Lucas PR. Spinal epidural abscess in adults. J Am Acad Orthop Surg 2004;12:155–163.
31. Ozaras R, Celik AD, Zengin K, et al. Is laparotomy necessary in the diagnosis of fever of unknown origin? Acta Chir Belg 2005;105:89–92.
32. Knockaert DC, Mortelmans LA, De Roo MC, et al. Clinical value of gallium-67 scintigraphy in evaluation of fever of unknown origin. Clin Infect Dis 1994;18:601–605.
33. Syrjala MT, Valtonen V, Liewendahl K, et al. Diagnostic significance of indium-111 granulocyte scintigraphy in febrile patients. J Nucl Med 1987;28:155–160.
34. Peters AM. Nuclear medicine imaging in fever of unknown origin. Q J Nucl Med 1999;43:61–73.
35. Kjaer A, Lebech AM. Diagnostic value of (111)In-granulocyte scintigraphy in patients with fever of unknown origin. J Nucl Med 2002;43: 140–144.
36. Peters AM. The utility of [99mTc]HMPAO-leukocytes for imaging infection. Semin Nucl Med 1994;24:110–127.

37. Gallowitsch HJ, Heinisch M, Mikosch P, et al. [Tc-99m ciprofloxacin in clinically selected patients for peripheral osteomyelitis, spondylodiscitis and fever of unknown origin–preliminary results]. Nuklearmedizin 2002; 41:30–36.

38. Meller J, Ivancevic V, Conrad M, et al. Clinical value of immunoscintigraphy in patients with fever of unknown origin. J Nucl Med 1998;39: 1248–1253.

39. Maugeri D, Santangelo A, Abbate S, et al. A new method for diagnosing fever of unknown origin (FUO) due to infection of muscular-skeletal system in elderly people: leukoscan Tc-99m labelled scintigraphy. Eur Rev Med Pharmacol Sci 2001;5:123–126.

40. Ak I, Stokkel MP, Pauwels EK. Positron emission tomography with 2–[18F] fluoro-2–deoxy-D-glucose in oncology. Part II. The clinical value in detecting and staging primary tumours. J Cancer Res Clin Oncol 2000;126:560–574.

41. Hawkins RA, Choi Y, Huang SC, et al. Quantitating tumor glucose metabolism with FDG and PET. J Nucl Med 1992;33:339–344.

42. Avril N, Menzel M, Dose J, et al. Glucose metabolism of breast cancer assessed by 18F-FDG PET: histologic and immunohistochemical tissue analysis. J Nucl Med 2001;42:9–16.

43. Warburg O. On the origin of cancer cells. Science 1956;123:309–314.

44. Bakheet SM, Powe J. Benign causes of 18–FDG uptake on whole body imaging. Semin Nucl Med 1998;28:352–358.

45. Chakrabarti R, Jung CY, Lee TP, et al. Changes in glucose transport and transporter isoforms during the activation of human peripheral blood lymphocytes by phytohemagglutinin. J Immunol 1994;152:2660–2668.

46. Gamelli RL, Liu H, He LK, et al. Augmentations of glucose uptake and glucose transporter-1 in macrophages following thermal injury and sepsis in mice. J Leukoc Biol 1996;59:639–647.

47. Ahmed N, Kansara M, Berridge MV. Acute regulation of glucose transport in a monocyte-macrophage cell line: Glut-3 affinity for glucose is enhanced during the respiratory burst. Biochem J 1997;327(pt 2):369–375.

48. Tan AS, Ahmed N, Berridge MV. Acute regulation of glucose transport after activation of human peripheral blood neutrophils by phorbol myristate acetate, fMLP, and granulocyte-macrophage colony-stimulating factor. Blood 1998;91:649–655.

49. Sorbara LR, Maldarelli F, Chamoun G, et al. Human immunodeficiency virus type 1 infection of H9 cells induces increased glucose transporter expression. J Virol 1996;70:7275–7279.

50. Kubota R, Yamada S, Kubota K, et al. Intratumoral distribution of fluorine-18–fluorodeoxyglucose in vivo: high accumulation in macrophages and granulation tissues studied by microautoradiography. J Nucl Med 1992;11:1972–1980.

51. Brown RS, Leung JY, Fisher SJ, et al. Intratumoral distribution of tritiated fluorodeoxyglucose in breast carcinoma: I. Are inflammatory cells important? J Nucl Med 1995;36:1854–1861.

52. Kostakoglu L, Agress H Jr, Goldsmith SJ. Clinical role of FDG PET in evaluation of cancer patients. Radiographics 2003;23:315–340; quiz 533.

53. Divgi C. Imaging: Staging and evaluation of lymphoma using nuclear medicine. Semin Oncol 2005;32:11–18.

54. Kazama T, Faria SC, Varavithya V, et al. FDG PET in the evaluation of treatment for lymphoma: clinical usefulness and pitfalls. Radiographics 2005;25:191–207.

55. Hudson MM, Krasin MJ, Kaste SC. PET imaging in pediatric Hodgkin's lymphoma. Pediatr Radiol 2004;34:190–198.

56. Zhuang H, Alavi A. 18–fluorodeoxyglucose positron emission tomographic imaging in the detection and monitoring of infection and inflammation. Semin Nucl Med 2002;32:47–59.

57. El-Haddad G, Zhuang H, Gupta N, et al. Evolving role of positron emission tomography in the management of patients with inflammatory and other benign disorders. Semin Nucl Med 2004;34:313–329.

58. Zhuang H, Duarte PS, Pourdehand M, et al. Exclusion of chronic osteomyelitis with F-18 fluorodeoxyglucose positron emission tomographic imaging. Clin Nucl Med 2000;25:281–284.

59. Guhlmann A, Brecht-Krauss D, Suger G, et al. Fluorine-18–FDG PET and technetium-99m antigranulocyte antibody scintigraphy in chronic osteomyelitis. J Nucl Med 1998;39:2145–2152.

60. Guhlmann A, Brecht-Krauss D, Suger G, et al. Chronic osteomyelitis: detection with FDG PET and correlation with histopathologic findings. Radiology 1998;206:749–754.

61. Meller J, Koster G, Liersch T, et al. Chronic bacterial osteomyelitis: prospective comparison of (18)F-FDG imaging with a dual-head coincidence camera and (111)In-labelled autologous leucocyte scintigraphy. Eur J Nucl Med Mol Imaging 2002;29:53–60.

62. Erdman WA, Tamburro F, Jayson HT, et al. Osteomyelitis: characteristics and pitfalls of diagnosis with MR imaging. Radiology 1991;180:533–539.

63. Crim JR, Seeger LL. Imaging evaluation of osteomyelitis. Crit Rev Diagn Imaging 1994;35:201–256.

64. Zhuang H, Sam JW, Chacko TK, et al. Rapid normalization of osseous FDG uptake following traumatic or surgical fractures. Eur J Nucl Med Mol Imaging 2003;30:1096–1103.

65. Koort JK, Makinen TJ, Knuuti J, et al. Comparative 18F-FDG PET of experimental Staphylococcus aureus osteomyelitis and normal bone healing. J Nucl Med 2004;45:1406–1411.

66. Zhuang H, Duarte PS, Pourdehnad M, et al. The promising role of 18F-FDG PET in detecting infected lower limb prosthesis implants. J Nucl Med 2001;42:44–48.

67. Keidar Z, Militianu D, Melamed E, et al. The diabetic foot: initial experience with 18F-FDG PET/CT. J Nucl Med 2005;46:444–449.

68. O'Doherty MJ, Barrington SF, Campbell M, et al. PET scanning and the human immunodeficiency virus-positive patient. J Nucl Med 1997;38:1575–1583.

69. Heald AE, Hoffman JM, Bartlett JA, et al. Differentiation of central nervous system lesions in AIDS patients using positron emission tomography (PET). Int J STD AIDS 1996;7:337–346.

70. Dubey N, Miletich RS, Wasay M, et al. Role of fluorodeoxyglucose positron emission tomography in the diagnosis of neurosarcoidosis. J Neurol Sci 2002;205:77–81.

71. Milman N, Mortensen J, Sloth C. Fluorodeoxyglucose PET scan in pulmonary sarcoidosis during treatment with inhaled and oral corticosteroids. Respiration 2003;70:408–413.

72. Walter MA, Melzer RA, Schindler C, et al. The value of [(18)F]FDG-PET in the diagnosis of large-vessel vasculitis and the assessment of activity and extent of disease. Eur J Nucl Med Mol Imaging 2005;(6):674–681.

73. Moosig F, Czech N, Mehl C, et al. Correlation between 18–fluorodeoxyglucose accumulation in large vessels and serological markers of inflammation in polymyalgia rheumatica: a quantitative PET study. Ann Rheum Dis 2004;63:870–873.

74. Neurath MF, Vehling D, Schunk K, et al. Noninvasive assessment of Crohn's disease activity: a comparison of 18F-fluorodeoxyglucose positron emission tomography, hydromagnetic resonance imaging, and granulocyte scintigraphy with labeled antibodies. Am J Gastroenterol 2002; 97:1978–1985.

75. Pio BS, Byrne FR, Aranda R, et al. Noninvasive quantification of bowel inflammation through positron emission tomography imaging of 2–deoxy-2–[18F]fluoro-D-glucose-labeled white blood cells. Mol Imaging Biol 2003;5:271–277.

76. Roivainen A, Parkkola R, Yli-Kerttula T, et al. Use of positron emission tomography with methyl-11C-choline and 2–18F-fluoro-2–deoxy-D-glucose in comparison with magnetic resonance imaging for the assessment of inflammatory proliferation of synovium. Arthritis Rheum 2003; 48:3077–3084.

77. Beckers C, Ribbens C, Andre B, et al. Assessment of disease activity in rheumatoid arthritis with (18)F-FDG PET. J Nucl Med 2004;45:956–964.

78. Bleeker-Rovers CP, Jager G, Tack CJ, et al. F-18–fluorodeoxyglucose positron emission tomography leading to a diagnosis of septic thrombophlebitis of the portal vein: description of a case history and review of the literature. J Intern Med 2004;255:419–423.

79. Miceli M, Atoui R, Walker R, et al. Diagnosis of deep septic thrombophlebitis in cancer patients by fluorine-18 fluorodeoxyglucose positron emission tomography scanning: a preliminary report. J Clin Oncol 2004; 22:1949–1956.

80. Miceli MH, Jones Jackson LB, Walker RC, et al. Diagnosis of infection of implantable central venous catheters by [18F]fluorodeoxyglucose positron emission tomography. Nucl Med Commun 2004;25:813–818.

81. Duysinx B, Nguyen D, Louis R, et al. Evaluation of pleural disease with 18–fluorodeoxyglucose positron emission tomography imaging. Chest 2004;125:489–493.

82. Sugawara Y, Gutowski TD, Fisher SJ, et al. Uptake of positron emission tomography tracers in experimental bacterial infections: a comparative biodistribution study of radiolabeled FDG, thymidine, L-methionine, 67Ga-citrate, and 125I-HSA. Eur J Nucl Med 1999;26: 333–341.

83. Blockmans D, Knockaert D, Maes A, et al. Clinical value of [(18)F]fluorodeoxyglucose positron emission tomography for patients with fever of unknown origin. Clin Infect Dis 2001;32:191–196.

84. de Winter F, van de Wiele C, Vogelaers D, et al. Fluorine-18 fluorodeoxyglucose-position emission tomography: a highly accurate imaging modality for the diagnosis of chronic musculoskeletal infections. J Bone Joint Surg Am 2001;83–A:651–660.

85. Kalicke T, Schmitz A, Risse JH, et al. Fluorine-18 fluorodeoxyglucose PET in infectious bone diseases: results of histologically confirmed cases. Eur J Nucl Med 2000;27:524–528.

86. Xiu Y, Yu XQ, Cheng E, et al. Sarcoidosis demonstrated by FDG PET imaging with negative findings on gallium scintigraphy. Clin Nucl Med 2005;30:193–195.

87. Porceddu SV, Jarmolowski E, Hicks RJ, et al. Utility of positron emission tomography for the detection of disease in residual neck nodes after (chemo)radiotherapy in head and neck cancer. Head Neck 2005;27: 175–181.

88. Buls N, de Mey J, Covens P, et al. Health screening with CT: prospective assessment of radiation dose and associated detriment. JBR-BTR 2005;88: 12–16.

89. Asif A, Epstein M. Prevention of radiocontrast-induced nephropathy. Am J Kidney Dis 2004;44:12–24.

90. Cochran ST. Anaphylactoid reactions to radiocontrast media. Curr Allergy Asthma Rep 2005;5:28–31.

91. Dadparvar S, Anderson GS, Bhargava P, et al. Paraneoplastic encephalitis associated with cystic teratoma is detected by fluorodeoxyglucose positron emission tomography with negative magnetic resonance image findings. Clin Nucl Med 2003;28:893–896.

92. Yap JT, Carney JP, Hall NC, et al. Image-guided cancer therapy using PET/CT. Cancer J 2004;10:221–233.

93. El-Haddad G, Alavi A, Mavi A, et al. Normal variants in [18F]-fluorodeoxyglucose PET imaging. Radiol Clin North Am 2004;42: 1063–1081, viii.

94. Torizuka T, Tamaki N, Inokuma T, et al. In vivo assessment of glucose metabolism in hepatocellular carcinoma with FDG-PET. J Nucl Med 1995;36:1811–1817.

95. Delbeke D, Pinson CW. Pancreatic tumors: role of imaging in the diagnosis, staging, and treatment. J Hepatobiliary Pancreat Surg 2004;11: 4–10.

96. Takamochi K, Yoshida J, Murakami K, et al. Pitfalls in lymph node staging with positron emission tomography in non-small cell lung cancer patients. Lung Cancer 2005;47:235–242.

97. Lee FY, Yu J, Chang SS, et al. Diagnostic value and limitations of fluorine-18 fluorodeoxyglucose positron emission tomography for cartilaginous tumors of bone. J Bone Joint Surg Am 2004;86–A:2677–2685.

98. Friedman KP, Wahl RL. Clinical use of positron emission tomography in the management of cutaneous melanoma. Semin Nucl Med 2004;34: 242–253.

99. Hoshino A, Kawada E, Ukita T, et al. Usefulness of FDG-PET to diagnose intravascular lymphomatosis presenting as fever of unknown origin. Am J Hematol 2004;76:236–239.

100. Sugawara Y, Braun DK, Kison PV, et al. Rapid detection of human infections with fluorine-18 fluorodeoxyglucose and positron emission tomography: preliminary results. Eur J Nucl Med 1998;25:1238–1243.

101. Zhuang HM, Cortes-Blanco A, Pourdehnad M, et al. Do high glucose levels have differential effect on FDG uptake in inflammatory and malignant disorders? Nucl Med Commun 2001;22:1123–1128.

102. Meller J, Altenvoerde G, Munzel U, et al. Fever of unknown origin: prospective comparison of [18F]FDG imaging with a double-head coincidence camera and gallium-67 citrate SPET. Eur J Nucl Med 2000;27: 1617–1625.

103. Lorenzen J, Buchert R, Bohuslavizki KH. Value of FDG PET in patients with fever of unknown origin. Nucl Med Commun 2001;22:779–783.

104. Bleeker-Rovers CP, de Kleijn EM, Corstens FH, et al. Clinical value of FDG PET in patients with fever of unknown origin and patients suspected of focal infection or inflammation. Eur J Nucl Med Mol Imaging 2004;31: 29–37.

105. Buysschaert I, Vanderschueren S, Blockmans D, et al. Contribution of (18)fluoro-deoxyglucose positron emission tomography to the work-up of patients with fever of unknown origin. Eur J Intern Med 2004;15: 151–156.
106. Kjaer A, Lebech AM, Eigtved A, et al. Fever of unknown origin: prospective comparison of diagnostic value of 18F-FDG PET and 111In-granulocyte scintigraphy. Eur J Nucl Med Mol Imaging 2004;31:622–626.

24

Infection and Inflammation

Marc P. Hickeson

Positron emission tomography (PET) with fluorine-18 (^{18}F)-fluoro-2-deoxyglucose (FDG) has been proven to be a valuable noninvasive imaging modality for the diagnosis, staging, and monitoring of therapy for various malignancies. In addition, studies are demonstrating the value of FDG-PET for the evaluation of nononcologic conditions. Based on the literature, conditions such as osteomyelitis, fever of unknown origin (FUO), acquired immunodeficiency syndrome (AIDS), vasculitis, and inflammatory bowel disease can be successfully imaged with FDG-PET. With the approval of additional PET radiotracers in the future, there will be more widespread applications of PET for inflammatory and infectious disorders.

Unlike anatomic imaging modalities such as computed tomography (CT), magnetic resonance imaging (MRI), and ultrasound, PET is a molecular imaging modality that detects metabolic abnormalities present in the disease before structural abnormalities become evident. In addition to FDG, other radiopharmaceuticals are available for scintigraphic imaging such as technetium-99m (^{99m}Tc)-hexamethylpropylene-amine-oxime (HMPAO)-labeled leukocytes, indium-111 (^{111}In)-oxime labeled leukocytes, gallium-67 (^{67}Ga) citrate, ^{99m}Tc-labeled antigranulocyte monoclonal antibodies, and ^{99m}Tc-labeled immunoglobulins. Advantages of FDG-PET as compared with the aforementioned radiopharmaceuticals for the imaging of inflammation and infection include the ability to provide a result as early as $1\frac{1}{2}$ to 2 hours after tracer injection, the relatively low radiation dose, and the excellent spatial resolution and lesion-to-background contrast. These advantages contribute to the superior accuracy of FDG-PET for the diagnosis or exclusion of infections.

Clinical Applications of FDG-PET

The specific clinical applications of FDG-PET are as follows:

1. Osteomyelitis
2. Fever of unknown origin (FUO) (discussed in Chapter 23)

3. Acquired immunodeficiency syndrome (AIDS)
4. Vasculitis
5. Inflammatory bowel disease (IBD)
6. Thyroiditis
7. Chronic granulomatous disease (CGD)

Osteomyelitis

Although there is limited literature about FDG-PET imaging of osteomyelitis specifically in the pediatric population, FDG-PET has been shown to have a promising role for imaging bone infection in the general population (1–5). This is due to the high metabolic state and increase glucose accumulation by the inflammatory cells (6).

Unlike in adults, osteomyelitis in children usually results from hematogenous spread of microorganisms to bones. Infection usually affects a single bone and typically involves the metaphysis of long bone, most commonly the tibia, femur, or humerus. The clinical presentation of osteomyelitis includes local pain and swelling, fever, chills, and malaise. The most common infecting organisms are streptococci and *Staphylococcus aureus* in neonates, and *S. aureus* in the pediatric population. The diagnosis can usually be established with positive triple-phase bone scintigraphy and blood culture.

Although bone scintigraphy is highly sensitive and specific for the diagnosis of osteomyelitis in intact bone, interpretation is complicated in the presence of a coexisting fracture and surgical intervention at the site of suspected osteomyelitis. In this latter setting, further imaging using an infection radiotracer such as ^{67}Ga, ^{111}In-labeled leukocytes, and ^{18}F-FDG is often necessary to increase the specificity for osteomyelitis. The most specific method is with ^{111}In-labeled leukocytes; however, this is sensitive only for acute infection. ^{67}Ga is preferred to ^{111}In-labeled leukocytes for the detection of chronic infection (7,8). Fluorodeoxyglucose-PET also shows promise for the evaluation of chronic osteomyelitis. Unlike other nuclear medicine imaging modalities, FDG-PET provides good spatial resolution and intrinsic tomographic images, which allow differentiation of soft tissue infection from osteomyelitis. It also provides results within 3 hours after FDG injection, which is shorter than the few days required with ^{67}Ga imaging. It is also known that hypermetabolism seen on FDG-PET at the site of fractures normalizes relatively rapidly. A fracture may be associated with increased FDG uptake for up to 3 months (9). For this reason, FDG-PET facilitates differentiation of a noncomplicated fracture of greater than 3 months from a pathologic fracture (i.e., infection), and thus is not useful before 3 months. A negative FDG-PET study essentially rules out osteomyelitis (5). Fluorodeoxyglucose-PET also has promise for the monitoring the response to antimicrobial therapy (3).

In summary, FDG-PET is a functional imaging modality with high sensitivity for diagnosis of acute and chronic osteomyelitis. The value of PET is limited for the evaluation of acute uncomplicated osteomyelitis. However, in the minority of the cases of osteomyelitis involving nonintact bone, FDG-PET has great promise for diagnosis and for monitoring the response to antimicrobial therapy.

Acquired Immunodeficiency Syndrome

Acquired immunodeficiency syndrome (AIDS) is an infectious disease caused by human immunodeficiency virus (HIV). Morbidity and mortality from HIV infection most commonly occur not from the HIV infection itself but from the malignancies and opportunistic pathogens associated with AIDS.

O'Doherty et al. (10) studied the role of PET scanning in patients infected with HIV. Fluorodeoxyglucose-PET scan had a sensitivity and specificity of 92% and 94%, respectively, for the localization of focal pathology requiring treatment. The positive predictive value was greater than for hypermetabolic foci on FDG-PET with intensity greater than that of the liver. Fluorodeoxyglucose-PET can help localize a wide variety of infections such as *Cryptococcus neoformans, Pneumocystis carinii* pneumonia, *Pseudomonas aeruginosa, Mycobacterium tuberculosis,* and *Mycobacterium avium intracellulare* (Fig. 24.1). Furthermore, imaging with FDG using a dual-head coincidence imaging system was shown to provide a higher sensitivity than with ^{67}Ga imaging for the demonstration of a focus of infection in patients with AIDS (11).

Positron emission tomography has played a major role in the management of AIDS with central nervous system (CNS) lesions. Patients with HIV who present with a change in mental status or abnormal neurologic signs often have CNS lesions demonstrated on a CT scan or MRI. Toxoplasmosis is the most common infectious etiology of focal CNS lesions, and malignant lymphoma is the most common CNS malignancy in HIV-infected patients. Thallium-201 (^{201}Tl) and ^{99m}Tc-sestamibi have been used for the differentiation of toxoplasmosis and lymphoma in HIV-infected patients presenting with intracranial mass lesions. Heald et al. (12) reported that FDG-PET has a high accuracy

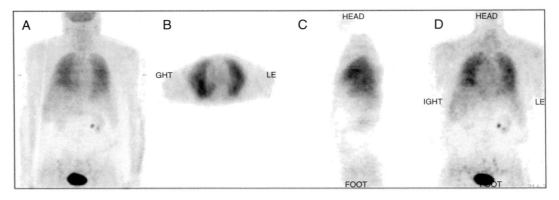

Figure 24.1. Fluorodeoxyglucose (FDG)-PET attenuation corrected imaging demonstrates diffuse and bilateral increased FDG uptake in the lungs. Maximal intensity projection (A), transaxial (B), sagittal (C), and coronal (D) are shown. The final diagnosis was *Pneumocystis carinii* pneumonia established by bronchoalveolar lavage.

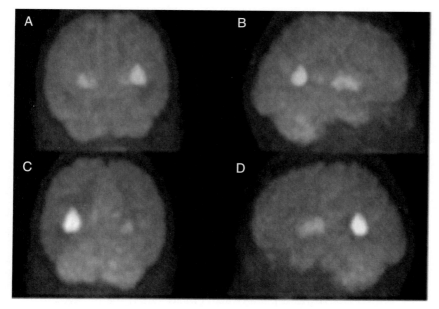

Figure 24.2. Biopsy-proven central nervous system (CNS) lymphoma involving the left parietal lobe shown on FDG-PET maximal intensity projection images in the anterior (A), right lateral (B), posterior (C) and left lateral (D) projections.

for the differentiation of CNS lymphoma from infections in the setting of brain mass lesions (Fig. 24.2). Lymphoma is associated with intense hypermetabolism as compared to infections. In that study, there were two false-positive cases due to progressive multifocal leukoencephalopathy demonstrating intense hypermetabolism on FDG-PET. Studies are currently under way to assess the accuracy of FDG-PET for the characterization of brain lesion in patients with AIDS (Fig. 24.2).

Fluorodeoxyglucose-PET has great promise to become a standard modality for localization, for the determination of the extent of opportunistic infections, and for the differentiation of CNS lymphoma from opportunistic infection in patients with brain mass lesions associated with AIDS.

Vasculitis

Vasculitis is defined as an inflammatory process associated with accumulation of leukocytes in the blood vessel wall and reactive damage to the mural structures. It is typically classified by the size of vessels most commonly involved by the disease. In several studies, FDG-PET has been shown to be useful for the evaluation of large vessel vasculitides, such as Takayasu disease and giant cell arteritis in arteries measuring more than 4mm in diameter (13–21), particularly for the initial diagnosis and for the assessment of response to treatment.

In children, Kawasaki disease (KD) and Henoch-Schönlein purpura are the most common vasculitides. Kawasaki disease is a vascular inflammatory disorder of unknown etiology that is usually self-limited.

The clinical manifestations include fevers, erythema, edema, mucositis, lymphadenopathy, and conjunctivitis. Diagnosis is usually established by history and physical examination. The most serious complication is myocardial infarction, for which echocardiogram is used for the evaluation of KD. Fluorodeoxyglucose-PET has been shown to be helpful for the evaluation for myocardial viability in patients with KD and previous myocardial infarct (22). Henoch-Schönlein purpura is a small vessel inflammatory disease to the skin, kidneys, gastrointestinal tract, lungs, and CNS. Because the small vessels are the predominant sites of involvement, FDG-PET is not expected to be a sensitive modality for the diagnosis of Henoch-Schönlein purpura.

In the adolescence population, Takayasu arteritis (TA) is the most common cause of vasculitis. It is a large vessel granulomatous inflammatory process affecting the aorta and its major branches. The signs and symptoms are nonspecific, such as fevers, weight loss, and lethargy. Because of the nonspecificity of these symptoms, TA may be undiagnosed for several months to years. Complications include aortic aneurysms, rupture, stenosis and thrombus, congestive heart failure, ischemic strokes, and end-organ infarcts. The diagnosis of TA is established by invasive angiography or MR angiography. However, diagnosis is difficult because the structural changes seen by contrast angiography are only seen late during the disease. Magnetic resonance angiography is currently becoming the modality of choice for diagnosis early in the disease. It would demonstrate the inflammatory wall thickening of the involved vessel in the early phases of the disease. Positron emission tomography with FDG also has promise in the evaluation of patients with TA. Hara et al. (23) reported a case of early TA in which the involved vessels demonstrated increased FDG uptake on PET imaging. Meller et al. (24) have shown subsequently in a study of five patients that FDG-PET is a suitable modality for the diagnosis of early TA (Fig. 24.3). In another study that included 15 patients, one with TA, FDG-PET detected more vascular areas involved by the inflammatory process than did the MRI (25). Fluorodeoxyglucose-PET has also been shown to be a promising modality for the early evaluation of the response to treatment of vasculitis (15,17) as the FDG-PET scan normalizes following successful treatment. Fluorodeoxyglucose-PET shows the potential to have an important role in the early diagnosis and monitoring treatment of patients with large and medium vessel vasculitis (Fig. 24.3).

Inflammatory Bowel Disease

Inflammatory bowel disease (IBD) is an inflammatory disease that affects the gastrointestinal tract. The etiology is uncertain but is probably immune-mediated. There are two main categories of IBD: Crohn's disease and ulcerative colitis. Crohn's disease can involve any region along the gastrointestinal tract from the mouth to the anus, and typically presents with diarrhea, abdominal pain, and weight loss. Ulcerative colitis involves the rectum and extends proximally, is limited to the

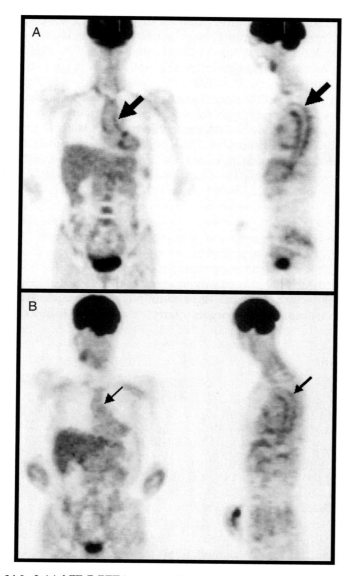

Figure 24.3. Initial FDG-PET images in the coronal and sagittal planes demonstrating intense FDG activity in the thoracic aorta (large arrows). Follow-up study demonstrated normalization in the ascending aorta (small arrow) and partial resolution in the descending aorta (medium arrow). [*Source:* Meller et al. (25), with permission of Springer.]

large intestine, and typically presents with bloody diarrhea, abdominal pain, and tenesmus. There are several extraintestinal manifestations of IBD, which include ocular manifestations, nephrolithiasis, arthropathy most commonly affecting large joints, primary sclerosing cholangitis, and erythema nodosum.

Positron emission tomography is a noninvasive modality that was reported to be helpful for the detection of disease activity in patients with IBD (26). However, the presence of physiologic FDG activity in the large intestine can affect the sensitivity and specificity of PET for the evaluation of IBD. Despite this limitation of FDG-PET, Neurath et al. (27) reported a sensitivity of 85% with FDG-PET for the demonstration of disease activity in Crohn's disease, which was significantly superior to that of other noninvasive imaging methods including MRI and leukocyte scintigraphy, and a specificity of greater than 89%.

Recently, investigators demonstrated clinically feasible methods of labeling FDG with leukocytes (28). The PET images with FDG-labeled leukocytes demonstrate minimal tracer activity in the healthy gastrointestinal and urinary tract as compared to FDG-PET images. Therefore, PET with FDG-labeled leukocytes provides abdominopelvic images with minimal hindrance from physiologic distribution of the radiotracer. The intensity of foci of FDG-labeled leukocytes activity correlated well with the degree of inflammation on histology (28).

In brief, FDG-PET is a noninvasive modality that has shown great promise for the detection of inflamed segments in patients with IBD. Studies are currently under way to assess the accuracy of FDG-labeled leukocytes, which will provide abdominopelvic images that are not hindered by normal physiologic activity in the gastrointestinal and urinary tract.

Thyroiditis

Thyroiditis is defined as an inflammatory process involving the thyroid. Although it is most prevalent between the third and fifth decades of life, it has been reported at all ages. Several types of thyroiditis exist, most commonly chronic lymphocytic (Hashimoto's) thyroiditis, subacute thyroiditis, and silent thyroiditis.

Thyroiditis can present incidentally as diffuse hypermetabolism involving the thyroid gland on FDG-PET (29–31). The differential diagnosis for diffuse hypermetabolism in the thyroid glands includes Graves' disease (32) and subclinical hypothyroidism associated with elevated serum thyroid-stimulating hormone (TSH) without any other thyroid pathology (33). Thyroiditis can be distinguished from thyroid cancer, which usually demonstrates focal hypermetabolism in the nodule.

In summary, the presence of diffuse hypermetabolism of the thyroid should raise the suspicion of subclinical hypothyroidism or thyroiditis in patients without symptoms of hyperthyroidism.

Chronic Granulomatous Disease

Chronic granulomatous disease (CGD) is a rare primary immunodeficiency disorder that results in recurrent, often life-threatening, bacterial and fungal infections. The vast majority of patients first presents during infancy or childhood. Chronic granulomatous disease is suspected to result from the inability of the phagocytes to produce adequate quantities of superoxide radicals to kill catalase positive bacteria and fungi. The diagnosis is established by determining the phagocytic cells' oxidase activity. Treatments for patients with CGD include aggressive treatment of infection, lifelong antibiotic prophylaxis, and γ-interferon therapy. This disease can be cured by bone marrow transplantation, provided that the patient does not have any underlying infection at the time of transplant (34).

Computed tomography scan has a valuable role in localizing the sites and extent of infectious foci in CGD patients. However, it cannot differentiate active lesions from chronic inactive lesions. Fluorodeoxyglucose-PET is a suitable imaging modality that can differentiate active infectious lesions from chronic inactive lesions by the presence of increased FDG accumulation in inflammatory tissues (6,26). In a study involving seven children with CGD, FDG-PET was compared with CT scan for the accuracy of the detection of infective foci (35). The number of lesions detected by FDG-PET and CT scan was 116 and 126, respectively. Fifty-nine lesions suspicious for active infection on CT scan were excluded by PET, and an additional 49 infectious lesions not seen on CT were detected by PET. The infectious agents were identified in all seven patients based on the FDG-PET results. Early identification of active lesions and differentiation of active lesions from chronic inactive lesions with therapy are important to prevent drug-related toxicities from ineffective or inappropriately prolonged treatment (Fig. 24.4).

In summary, FDG-PET is useful for the management of patient with CGD. It provides the ability to differentiate active infection from chronic inactive granuloma. A positive PET scan indicates that infection is present and that the abnormal hypermetabolic focus can be biopsied. A negative PET scan indicates that there is no evidence of infection. This would justify the discontinuation of aggressive,

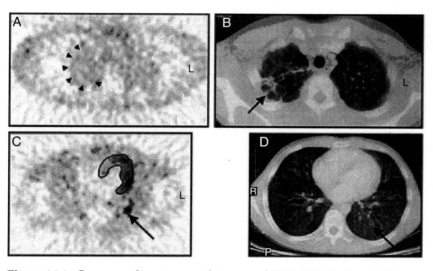

Figure 24.4. Corresponding transaxial images of FDG-PET (A,C) and CT scan (B,D) showing inactive lesion (A,B) and active lesions (C,D) due to *Actinomyces naeslundii*. [*Source:* Gungor et al. (35), with permission from the BMJ Publishing Group.]

potentially toxic antimicrobial treatment and qualify the patient to be a candidate for bone marrow transplantation.

Differentiation of Infectious or Inflammatory Processes from Malignancy

[18]F-fluoro-2-deoxyglucose is a glucose analogue. Its accumulation is not specific to tumors. It has been demonstrated that tumors as well as inflammatory and infectious processes frequently accumulate FDG (5,36), which may result in false-positive interpretation of FDG-PET for the presence of tumors. Tumors typically exhibit more intense FDG activity than inflammatory and infectious lesions. The standard uptake value (SUV) is a semiquantitative measurement of the intensity of uptake (see below). However, there is considerable overlap of the SUV of benign and malignant lesions. This makes the differentiation of benign from malignant lesions difficult if only one time point is used for imaging, particularly for lesions with mild to moderate FDG intensities (SUVs ranging from 1 to 5). The SUV can be calculated as follows:

$$SUV = \frac{Activity \ in \ MBq/mL \times (Decay \ factor \ of \ ^{18}F \ after \ injection)^{-1}}{Injected \ dose \ in \ MBq \times Body \ weight \ in \ g}$$

It has been demonstrated that the intensity of FDG accumulation in inflammatory tissues is maximal at approximately 60 minutes after injection and gradually decreases afterward (37). Lodge et al. (38) subsequently reported significantly different time-activity responses of benign and malignant lesions. Benign lesion peak FDG activity occurred within 30 minutes, whereas malignant lesions' maximal activity occurred at approximately 4 hours after injection. The different FDG uptake patterns may be attributed to the different enzymatic expression of hexokinase and glucose-6-phosphatase in benign and in malignant lesions. Tumors typically exhibit decreased glucose-6-phosphatase activity as compared to benign lesions (39,40). As a result, the hexokinase/glucose-6-phosphatase ratio is increased in tumors, which may explain why tumors demonstrate increasing FDG accumulation over a longer period of time after injection. Unlike tumors, mononuclear cells, which predominate in chronic inflammatory processes, have increased glucose-6-phosphatase activity (41). This may account for the shorter time to peak FDG accumulation after injection as compared with tumors. For this reason, dual-time point imaging is sometimes helpful for the differentiation of benign from malignant lesions.

Dual-time point imaging with FDG-PET is a technique that has been found to be helpful for distinguishing tumors from benign lesions in various conditions (42–45). In this technique, the first scan is performed using the same method as in single-time point imaging. The second scan is performed in the site of the lesion in question. Factors affecting the accuracy of this technique are the time of the first scan after injection and the time interval between the first and second scans. Because

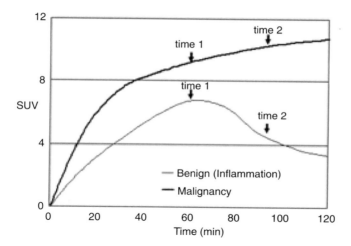

Figure 24.5. Plot of standard uptake value (SUV) versus time after FDG injection for inflammatory and malignant lesions.

FDG uptake by inflammatory cells peaks in intensity at about 60 minutes after injection, the suggested time of the first scan should be at least 60 minutes after FDG administration. The time interval between the first and second scans should be at least 30 minutes to provide adequate additional accumulation of FDG in tumors and differentiation between benign lesions and tumors (Fig. 24.5) (45). The positive interpretation criterion of this technique is an increase in SUV by at least 10% between the first to second scans (43).

Dual-time point imaging is a helpful technique for differentiating benign from malignant lesions, particularly for those with mild or moderate FDG accumulation. Malignant lesions increase in intensity on delayed imaging, and benign lesions demonstrate stable or decreasing intensity on delayed imaging.

Conclusion

Positron emission tomography is a noninvasive modality that shows great promise for the evaluation of patients with infections. The most commonly used radiopharmaceutical is FDG. With the availability of further studies, infection and inflammation may become a major clinical indication for FDG-PET in the clinical practice of medicine.

References

1. Robiller FC, Stumpe KD, Kossmann T, Weisshaupt D, Bruder E, von Schulthess GK. Chronic osteomyelitis of the femur: value of PET imaging. Eur Radiol 2000;10(5):855–858.
2. De Winter F, Vogelaers D, Gemmel F, Dierckx RA. Promising role of 18-F-fluoro-D-deoxyglucose positron emission tomography in clinical infectious diseases. Eur J Clin Microbiol Infect Dis 2002;21(4):247–257.

3. Kalicke T, Schmitz A, Risse JH, et al. Fluorine-18 fluorodeoxyglucose PET in infectious bone diseases: results of histologically confirmed cases. Eur J Nucl Med 2000;27(5):524–528.

4. Zhuang H, Alavi A. 18-fluorodeoxyglucose positron emission tomographic imaging in the detection and monitoring of infection and inflammation. Semin Nucl Med 2002;32(1):47–59.

5. Zhuang H, Duarte PS, Pourdehand M, Shnier D, Alavi A. Exclusion of chronic osteomyelitis with F-18 fluorodeoxyglucose positron emission tomographic imaging. Clin Nucl Med 2000;25(4):281–284.

6. Kubota R, Yamada S, Kubota K, Ishiwata K, Tamahashi N, Ido T. Intratumoral distribution of fluorine-18-fluorodeoxyglucose in vivo: high accumulation in macrophages and granulation tissues studied by microautoradiography. J Nucl Med 1992;33(11):1972–1980.

7. Alazraki NP. Radionuclide imaging in the evaluation of infections and inflammatory disease. Radiol Clin North Am 1993;31(4):783–794.

8. Saitoh-Miyazaki C, Itoh K. Comparative findings between 111-indium-labeled leukocytes and 67-gallium scintigraphy for patients with acute and chronic inflammatory diseases. Prog Clin Biol Res 1990;355:141–150.

9. Zhuang H, Sam JW, Chacko TK, et al. Rapid normalization of osseous FDG uptake following traumatic or surgical fractures. Eur J Nucl Med Mol Imaging 2003;30(8):1096–1103.

10. O'Doherty MJ, Barrington SF, Campbell M, Lowe J, Bradbeer CS. PET scanning and the human immunodeficiency virus-positive patient. J Nucl Med 1997;38(10):1575–1583.

11. Santiago JF, Jana S, Gilbert HM, et al. Role of fluorine-18–fluorodeoxyglucose in the work-up of febrile AIDS patients. Experience with dual head coincidence imaging. Clin Positron Imaging 1999;2(6):301–309.

12. Heald AE, Hoffman JM, Bartlett JA, Waskin HA. Differentiation of central nervous system lesions in AIDS patients using positron emission tomography (PET). Int J STD AIDS 1996;7(5):337–346.

13. Belhocine T. 18FDG imaging of giant cell arteritis: usefulness of whole-body plus brain PET. Eur J Nucl Med Mol Imaging 2004;31(7):1055–1056.

14. Brodmann M, Passath A, Aigner R, Seinost G, Stark G, Pilger E. F18-FDG-PET as a helpful tool in the diagnosis of giant cell arteritis. Rheumatology (Oxf) 2003;42(10):1264–1266.

15. Bleeker-Rovers CP, Bredie SJ, van der Meer JW, Corstens FH, Oyen WJ. F-18-fluorodeoxyglucose positron emission tomography in diagnosis and follow-up of patients with different types of vasculitis. Neth J Med 2003;61(10):323–329.

16. Bleeker-Rovers CP, Bredie SJ, van der Meer JW, Corstens FH, Oyen WJ. Fluorine 18 fluorodeoxyglucose positron emission tomography in the diagnosis and follow-up of three patients with vasculitis. Am J Med 2004;116(1):50–53.

17. Webb M, Chambers A, A AL-N, et al. The role of 18F-FDG PET in characterising disease activity in Takayasu arteritis. Eur J Nucl Med Mol Imaging 2004;31(5):627–634.

18. Moosig F, Czech N, Mehl C, et al. Correlation between 18-fluorodeoxyglucose accumulation in large vessels and serological markers of inflammation in polymyalgia rheumatica: a quantitative PET study. Ann Rheum Dis 2004;63(7):870–873.

19. Wenger M, Gasser R, Donnemiller E, et al. Images in cardiovascular medicine. Generalized large vessel arteritis visualized by 18-

fluorodeoxyglucose-positron emission tomography. Circulation 2003; 107(6):923.

20. Andrews J, Al-Nahhas A, Pennell DJ, et al. Non-invasive imaging in the diagnosis and management of Takayasu's arteritis. Ann Rheum Dis 2004;63(8):995–1000.

21. Blockmans D. The use of (18F)fluoro-deoxyglucose positron emission tomography in the assessment of large vessel vasculitis. Clin Exp Rheumatol 2003;21(6 suppl 32):S15–22.

22. Yoshibayashi M, Tamaki N, Nishioka K, et al. Regional myocardial perfusion and metabolism assessed by positron emission tomography in children with Kawasaki disease and significance of abnormal Q waves and their disappearance. Am J Cardiol 1991;68(17):1638–1645.

23. Hara M, Goodman PC, Leder RA. FDG-PET finding in early-phase Takayasu arteritis. J Comput Assist Tomogr 1999;23(1):16–18.

24. Meller J, Grabbe E, Becker W, Vosshenrich R. Value of F-18 FDG hybrid camera PET and MRI in early Takayasu aortitis. Eur Radiol 2003;13(2): 400–405.

25. Meller J, Strutz F, Siefker U, et al. Early diagnosis and follow-up of aortitis with [(18)F]FDG PET and MRI. Eur J Nucl Med Mol Imaging 2003; 30(5):730–736.

26. Bicik I, Bauerfeind P, Breitbach T, von Schulthess GK, Fried M. Inflammatory bowel disease activity measured by positron-emission tomography. Lancet 1997;350(9073):262.

27. Neurath MF, Vehling D, Schunk K, et al. Noninvasive assessment of Crohn's disease activity: a comparison of 18F-fluorodeoxyglucose positron emission tomography, hydromagnetic resonance imaging, and granulocyte scintigraphy with labeled antibodies. Am J Gastroenterol 2002;97(8): 1978–1985.

28. Pio BS, Byrne FR, Aranda R, et al. Noninvasive quantification of bowel inflammation through positron emission tomography imaging of 2-deoxy-2-[18F]fluoro-D-glucose-labeled white blood cells. Mol Imaging Biol 2003; 5(4):271–277.

29. Schmid DT, Kneifel S, Stoeckli SJ, Padberg BC, Merrill G, Goerres GW. Increased 18F-FDG uptake mimicking thyroid cancer in a patient with Hashimoto's thyroiditis. Eur Radiol 2003;13(9):2119–2121.

30. Yasuda S, Shohsu A, Ide M, Takagi S, Suzuki Y, Tajima T. Diffuse F-18 FDG uptake in chronic thyroiditis. Clin Nucl Med 1997;22(5):341.

31. Yasuda S, Shohtsu A, Ide M, et al. Chronic thyroiditis: diffuse uptake of FDG at PET. Radiology 1998;207(3):775–778.

32. Santiago JF, Jana S, El-Zeftawy H, Naddaf S, Abdel-Dayem HM. Increased F-18 fluorodeoxyglucose thyroidal uptake in Graves' disease. Clin Nucl Med 1999;24(9):714–715.

33. El-Haddad G, Zhuang H, Gupta N, Alavi A. Evolving role of positron emission tomography in the management of patients with inflammatory and other benign disorders. Semin Nucl Med 2004;34(4):313–329.

34. Ozsahin H, von Planta M, Muller I, et al. Successful treatment of invasive aspergillosis in chronic granulomatous disease by bone marrow transplantation, granulocyte colony-stimulating factor-mobilized granulocytes, and liposomal amphotericin-B. Blood 1998;92(8):2719–2724.

35. Gungor T, Engel-Bicik I, Eich G, et al. Diagnostic and therapeutic impact of whole body positron emission tomography using fluorine-18-fluoro-2-deoxy-D-glucose in children with chronic granulomatous disease. Arch Dis Child 2001;85(4):341–345.

36. Sugawara Y, Braun DK, Kison PV, Russo JE, Zasadny KR, Wahl RL. Rapid detection of human infections with fluorine-18 fluorodeoxyglucose and positron emission tomography: preliminary results. Eur J Nucl Med 1998; 25(9):1238–1243.

37. Yamada S, Kubota K, Kubota R, Ido T, Tamahashi N. High accumulation of fluorine-18-fluorodeoxyglucose in turpentine-induced inflammatory tissue. J Nucl Med 1995;36(7):1301–1306.

38. Lodge MA, Lucas JD, Marsden PK, Cronin BF, O'Doherty MJ, Smith MA. A PET study of 18FDG uptake in soft tissue masses. Eur J Nucl Med 1999;26(1):22–30.

39. Gallagher BM, Fowler JS, Gutterson NI, MacGregor RR, Wan CN, Wolf AP. Metabolic trapping as a principle of radiopharmaceutical design: some factors responsible for the biodistribution of [18F] 2-deoxy-2-fluoro-D-glucose. J Nucl Med 1978;19(10):1154–1161.

40. Nelson CA, Wang JQ, Leav I, Crane PD. The interaction among glucose transport, hexokinase, and glucose-6-phosphatase with respect to 3H-2-deoxyglucose retention in murine tumor models. Nucl Med Biol 1996; 23(4):533–541.

41. Suzuki S, Toyota T, Suzuki H, Goto Y. Partial purification from human mononuclear cells and placental plasma membranes of an insulin media-tor which stimulates pyruvate dehydrogenase and suppresses glucose-6-phosphatase. Arch Biochem Biophys 1984;235(2):418–426.

42. Sahlmann CO, Siefker U, Lehmann K, Meller J. Dual time point 2-[18F]fluoro-2'-deoxyglucose positron emission tomography in chronic bac-terial osteomyelitis. Nucl Med Commun 2004;25(8):819–823.

43. Matthies A, Hickeson M, Cuchiara A, Alavi A. Dual time point 18F-FDG PET for the evaluation of pulmonary nodules. J Nucl Med 2002;43(7): 871–875.

44. Zhuang H, Pourdehnad M, Lambright ES, et al. Dual time point 18F-FDG PET imaging for differentiating malignant from inflammatory processes. J Nucl Med 2001;42(9):1412–1417.

45. Hustinx R, Shiue CY, Alavi A, et al. Imaging in vivo herpes simplex virus thymidine kinase gene transfer to tumour-bearing rodents using positron emission tomography and. Eur J Nucl Med 2001;28(1):5–12.

25

Inflammatory Bowel Disease

Jean-Louis Alberini and Martin Charron

In the 1970s, research with positron emission tomography (PET) expanded in the fields of cardiology and neurology, but since the 1990s a dramatic upsurge of PET occurred in oncology applications using mostly fluorodeoxyglucose (FDG). This development can be explained by the ability to obtain whole-body acquisition and good image quality and by an improvement of the availability of FDG. However, FDG is not tumor specific. False-positive FDG-PET results in cases of infection and inflammation are well known (1,2). The first report of PET use in infection was the description of FDG uptake in abdominal abscesses in 1989 (3). This led some to consider PET with FDG as a useful tool for rapid detection of infectious processes (4). This property was considered as an opportunity to use FDG-PET in the diagnosis and follow-up of infectious or inflammatory processes, where it can replace other investigations, for instance, using white blood cell scintigraphy as well as Ga-67.

Another potential source of nonmalignant increased FDG uptake is the presence of physiologic activity (in brown fat tissue, muscles, glands, lymphoid tissue). Development of PET–computed tomography (CT) scanners in 2001 allowed decreased acquisition time and improved image analysis by limiting false-positive results due to these physiologic activities. Localization of increased FDG uptake is improved when PET and CT images are co-registered, and PET and CT interpretations can be improved when they are associated.

Physiologic FDG Colonic Activity

Although the FDG uptake pattern in the normal colon and intestine is usually mild to moderate, there can be instances of more intense uptake. Segmental and intense colonic increased uptake can be related to inflammation, but uptake in the cecum and descending colon is common in patients without inflammatory bowel disease with a rate estimated to be 11% in a series of 1068 patients (5). The presence of irregular or focal intense accumulation was reported in asymptomatic patients (6). Different kind of colitis associated with FDG increased uptake have been reported (7–9). Causes of uptake are not clear, but several hypotheses have been suggested (10–12). It could be caused by any of the following:

- Smooth muscle activity in relation with peristaltism (6,10–12)
- Accumulation of FDG in superficial mucosal cells and a possible shedding of FDG in the stool (13)
- Intraluminal leak of FDG through tight junctions between epithelial cells related to an increased permeability (6) or maybe related to the presence of WBC (13)
- Presence of lymphoid tissue (14)
- Bacterial uptake (15)

The published data for the increased uptake associated with peristaltism are contradictory. The use of drugs with antiperistaltic effects (atropine, sincalide) has not shown any difference of the level of intestinal FDG uptake with the baseline state in five young volunteers (16). In another study (17), the use of N-butylscopolamine enabled bowel FDG uptake to decrease. A higher incidence of colonic uptake, especially in the descending colon, was associated with constipation (6). This increased uptake can be explained by a stercoral stasis, which may be responsible for stool accumulation and for an increase of peristaltic motion. Presence of FDG was noted in stools (6). This has led to the proposal of an intestinal preparation with iso-osmotic solution (13). Another hypothesis to explain increased colic uptake was the presence of lymphoid tissue in the cecum walls (14) because it is known that FDG can accumulate in other sites of lymphoid tissue as well as tonsils and adenoids in the Waldeyer ring (18). Finally, it is difficult to determine the mechanism originally responsible for increased uptake.

PET Imaging Compared to Other Nuclear Imaging Techniques

Endoscopic and radiologic methods of disease localization are more invasive when compared with the technetium-99m (^{99m}Tc)–white blood cell (WBC) scan and tend to produce more discomfort as a result of the instrumentation and preparation for the procedure (e.g., bowel cleansing). Moreover, several studies are needed to analyze the entire bowel, because colonoscopy cannot evaluate the entire small bowel. There is a need for a noninvasive technique that can be utilized in the follow-up of pediatric patients. The ^{99m}Tc-WBC scan seems ideally suited to obtain a precise temporal snapshot of the distribution and intensity of inflammation, whereas radiographic modalities of investigation tend to represent more chronic changes. An additional advantage is high patient acceptability, especially in children. Patients prefer the ^{99m}Tc-WBC scintigraphy to barium study or enteroclysis. The effective dose equivalent for a ^{99m}Tc-WBC study is approximately 3 mSv, whereas it is on the order of 6 mSv for a barium small bowel follow-through or 8.5 mSv for a barium enema. A high yield (percent of positive studies) is noted at 30 minutes (88%). The test and acquisition can be terminated if there is a clinical need to shorten the examination time.

Scintigraphy with ^{99m}Tc-WBC has been reported to be sensitive for the detection of inflammation in adults. The correlation between scintigraphic and endoscopic findings is close enough that scintigraphy can supplement left-sided colonoscopy in the event that total colonoscopy is technically impossible in a selected case. It appears likely that the ^{99m}Tc-WBC scan can be used as a monitoring tool for inflammatory activity in place of colonoscopy. Scintigraphy can also be used to document the proximal extension of ulcerative proctosigmoiditis or post-operative recurrence of Crohn's disease (CD). The ^{99m}Tc-WBC scan is occasionally useful to assess the inflammatory component of a stricture seen on a small bowel follow-through.

However, ^{99m}Tc-WBC scintigraphy has limitations. It is not useful in defining anatomic details such as strictures, prestenotic dilations, or fistulas, which are best evaluated by barium radiographic studies. Occasionally, in a patient with CD, it can be difficult to distinguish the large bowel from small bowel if the uptake is focal, because landmarks disappear. The presence of gastrointestinal (GI) bleeding occurring at the same time as the ^{99m}Tc-WBC study can complicate the interpretation of findings.

The value of WBC scintigraphy is well established in the diagnosis of inflammatory bowel disease in children (19–22). Theoretically, FDG-PET offers some advantages compared to other radionuclide imaging methods. First, it allows noninvasive study of children and avoids some drawbacks inherent in WBC scintigraphy performed with indium 111 (^{111}In) or ^{99m}Tc-labeled leukocytes or granulocytes (23). Second, WBC scintigraphy is a time-consuming technique due to the delay for labeling (approximately 2 hours) and the required interval between injection and image acquisition. Delayed images performed approximately 4 hours after injection or later are recommended and probably essential (24). This delay should be compared to the 2- to 3-hour delay required for an FDG-PET scan. Third, WBC scintigraphy exposes the patient to the risk of contamination by infectious agents from the manipulation of blood samples for the labeling and may require a certain amount of blood sample in younger children. The biodistribution of activities in the liver, the urinary tract, and the bone marrow may generate difficulties for the analysis. On the other hand, radiation protection is always a concern in pediatrics; the dose delivered is more favorable with WBC scintigraphy than with FDG-PET (3 mSv vs. 6 mSv) (23).

However, WBC scintigraphy was shown to be sensitive and able to provide semiquantitative data on the severity and the extent of involved segments by inflammation (19–23,25) with a good correlation with endoscopic findings and clinical index. It was shown that WBC scintigraphy helps to differentiate continuous and discontinuous colitis (between Crohn's disease and ulcerative colitis) (26). Lack of anatomic information is no longer a limitation for this technique because of the introduction of combined single photon emission computed tomography (SPECT) and CT systems, but the role of the co-registration in this situation is not yet validated. However, this technique increases the dose delivered to the patient. In published studies using WBC scintigraphy, imaging was performed classically with static views (19–23,25), but it was shown that SPECT can improve the quantification (25). However, γ-emitter imaging lacks spatial resolution, and its assessment of the intensity of the bowel activity is only semiquantitative. The main advantage of PET imaging in this field is the opportunity to obtain three-dimensional (3D) slices in one procedure in a shorter time than SPECT takes and with a better image quality. Furthermore, PET imaging allows a more accurate semiquantitative analysis using standard uptake values (SUVs). In the first two published studies (27,28), the method for the semiquantitative analysis of FDG uptake was a measure of a ratio of maximum uptake between intestine and vertebral body. Now most of the PET scans are performed with correction attenuation using external γ-emitters sources or CT; SUV data are easily available. Currently no data show that the use of PET-CT for this indication can improve the performance of PET by the association of anatomic and metabolic data.

The role of PET in inflammatory bowel disease is not clearly established even if some publications have shown promising results with FDG. However, the presence of physiologic colonic activity is a challenge in this situation and leads to the conclusion that FDG is probably not the best-suited tracer in inflammatory bowel disease. It is not yet shown that FDG-PET is superior to WBC scintigraphy. New tracers are under investigation or will be developed in order to investigate inflammation more specifically. The role of PET imaging in the evaluation of treatment efficacy has not been yet evaluated.

The first studies suggesting that FDG-PET may be a useful tool to identify active inflammation in inflammatory bowel disease in adults and in children were published in *Lancet* (27,28). In the first study, FDG-PET was used to assess the treatment efficacy on a long-term follow-up in six patients. A correlation between PET and endoscopic findings was found in five patients with true-positive PET results; PET and endoscopy were negative in one patient. In the second study, performed in a pediatric population affected by inflammatory bowel disease in 18 cases and presenting nonspecific abdominal symptoms in seven cases, sensitivity and specificity were 81% and 85%, respectively, on a per-patient analysis and 71% and 81%, respectively, on a per-segment analysis. More recently, performances of FDG-PET were compared to those of hydro–magnetic resonance imaging (MRI) and antigen-95 granulocyte antibodies in a prospective study including 91 patients (29). In this population, 59 patients had Crohn's disease and 32 patients served as controls (12 irritable bowel syndrome and 20 tumor patients). Positron emission tomography sensitivity was higher than that of MRI or granulocyte antibodies (85.5%, 40.9%, and 66.7%, respectively), but specificity was lower (89%, 93%, and 100%, respectively). Positron emission tomography showed more findings correlated with histopathologic findings than hydro-MRI or granulocyte antibodies. Intensity of FDG uptake used in this study was estimated by the measures of SUV_{max}. No correlation was found among SUV_{max}, Crohn's Disease Activity Index, C-reactive protein, and the number of involved segments. N-butylscopolamine was used in this study in order to decrease motion artifacts. This can explain why no intestinal increased FDG uptake was found in the control group of patients with irritable bowel syndrome.

The most exciting application of PET imaging is the opportunity to use FDG-labeled leukocytes for this indication, as developed by Forstrom and colleagues (30). The labeling procedure resulted in a satisfactory yield (80%) after a leukocyte incubation with FDG for 10 to 20 minutes in a heparin-saline solution at 37°C. The activity was found more in the granulocyte (78.5% ± 1.4%) than in the lymphocyte-platelet fraction (12.6% ± 1.9%) or in the plasma (5.8% ± 1.8%). The cells' viability and the stability of labeling were excellent (30). Fluorodeoxyglucose-labeled autologous leukocyte scintigraphy performed in four normal volunteers has shown a predominant uptake in the reticuloendothelial system similar to that of other radiolabeled leukocytes and no gastrointestinal uptake (31). Injection of FDG-labeled leukocytes using 250 MBq (225–315 MBq) exposes to a dose of 3 to 4 mGy approximately, similar to the dose delivered by ^{111}In-labeled WBC scintigraphy. Pio and colleagues (32) have shown that PET imaging using FDG-labeled WBC was feasible and facilitated assessment of bowel inflammation accurately and rapidly in murine and human subjects. In animal models, inflammatory bowel disease was present in Gi2α-deficient mice (lacking the signal transducing G-protein) or induced by an injection of exogenous leukocytes. A correlation between intestinal segments with increased uptake of FDG-labeled WBC and histopathologic and colonoscopic findings was found. Their intensity was correlated with the degree of inflammation measured on the pathologic analysis performed on necropsied mice and used as the gold standard. The acquisition protocol used in this study seems very simple because acquisition was started 40 minutes after injection and lasted 30 minutes.

PET and Cancers in Patients with Inflammatory Bowel Disease

Patients with inflammatory bowel disease are exposed to a higher risk of colorectal cancer than the general population; for patients with ulcerative colitis this risk can reach a factor of 2. Colorectal cancer is overall observed in 5.5% to 13.5% of patients with ulcerative colitis and in 0.4% to 0.8% in patients with Crohn's disease (33). Colorectal cancer can account for approximately 15% of all deaths in these patients (34,35). However, the increased risk of colorectal cancer is not well known (34), especially in Crohn's disease patients (36). Established risk factors include long duration (34), large extent and severity of the disease (37), early disease onset, presence of complicating primary sclerosing cholangitis or stenotic disease, (33) and perhaps a family history of colorectal cancer (38).

Although this risk does not usually involve children during their childhood because colorectal cancer occurs after several years of the disease onset, it was shown in a meta-analysis (34) that the cumulative probabilities of any child developing cancer were estimated to be 5.5% at 10 years of duration, 10.8% at 20 years, and 15.7% at 30 years. The average age of onset of ulcerative colitis was 10 years in several studies. All these data mean that this child population will require permanent surveillance for early detection of colorectal cancer.

The current surveillance strategy includes colonoscopic examinations (39), but its impact on survival in patients with extensive disease is still under debate (40). It seems in different studies that dying by colorectal cancer in the group of patients with colonoscopic surveillance was lower than in the no-surveillance group (40). It is logical to consider that surveillance will facilitate detection of advanced adenomas, adenomas with appreciable villous tissue or high-grade dysplasia, or cancer at an early stage. The optimal interval between surveillance procedures is not established, but a delay of approximately 3 years seems to be cost-effective (41). Because the estimated incidence of colorectal cancer in ulcerative colitis patients can reach 27% over a 30-year period, prevention can lead to the proposal of a prophylactic colectomy. This attitude is questionable considering the complications risk and the consequences on the quality of life (41), but the cumulative colectomy rate can be high after a long duration of disease (42). It was proposed to start this surveillance 7 or 8 years after the disease onset in case of total colitis (33) or immediately in patients with primary sclerosing cholangitis (38).

Finally, because of the better acceptance of noninvasive techniques by patients, FDG-PET has a role to play in the surveillance workup in children (when the disease onset is early) or in young adults. Indeed it was shown that FDG-PET is a sensitive tool to detect premalignant colonic lesions (43–46). The presence of colonic nodular-focal FDG findings detected by FDG-PET is suggestive of a premalignant lesion. In a series of 20 patients with nodular colonic FDG uptake on a routine PET-CT scan, we found that these foci were associated with colonoscopic lesions in 75% of the patients (15/20 patients) and in 67% of the total amount of FDG findings (14/21 areas) (47). Histopathologic findings revealed advanced neoplasms in 13 patients (13 villous adenomas and three carcinomas) and two cases of hyperplastic polyps. Co-registration of PET and CT data improved the analysis of colonic FDG uptake by avoiding confusion between abnormal focal uptake and physiologic activity, especially in case of fecal stasis. These results were in agreement with a recent paper (48) in which the authors found nine colorectal carcinomas and 27 adenomas. Among these adenomas, seven were high-grade dysplasia adenomas. Inflammatory lesions were reported in 12 of 69 patients (17%), and the diagnostic was confirmed by endoscopy. There were four cases of diffuse colonic uptake related to three active colitis and one reactivation of ulcerative colitis, and eight cases of segmental colonic uptake with one identified pseudomembranous colitis. This may suggest that PET or PET-CT can play a role in the diagnostic procedure in the surveillance strategy of patients with inflammatory bowel disease in order to detect early lesions susceptible to easy removal, that is, neoplasia at a surgically curative stage or, better yet, at a dysplastic, still noninvasive stage.

Another situation that exposes inflammatory bowel disease patients to a higher risk of malignant lesion is the presence of primary sclerosing cholangitis. Because of its poor prognosis when diagnosed at an advanced stage (49), early detection of cholangiocarcinoma lesions is crucial. Surgical resection and liver transplantation are the only curative treatments. A study has shown that FDG-PET has the potential to detect small cholangiocarcinoma tumors in nine patients with primary sclerosing cholangitis (50) in spite of its limited spatial resolution. A more recent study (51) in 50 patients with biliary tract cancers of whom 36 had cholangiocarcinoma was not so optimistic on the value of PET in diagnosis of cholangiocarcinoma; PET sensitivity was much higher in the nodular rather than the infiltrating form (85% vs. 18%), and there was a false-positive result in a patient with primary sclerosing cholangitis associated with an acute cholangitis. Its sensitivity to identifying carcinomatosis was very poor, with three false-negative results out of three patients. However, detection of unsuspected distant metastases led to a change in surgical management in 31% (11/36). The FDG-PET performances to detect carcinomatosis or pulmonary metastases were really better in other series (52,53). To conclude, FDG-PET is a useful tool in the diagnosis of cholangiocarcinoma especially for the nodular form, but it can fail to differentiate cholangiocarcinoma from cholangitis. Its value in the preoperative workup to confirm that cholangiocarcinoma lesions are only localized in the liver seems limited, but further studies are required.

Conclusions

The main advantages of nuclear medicine methods are their capability to explore metabolic processes at a molecular level, with a quantitative approach, and the potential to label molecules and antibodies that can be proposed as treatments. Ultrasonography, CT, and MRI are suited for the diagnosis of inflammatory bowel disease complications, but the latest technologic improvements have allowed exploration of the intestinal wall with nonirradiating techniques. Although [111]In- or ^{99m}Tc-labeled WBC scintigraphy remains a reliable method for diagnosis of inflammatory bowel disease, it cannot replace colonoscopy. Positron emission tomography as a new nuclear imaging modality offers significant advantages in the diagnosis and follow-up in inflammatory bowel disease because of its better spatial resolution, its volumetric acquisition in one step, the high signal-to-background ratio, the opportunity to quantify signal intensity, its good availability, and the lack of side effects. Although some studies have shown good performance with FDG, it does not seem to be the best suited tracer because of the physiologic colonic uptake. One challenge for FDG-PET imaging in inflammatory bowel disease is to determine if it can be included in the surveillance of patients with ulcerative colitis because of a higher risk of colorectal cancer and cholangiocarcinoma in this population. Several studies have shown that FDG-PET is a sensitive and noninvasive method to detect premalignant colonic lesions, especially high-grade dysplasia adenomas. Its place beside the repeated colonoscopic investigations has to be evaluated.

Development of new tracers in order to study different metabolisms, inflammatory reactions, and probably immunologic reactions involved in inflammatory bowel disease will be a challenge. The opportunity to label new drugs with positron emitters should be investigated in order to propose clinical tools to evaluate therapeutic efficacy. At the moment, the preliminary results obtained with FDG-labeled leukocytes in humans are very promising.

References

1. Zhuang H, Alavi A. 18-fluorodeoxyglucose positron emission tomographic imaging in the detection and monitoring of infection and inflammation. Semin Nucl Med 2002;32(1):47–59.
2. Zhuang H, Yu JQ, Alavi A. Applications of fluorodeoxyglucose-PET imaging in the detection of infection and inflammation and other benign disorders. Radiol Clin North Am 2005;43(1):121–134.
3. Tahara T, Ichiya Y, Kuwabara Y, et al. High [18F]-fluorodeoxyglucose uptake in abdominal abscesses: a PET study. J Comput Assist Tomogr 1989;13(5):829–831.
4. Sugawara Y, Braun DK, Kison PV, Russo JE, Zasadny KR, Wahl RL. Rapid detection of human infections with fluorine-18 fluorodeoxyglucose and positron emission tomography: preliminary results. Eur J Nucl Med 1998;25(9):1238–1243.
5. Yasuda S, Takahashi W, Takagi S, Fujii H, Ide M, Shohtsu A. Factors influencing physiological FDG uptake in the intestine. Tokai J Exp Clin Med 1998;23(5):241–244.
6. Kim S, Chung JK, Kim BT, et al. Relationship between gastrointestinal F-18–fluorodeoxyglucose accumulation and gastrointestinal symptoms in whole-body PET. Clin Positron Imaging 1999;2(5):273–279.
7. Meyer MA. Diffusely increased colonic F-18 FDG uptake in acute enterocolitis. Clin Nucl Med 1995;20(5):434–435.
8. Hannah A, Scott AM, Akhurst T, Berlangieri S, Bishop J, McKay WJ. Abnormal colonic accumulation of fluorine-18–FDG in pseudomembranous colitis. J Nucl Med 1996;37(10):1683–1685.
9. Kresnik E, Gallowitsch HJ, Mikosch P, et al. (18)F-FDG positron emission tomography in the early diagnosis of enterocolitis: preliminary results. Eur J Nucl Med Mol Imaging 2002;29(10):1389–1392.
10. Engel H, Steinert H, Buck A, Berthold T, Huch Boni R, von Schulthess G. Whole-body PET: physiological and artifactual fluorodeoxyglucose accumulations. J Nucl Med 1996;37(3):441–446.
11. Strauss LG. Fluorine-18 deoxyglucose and false-positive results: a major problem in the diagnostics of oncological patients. Eur J Nucl Med 1996;23(10):1409–1415.
12. Delbeke D. Oncological applications of FDG PET imaging: brain tumors, colorectal cancer, lymphoma and melanoma. J Nucl Med 1999;40(4):591–603.

13. Miraldi F, Vesselle H, Faulhaber PF, Adler LP, Leisure GP. Elimination of artifactual accumulation of FDG in PET imaging of colorectal cancer. Clin Nucl Med 1998;23(1):3–7.
14. Cook GJ, Fogelman I, Maisey MN. Normal physiological and benign pathological variants of 18–fluoro-2–deoxyglucose positron-emission tomography scanning: potential for error in interpretation. Semin Nucl Med 1996;26(4):308–314.
15. Shreve PD, Anzai Y, Wahl RL. Pitfalls in oncologic diagnosis with FDG PET imaging: physiologic and benign variants. Radiographics 1999;19(1):61–77; quiz 150–151.
16. Jadvar H, Schambye RB, Segall GM. Effect of atropine and sincalide on the intestinal uptake of F-18 fluorodeoxyglucose. Clin Nucl Med 1999;24(12):965–967.
17. Stahl A, Weber WA, Avril N, Schwaiger M. Effect of N-butylscopolamine on intestinal uptake of fluorine-18–fluorodeoxyglucose in PET imaging of the abdomen. Nuklearmedizin 2000;39(8):241–245.
18. Jabour BA, Choi Y, Hoh CK, et al. Extracranial head and neck: PET imaging with 2–[F-18]fluoro-2–deoxy-D-glucose and MR imaging correlation. Radiology 1993;186(1):27–35.
19. Jewell F, Davies A, Sandhu B, Duncan A, Grier D. Technetium-99m-HMPAO labelled leucocytes in the detection and monitoring of inflammatory bowel disease in children. Br J Radiol 1996;69:508–514.
20. Jobling J, Lindley K, Yousef Y, Gordon I, Milla P. Investigating inflammatory bowel disease—white cell scanning, radiology, and colonoscopy. Arch Dis Child 1996;74:22–26.
21. Papos M, Varkonyi A, Lang J, et al. HM-PAO-labeled leukocyte scintigraphy in pediatric patients with inflammatory bowel disease. J Pediatr Gastroenterol Nutr 1996;23:547–552.
22. Shah D, Cosgrove M, Rees J, Jenkins H. The technetium white cell scan as an initial imaging investigation for evaluating suspected childhood inflammatory bowel disease. J Pediatr Gastroenterol Nutr 1997;25:524–528.
23. Alberini J, Badran A, Freneaux E, et al. Technetium-99m HMPAO-labelled leukocyte imaging compared with endoscopy, ultrasonography and contrast radiology in children with inflammatory bowel disease. JPGN 2001;32:278–286.
24. Charron M, del Rosario F, Kocoshis S. Comparison of the sensitivity of early versus delayed imaging with Tc-99m HMPAO WBC in children with inflammatory bowel disease. Clin Nucl Med 1998;23:649–653.
25. Charron M, del Rosario F, Kocoshis S. Pediatric inflammatory bowel disease: assessment with scintigraphy with 99mTc white blood cells. Radiology 1999;212:507–513.
26. Charron M, del Rosario F, Kocoshis S. Use of technetium-tagged white blood cells in patients with Crohn's disease and ulcerative colitis: is differential diagnosis possible? Pediatr Radiol 1998;28:871–877.
27. Bicik I, Bauerfeind P, Breitbach T, von Schulthess G, Fried M. Inflammatory bowel disease activity measured by positron-emission tomography. Lancet 1997;350:262.
28. Skehan S, Issenman R, Mernagh J, Nahmias C, Jacobson K. 18F-fluorodeoxyglucose positron tomography in diagnosis of pediatric inflammatory bowel disease. Lancet 1999;354:836–837.
29. Neurath MF, Vehling D, Schunk K, et al. Noninvasive assessment of Crohn's disease activity: a comparison of 18F-fluorodeoxyglucose positron emission tomography, hydromagnetic resonance imaging, and granulocyte

scintigraphy with labeled antibodies. Am J Gastroenterol 2002;97(8): 1978–1985.

30. Forstrom LA, Mullan BP, Hung JC, Lowe VJ, Thorson LM. 18F-FDG labelling of human leukocytes. Nucl Med Commun 2000;21(7):691–694.

31. Forstrom L, Dunn W, Mullan B, Hung J, Lowe V, Thorson L. Biodistribution and dosimetry of [18F]fluorodeoxyglucose labelled leukocytes in normal human subjects. Nucl Med Commun 2002;23:721–725.

32. Pio BS, Byrne FR, Aranda R, et al. Noninvasive quantification of bowel inflammation through positron emission tomography imaging of 2–deoxy-2–[18F]fluoro-D-glucose-labeled white blood cells. Mol Imaging Biol 2003;5(4):271–277.

33. Pohl C, Hombach A, Kruis W. Chronic inflammatory bowel disease and cancer. Hepatogastroenterology 2000;47(31):57–70.

34. Eaden J, Abrams K, Mayberry J. The risk of colorectal cancer in ulcerative colitis: a meta-analysis. Gut 2001;48(4):526–535.

35. Munkholm P. Review article: the incidence and prevalence of colorectal cancer in inflammatory bowel disease. Aliment Pharmacol Ther 2003; 18(suppl 2):1–5.

36. Jess T, Winther K, Munkholm P, Langholz E, Binder V. Intestinal and extraintestinal cancer in Crohn's disease: follow-up of a population-based cohort in Copenhagen County, Denmark. Aliment Pharmacol Ther 2004;19(3):287–293.

37. Rutter M, Saunders B, Wilkinson K, et al. Severity of inflammation is a risk factor for colorectal neoplasia in ulcerative colitis. Gastroenterology 2004;126(2):451–459.

38. Itzkowitz S, Harpaz N. Diagnosis and management of dysplasia in patients with inflammatory bowel diseases. Gastroenterology 2004;126(6):1634–1648.

39. Rutter M, Saunders B, Wilkinson K, et al. Cancer surveillance in long-standing ulcerative colitis: endoscopic appearances help predict cancer risk. Gut 2004;53(12):1813–1816.

40. Mpofu C, Watson A, Rhodes J. Strategies for detecting colon cancer and/or dysplasia in patients with inflammatory bowel disease. Cochrane Database Syst Rev 2004:CD000279.

41. Inadomi J. Cost-effectiveness of colorectal cancer surveillance in ulcerative colitis. Scand J Gastroenterol Suppl 2003;237:17–21.

42. Langholz E, Munkholm P, Davidsen M, Binder V. Colorectal cancer risk and mortality in patients with ulcerative colitis. Gastroenterology 1992; 103(5):1444–1451.

43. Yasuda S, Fujii H, Nakahara T, et al. 18F-FDG PET detection of colonic adenomas. J Nucl Med 2001;42(7):989–992.

44. Drenth JP, Nagengast FM, Oyen WJ. Evaluation of (pre-)malignant colonic abnormalities: endoscopic validation of FDG-PET findings. Eur J Nucl Med 2001;28(12):1766–1769.

45. Tatlidil R, Jadvar H, Bading JR, Conti PS. Incidental colonic fluorodeoxyglucose uptake: correlation with colonoscopic and histopathologic findings. Radiology 2002;224(3):783–787.

46. Chen YK, Kao CH, Liao AC, Shen YY, Su CT. Colorectal cancer screening in asymptomatic adults: the role of FDG PET scan. Anticancer Res 2003; 23(5b):4357–4361.

47. Gutman F, Alberini JL, Wartski M, et al. Incidental colonic focal lesions detected by FDG-PET/CT. AJR 2005;185;2:495–500.

48. Kamel EM, Thumshirn M, Truninger K, et al. Significance of incidental 18F-FDG accumulations in the gastrointestinal tract in PET/CT: correlation

with endoscopic and histopathologic results. J Nucl Med 2004;45(11): 1804–1810.

49. Yalcin S. Diagnosis and management of cholangiocarcinomas: a comprehensive review. Hepatogastroenterology 2004;51(55):43–50.

50. Keiding S, Hansen S, Rasmussen H, et al. Detection of cholangiocarcinoma in primary sclerosing cholangitis by positron emission tomography. Hepatology 1998;28(3):700–706.

51. Anderson C, Rice M, Pinson C, Chapman W, Chari R, Delbeke D. Fluorodeoxyglucose PET imaging in the evaluation of gallbladder carcinoma and cholangiocarcinoma. J Gastrointest Surg 2004;8(1):90–97.

52. Kluge R, Schmidt F, Caca K, et al. Positron emission tomography with [(18)F]fluoro-2–deoxy-D-glucose for diagnosis and staging of bile duct cancer. Hepatology 2001;33(5):1029–1035.

53. Kim Y, Yun M, Lee W, Kim K, Lee J. Usefulness of 18F-FDG PET in intrahepatic cholangiocarcinoma. Eur J Nucl Med Mol Imaging 2003;30(11): 1467–1472.

26A

Hyperinsulinism of Infancy: Noninvasive Differential Diagnosis

Maria-João Santiago-Ribeiro, Nathalie Boddaert, Pascale De Lonlay, Claire Nihoul-Fekete, Francis Jaubert, and Francis Brunelle

Hyperinsulinism (HI) is the most important cause of recurrent hypoglycemia in infancy. The hypersecretion of insulin induces profound hypoglycemias that require aggressive treatment to prevent the high risk of neurologic complications (1,2). Hyperinsulinism can be due to two different histopathologic types of lesions, a focal or a diffuse form (3,4), based on different molecular entities despite an indistinguishable clinical pattern (5–9). In focal HI, which represents about 40% of all cases (10), the pathologic pancreatic β cells are gathered in a focal adenoma, usually 2.5 to 7.5 mm in diameter. Conversely, diffuse HI corresponds to an abnormal insulin secretion of the whole pancreas with disseminated β cells showing enlarged abnormal nuclei (11). Finally, about 10% of HI cases are clinically atypical and could not be classified, having unknown molecular basis and histopathologic form (12).

The two histopathologic forms correspond to two distinct molecular entities most implicating the *SUR1* and *KIR6.2* genes. The focal HI is associated with a loss of a maternal allele from chromosome 11p15 in the lesion and a somatic reduction to homozygosity in the paternally inherited mutation in either of the genes encoding the two subunits of the K^+ ATP channel: the sulfonylurea receptor type 1 (SUR1, MIM-600509) and the inward-rectifying potassium-channel (KIR6.2, MIM-600937). The diffuse form of HI is more heterogeneous and its genetic basis has been recognized in only 50% of the cases. Diffuse HI involves the genes *SUR1* and *KIR6.2* in recessively inherited hyperinsulinism or, more rarely, dominantly inherited hyperinsulinism. The glucokinase gene or other loci are also involved in dominantly inherited hyperinsulinism. The glutamate dehydrogenase gene is concerned when hyperammonemia is associated with hyperinsulinism.

Control of HI is attempted through medical treatment with diazoxide, nifedipine, or octreotide (13–15), but pancreatectomy is the only option for patients resistant to these treatments (10,16). Therefore, the differential diagnosis between the two forms becomes of major importance because their surgical treatment and the outcome differ considerably. Focal HI is totally cured by the selective resection of the adenoma, whereas diffuse forms of HI require a subtotal pancreatectomy with severe iatrogenic diabetes as consequence (17,18).

The localization of insulin hypersecretion before surgery is only possible through pancreatic venous catheterization (PVC), allowing a pancreatic map of insulin concentrations, with an eventually additional pancreatic arterial calcium stimulation (PACS) (19–21). Pancreatic venous catheterization is invasive and technically difficult to perform and requires general anesthesia. The concentrations of plasmatic glucose must be maintained between 2 and 3 mmol/L before and during the PVC. Moreover, all medical treatments have to be stopped 5 days before the study. Therefore, it is of major interest to find another less invasive way to differentiate between focal and diffuse HI. This method should precisely localize the pathological area of focal HI to guide the surgeon.

L-dihydroxyphenylalanine (L-DOPA) is a precursor of catecholamines that is converted to dopamine by the aromatic amino acid decarboxylase (AADC) enzyme. In addition to its role as a precursor of noradrenaline and adrenaline, dopamine is a transmitter substance in the central and peripheral nervous system. The capacity to take up and decarboxylate amine precursors such as L-DOPA or 5-hydroxytryptophan (5-HTP) and store their amine biogenic (dopamine and serotonin) is characteristic of neuroendocrine cells.

Pancreatic cells contain markers usually associated with neuroendocrine cells, such as tyrosine hydroxylase, dopamine, neuronal dopamine transporter, vesicular dopamine transporter, and monoamine oxidases A and B (22–24). Pancreatic islets have been shown to take up L-DOPA and convert it to dopamine through the aromatic amino acid dopa decarboxylase (25–27).

The term *neuroendocrine tumors* comprises a wide variety of rare tumor entities that may originate either from pure endocrine organs (e.g., pituitary adenomas), from pure nerve structures (e.g., neuroblastomas), or from elements of the diffuse (neuro)endocrine system as all endocrine tumors of the gastroenteropancreatic (GEP) tract. These neuroendocrine disordered cells share similar cytochemical and ultrastructural characteristics. They have the capacity to take up and convert dopamine precursors to amines or peptides, or both, which they store in secretory granules in the cytoplasm. Yet, it has been discovered that other cells throughout the body share this ability of amine precursor uptake and decarboxylation (APUD). The term APUD has lately been found to be inadequate, because several cell types included in the system do not metabolize amines. Furthermore, there is evidence that some APUD cell types are not of neural crest origin but are derived from endoderm (28).

Positron emission tomography (PET) performed with fluorine-18 (^{18}F)-fluoro-L-dihydroxyphenylalanine (^{18}F-fluoro-L-DOPA) has been extensively used to study the central dopaminergic system. Nevertheless, several recent studies have demonstrated the usefulness of this radiotracer to detect neuroendocrine tumors as pheochromocytomas, thyroid medullar carcinomas, or gastrointestinal carcinoid tumors that usually contain secretory granules and have the ability to produce biogenic amines (29,30).

Technique

Data Acquisition and Processing

The patients fasted for at least 6 hours prior to the PET study, and their medications were stopped for at least 72 hours. During all PET studies, normoglycemia is maintained by glucose infusion, which is carefully adjusted according to frequent blood glucose monitoring. Maximal glucose infusion rates between 6.4 and 13.2 mg/kg/min are needed. Positron emission tomography acquisition is performed under light sedation (pentobarbital associated or not with chloral).

Patients are placed in the supine position in the tomograph using a three-dimensional (3D) laser alignment. To ensure the optimal position in the scanner and to avoid movement artifacts, children should be comfortably immobilized during the study acquisition by placing them in a vacuum mattress. Intravenous bolus injection of a mean of 4.0 MBq/kg ^{18}F-fluoro-L-DOPA is done 30 to 50 minutes before transmission acquisition.

Tissue attenuation is measured postinjection and before emission acquisition. Transmission scans (2D acquisition mode) lasted 2.5 minutes per bed position (field of view of 15 cm), with two or three steps, according to the height of the patient, from the neck to the hip. After segmentation, they are used for subsequent correction of attenuation of emission scans. Thorax-abdomen emission scans (3D acquisition mode) start between 45 to 65 minutes after the radiotracer injection; 2.5-minute step acquisition, two or three steps for one scan, is acquired over 30 minutes.

The emission sets are corrected for scatter using a model-based correction, allowing the simulation of the map of single scatter events. The images are reconstructed using an attenuation weighted ordered subset expectation maximization iterative algorithm with four iterations and six subsets.

Data Analysis

The reconstructed images are evaluated in a 3D display using axial, coronal, and sagittal views to define pancreas, which invariably has a sufficiently high uptake of ^{18}F-fluoro-L-DOPA to distinguish it from the surrounding organs in the upper abdomen. Variable uptake is also seen in the gallbladder, biliary duct, and duodenum; nevertheless all of them could be discerned from pancreatic target tissue uptake.

For each patient, all thorax-abdomen emission scans are assembled with bed position overlap. A gaussian filter was used to smooth the images. This assembled image could be recalculated to provide the standard uptake value (SUV) where the radioactivity concentration in each pixel is divided by the total injected dose of ^{18}F-fluoro-L-DOPA at the beginning of the emission acquisition and the body weight. However, this imaging sequence is not crucial, and only one thorax-abdomen emission scan can be done 60 minutes postinjection. In fact, pancreas uptake of ^{18}F-fluoro-L-DOPA is constant during the emission acquisition (30 minutes).

Eighteen children with HI were studied using PET and ^{18}F-fluoro-L-DOPA. Five of them presented an abnormal focal radiotracer uptake whereas a diffuse uptake pattern was observed in the pancreatic area of the other patients. All patients with focal radiotracer uptake were submitted to surgery, and the localization of the focal form characterized by PET was confirmed by histologic samples. Figure 26A.1 illustrates an example of a typical focal form of HI. A diffuse accumulation pattern of ^{18}F-fluoro-L-DOPA was observed in the whole pancreas for patients with diffuse insulin secretion (Fig. 26A.2). Diffuse HI forms resistant to medical treatment (four patients) were operated and PET results were supported by the data from histologic analysis after subtotal pancreatectomy.

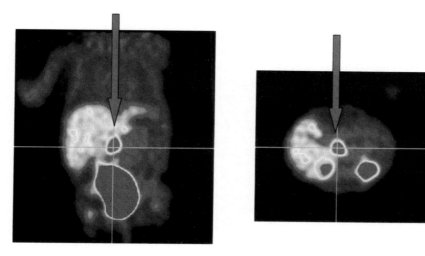

Figure 26A.1. Focal hyperinsulinism (HI). The abnormal focal increased uptake of the radiotracer is visualized in the pancreas on coronal and axial projections (arrows). Physiologic distribution of the radiotracer with higher accumulation in the kidneys and the urinary bladder and a lower accumulation in the liver is also observed.

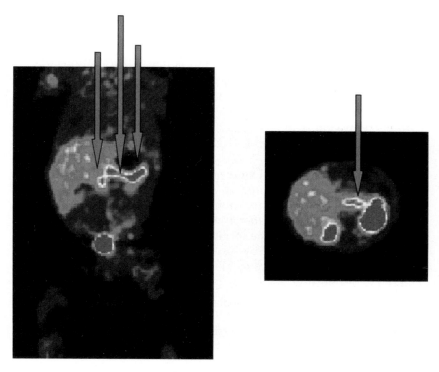

Figure 26A.2. Diffuse HI. The abnormaldiffuse increased uptake of the radio-tracer is visualized in all the pancreas on coronal and axial projections (arrows).

References

1. Stanley CA, Lieu YK, Hsu BY, et al. Hyperinsulinemia and hyperam-monemia in infants with regulatory mutations of the glutamate dehydro-genase gene. N Engl J Med 1998;338:1352–1357.
2. Menni F, de Lonlay P, Sevin C, et al. Neurologic outcomes of 90 neonates and infants with persistent hyperinsulinemic hypoglycemia. Pediatrics 2001;107:476–479.
3. Rahier J, Falt K, Muntefering H, Becker K, Gepts W, Falkmer S. The basic structural lesion of persistent neonatal hypoglycaemia with hyperinsulin-ism: deficiency of pancreatic D cells or hyperactivity of B cells? Diabetolo-gia 1984;26:282–289.
4. Goossens A, Gepts W, Saudubray JM, et al. Diffuse and focal nesidioblas-tosis. A clinicopathological study of 24 patients with persistent neonatal hyperinsulinemic hypoglycemia. Am J Surg Pathol 1989;13:766–775.
5. Thomas PM, Cote GJ, Wohllk N, et al. Mutations in the sulfonylurea recep-tor gene in familial persistent hyperinsulinemic hypoglycemia of infancy. Science 1995;268:426–429.
6. Nestorowicz A, Wilson BA, Schoor KP, et al. Mutations in the sulfonylurea receptor gene are associated with familial hyperinsulinism in Ashkenazi Jews. Hum Mol Genet 1996;5:1813–1822.
7. De Lonlay P, Fournet JC, Rahier J, et al. Somatic deletion of the imprinted 11p15 region in sporadic persistent hyperinsulinemic hypoglycemia of

infancy is specific of focal adenomatous hyperplasia and endorses partial pancreatectomy. J Clin Invest 1997;100:802–807.

8. Verkarre V, Fournet JC, de Lonlay P, et al. Paternal mutation of the sulfonylurea receptor (SUR1) gene and maternal loss of 11p15 imprinted genes lead to persistent hyperinsulinism in focal adenomatous hyperplasia. J Clin Invest 1998;102:1286–1291.

9. Fournet JC, Mayaud C, de Lonlay P, et al. Unbalanced expression of 11p15 imprinted genes in focal forms of congenital hyperinsulinism: association with a reduction to homozygosity of a mutation in ABCC8 or KCNJ11. Am J Pathol 2001;158:2177–2184.

10. De Lonlay-Debeney P, Poggi-Travert F, Fournet JC, et al. Clinical features of 52 neonates with hyperinsulinism. N Engl J Med 1999;340:1169–1175.

11. Sempoux C, Guiot Y, Lefevre A, et al. Neonatal hyperinsulinemic hypoglycemia: heterogeneity of the syndrome and keys for differential diagnosis. J Clin Endocrinol Metab 1998;83:1455–1461.

12. De Lonlay P, Benelli C, Fouque F, et al. Hyperinsulinism and hyperammonemia syndrome: report of twelve unrelated patients. Pediatr Res 2001;50:353–357.

13. Hirsch HJ, Loo S, Evans N, Crigler JF, Filler RM, Gabbay KH. Hypoglycemia of infancy and nesidioblastosis. Studies with somatostatin. N Engl J Med 1977;296:1323–1326.

14. Glaser B, Hirsch HJ, Landau H. Persistent hyperinsulinemic hypoglycemia of infancy: long-term octreotide treatment without pancreatectomy. J Pediatr 1993;123:644–650.

15. Thornton PS, Alter CA, Katz LE, Baker L, Stanley CA. Short- and long-term use of octreotide in the treatment of congenital hyperinsulinism. J Pediatr 1993;123:637–643.

16. De Lonlay P, Fournet JC, Touati G, et al. Heterogeneity of persistent hyperinsulinaemic hypoglycaemia. A series of 175 cases. Eur J Pediatr 2002;161:37–48.

17. Filler RM, Weinberg MJ, Cutz E, Wesson DE, Ehrlich RM. Current status of pancreatectomy for persistent idiopathic neonatal hypoglycemia due to islet cell dysplasia. Prog Pediatr Surg 1991;26:60–75.

18. Fekete CN, de Lonlay P, Jaubert F, Rahier J, Brunelle F, Saudubray JM. The surgical management of congenital hyperinsulinemic hypoglycemia in infancy. J Pediatr Surg 2004;39:267–269.

19. Brunelle F, Negre V, Barth MO, et al. Pancreatic venous samplings in infants and children with primary hyperinsulinism. Pediatr Radiol 1989;19:100–103.

20. Dubois J, Brunelle F, Touati G, et al. Hyperinsulinism in children: diagnostic value of pancreatic venous sampling correlated with clinical, pathological and surgical outcome in 25 cases. Pediatr Radiol 1995;25:512–516.

21. Chigot V, De Lonlay P, Nassogne MC, et al. Pancreatic arterial calcium stimulation in the diagnosis and localisation of persistent hyperinsulinemic hypoglycaemia of infancy. Pediatr Radiol 2001;31:650–655.

22. Lemmer K, Ahnert-Hilger G, Hopfner M, et al. Expression of dopamine receptors and transporter in neuroendocrine gastrointestinal tumor cells. Life Sci 2002;11:667–678.

23. Rodriguez MJ, Saura J, Finch CC, Mahy N, Billet EE. Localization of monoamine oxidase A and B in human pancreas, thyroid and adrenal glands. J Histochem Cytochem 2000;48:147–151.

24. Orlefors H, Sundin A, Fasth KJ, et al. Demonstration of high monoaminoxidase-A levels in neuroendocrine gastroenteropancreatic tumors in vitro

and in vivo-tumor visualization using positron emission tomography with ^{11}C-harmine. Nucl Med Biol 2003;30:669–679.

25. Oei HK, Gazdar AF, Minna JD, Weir GC, Baylin SB. Clonal analysis of insulin and somatostatin secretion and L-dopa decarboxylase expression by a rat islet cell tumor. Endocrinology 1983;112:1070–1075.
26. Lindstrom P. Aromatic-L-amino-acid decarboxylase activity in mouse pancreatic islets. Biochim Biophys Acta 1986;884:276–281.
27. Borelli MI, Villar MJ, Orezzoli A, Gagliardino JJ. Presence of DOPA decarboxylase and its localisation in adult rat pancreatic islet cells. Diabetes Metab 1997;23:161–163.
28. Oei HK, De Jong M, Krenning EP. Gastroenteropancreatic neuroendocrine tumors. In: Feinendegen LE, Shreeve WW, Eckelman WC, Bahk YW, Wagner HN, eds. Molecular Nuclear Medicine. Heidelberg: Springer-Verlag, 2003:385–397.
29. Hoegerle S, Altehoefer C, Ghanem N, et al. Whole-body ^{18}F DOPA PET for detection of gastrointestinal carcinoid tumors. Radiology 2001;220:373–380.
30. Hoegerle S, Nitzche E, Altehoefer C, et al. Pheochromocytomas: detection with ^{18}F DOPA whole-body PET-initial results. Radiology 2002;222:507–512.

Hyperinsulinism of Infancy: Localization of Focal Forms

Olga T. Hardy and Charles A. Stanley

Congenital Hyperinsulinism

Congenital hyperinsulinism is the most common cause of persistent hypoglycemia in infants and children (1). Infants with severe forms of the disorder (formerly termed nesidioblastosis) present with hypoglycemia in the newborn period and are at high risk of seizures, permanent brain damage, and retardation. Infants with congenital hyperinsulinism may have either focal or diffuse abnormalities of the pancreatic β cells. In cases with diffuse disease, an underlying defect in the β-cell adenosoine triphosphate (ATP)-dependent potassium channel may be present, caused by recessive loss of function mutations of the two genes encoding the KATP channel, *SUR1* or *Kir6.2* (1,2). These mutations may also cause focal hyperinsulinism in which there is an area of β-cell adenomatosis due to loss of heterozygosity for the maternal 11p region and expression of a paternally derived KATP channel mutation (3). Most of the cases with severe hyperinsulinism do not respond to medical therapy with diazoxide, octreotide (Fig. 26B.1), or continuous feedings and require near-total pancreatectomy to control hypoglycemia. However, cases of focal hyperinsulinism can be treated effectively with partial pancreatectomy. The surgical approach and therapeutic outcome for the infants depends on preoperatively distinguishing between focal and diffuse forms of hyperinsulinism. This chapter describes the focal lesions of hyperinsulinism, the pancreatectomy procedure, previous methods of determining the site of focal lesions, and the rationale for using positron emission tomography (PET) scans with ^{18}F-fluoro-L-DOPA.

Focal Hyperinsulinism

Histologically, focal hyperinsulinism has the appearance of β-cell adenomatosis (Fig. 26B.2) but does not affect pancreatic architecture and is invisible to the naked eye. Focal hyperinsulinism is clonal in origin

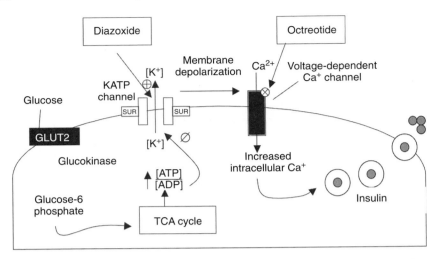

Figure 26B.1. Pathways of insulin secretion in the β cell. Glucose is metabolized through GLUT2 and glucokinase to increase adenosine triphosphate (ATP) formation. The elevation of the ATP/adenosine diphosphate (ADP) ratio leads to closure of KATP channels, depolarization of the membrane, opening of voltage-gated Ca^{2+} channels, and an increase in intracellular Ca^{2+}, which triggers the exocytosis of insulin granules. Because diazoxide suppresses insulin secretion by opening KATP channels, infants with diffuse or focal HI due to KATP mutations can not respond to treatment with diazoxide.

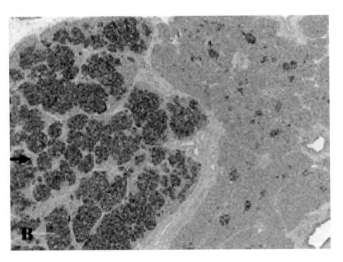

Figure 26B.2. Gross and histopathologic section of focal hyperinsulinism. This is an area of focal adenomatosis characterized by a pattern of crowded islets and limited exocrine tissue present in the surrounding periphery. Normal neighboring tissue to the right has an appropriate amount of islets present.

and the result of a specific loss of maternal alleles (loss of heterozygosity, LOH) in the p15 region of chromosome 11 (4) where the two KATP channel genes, *SUR1* and *Kir6.2*, are located. The maternal LOH results in loss of one or more maternally expressed tumor suppressor genes *p57KIP2* and *H19* as well as isodisomy for the paternally expressed insulin-like growth factor 2 gene (4). The loss of the maternal 11p thus leads to expansion of a clone of β cells that expresses a paternally derived KATP channel defect. These focal lesions are treatable with focal resection of the affected pancreatic area.

Pancreatectomy

Infants with congenital hyperinsulinism that fail medical management require partial or near-total pancreatectomy. During this operation, biopsies from the pancreatic head, body, and tail are examined for β cells with large nuclei and abundant cytoplasm suggestive of diffuse disease. When frozen sections demonstrate the absence of nuclear enlargement in biopsies from the head, body, and tail of the pancreas, further search for a focal lesion is conducted using additional biopsies until the focal lesion is found. Infants in whom frozen sections demonstrate diffuse disease, as evidenced by islet nuclear enlargement in all areas of the pancreas, undergo near-total pancreatectomy, removing approximately 98% of the organ. Many of these children subsequently develop iatrogenic diabetes. Preoperative differentiation between diffuse and focal disease and localization of a potential focal lesion is important to guide the surgical approach and improve surgical outcome.

Localization of Focal Pancreatic Lesions

Previous efforts to image focal congenital hyperinsulinism have been unsuccessful, including computed tomography (CT), magnetic resonance imaging (MRI), ultrasonography (preoperative and intraoperative), and radiolabeled octreotide scans (5). As discussed below, pharmacologic tests and techniques using interventional radiology have had limited success.

Pharmacologic Tests

Children with diffuse hyperinsulinism associated with the two most common mutations of *SUR1* display abnormal positive acute insulin responses (AIRs) to calcium and abnormal negative AIR to the KATP channel antagonist tolbutamide as well as an impaired insulin response to glucose (6). It was hypothesized that infants with diffuse and focal diazoxide-unresponsive hyperinsulinism could be distinguished by their AIRs to calcium and tolbutamide stimulation. That is, both types would respond to calcium, but only focal lesions would respond to tolbutamide. This hypothesis was tested in a group of 30 focal and 13 diffuse cases. Only two thirds of these cases responded to calcium;

although most focal cases responded to tolbutamide, half of the diffuse cases responded as well (7). This probably reflects the fact that some of the disease-causing mutations retain some partial function of the KATP channel (8). As a consequence, preoperative AIR tests cannot be used to distinguish focal vs. diffuse disease.

Interventional Radiology

Over the past 5 years, we have used the procedure of selective pancreatic arterial calcium stimulation with hepatic vein sampling (ASVS) for localization of focal hyperinsulinism lesions. It relies on the hypothesis that hypersensitivity to calcium stimulation in children with both diffuse and focal hyperinsulinism would make it possible to use selective pancreatic arterial stimulation with hepatic venous insulin sampling to differentiate focal from diffuse disease and to localize focal lesions. The ASVS procedure is carried out under general anesthesia, and plasma glucose levels must be maintained between 60 and 90 mg/dL. A positive response to the ASVS test is defined as a twofold or greater rise in plasma insulin after calcium infusion. A positive response from a single region of the pancreas is taken as evidence of focal disease. Results from a study looking at ASVS in 50 children revealed that ASVS localized the lesion in 24 of 33 focal cases (73%) but correctly diagnosed diffuse disease in only four of 13 cases. The ASVS test has about the same accuracy as transhepatic portal venous insulin sampling (THPVS), which correctly identified the region of focal lesions in only 76% of 45 cases (3). Both of these tests are technically difficult to perform and are associated with significant risks of general anesthesia and intubation, hypoglycemia, femoral artery catheterization and thrombosis, radiation exposure, and need for transfusion due to blood sampling.

PET Using ^{18}F-fluoro-L-DOPA for Focal Hyperinsulinism

Fluorine-18 (^{18}F)-labeled L-fluoro-DOPA has been used successfully to detect neuroendocrine tumors, such as carcinoids and endocrine pancreatic tumors in adults (9). Neuroendocrine tumors belong to the amine precursor uptake and decarboxylation (APUD) cell system and have the capacity to take up and to decarboxylate amine precursors, transform them into biogenic amines, and store them in vesicles. Thus, these cells can take up radioactively labeled ^{18}F-fluoro-L-DOPA to store as dopamine, which can be detected by PET imaging. ^{18}F-fluoro-L-DOPA-PET was not successful in localizing insulinomas but was accurate in localizing focal lesions of hyperinsulinism (10).

Researchers in France recently published their experience with ^{18}F-fluoro-L-DOPA PET scan on infants with congenital hyperinsulinism (11). They studied 15 patients with hyperinsulinism based on clinical diagnosis. Under conscious sedation, they injected a mean dose of 4 MBq/kg ^{18}F-labeled L-fluoro-DOPA intravenously 30 to 50 minutes before transmission acquisition. They observed an abnormal focal pancreatic uptake of ^{18}F-fluoro-L-DOPA in five patients and a diffuse uptake in the other 10 patients. All five of the patients with focal uptake

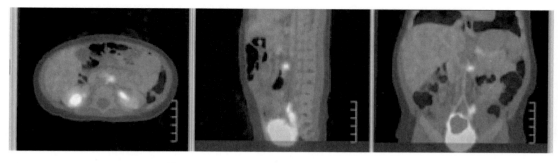

Figure 26B.3. Focal uptake of ^{18}F-labeled L-fluoro-DOPA believed to be behind the superior mesenteric artery (SMA).

and four of the patients with diffuse uptake underwent surgery. The histopathologic results were consistent with the PET findings in these nine cases.

The results from France, as well as preliminary data from a research group in Finland, suggest that ^{18}F-labeled L-fluoro-DOPA is an accurate noninvasive technique to distinguish between focal and diffuse forms of hyperinsulinism and to localize areas of focal lesions. As described in abstracts presented at the Endocrine Society meeting and the International Pediatric Endocrinology conference, our group at the Children's Hospital of Philadelphia has accumulated preliminary data using ^{18}F-fluoro-L-DOPA-PET in children with congenital hyperinsulinism (Fig. 26B.3). The very encouraging results suggest that this test is 100% accurate in distinguishing diffuse from focal disease and in localizing the site of the focal lesion.

Conclusion

Focal hyperinsulinism is an important cause of hypoglycemia in young infants and is potentially curable by surgery. Preliminary information about the success of ^{18}F-fluoro-L-DOPA PET suggests that this may be a method of choice for preoperative identification of focal lesions. An advantage to this technique is that it may be used to select out patients with diffuse disease who may be candidates for nonsurgical treatment. More important, the information acquired using ^{18}F-fluoro-L-DOPA-PET should make it possible for the surgeon to cure focal hyperinsulinism by local excision.

Acknowledgment

This work was supported in part by National Institutes of Health (NIH) grants RO1 DK 56268 (to C.A.S.) and MO1 RR 00240. O.T.H. was supported by NIH training grant T32 DK63688 (C.A.S.).

References

1. Stanley CA. Hyperinsulinism in infants and children. Pediatr Clin North Am 1997;44:363.
2. Glaser B, Thornton P, Otonkoski T, Junien C. Genetics of neonatal hyperinsulinism. Arch Dis Child (Fetal Neonatal Ed) 2000;82:F79.
3. de Lonlay-Debeney P, Poggi-Travert F, Fournet JC, et al. Clinical features of 52 neonates with hyperinsulinism. N Engl J Med 1999;340:1169–1175.
4. Verkarre V, Fournet JC, de Lonlay P, et al. Paternal mutation of the sulfonylurea receptor (SUR1) gene and maternal loss of 11p15 imprinted genes lead to persistent hyperinsulinism in focal adenomatous hyperplasia. J Clin Invest 1998;102:1286–1291.
5. Adzick NS, Thornton PS, Stanley CA, Kaye RD, Ruchelli E. A multidisciplinary approach to the focal form of congenital hyperinsulinism leads to successful treatment by partial pancreatectomy. J Pediatr Surg 2004;39: 270–275.
6. Grimberg A, Ferry RJ, Kelly A, et al. Dysregulation of insulin secretion in children with congenital hyperinsulinism due to sulfonylurea receptor mutations. Diabetes 2001;50:322–328.
7. Stanley CA, Thornton PS, Ganguly A, et al. Preoperative evaluation of infants with focal or diffuse congenital hyperinsulinism by intravenous acute insulin response tests and selective pancreatic arterial calcium stimulation. J Clin Endocrinol Metab 2004;89:288–296.
8. Henwood M, Kelly A, MacMullen C, et al. Genotype-phenotype correlations in children with congenital hyperinsulinism due to recessive mutations of the adenosine triphosphate-sensitive potassium channel genes. J Clin Endocrinol Metab 2005;90:789–794.
9. Erikkson B, Bergstrom M, Orlefors H, Sundin A, Oberg K, Langstrom B. PET for clinical diagnosis and research in neuroendocrine tumors. In: Sandler, Coleman, Patton, Wackers, Gottschalk, eds. Diagnostic Nuclear Medicine, 4th ed. Philadelphia: Lippincott Williams & Wilkins, 2003:747–754.
10. Boddaert N, Riberio MJ, Nuutila P, et al. ^{18}F-fluoro-L-DOPA PET SCAN in focal forms of hyperinsulinism of infancy. Presented at the 40th annual congress of the European Society of Paediatric Radiology, June 2003, Genoa, Italy.
11. Ribeiro M, De Lonlay P, Delzescaux T, et al. Characterization of hyperinsulinism in infancy assessed with PET and 18F-Fluoro-L-DOPA. J Nucl Med 2005;46:560–566.

27

Multimodal Imaging Using PET and MRI

Thomas Pfluger and Klaus Hahn

Magnetic resonance imaging (MRI) and positron emission tomography (PET) are diagnostic imaging modalities that facilitate visualization of morphologic as well as functional features of different diseases in childhood. Both modalities are often used separately or even in competition. Some of the most important indications for both PET and MRI lie in the field of pediatric oncology. The malignant diseases in children are leukemia, brain tumors, lymphomas, neuroblastoma, soft tissue sarcomas, Wilms' tumor, and bone sarcomas. Apart from leukemia, correct assessment of tumor expansion with modern imaging techniques, mainly consisting of ultrasonography, computed tomography (CT), MRI, and PET, is essential for cancer staging, for the choice of the best therapeutic approach, and for restaging after therapy or in recurrence (1,2).

Indications for MRI in Children

Magnetic resonance imaging is an excellent tool for noninvasive evaluation of tumor extent, and it has become the study of choice for evaluating therapy-induced regression in the size of musculoskeletal sarcomas. It directly demonstrates the lesion in relationship to surrounding normal structures with exquisite anatomic detail (3,4).

Especially in children, MRI offers several fundamental advantages compared to CT examinations and other whole-body imaging modalities, such as the absence of radiation exposure; the nonuse of iodinated, potential nephrotoxic contrast agents; a high intrinsic contrast for soft tissue and bone marrow; and accurate morphologic visualization of internal structure. All of these advantages are decisive factors in tumor staging (5–7). Due to its much higher intrinsic soft tissue contrast compared to CT, MRI has been shown to be advantageous in neuroradiologic, musculoskeletal, cardiac, and oncologic diseases (2,6). On the other hand, CT plays a major role in the assessment of thoracic lesions and masses due to a lower frequency of movement artifacts.

Because structural abnormalities are detected with high accuracy, MRI generally has a high sensitivity for detecting structural alterations but a low specificity for further characterization of these abnormalities (8). Frequently, these structural abnormalities are not reliable indicators of viable tumor tissue, especially after treatment (4).

T2-weighted MRI sequences visualize fluid-equivalent changes with high sensitivity. This is of special importance in detection of cysts and edema in the diagnosis of inflammatory and tumorous diseases. High signal intensity on T1-weighted MRI sequences facilitates the differentiation of adipose tissue and hemorrhage. Depiction of soft tissue or lesion perfusion can be achieved by the use of paramagnetic contrast agents like gadolinium–diethylenetriamine pentaacetic acid (Gd-DTPA).

Modern fast and ultrafast sequences permit monitoring of contrast medium perfusion over time, which improves recognition of lesions. These rapid sequences are especially widespread in contrast-enhanced MR angiography (MRA), which provides high-resolution selective arterial and venous vascular imaging. A further improvement in the contrast medium effect has been achieved by suppression of the signal from adipose tissue in T1-weighted sequences. These fat-suppressed, contrast-enhanced sequences are currently considered "state of the art" in the workup of tumors and inflammatory processes.

Necessary Components for Multimodality Imaging

Three basic components are required for multimodal imaging. First, multiple imaging modalities, often including one nuclear medical [PET, single photon emission computed tomography (SPECT)] and one radiologic (CT, MRI) cross-sectional imaging method, must be available. Second, there must be simple and prompt access to the corresponding images or image data sets. Adequate multimodal imaging requires a clinic-wide computer network, a digital archive of radiologic and nuclear medical studies, multimodal image viewing workstations, and appropriate software for image correlation and fusion (9,10). These requirements are currently satisfied to only a limited extent in hospital departments of radiology and nuclear medicine and in private practices. Third, and probably most important, is the competence of the physician in evaluating these different nuclear medical and radiologic data sets. Because each individual modality can yield false-negative findings, a careful and time-consuming separate analysis of each individual modality prior to multimodal processing is essential. In combined multimodal image evaluation, there is a tendency to depend primarily on the findings of PET, which usually identifies pathologic processes more rapidly. In doing so, one runs the risk of missing diagnoses that would be seen on MRI because of the reliance on false-negative PET scans. Therefore, a mainly PET-guided analysis of MRI should be avoided.

Algorithms and Accuracy of Combined Image Analysis and Image Registration

The retrospective registration and superimposition of multimodal image data can be done using different approaches and algorithms, which, in general, can be broken down into feature- and volume-based techniques. The image transformation can be static (displacement and rotation in all three spatial axes) or nonlinear (e.g., additional stretching or compression in order to compensate for respiratory movements) (11). The classic example of a feature-based method is the "surface matching" or Pelizzari algorithm, which uses organ surfaces as a property (12). The disadvantages of this technique are the requirement for a potentially quite extensive segmentation of the organ surface in the different modalities and the fact that image registration is based on only the extracted portions of the image (surface pixels).

Simply stated, volume-based techniques analyze similarities of pixel distribution in the two imaging modalities (11). The representative of this algorithm group enjoying the widest current application is the "mutual information" algorithm in which two-dimensional gray-scale histograms of the individual modalities and a combined histogram are analyzed and compared in various image transformations (13,14). Advantages of the volume-based techniques include the fully automatic application, their robustness compared to a different "field of view," and the higher degree of precision in image registration (11).

A meta-analysis by Hutton and Braun (10) quantified the exactness of software-based cerebral image registration at less than 3mm (10). For extracerebral applications, the PET and CT registration of pulmonary focal lesions showed a comparable exactness (average position of center of the lesion) of 6.2mm for separate modalities (15) and of 7.6mm for combined PET/CT scanners (16).

Analysis and Presentation of Multimodality Images

The evaluation of multimodal imaging data consists of three stages. The first stage corresponds to the separate analysis of the multimodal data in nuclear medicine and diagnostic radiology with subsequent comparison of the reported findings. In the case of discrepancies, a separate reevaluation of the imaging data is performed with comparison of the other imaging modality. This is currently the most widely used method, and it has the advantage of minimum requirements in terms of hardware and software, together with restricted logistic, temporal, and personnel requirements. The very great disadvantage is the lack of an exact anatomic-functional comparison of both methods. This disadvantage can be decisive in the recognition and delineation of physiologic changes.

The second stage consists of simultaneous interpretation of the multimodal data sets at the same site. Although this is possible using conventional films, it is more practicable when performed at viewing workstations having picture archiving and communication system (PACS) access. Although this method enhances the capacity for

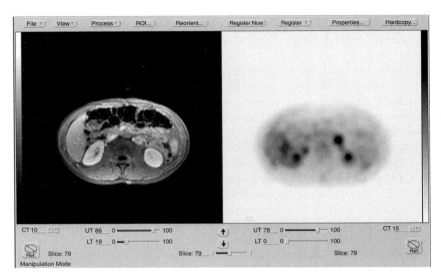

Figure 27.1. Multimodality display on a Hermes workstation (Nuclear Diagnostics AB, Haegersten, Sweden) demonstrating a left-sided paravertebral lymph node metastasis from a yolk sack tumor on magnetic resonance imaging (MRI) (left image) and positron emission tomography (PET) (right image).

morphologic correlation, because of the associated significant increase in personnel, cost, and time requirements, it is advisable to progress directly to the third stage.

In the third stage, analysis of spatially synchronized image data is performed simultaneously at a single workstation (Fig. 27.1). Synchronization may be interactive or partially or fully automatic with help of a fusion algorithm (17). These conditions provide for optimum spatial correlation of findings. Also useful is a common cursor that points to the corresponding location in both modalities, which are displayed side by side (11). This exact synchronization of data sets with appropriate software provides the additional capacity for image fusion with superimposition of both sets of imaging data in one image. In addition, a three-dimensional reconstruction of the fused imaging data can be used for therapy planning (Fig. 27.2, see color insert). When

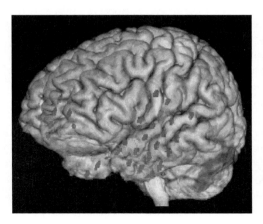

Figure 27.2. Three-dimensional (3D) reconstruction of a registered image data set. The cortical surface was rendered from MRI and red dots represent subdural EEG electrodes that were imaged with CT. The functional epileptogenic focus (orange) was defined by interictal fluorodeoxyglucose (FDG)-PET and ictal ECD–single photon emission computed tomography (SPECT). (See color insert.)

using a fused image, it is important to note that original information from the two individual imaging modalities may be partially lost, meaning that the original images of each modality should also be simultaneously displayed (Fig. 27.3, see color insert) (11).

Following image analysis comes the presentation of multimodal images to one's clinical colleagues, for whom the display of the fused imaging data sets moves to the foreground. Here, image fusion and three-dimensional reconstruction often represent decisive building blocks for understanding the pathology and for further therapeutic planning (Fig. 27.2).

Combination of MRI and PET

In combined imaging, morphologic information from MRI is complemented and extended by the functional information supplied by PET about glucose metabolism of the respective lesions. An important advantage of fluorodeoxyglucose (FDG)-PET, especially in the staging of malignant disease, is the capacity for examining the entire body or whole-body regions, whereas MRI is usually able to image only fractions of the same area during a single session (Fig. 27.4). Most publications of clinical applications and usefulness of multimodal diagnostic imaging concern oncologic imaging and multimodal diagnosis of epilepsy (7,18–27).

The major concentration of fluorine-18 (^{18}F)-FDG-PET is in oncologic diagnostics, where the evaluation of glucose metabolism in the tumor provides information on its viability. For this reason, PET in many cases has a higher specificity, sometimes even a higher sensitivity, than morphologic imaging modalities (MRI and CT) (28–33). Furthermore, a review of the literature shows PET imaging to be suitable for the majority of pediatric malignancies (1,34–42). Advances in these two anatomic and functional diagnostic imaging technologies have significantly influenced the staging and treatment approaches for pediatric tumors (8,38). The methods provide complementary information and have become essential in modern cancer therapy. Thus, anatomic and functional noninvasive technologies should be viewed as complementary rather than competitive. To identify a change in function without knowing accurately where it is localized, or, equivalently, to know there is an anatomic change without understanding the nature of the underlying cause compromises the clinical efficacy of both anatomic and functional imaging techniques (8,38,43). Combination of whole-body PET and state-of-the-art MRI offers accurate registration of metabolic and molecular aspects of a disease with exact correlation to anatomic findings, improving the diagnostic value of PET and MRI in identifying and characterizing malignancies and in tumor staging. Positron emission tomography can be used to detect areas of malignancies, tumor growth, therapeutic response, and recurrence. Malignancies with low or normal metabolic activity may show clearly positive or suspicious findings in the MRI (6). In a comparative study demonstrating the potential of combined PET-MRI diagnostics in 42 pediatric examinations, the sensitivity and specificity in detecting viable tumor

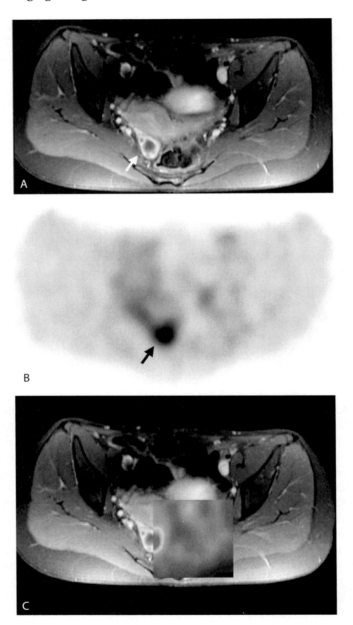

Figure 27.3. Histologically proven nonaffected cystic ovary in a patient with a recurrent yolk sack tumor: T1-weighted, fat-suppressed MR sequence after application of gadolinium–diethylenetriamine pentaacetic acid (Gd-DTPA) (A) depicts a physiologic-appearing cystic ovary (arrow). Corresponding PET (B) revealed a false-positive finding with an increased glucose uptake (arrow) suspect of a recurrent disease. Multimodality display of registered images (C) shows exact spatial correlation between the cystic ovary in MRI and increased glucose uptake in PET. (See color insert.)

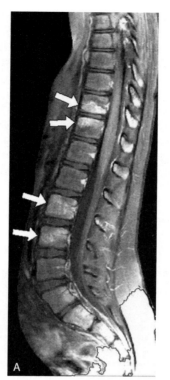

35   68   71

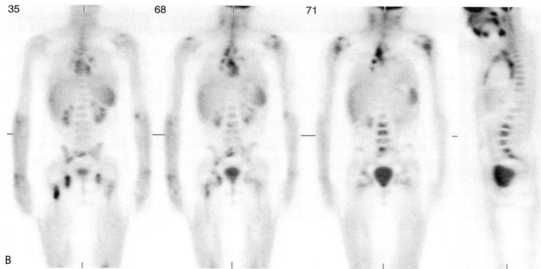

B

Figure 27.4. Non-Hodgkin's lymphoma in a 12-year-old girl with back pain. A: MRI shows a strong contrast enhancement in vertebral bodies of the thoracic and lumbar spine (arrows). A clear distinction between inflammatory and tumoral lesions was not possible. B: PET as a whole-body examination tool shows multiple bone and mediastinal lesions with the typical distribution pattern of a malignant lymphoma.

were significantly increased with combined analysis (44). The main reasons for false-positive PET findings when looking at suspected solitary tumor lesions in children are inflammatory or reactive changes in lymph nodes without tumor infiltration, normal bone marrow after chemotherapy, and physiologic FDG uptake of the intestine, the ovary (Fig. 27.3), the ureter, and brown adipose tissue. False-negative findings in FDG-PET primarily occur in bone metastases and tumor-affected lymph nodes due to low glucose metabolism or small size (Fig. 27.5). One reason is the limited spatial resolution of PET, which leads to false-negative findings in very small lesions (45). Under chemotherapy, active bone metastases may temporarily become PET-negative (Table 27.1) (35).

In MRI, the main reasons for false-positive findings are enlarged lymph nodes and bone marrow edema without tumor involvement.

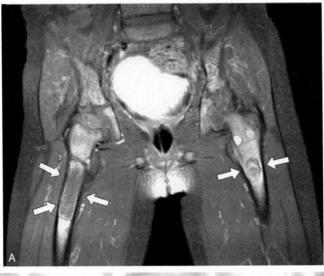

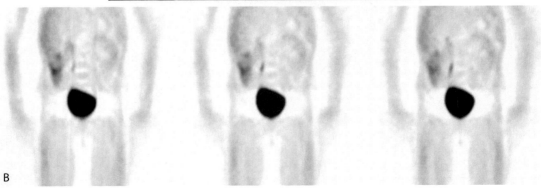

Figure 27.5. Histologically proven metastases of a Ewing sarcoma in the proximal femoral bone on both sides. A: T1-weighted fat-suppressed MR sequence shows hypointense lesions within the bone (arrows). B: Corresponding PET revealed a false-negative finding with no signs of metastatic spread in either femoral bone.

Table 27.1. Possible sources of false-positive and false-negative findings in MRI and FDG-PET

False-positive PET:	Brown adipose tissue; physiologic uptake in the muscles, bowel, ureter, and ovary; inflammatory changes (i.e., in lymph nodes); normal bone marrow after chemotherapy
False-positive MRI:	Posttherapeutic changes (i.e., persisting bone marrow edema in treated metastases), enlarged lymph nodes without tumor affection
False-negative PET:	Metastases with a small size and/or low glucose metabolism, tumor lesions under chemotherapy
False-negative MRI:	Small lymph node and bone metastases, lesions in the neighborhood of the bowel

Small bone and lymph node metastases can also be responsible for false-negative findings. Tumor lesions adjacent to normal bowel structures quite often cannot be distinguished from the bowel and consequently cannot be detected with MRI (Fig. 27.6). In the diagnosis of lymph nodes, a diameter of more than 1 cm is the leading parameter for the diagnosis of a metastasis. Therefore, lymph node metastases smaller than this and reactive lymph node enlargement are misinterpreted. Lesion size is not a reliable parameter for metastatic involvement (46). After successful tumor therapy, bone marrow edema often persists for a long time in MRI and may be responsible for false-positive findings. In summary, MRI is highly sensitive, but not very specific (Table 27.1) (35,45,47,48).

When combining FDG-PET and MRI in pediatric oncology, PET as a whole-body imaging tool plays a major role in assessing MRI-positive lesions. The most important benefit of MRI is to distinguish PET-positive tumor lesions from physiologically increased glucose uptake. In addition, MRI is indispensable for surgical and biopsy planning (Fig. 27.7). The combination of PET and MRI improves the diagnostic value of PET and MRI in identifying and characterizing tumor tissue, respectively (4,6,49).

Positron emission tomography is also used in the workup of inflammatory disease, though far less frequently than for oncologic indications. It is the method of choice in the search for a focus of inflammation in a patient with fever of unknown origin and/or unclear sepsis (50–54). Lesions detected with PET can be further delineated with MRI, which may also be useful for further therapy planning.

^{18}F-fluorodeoxyglucose-PET is also very useful in the presurgical focus localization in the workup of epilepsy. An exact integration of the findings of morphologic, electrophysiologic, and nuclear medical examinations is of great importance in the planning of surgical procedures for the treatment of epilepsy and for determination of the borders of resection, again underscoring the role of integrative diagnostics (55,56).

In patients with epilepsy, functional diagnostic methods include EEG and nuclear medical methods for visualizing cerebral metabolism and

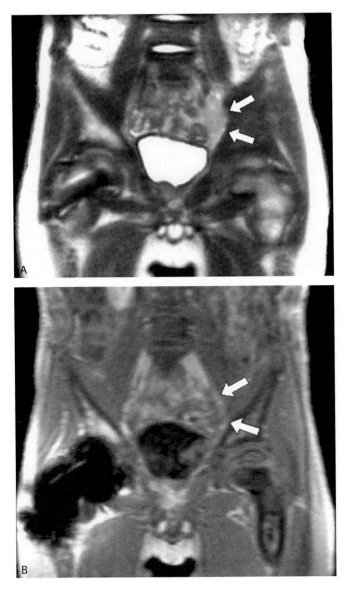

Figure 27.6. Recurrent tumor of a rhabdomyosarcoma lateral and superior to the urine bladder (arrows) in a 6-year-old boy. This recurrent lesion cannot be distinguished from the adjacent bowel either in T2-weighted MRI (A) or in the T1-weighted sequence after application of Gd-DTPA (B), thereby leading to a false-negative finding. PET clearly depicts an increased glucose metabolism in the corresponding region resulting in true-positive finding (C). Furthermore, postoperative metal artifacts in the right proximal femoral bone can be seen in MRI (A,B). PET and MRI show a metastasis of the left proximal femoral bone as well.

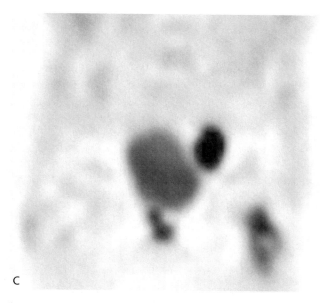

C

Figure 27.6. *Continued.*

perfusion. Frequently, ictal technetium-99m ECD-SPECT is combined with interictal FDG-PET, which permits more exact identification of the seizure focus with typical hypometabolism seen on PET (57–60). Beside conventional EEG leads, subdural electrodes may be implanted prior to the actual surgical procedure for direct measurement of the EEG signal from the cortical surface. These subdural electrodes can also be used for cortical stimulation. This permits delineation of functionally important areas that must be protected during a resective procedure. Knowledge of the exact position of the individual electrode points is important for demarcation of the resection boundaries. Because only CT can visualize these electrode points with sufficient accuracy, integration of CT information into the combined PET-MRI analysis is also necessary (56). Demarcation of resection boundaries, therefore, requires integration of all four described modalities: MRI for brain morphology, CT to establish the position of the subdural EEG electrodes, PET for visualization of brain metabolism, and SPECT for visualization of hyperperfusion. This is best achieved with three-dimensional image fusion, which permits exact spatial integration (Fig. 27.2). Here, registration of images is possible within 1.5 mm, which is adequate for clinical application (61). This method has also been shown to be superior to localization of electrodes using a conventional radiograph (56). The resulting reconstructed three-dimensional data set provides the neurosurgeon with the information needed for exact preoperative planning, including functional information on the focus of the seizure and important (especially language-related) brain areas that must be protected during resection.

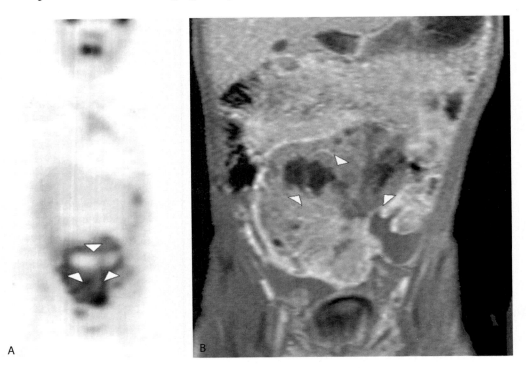

Figure 27.7. Rhabdomyosarcoma of the lower abdomen in a 6-year-old boy. A: FDG-PET demonstrates a large area with increased glucose uptake correlating to the primary tumor and a central photopenic defect (arrowheads). B: This photopenic defect correlates well to central necrosis visible in the T1-weighted, contrast-enhanced MR sequence (arrowheads). C: For operative planning, a T2-weighted short-time inversion recovery (STIR) sequence is necessary for the delineation of tumor borders and course of vessels.

Conclusion

It is important to emphasize that MRI and PET are not competing modalities. Instead, these two methods in combination can produce a synergy between function and morphology. For planning of biopsies and resective surgery, the knowledge of function (i.e., tumor viability) provided by PET and of the exact morphology of the tumor provided by MRI is often crucial. In patients with cerebral lesions, the whole spectrum of digital image fusion with direct superimposition of several modalities and subsequent three-dimensional reconstruction should be applied. This provides the surgeon with the tools for exact planning of approach and resection boundaries.

Direct image superimposition is not necessary for extracranial questions because information from individual modalities may be partially lost during fusion. The simultaneous evaluation of both modalities is to be emphasized. Having corresponding slices from both modalities displayed at a single workstation for synchronized evaluation is very

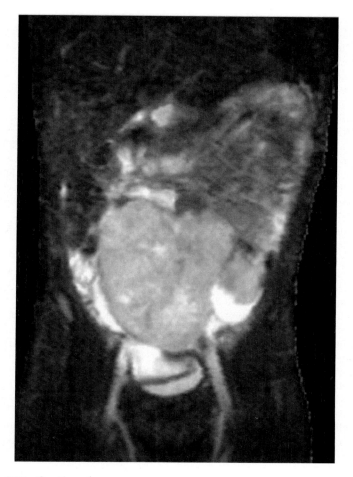

Figure 27.7. *Continued.*

useful. This is the most reliable method of immediately and efficiently correlating pathologic and especially unclear findings with the corresponding slice on the other imaging method. Because of MRI's low specificity in oncologic staging and at follow-up monitoring, the addition of PET for evaluating tumor vitality is essential.

References

1. Connolly LP, Drubach LA, Ted Treves S. Applications of nuclear medicine in pediatric oncology. Clin Nucl Med 2002;27(2):117–125.
2. Schmidt GP, Baur-Melnyk A, Tiling R, Hahn K, Reiser MF, Schoenberg SO. Comparison of high resolution whole-body MRI using parallel imaging and PET-CT. First experiences with a 32–channel MRI system. Radiologe 2004;44(9):889–898.

3. Bloem JL, van der Woude HJ, Geirnaerdt M, Hogendoorn PC, Taminiau AH, Hermans J. Does magnetic resonance imaging make a difference for patients with musculoskeletal sarcoma? Br J Radiol 1997;70(832):327–337.

4. Bredella MA, Caputo GR, Steinbach LS. Value of FDG positron emission tomography in conjunction with MR imaging for evaluating therapy response in patients with musculoskeletal sarcomas. AJR 2002;179(5): 1145–1150.

5. Antoch G, Vogt FM, Bockisch A, Ruehm SG. Whole-body tumor staging: MRI or FDG-PET/CT? Radiologe 2004;44(9):882–888.

6. Gaa J, Rummeny EJ, Seemann MD. Whole-body imaging with PET/MRI. Eur J Med Res 2004;9(6):309–312.

7. Pfluger T, Schmied C, Porn U, et al. Integrated imaging using MRI and 123I metaiodobenzylguanidine scintigraphy to improve sensitivity and specificity in the diagnosis of pediatric neuroblastoma. AJR 2003;181(4): 1115–1124.

8. Czernin J. Clinical applications of FDG-PET in oncology. Acta Med Austriaca 2002;29(5):162–170.

9. Alyafei S, Inoue T, Zhang H, et al. Image fusion system using PACS for MRI, CT, and PET images. Clin Positron Imaging 1999;2(3):137–143.

10. Hutton BF, Braun M. Software for image registration: algorithms, accuracy, efficacy. Semin Nucl Med 2003;33(3):180–192.

11. Slomka PJ. Software approach to merging molecular with anatomic information. J Nucl Med 2004;45(suppl 1):36S–45S.

12. Pelizzari CA, Chen GT, Spelbring DR, Weichselbaum RR, Chen CT. Accurate three-dimensional registration of CT, PET, and/or MR images of the brain. J Comput Assist Tomogr 1989;13(1):20–26.

13. Maes F, Collignon A, Vandermeulen D, Marchal G, Suetens P. Multimodality image registration by maximization of mutual information. IEEE Trans Med Imaging 1997;16(2):187–198.

14. Wells WM 3rd, Viola P, Atsumi H, Nakajima S, Kikinis R. Multi-modal volume registration by maximization of mutual information. Med Image Anal 1996;1(1):35–51.

15. Skalski J, Wahl RL, Meyer CR. Comparison of mutual information-based warping accuracy for fusing body CT and PET by 2 methods: CT mapped onto PET emission scan versus CT mapped onto PET transmission scan. J Nucl Med 2002;43(9):1184–1187.

16. Cohade C, Osman M, Marshall LN, Wahl RN. PET-CT: accuracy of PET and CT spatial registration of lung lesions. Eur J Nucl Med Mol Imaging 2003;30(5):721–726.

17. Stokking R, Zubal IG, Viergever MA. Display of fused images: methods, interpretation, and diagnostic improvements. Semin Nucl Med 2003; 33(3):219–227.

18. Aquino SL, Asmuth JC, Alpert NM, Halpern EF, Fischman AJ. Improved radiologic staging of lung cancer with 2-(18F)-fluoro-2-deoxy-D-glucose-positron emission tomography and computed tomography registration. J Comput Assist Tomogr 2003;27(4):479–484.

19. Cohade C, Wahl RL. Applications of positron emission tomography/computed tomography image fusion in clinical positron emission tomography—clinical use, interpretation methods, diagnostic improvements. Semin Nucl Med 2003;33(3):228–237.

20. Coleman RE, Hawk TC, Hamblen SM, Laymon CM, Turkington TG. Detection of recurrent brain tumor. Comparison of MR registered camera-based and dedicated PET images. Clin Positron Imaging 1999;2(1):57–61.

21. Dresel S, Grammerstorff J, Schwenzer K, et al. (18F)FDG imaging of head and neck tumours: comparison of hybrid PET and morphological methods. Eur J Nucl Med Mol Imaging 2003;30(7):995–1003.

22. Keidar Z, Israel O, Krausz Y. SPECT/CT in tumor imaging: technical aspects and clinical applications. Semin Nucl Med 2003;33(3):205–218.

23. Murphy M, O'Brien TJ, Morris K, Cook MJ. Multimodality image-guided epilepsy surgery. J Clin Neurosci 2001;8(6):534–538.

24. So EL. Role of neuroimaging in the management of seizure disorders. Mayo Clin Proc 2002;77(11):1251–1264.

25. Tsai CC, Tsai CS, Ng KK, et al. The impact of image fusion in resolving discrepant findings between FDG-PET and MRI/CT in patients with gynaecological cancers. Eur J Nucl Med Mol Imaging 2003;21:21.

26. Visvikis D, Ell PJ. Impact of technology on the utilisation of positron emission tomography in lymphoma: current and future perspectives. Eur J Nucl Med Mol Imaging 2003;30(suppl 1):S106–116.

27. Zhang W, Simos PG, Ishibashi H, et al. Multimodality neuroimaging evaluation improves the detection of subtle cortical dysplasia in seizure patients. Neurol Res 2003;25(1):53–57.

28. Anderson H, Price P. What does positron emission tomography offer oncology? Eur J Cancer 2000;36(16):2028–2035.

29. Bar-Shalom R, Valdivia AY, Blaufox MD. PET imaging in oncology. Semin Nucl Med 2000;30(3):150–185.

30. Czech N, Brenner W, Kampen WU, Henze E. [Diagnostic value of positron emission tomography (PET) in clinical oncology.] Dtsch Med Wochenschr 2000;125(18):565–567.

31. Delbeke D, Martin WH. Positron emission tomography imaging in oncology. Radiol Clin North Am 2001;39(5):883–917.

32. Mankoff DA, Bellon JR. Positron-emission tomographic imaging of cancer: glucose metabolism and beyond. Semin Radiat Oncol 2001;11(1):16–27.

33. Scott AM. Current status of positron emission tomography in oncology. Intern Med J 2001;31(1):27–36.

34. Brisse H, Ollivier L, Edeline V, et al. Imaging of malignant tumours of the long bones in children: monitoring response to neoadjuvant chemotherapy and preoperative assessment. Pediatr Radiol 2004;34(8):595–605.

35. Daldrup-Link HE, Franzius C, Link TM, et al. Whole-body MR imaging for detection of bone metastases in children and young adults: comparison with skeletal scintigraphy and FDG PET. AJR 2001;177(1):229–236.

36. Franzius C, Daldrup-Link HE, Wagner-Bohn A, et al. FDG-PET for detection of recurrences from malignant primary bone tumors: comparison with conventional imaging. Ann Oncol 2002;13(1):157–160.

37. Hawkins DS, Rajendran JG, Conrad EU 3rd, Bruckner JD, Eary JF. Evaluation of chemotherapy response in pediatric bone sarcomas by (F-18)-fluorodeoxy-D-glucose positron emission tomography. Cancer 2002;94(12):3277–3284.

38. Hudson MM, Krasin MJ, Kaste SC. PET imaging in pediatric Hodgkin's lymphoma. Pediatr Radiol 2004;34(3):190–198.

39. Montravers F, McNamara D, Landman-Parker J, et al. ((18)F)FDG in childhood lymphoma: clinical utility and impact on management. Eur J Nucl Med Mol Imaging 2002;29(9):1155–1165.

40. O'Hara SM, Donnelly LF, Coleman RE. Pediatric body applications of FDG PET. AJR 1999;172(4):1019–1024.

41. Shulkin BL. PET imaging in pediatric oncology. Pediatr Radiol 2004;34(3): 199–204.
42. Shulkin BL, Mitchell DS, Ungar DR, et al. Neoplasms in a pediatric population: 2–(F-18)-fluoro-2–deoxy-D-glucose PET studies. Radiology 1995; 194(2):495–500.
43. Townsend DW, Cherry SR. Combining anatomy and function: the path to true image fusion. Eur Radiol 2001;11(10):1968–1974.
44. Pfluger T, Vollmar C, Porn U, et al. Combined PET/MRI in cerebral and pediatric diagnostics. Der Nuklearmediziner 2002;25(2):122–127.
45. Hueltenschmidt B, Sautter-Bihl ML, Lang O, et al. Whole body positron emission tomography in the treatment of Hodgkin disease. Cancer 2001; 91(2):302–310.
46. Torabi M, Aquino SL, Harisinghani MG. Current concepts in lymph node imaging. J Nucl Med 2004;45(9):1509–1518.
47. Ilias I, Pacak K. Current approaches and recommended algorithm for the diagnostic localization of pheochromocytoma. J Clin Endocrinol Metab 2004;89(2):479–491.
48. Korholz D, Kluge R, Wickmann L, et al. Importance of F18–fluorodeoxy-D-2–glucose positron emission tomography (FDG-PET) for staging and therapy control of Hodgkin's lymphoma in childhood and adolescence— consequences for the GPOH-HD 2003 protocol. Onkologie 2003;26(5): 489–493.
49. Popperl G, Lang S, Dagdelen O, et al. Correlation of FDG-PET and MRI/ CT with histopathology in primary diagnosis, lymph node staging and diagnosis of recurrency of head and neck cancer. Rofo 2002;174(6):714– 720.
50. Blockmans D, Knockaert D, Maes A, et al. Clinical value of ((18)F)fluoro-deoxyglucose positron emission tomography for patients with fever of unknown origin. Clin Infect Dis 2001;32(2):191–196.
51. Kapucu LO, Meltzer CC, Townsend DW, Keenan RJ, Luketich JD. Fluorine-18–fluorodeoxyglucose uptake in pneumonia. J Nucl Med 1998;39(7): 1267–1269.
52. Kresnik E, Mikosch P, Gallowitsch HJ, Heinisch M, Lind P. F-18 fluo-rodeoxyglucose positron emission tomography in the diagnosis of inflammatory bowel disease. Clin Nucl Med 2001;26(10):867.
53. Meller J, Becker W. [Nuclear medicine diagnosis of patients with fever of unknown origin (FUO).] Nuklearmedizin 2001;40(3):59–70.
54. Weiner GM, Jenicke L, Buchert R, Bohuslavizki KH. [FDG PET for the localization diagnosis in inflammatory disease of unknown origin—two case reports.] Nuklearmedizin 2001;40(4):N35–38.
55. Barnett GH, Kormos DW, Steiner CP, Morris H. Registration of EEG electrodes with three-dimensional neuroimaging using a frameless, armless stereotactic wand. Stereotact Funct Neurosurg 1993;61(1):32–38.
56. Winkler PA, Vollmar C, Krishnan KG, Pfluger T, Brückmann H, Noachtar S. Usefulness of 3–D reconstructed images of the human cerebral cortex for localization of subdural electrodes in epilepsy surgery. Epilepsy Res 2000;41(7):169–178.
57. Carreras JL, Perez-Castejon MJ, Jimenez AM, Domper M, Montz R. [Neuroimaging in epilepsy. Advances in SPECT and PET in epilepsy.] Rev Neurol 2000;30(4):359–363.
58. Matheja P, Kuwert T, Stodieck SR, et al. PET and SPECT in medically non-refractory complex partial seizures. Temporal asymmetries of glucose consumption, benzodiazepine receptor density, and blood flow. Nuklearmedizin 1998;37(7):221–226.

59. Noachtar S, Arnold S, Yousry TA, Bartenstein P, Werhahn KJ, Tatsch K. Ictal technetium-99m ethyl cysteinate dimer single-photon emission tomographic findings and propagation of epileptic seizure activity in patients with extratemporal epilepsies. Eur J Nucl Med 1998;25(2):166–172.
60. Oliveira AJ, da Costa JC, Hilario LN, Anselmi OE, Palmini A. Localization of the epileptogenic zone by ictal and interictal SPECT with 99mTc-ethyl cysteinate dimer in patients with medically refractory epilepsy. Epilepsia 1999;40(6):693–702.
61. Pfluger T, Vollmar C, Wismuller A, et al. Quantitative comparison of automatic and interactive methods for MRI-SPECT image registration of the brain based on 3-dimensional calculation of error. J Nucl Med 2000; 41(11):1823–1829.

28

Current Research Efforts

Fabio Ponzo and Martin Charron

Over the past 20 years, as clinical applications have been gradually expanding, positron emission tomography (PET) has become an indispensable imaging technique in several medical fields such as oncology, neurology, and cardiology. Application of PET in pediatrics is still very limited, likely due to the smaller number of clinical reports involving PET in pediatric as compared to adult medicine and to the lesser availability of PET scanners in pediatric facilities. However, the recent expansion of the regional availability of the most common PET radiotracer, fluorine-18 fluorodeoxyglucose (^{18}F-FDG) and, more importantly, the recent appearance of the dual-modality PET–computed tomography(CT) imaging system have provided new opportunities of expansion of PET to the pediatric field. The recent mechanical coupling of CT to PET in the same imaging device for attenuation correction permits precise localization of metabolic findings on anatomic images and shortens the total acquisition time. Both qualities are particularly important in pediatric imaging, making the study more acceptable to patients and parents and less cumbersome for personnel. Moreover, the shortened acquisition time reduces the probability of motion artifacts on reconstructed images. This chapter briefly summarizes the state of clinical applications of PET in the pediatric field and discusses potential new research approaches and new clinical applications of PET and PET-CT in pediatric patients.

Patient Preparation

Preparation of children and parents for PET imaging is critical, and its importance has already been the object of discussion (1,2). The importance of NPO (nothing by mouth) status for 4 to 6 hours prior to FDG administration needs to be emphasized and coordinated with family members and personnel taking care of the pediatric patient, especially in the case of children on total parenteral nutrition or undergoing chemotherapeutic therapy intravenously if dextrose is present in the intravenous fluids. Reliable intravenous access is fundamental, and bladder catheterization is needed to avoid reconstruction artifacts in the pelvis and the possibility of voiding and contamination during image acquisition (3,4).

Sedation protocols vary, and several guidelines are available (5–7). Sedatives may affect cerebral metabolism but sometimes are required for completion of the study because light sedation is rarely helpful (8). Especially in case of sedated patients, PET-CT devices are quite valuable; spiral CT takes less than a minute, and the three-dimensional (3D) mode of acquisition of emission data reduces the emission imaging time to 4 to 5 minutes per bed position. Moreover, CT scans performed for attenuation correction are obtained with reduced milliamperes (mA), decreasing the absorbed dose to the patient without loss of image quality. Imaging protocols for PET-CT are a compromise between the desired combination of CT scans of different portions of the body and the patient's tolerance. For this reason, the acquisition of CT images for the purpose of attenuation correction follows a simpler protocol (9–13). For example, PET-CT scans are done with free breathing, in contrast to diagnostic CT examination of the chest, which is often performed with the breath-hold technique. Breath holding with PET-CT can contribute to misregistration between CT and PET data.

Both intravenous and oral contrast can be used in pediatrics with PET-CT without significant untoward effects on image quality. Oral contrast must be taken with sugar-free beverages to avoid competition in uptake of FDG and cannot be administered before the PET-CT study in case of general anesthesia.

Contrast can improve interpretation of PET-CT images when evaluating small children with limited retroperitoneal fat (14,15), although semiquantitative measures such as the standard uptake value (SUV) may be affected (15–17). Future studies are needed to compare the diagnostic accuracy of PET-CT scans done after administration of intravenous (IV) or oral contrast and nonenhanced PET-CT scans. Better delineation of blood vessels may be critical in some cases, such as in lymphomas where better delineation of involved lymph nodes may result in a change in patient management. Administration of IV contrast may cause artifacts, especially in the lower neck, a region already complicated by the common presence of activated brown fat in children. The timing between contrast injection and imaging must be carefully observed on a patient-by-patient basis. Possible effects on SUV analysis by contrast dye still need to be evaluated.

Neurology

Normal Brain Development

The first structures to show glucose metabolism immediately after birth are the sensorimotor cortex, thalamus, brainstem, and cerebellar vermis, followed by the basal ganglia and the parietal, temporal, calcarine, and cerebellar cortices in the next 3 months of life and the frontal cortex and the dorsolateral cortex during the second 6 months of life (18–20).

Recently, co-registration of PET and magnetic resonance imaging (MRI) has allowed identification of fetal organs and demonstrated that ^{18}F-FDG readily crosses the placenta and that ^{18}F accumulates in both maternal and fetal brain in a nonhuman primate animal model. This study demonstrates the potential for noninvasively measuring the transfer of drugs across the placenta and for measuring the fetal drug distribution (21).

Epilepsy

Nearly all studies in children with epilepsy have been performed during interictus, given the relatively short half-life of ^{18}F. The approximately 30-minute uptake time of FDG may also depict a combination of the areas of seizure propagation and the actual seizure focus. Nevertheless, in patients with continuous or frequent seizures, ictal PET has been shown to be able to localize extratemporal seizures (22). Interictal FDG-PET has proven useful in the localization of the epileptogenic region, which is indicated by regional hypometabolism (22,23). Among the available imaging modalities, FDG-PET is superior to CT and MRI alone in preoperative evaluation when combined with EEG data (22,24–26). Results from FDG-PET also have good correlation with those of MR spectroscopy (27).

Poor prognosis has been associated with bitemporal hypometabolism on FDG-PET. These patients are typically not candidates for resective surgery (28–31). Children with infantile spasms may also benefit from evaluation with FDG-PET (32). Other PET radiotracers have also been applied in epilepsy diagnosis. Reduced uptake of carbon-11 (^{11}C)-flumazenil and of ^{11}C-labeled (S)-(N-methyl)-ketamine corresponds to the epileptogenic region. A relative increase in uptake of ^{11}C-carfentanil and ^{11}C-deprenyl may also help in identifying epileptogenic foci (33–39). In patients with tuberous sclerosis, α-^{11}C–methyl-L-tryptophan may also differentiate between epileptogenic and nonepileptogenic tubers (40).

6-^{18}F-L-3,4-Fluorodihydroxyphenylalanine (^{18}F-fluoro-L-DOPA) recently has been shown to be a promising agent in evaluation of control circuits of epilepsy. ^{18}F-fluoro-L-DOPA permits measurements of presynaptic dopaminergic function and has been frequently used in studies of Parkinson's disease. In drug-resistant epileptic patients with ring chromosome 20, ^{18}F-fluoro-L-DOPA has shown involvement of the basal ganglia (41).

The role of dopamine function in other types of drug-resistant epileptic syndromes has been recently evaluated by Bouilleret et al. (42). In an experimental study, three groups of children, the first composed of drug-resistant epileptic patients with ring chromosome 20, the second composed of patients with resistant, generalized "absence-like" epilepsy, and the third composed of patients with drug-resistant temporal lobe epilepsy with hippocampal sclerosis, were studied with ^{18}F-fluoro-L-DOPA PET. The researchers used two strategies of analysis of the ^{18}F-fluoro-L-DOPA uptake in basal ganglia: a multiple-time graphical analysis with regions of interest, and an all-brain statistical parametric mapping analysis using a voxel-by-voxel statistical t-test. Each epileptic group was compared with a group of healthy volunteers. The results showed that a decrease of uptake value was observed in the striatum in all groups of patients with both types of analysis. Multiple-time graphical analysis showed a reduction of uptake over each basal ganglion in both generalized (groups 1 and 2) and focal (group 3) epilepsies, confirming the involvement of the basal ganglia in patients with r20 epilepsy.

More interestingly, a unilateral decrease of uptake was detected using statistical parametric mapping (SPM) analysis. This decrease was ipsilateral to the seizure side in patients with focal temporal lobe epilepsy. Moreover, SPM analysis showed a decrease of ^{18}F-fluoro-L-DOPA uptake in the substantia nigra bilaterally. This result confirms the involvement of dopamine neurotransmission in seizure control and demonstrates that this involvement is not specific to epileptic patients with ring chromosome 20. Further studies are needed to determine whether the decrease of ^{18}F-fluoro-L-DOPA uptake is a cause or a consequence of seizures and to evaluate the specific role of substantia nigra in the control of different forms of seizures.

The dopamine system modulation may have a potential role in controlling epileptic foci; this opens new possibilities of pharmacologic treatment of drug-resistant epilepsy (42).

Cerebral Inflammatory Diseases

Rasmussen's encephalitis in infants has been investigated using FDG-PET. It is characterized by unilateral cerebral decreased FDG uptake corresponding to regions of cerebral atrophy seen at MRI, increasing the specificity of MRI findings (43,44). Abnormal FDG uptake may also precede clinical symptoms in HIV-1–infected children born to seropositive mothers (45).

Other Neurologic Applications

In term newborns, perinatal asphyxia may cause hypoxic-ischemic encephalopathy, which has been studied with FDG PET. The impairment of cerebral glucose metabolism correlates well with the severity of encephalopathy and short-term clinical outcome (40,46–48). A change in cerebral glucose metabolism has been demonstrated in other childhood brain disorders such as traumatic brain injury, autism, attention-deficit/hyperactivity disorder, schizophrenia, sickle cell encephalopathy, and anorexia and bulimia nervosa (49–57).

Prader-Willi syndrome (PWS) has been recently studied with FDG-PET (58). This syndrome is a neurogenetic disorder caused by lack of expression of paternal genes in the 15q11-q13 region, and is the most common form of human syndromic obesity. Along with compulsive hyperphagia, children affected with PWS present hypothalamic hypogonadism and mental retardation. In this study, nine children affected with PWS underwent resting brain FDG-PET, and the results showed decreased glucose metabolism in regions associated with taste perception and food reward such as the superior temporal gyrus and insula. There was increased FDG uptake in areas involved in cognitive functions related to eating or obsessive-compulsive behavior such as the orbitofrontal and middle frontal gyrus, left cingulate gyrus, and right uncus. Interestingly, the hypothalamus, the brain region usually involved in energy intake, did not show abnormal metabolism.

Patients with hereditary spastic paraplegia (HSP), a rare hereditary autosomal-recessive disorder, suffer slowly progressive retrograde axonal degeneration of the corticospinal tracts and dorsal columns. Symptoms are ataxia, dysarthria, unipolar depression, epilepsy, migraine, and cognitive impairment. The disease is linked to the SPG4 locus on chromosome 2p (59). Oxygen-15–radiolabeled water (^{15}O-H$_2$O) PET has been used to study regional cerebral blood flow in patients with HSP. ^{15}O-H$_2$O PET showed significantly relative decreased blood flow in frontotemporal and thalamic regions at rest. Ongoing studies are being performed for the evaluation of cerebral activation response after motor stimuli.

Cardiology

Only a few papers have been published investigating the role of PET in pediatric cardiology (60,61). Positron emission tomography with nitrogen-13 (^{13}N)-ammonia has been employed to measure myocardial perfusion in infants after anatomic repair of congenital heart defects and after Norwood palliation for hypoplastic left heart syndrome (62,63). Positron emission tomography has also been used to assess myocardial blood flow and impaired coronary flow reserve after coronary reimplantation in patients with Fontan-like operations (64,65).

Gated FDG-PET has been proved useful in the evaluation of regional glucose metabolism and contractile function in children after arterial switch operation and suspected myocardial infarction (66). In children with Kawasaki disease, combined assessment of cardiac flow and metabolism with PET showed abnormalities in more than 40% of patients during the acute and the convalescent stage of disease (67). Positron emission tomography with ^{11}C-acetate has demonstrated reduced Krebs' cycle activity in children with mitochondrial cardiomyopathy despite normal myocardial perfusion (68).

Inflammatory Disease

Potential new application of FDG-PET in the study of inflammatory diseases can be hypothesized because FDG accumulation is not specific for tumors. Neutrophils and macrophages also exhibit increased glucose metabolism at the site of inflammation and infection. At the present time, only a limited number of publications address the role of FDG-PET in detecting inflammatory diseases in infants and children.

Fluorodeoxyglucose-PET was proven useful in the assessment of children with suspected inflammatory bowel disease (69). Potential advantages of FDG-PET include its noninvasiveness, its repeatability, and its capability to localize the segment involved and to quantify disease activity in view of the assessment of therapeutic efficacy. The sensitivity and accuracy of FDG-PET have not yet been compared with those of other diagnostic techniques such as abdominal ultrasound, small bowel follow through, and endoscopy/histology. However, FDG-PET has already demonstrated higher sensitivity than CT in detecting active infective foci in children with chronic granulomatous disease (70).

Other authors have reported the clinical usefulness of FDG-PET in detecting occult infectious foci (71), identifying infectious mononucleosis lesions (72), and monitoring therapy in patients with aspergillosis (73). An overview of the literature with regard to the value of PET in pediatric lung diseases was published by Richard et al. (74).

In acute pneumonia, neutrophils are the primary cell type responsible for the increase in ^{18}F-FDG tissue uptake, 10 to 40 times above values obtained in normal subjects (75–78).

^{18}F-Fluorodeoxyglucose-PET has shown different rates of glucose uptake in the lungs in different patient groups, despite the presence of airway neutrophilia in each, according to the presence of acute or chronic inflammatory disease (75,79,80). More reliable quantification of pulmonary inflammation than the mere number of neutrophils present in the tissue has also been obtained in experimental allergen-induced airway inflammation in asthmatics (81) and in a neonatal model of acute lung injury in piglets (82) using FDG-PET.

Cystic fibrosis (CF) is the most common inherited disease of Caucasians; it is autosomal recessive and occurs in approximately 1 in 2500 to 3000 live births. The life expectancy of a child born with CF has gradually improved and is now approaching 32 years (83). The morbidity and mortality in this disease result from airway infection and inflammation. The intense and persistent host inflammatory response is thought to account for progressive, suppurative pulmonary disease (84), the neutrophils being the prominent inflammatory cells (85). Only preliminary data are available regarding the use of FDG-PET in CF (86), but a recent report has compared the ability of FDG-PET in monitoring disease activity in children with CF (87). At the present time bronchoalveolar lavage is the only available method to quantify airway inflammation directly, but it is invasive and samples only limited volume of the lungs. Preliminary data from Chen et al. (87) have shown that the calculated plasma/activity ratio from a dynamic PET scan on a region of interest placed over the entire lung positively correlates with the mean neutrophil count from bronchoalveolar lavage. Therefore, FDG-PET seems to be an effective, noninvasive tool to measure neutrophilic inflammation in CF. It may also have an important role in monitoring the response to therapy, as already reported in the setting of sarcoidosis treated with corticosteroids (88). It might be also useful as a noninvasive method of testing new antiinflammatory therapies in children with inflammatory lung disease.

Oncology

Potential Causes of Misinterpretation of FDG-PET in Children

Fluorodeoxyglucose distribution may be altered in children because of areas of physiologically increased glucose metabolism; this is particularly evident in the thymus (89,90) and in the skeletal growth centers, mostly in the long bone physes. As in adults, other potential pitfalls include variable FDG uptake in working skeletal muscles, brown fat, myocardium, thyroid gland, and the gastrointestinal tract. Fluorodeoxyglucose is also always present in the renal pelvis, ureters, and bladder because of its renal excretion (91–95).

To decrease the incidence of interfering brown fat activity, the use of pharmacologic interventions has been described: propranolol or reserpine treatment seems to reduce FDG uptake (96); diazepam in low doses shows no effectiveness (97).

The recent use of PET-CT has significantly decreased the incidence of false-positive findings on PET, given the precise anatomic correlation of metabolic evidences on PET images. The most common equivocal areas on PET that can be further clarified as nonmalignant by PET-CT include brown fat, bowel, thymus muscle, ureters, stomach, and esophagus (98).

To further enhance the specificity of PET-CT, the use of intravenous contrast has been proposed but there is still insufficient evidence in the literature to support its use (99–101). Recent preliminary data have instead compared PET-CT with contrast enhanced CT in children with lymphoma (102). The authors have reported discrepant findings between the two techniques, mostly related to metabolically active subcentimeter lymph nodes and residual soft tissue in the mediastinum negative on PET-CT. Further studies are needed to compare the diagnostic accuracy of contrast-enhanced CT with non–contrast-enhanced PET-CT and to evaluate the impact of possible added value of contrast-enhanced CT over PET-CT on patient management.

Diffuse high FDG uptake in bone marrow and spleen following administration of hematopoietic stimulating factors (103,104) and of granulocyte colony-stimulating factor may also cause misinterpretation of FDG accumulation (103). Chemotherapy may also cause thymus hyperplasia with relative increased FDG metabolism (89,105). The coregistration technique of the new combined PET-CT imaging systems may also cause artifacts that are not limited to pediatric patients; they are caused by metallic objects, respiration, and oral and intravenous contrast agents (106).

Central Nervous System Tumors

Magnetic resonance imaging and CT are now the imaging modalities used for staging and follow-up of children with central nervous system (CNS) tumors, but the role of PET has been increasing in recent years. Increased FDG uptake can help distinguish viable tumor from post-therapeutic sclerotic changes (107–109) and correlates well with histopathology and clinical data (110–113). Preoperative planning, including a combination of MRI and PET data, improves the diagnostic yield of stereotactic brain biopsy in pediatric brain tumors and reduces tissue sampling in high-risk functional areas (114,115).

In children affected by neurofibromatosis type 1 who have low-grade astrocytomas, FDG-PET has good correlation with clinical outcome (116). Fluorodeoxyglucose uptake in brain tumors can be a better predictor of tumor growth than histopathology (117). Other positron-emitting tracers such as ^{18}F-α-methyltyrosine (118), ^{11}C-methionine (119), and ^{11}C-thymidine (120) have been reported to be useful in the study pediatric brain tumors. Recent initial results with O-(2-^{18}F-fluorethyl)-L-tyrosine (FET)-PET in 44 patients with primary bone tumors seem to indicate that tumor uptake is higher in high-grade tumors, and different uptake kinetics of FET may help in identifying a highly aggressive brain lesion (121).

A possible future application of PET in the evaluation of recurrent tumor may take advantage of the possibility of co-registration between PET images and MR images. The co-registration technique has been used already to improve the anatomic localization of metabolically active sites in pediatric tumors (122). Moreover, further characterization may be obtained using co-registration between metabolic information obtained with FDG-PET and anatomic and metabolic data obtained with proton magnetic resonance spectroscopy (MRS) imaging. Additional studies are still needed to compare enhanced glucose metabolism and choline/lactate ratios in brain tumors with different degrees of aggressiveness.

Lymphoma and Leukemia

Non-Hodgkin's and Hodgkin's lymphomas are the third most common type of malignancy in childhood, accounting for between 10% and 15% of pediatric malignancies. Lymphoblastic and small-cell tumors are the most common histologic types of non-Hodgkin's lymphoma. Nodular sclerosing and mixed cellularity are the most common histologic types of Hodgkin's disease. In adult patients, FDG has been shown to accumulate in non-Hodgkin's and Hodgkin's lymphomas (91,123–146), with more intense uptake in higher-grade lymphomas than in lower-grade lymphomas (130,132).

Fluorodeoxyglucose-PET has been reported to be highly effective in evaluating lymphomatous involvement for staging and patient management (127,128,133,134,147). Fluorodeoxyglucose uptake also has excellent predictive value for patient outcome in the follow-up period (148). Fluorodeoxyglucose-PET is useful in identifying the site of biopsy or in eliminating the need for biopsy at staging (128,140) and in assessing activity in posttherapy residual soft tissue masses (134,142).

The co-registration between PET and CT in the new PET-CT devices has been effective in the evaluation of lymphoma. A recent report found that 75% of FDG-PET-CT studies provided further information on patient disease status (149).

In summary, PET plays an increasingly important role in staging, evaluating tumor response, planning radiation treatment fields, and monitoring after completion of therapy in pediatric lymphoma (150–152). In he future, FDG-PET-CT may function as primary imaging modality in these patients. In addition, possible deficits of glucose metabolism after cranial radiation therapy have been studied with FDG-PET in children treated for acute lymphoblastic leukemia. Quantification of cerebral glucose uptake provided by PET demonstrated significant changes after cranial radiation therapy (153).

Neuroblastoma

Neuroblastoma is the most common extracranial solid malignant tumor in children. Up to 70% of patients have disseminated neuroblastoma at presentation. Proper staging is critical because localized neuroblastoma may be treated with surgery with or without preoperative chemotherapy, according to the degree of the local extension. Distant metastases are indicative of poor prognosis. Magnetic resonance imaging, CT, bone scintigraphy, and scintigraphy with meta-iodobenzylguanidine (mIBG) or indium-111-pentetreotide are currently used in clinical practice for the evaluation of disseminated disease (154). Neuroblastomas are metabolically active tumors that avidly concentrate FDG. However, FDG-PET has been shown to have disconcordant results when compared to mIBG and is not proved to be a better imaging technique in the delineation of residual disease (155). Therefore, at present, the primary role of FDG-PET is in the evaluation of known or suspected neuroblastomas that do not demonstrate mIBG uptake.

Children with high-risk neuroblastomas after resection of the primary tumor and in the absence or resolution of skull lesions may also be monitored using FDG-PET and bone marrow examinations without performing additional diagnostic tests (156).

The use of other radiopharmaceutical such as ^{11}C-hydroxyephedrine, ^{11}C-epinephrine, ^{18}F-3-iodobenzylguanidine, ^{18}F-fluoronorepinephrine, ^{18}F-flurometaraminol, ^{18}F-fluorodopamine, and iodine-124 (^{124}I)-mIBG have also been described as being useful in evaluating neuroblastoma (157–159).

Wilms' Tumor

Wilms' tumor is the most common renal malignancy of childhood, typically presenting as an asymptomatic abdominal mass. Other imaging modalities such as radiography, ultrasonography, CT, and MRI are commonly used in the definition of the local extent of Wilms' tumor in kidneys and soft tissue and in the detection of metastases. Fluorodeoxyglucose-PET has a limited role in the anatomic staging of primary tumor, given the renal excretion of FDG and the limited spatial resolution of PET. A potential role of FDG-PET is in the follow-up after radiation or chemotherapy for identification of residual disease (160).

Bone Tumors

Osteosarcoma and Ewing's sarcoma are the two primary bone malignancies of childhood. The treatment of choice for primary bone malignancies of an extremity is wide resection and limb-sparing surgery with chemotherapy pre- and postoperatively. Magnetic resonance imaging is currently used in anatomic staging of primary bone malignancies. However, MRI has shown variable results in assessing chemotherapeutic response (161–166).

The exact role of FDG-PET in osteosarcoma and Ewing's sarcoma is unclear. Semiquantification of FDG uptake using SUV analysis has been reported to provide useful information for the differentiation between benign and malignant bone tumors (167,168).

Several articles have evaluated the role of FDG-PET in comparison with other diagnostic techniques in the evaluation of metastatic disease in bone tumors. In a comparison of whole-body MRI, whole-body bone scan, and FDG-PET, Daldrup-Link et al. (169) have found the highest sensitivity for FDG-PET in the detection of osseous metastases from primary bone tumors. Franzius et al. (170) found spiral CT to be superior to FDG-PET in detecting pulmonary metastases and FDG-PET to be more sensitive, specific, and accurate than bone scintigraphy in identifying osseous metastases from Ewing's sarcoma. However, FDG-PET was less sensitive than bone scan for detecting metastases from osteosarcoma (171). For detection of recurrences from malignant primary bone tumors, Franzius et al. (172) also found FDG-PET to have higher sensitivity, specificity, and accuracy than conventional imaging modalities. Current experience suggests that, in patients with bone sarcomas, FDG-PET may play an important role in monitoring response to preoperative neoadjuvant chemotherapy (173–176). A decrease of FDG uptake in response to neoadjuvant chemotherapy correlates well with histopathologic findings and with disease-free survival after therapy.

As an alternative to bone scintigraphy and FDG-PET, the use of PET and PET-CT with ^{18}F-FNa (sodium fluoride) has been proposed by Even-Sapir et al. in assessing malignant osseous involvement and in differentiating malignant from benign bone lesions (177). In a series of 44 patients, the authors found ^{18}F-fluoride PET-CT both sensitive and specific for the detection of lytic and sclerotic malignant lesions. Positron emission tomography–CT also differentiated malignant from benign bone lesions, and, for most lesions, the anatomic data provided by the low-dose CT of the PET-CT study obviates the need for full-dose diagnostic CT for correlation purposes. The role of PET-CT with ^{18}F-FNa has not yet been evaluated in the pediatric population with bone tumors.

Osseous metastasis is the main adverse prognostic factor in patients with Ewing tumors. Recently, to evaluate osseous metastasis, a high-resolution animal PET scanner has been tested on an experimental mouse model for human Ewing tumor metastases. Both glucose metabolism and bone metabolism were assessed using ^{18}F-FDG and ^{18}F-FNa. Osteolytic lesions showed decreased ^{18}F-FNa uptake and increased ^{18}F-FDG uptake. The experimental mouse model and the high-resolution animal PET scanner may be used in future for the evaluation of new tracers for the diagnosis and monitoring of experimental therapies of Ewing tumor (178).

Rhabdomyosarcoma is the most common soft tissue malignancy of childhood. It can develop in any organ or tissue, most commonly in the head and neck and the genitourinary tract. Computed tomography or MRI is important for local staging. Radiation therapy and surgery are used to control local disease. Radiography, CT, and skeletal scintigraphy are used to identify metastases, which are treated with chemotherapy. Rhabdomyosarcomas show FDG uptake, and FDG-PET has been reported to have more clinical utility than standard imaging evaluation (8,173,179).

In soft tissue sarcomas, FDG-PET was able to distinguish high-grade soft tissue sarcoma from low-grade or benign tumors (180). Comparing the results of FDG-PET, MRI, and CT in 62 patients with soft tissue sarcomas, Lucas et al. (181) showed FDG-PET to be the best stand-alone modality for the assessment of local tumor recurrence and distant metastases.

For the evaluation of local recurrent disease in patients with musculoskeletal sarcomas, MRI has a prominent role. However, Bredella et al. (182) recently showed FDG-PET to be a useful adjunct to MRI in distinguishing viable tumor from scar tissue.

Pheochromocytoma

Pheochromocytoma and paraganglioma may occur at any age, but they are most common from early to mid-adulthood. For localization of primary tumor, MRI and CT are the diagnostic techniques in use. Scintigraphy with ^{131}I-mIBG has limited sensitivity. A possible role of PET in the staging and restaging of pheochromocytoma and paraganglioma has been hypothesized using 6-^{18}F-fluorodopamine. Preliminary results show that this technique is highly sensitive in pheochromocytoma localization (183).

Metastatic adrenal cortical carcinoma has very poor prognosis (184). The most common locations for distant metastases are the lung, liver, and skeleton. The preferred imaging methods (CT and MRI) are the screening methods for the most common lung and liver metastases (185). Fluorodeoxyglucose-PET imaging in adults seems to be able to differentiate malignant from benign adrenal lesions (186,187). Recently, a different cost-effective and noninvasive approach has been proposed in the evaluation of adrenocortical carcinomas in children: primary screening with PET, followed by morphologic imaging with CT or MRI (188).

Hepatoblastoma

Hepatoblastoma is a rare hepatic tumor of children. It is generally treated with surgical resection with perioperative use of chemotherapy. Posttreatment follow-up is generally achieved with serial monitoring of α-fetoprotein (AFP) levels and conventional radiologic imaging. Early detection of recurrent hepatoblastoma is not always possible with conventional imaging methods such as CT and MRI.

Philip et al. (189) have recently described the use of FDG-PET to locate the site of recurrence in the follow-up of three cases of pediatric patients with elevated AFP levels (189). In the first two patients, FDG-PET accurately located recurrent disease where it was not detected by conventional imaging modalities, including CT and MRI. In the third patient, FDG-PET imaging also located the recurrent disease in an MRI-identified adrenal metastasis. The technique of co-registration of PET with CT and MRI scans improved the anatomic localization of metabolically active sites and was particularly useful for determining the surgical approach. The results of this study seem to confirm the value of PET-CT and other co-registration techniques in the evaluation of early tumor recurrence or metastatic disease in hepatoblastoma. Additional studies are needed to evaluate the impact of FDG-PET-CT imaging in patient management.

Conclusion

The routine clinical use of PET in pediatric patients is still limited. This is partly because PET scanning in children is only supported when applicable to similar reimbursed adult conditions. Positron emission tomography–CT applications are still viewed with caution given the additional radiation dose delivered by the CT device used for attenuation purpose. Moreover, the number of pediatric institutions able to offer PET or PET-CT studies is still limited. Few pediatric centers can use cyclotron facilities, animal scanners, and dedicated personnel and researchers in the development of new radiotracer or devices suitable for pediatric diseases. However, given the actual conditions, it is remarkable to see the growing interest in pediatric applications of PET and the increasing number of clinical research projects involving PET in pediatric diseases. It is conceivable that in the future this number will rise even more, given the fast-growing importance PET-CT in the evaluation of adult neoplastic and inflammatory diseases. Finally, there is still need for a multiinstitutional, cooperative effort in this endeavor. A joint approach may help in the collection of data from different institutions and in directing combined efforts toward the most promising studies and applications.

References

1. Gordon I. Issues surrounding preparation, information, and handling the child and parent in nuclear medicine. J Nucl Med 1998;39:490–494.
2. Treves ST. Introduction. In: Treves ST, ed. Pediatric Nuclear Medicine, 2nd ed. New York: Springer-Verlag, 1995:1–11.
3. Shulkin BL. PET imaging in pediatric oncology. Pediatr Radiol 2004;34: 199–204.
4. Jadvar H, Alavi A, Mavi A, et al. PET imaging in pediatric diseases. Radiol Clin North Am 2005;43:135–152.
5. Mandell GA, Cooper JA, Majd M, et al. Procedure guidelines for pediatric sedation in nuclear medicine. J Nucl Med 1997;38:1640–1643.
6. American Academy of Pediatrics. Committee on Drugs. Guidelines for monitoring and management of pediatric patients during and after

sedation for diagnostic and therapeutic procedures. Pediatrics 1992;89: 1110–1115.

7. American Society of Anesthesiologists Task Force on Sedation and Analgesia by Non-anesthesiologists. Practice guidelines for sedation and analgesia by nonanesthesiologists. Anesthesiology 1996;84:459–471.

8. Shulkin BL. PET applications in pediatrics. Q J Nucl Med 1997;41:281–291.

9. Townsend DW, Beyer T. A combined PET-CT scanner: the path to true image fusion. Br J Radiol 2002;75(suppl):S24–30.

10. Kaste SC. Issues specific to implementing PET-CT for pediatric oncology: what we have learned along the way. Pediatr Radiol 2004;34:205–213.

11. Borgwardt L, Larsen HJ, Pedersen K, et al. Practical use and implementation of PET in children in a hospital PET center. Eur J Nucl Med Mol Imaging 2003;30(10):1389–1397.

12. Beyer T, Antoch G, Muller S, et al. Acquisition protocol considerations for combined PET/CT imaging. J Nucl Med 2004;45(suppl 1):25S–35S.

13. Cohade C, Wahl RL. Applications of positron emission tomography/computed tomography image fusion in clinical positron emission tomography—clinical use, interpretation methods, diagnostic improvements. Semin Nucl Med 2003;33(3):228–237.

14. Antoch G, Freudenberg LS, Strattus J, et al. Whole-body positron emission tomography-CT: optimized CT using oral and IV contrast materials. AJR 2002;179:1555–1560.

15. Dizendorf EV, Treyer V, von Schulthess GK, et al. Application of oral contrast media in coregistered positron emission tomography-CT. AJR 2002;179(12):477–481.

16. Visvikis D, Costa DC, Croasdale I, et al. CT-based attenuation correction in the calculation of semiquantitative indices of (18F)FDG uptake in PET. Eur J Nucl Med Mol Imaging 2003;30(3):344–353.

17. Nehmeh SA, Erdi YE, Kalaigian H, et al. Correction for oral contrast artifacts in CT attenuation-corrected PET images obtained by combined PET/CT. J Nucl Med 2003;44(12):1940–1944.

18. Chugani HT, Phelps ME. Maturational changes in cerebral function in infants determined by 18FDG positron emission tomography. Science 1986;231:840–843.

19. Chugani HT, Phelps ME, Mazziotta JC. Positron emission tomography study of human brain functional development. Ann Neurol 1987;22:487–497.

20. Chugani HT. Positron emission tomography. In: Berg BO, ed. Principles of Child Neurology. New York: McGraw-Hill, 1996:113–128.

21. Benveniste H, Fowler JS, Rooney WD. Maternal-fetal in vivo imaging: a combined PET and MRI study. J Nucl Med 2003;44(9):1522–1530.

22. Meltzer CC, Adelson PD, Brenner RP, et al. Planned ictal FDG PET imaging for localization of extratemporal epileptic foci. Epilepsia 2000; 41:193–200.

23. Snead III OC, Chen LS, Mitchell WG, et al. Usefulness of (18F) fluoro deoxyglucose positron emission tomography in pediatric epilepsy surgery. Pediatr Neurol 1996;14:98–107.

24. Fois A, Farnetani MA, Balestri P, et al. EEG, PET, SPET and MRI in intractable childhood epilepsies: possible surgical correlations. Childs Nerv Syst 1995;11:672–678.

25. Won HJ, Chang KH, Cheon JE, et al. Comparison of MR imaging with PET and ictal SPECT in 118 patients with intractable epilepsy. AJNR 1999;20: 593–599.

26. Muzik O, da Silva EA, Juhasz C, et al. Intracranial EEG versus flumazenil and glucose PET in children with extratemporal lobe epilepsy. Neurology 2000;54:171–179.

27. Holopainen IE, Lundbom NM, Metsahonkala EL, et al. Temporal lobe pathology in epilepsy: proton magnetic resonance spectroscopy and positron emission tomography study. Pediatr Neurol 1997;16:98–104.

28. Chugani HT, Shields WD, Shewmon DA, et al. Infantile spasms: I. PET identifies focal cortical dysgenesis in cryptogenic cases for surgical treatment. Ann Neurol 1990;27:406–413.

29. Chugani HT, Shewmon DA, Shields WD, et al. Surgery for intractable infantile spasms: neuroimaging perspectives. Epilepsia 1993;34:764–771.

30. Chugani HT, Da Silva E, Chugani DC. Infantile spasms: III. Prognostic implications of bitemporal hypometabolism on positron emission tomography. Ann Neurol 1996;39:643–649.

31. Chugani HT, Conti JR. Etiologic classification of infantile spasms in 140 cases: role of positron emission tomography. J Child Neurol 1996;11:44–48.

32. Hrachovy R, Frost J. Infantile spasms. Pediatr Clin North Am 1989;36:311–329.

33. Savic I, Svanborg E, Thorell JO. Cortical benzodiazepine receptor changes are related to frequency of partial seizures: a positron emission tomography study. Epilepsia 1996;37:236–244.

34. Arnold S, Berthele A, Drzezga A, et al. Reduction of benzodiazepine receptor binding is related to the seizure onset zone in extratemporal focal cortical dysplasia. Epilepsia 2000;41(7):818–824.

35. Richardson MP, Koepp MJ, Brooks DJ, et al. 11C-flumanezil PET in neocortical epilepsy. Neurology 1998;51:485–492.

36. Debets RM, Sadzot B, van Isselt JW, et al. Is 11C-flumazenil PET superior to 18-FDG-PET and 123I-iomazenial SPECT in presurgical evaluation of temporal lobe epilepsy? J Neurol Neurosurg Psychiatry 1997;62:141–150.

37. Kumlien E, Hartvig P, Valind S, et al. NMDA-receptor activity visualized with (S)-(N-methyl-11–C)ketamine and positron emission tomography in patients with medial temporal epilepsy. Epilepsia 1999;40:30–37.

38. Mayberg HS, Sadzot B, Meltzer CC, et al. Quantification of mu and non-mu opiate receptors in temporal lobe epilepsy using positron emission tomography. Ann Neurol 1991;30:3–11.

39. Kumlien E, Bergstrom M, Lilja A, et al. Positron emission tomography with (C-11)deuterium deprenyl in temporal lobe epilepsy. Epilepsia 1995;36:712–721.

40. Chuagani DC, Chugani HT, Muzik O, et al. Imaging epileptogenic tubers in children with tuberous sclerosis complex using alpha-(C-11)methyl-L-tryptophan positron emission tomography. Ann Neurol 1998;44:858–866.

41. Biraben A, Semah F, Ribeiro MJ, et al. PET evidence for the role of the basal ganglia in patients with ring chromosome 20 epilepsy. Neurology 2004;63:73–77.

42. Bouilleret V, Semah F, Biraben A Involvement of the basal ganglia in refractory epilepsy: an 18F-fluoro-L-DOPA PET study using 2 methods of analysis. J Nucl Med 2005;46(3):540–547.

43. Fiorella DJ, Provenzale JM, Coleman RE, et al. (18)F fluorodeoxyglucose positron emission tomography and MR imaging findings in Rasmussen encephalitis. AJNR 2001;22:1291–1299.

44. Lee JS, Juhasz C, Kaddurah AK, et al. Patterns of cerebral glucose metabolism in early and late stages of Rasmussen's syndrome. J Child Neurol 2001;16:798–805.

45. Depas G, Chiron C, Tardieu M, et al. Functional brain imaging in HIV-1–infected children born to seropositive mothers. J Nucl Med 1995;36: 2169–2174.

46. Thorngren-Jerneck K, Ohlsson T, et al. Cerebral glucose metabolism measured by positron emission tomography in term newborn infants with hypoxic ischemic encephalopathy. Pediatr Res 2001;49:495–501.

47. Volpe JJ, Herscovitch P, Perlman JM, et al. Positron emission tomography in the newborn: extensive impairment of regional cerebral blood flow with intraventricular hemorrhage and hemorrhagic intracerebral involvement. Pediatrics 1983;72(5):589–601.

48. Volpe JJ, Herscovitch P, Perlman JM, et al. Positron emission tomography in the asphyxiated term newborn: parasagittal impairment of cerebral blood flow. Ann Neurol 1985;17(3):287–296.

49. Zilbovicius M, Boddaert N, Belin P, et al. Temporal lobe dysfunction in childhood autism: a PET study. Am J Psychiatry 2000;157(12):1988–1993.

50. Ernst M, Zametkin AJ, Matochik JA, et al. High midbrain (18F)DOPA accumulation in children with attention deficit hyperactivity disorder. Am J Psychiatry 1999;156(8):1209–1215.

51. Jacobson LK, Hamburger SD, Van Horn JD, et al. Cerebral glucose metabolism in childhood onset schizophrenia. Psychiatry Res 1997;75(3):131–144.

52. Reed W, Jagust W, Al-Mateen M, et al. Role of positron emission tomography in determining the extent of CNS ischemia in patients with sickle cell disease. Am J Hematol 1999;60(4):268–272.

53. Delvenne V, Lotstra F, Goldman S, et al. Brain hypometabolism of glucose in anorexia nervosa: a PET scan study. Biol Psychiatry 1995;37(3):161–169.

54. Delvenne V, Goldman S, Simon Y, et al. Brain hypometabolism of glucose in bulimia nervosa. Int J Eat Disord 1997;21(4):313–320.

55. Worley G, Hoffman JM, Paine SS, et al. 18–fluorodeoxyglucose positron emission tomography in children and adolescents with traumatic brain injury. Dev Med Child Neurol 1995;37(3):213–220.

56. Yanai K, Iinuma K, Matsuzawa T, et al. Cerebral glucose utilization in pediatric neurological disorders determined by positron emission tomography. Eur J Nucl Med 1987;13(6):292–296.

57. Mohan KK, Chugani DC, Chugani HT. Positron emission tomography in pediatric neurology. Semin Pediatr Neurol 1999;6(2):111–119.

58. Cho S, Jin DK, Kim SE. Regional brain metabolic abnormality in Prader-Willi syndrome studied with FDG PET: plausible neural substrates of its psychobehavioral symptoms. Presented at the 51st annual meeting of the Society of Nuclear Medicine, 2004:864.

59. Nielsen JE, Johnsen B, Koefoed P, et al. Hereditary spastic paraplegia with cerebellar ataxia: a complex phenotype associated with a new SPG4 gene mutation. Eur J Neurol 2004;11(12):817–824.

60. Schelbert HR, Schwaiger M, Phelps ME. Positron computed tomography and its applications in the young. J Am Coll Cardiol 1985;5(1 suppl): 140S–149S.

61. Quinlivan RM, Robinson RO, Maisey MN. Positron emission tomography in pediatric cardiology. Arch Dis Child 1998;79(6):520–522.

62. Donnelly JP, Raffel DM, Shulkin BL, et al. Resting coronary flow and coronary flow reserve in human infants after repair or palliation of congenital heart defects as measured by positron emission tomography. J Thorac Cardiovasc Surg 1998;115(1):103–110.

63. Yates RW, Marsden PK, Badawi RD, et al. Evaluation of myocardial perfusion using positron emission tomography in infants following a neonatal arterial switch operation. Pediatr Cardiol 2000;21(2):111–118.

64. Hauser M, Bengel FM, Kuhn A, et al. Myocardial perfusion and coronary flow reserve assessed by positron emission tomography in patients after Fontan-like operations. Pediatr Cardiol 2003;24(4):386–392.

65. Hauser M, Bengel FM, Kuhn A, et al. Myocardial blood flow and flow reserve after coronary reimplantation in patients. Circulation 2001;103: 1875–1880.

66. Rickers C, Sasse K, Buchert R, et al. Myocardial viability assessed by positron emission tomography in infants and children after the arterial switch operation and suspected infarction. J Am Coll Cardiol 2000; 36(5):1676–1683.

67. Hwang B, Liu RS, Chu LS, et al. Positron emission tomography for the assessment of myocardial viability in Kawasaki disease using different therapies. Nucl Med Commun 2000;21(7):631–636.

68. Litvinova I, Litvinov M, Loeonteva I, et al. PET for diagnosis of mitochondrial cardiomyopathy in children. Clin Positron Imaging 2000;3(4): 172.

69. Skehan SJ, Issenman R, Mernagh J, et al. 18F-fluorodeoxyglucose positron tomography in diagnosis of pediatric inflammatory bowel disease. Lancet 1999;354:836–837.

70. Gungor T, Engel-Bicik I, Eich G, et al. Diagnostic and therapeutic impact of whole body positron emission tomography using fluorine-18-fluoro-2-deoxy-D-glucose in children with chronic granulomatous disease. Arch Dis Child 2001;85:341–345.

71. Muller AE, Kluge R, Biesold M, et al. Whole body positron emission tomography detected occult infectious foci in a child with acute myeloid leukaemia. Med Pediatr Oncol 2002;38:58–59.

72. Tomas MB, Tronco GG, Karayalcin G, et al. FDG uptake in infectious mononucleosis. Clin Positron Imaging 2000;3:176.

73. Franzius C, Biermann M, Hulskamp G, et al. Therapy monitoring in aspergillosis using F-18 FDG positron emission tomography. Clin Nucl Med 2001;26:232–233.

74. Richard JC, Chen DL, Ferkol T, et al. Molecular imaging for pediatric lung diseases. Pediatr Pulmonol 2004;37(4):286–296.

75. Jones H, Sriskandan S, Peters A, et al. Dissociation of neutrophil emigration and metabolic activity in lobar pneumonia and bronchiectasis. Eur Respir J 1997;10:795–803.

76. Jones HASJ, Krausz T, Boobis AR, et al. Pulmonary fibrosis correlates with duration of tissue neutrophil activation. Am J Respir Crit Care Med 1998;158:620–628.

77. Jones HA, Clark RJ, Rhodes CG, et al. In vivo measurement of neutrophil activity in experimental lung inflammation. Am J Respir Crit Care Med 1994;149:1635–1639.

78. Kapucu L, Meltzer C, Townsend DV, et al. Fluorine-18–fluorodeoxyglucose uptake in pneumonia. J Nucl Med 1998;39:1267–1269.

79. Jones H, Marino P, Shakur B, et al. In vivo assessment of lung inflammatory cell activity in patients with COPD and asthma. Eur Respir J 2003;21: 567–573.

80. Pantin CF, Valind SO, Sweatman M, et al. Measures of the inflammatory response in cryptogenic fibrosing alveolitis. Am Rev Respir Dis 1988;138: 1234–1241.

81. Taylor I, Hill A, Hayes M, et al. Imaging allergen-invoked airway inflammation in atopic asthma with (18F)-fluorodeoxyglucose and positron emission tomography. Lancet 1996;347:937–940.

82. Kirpalani H, Abubakar K, Nahmias C, et al. (18F)fluorodeoxyglucose uptake in neonatal acute lung injury measured by positron emission tomography. Pediatr Res 1997;41:892–896.

83. FitzSimmons S. The changing epidemiology of cystic fibrosis. J Pediatr 1993;122:1–9.

84. Richard JC, Chen DL, Ferkol T, et al. Molecular imaging for pediatric lung diseases. Pediatr Pulmonol 2004;37(4):286–296.

85. Konstan M, Hilliard K, Norvell T, et al. Bronchoalveolar lavage findings in cystic fibrosis patients with stable, clinically mild lung disease suggest ongoing infection and inflammation. Am J Respir Crit Care Med 1994; 150:448–454.

86. Chen D,Wilson K, Mintun M, et al. Evaluating pulmonary inflammation with 18F-fluorodeoxyglucose and positron emission tomography in patients with cystic fibrosis. Am J Respir Crit Care Med 2003;167: 323.

87. Chen DL, Pittman JE, Rosembluth DB. Evaluating pulmonary inflammation with 18F-fluorodeoxyglucose and positron emission tomography in patients with cystic fibrosis Presented at the 51st annual meeting of the Society of Nuclear Medicine 2004:534.

88. Brudin LH, Valind SO, Rhodes CG, et al. Fluorine-18 deoxyglucose uptake in sarcoidosis measured with positron emission tomography. Eur J Nucl Med 1994;21:297–305.

89. Weinblatt ME, Zanzi I, Belakhlef A, et al. False-positive FDG-PET imaging of the thymus of a child with Hodgkin's disease. J Nucl Med 1997;38: 888–890.

90. Patel PM, Alibazoglu H, Ali A, et al. Normal thymic uptake of FDG on PET imaging. Clin Nucl Med 1996;21:772–775.

91. Delbeke D. Oncological applications of FDG-PET imaging: colorectal cancer, lymphoma, and melanoma. J Nucl Med 1999;40:591–603.

92. Yeung HW, Grewal RK, Gonen M, et al. Patterns of (18)F-FDG uptake in adipose tissue and muscle: a potential source of false-positives for PET. J Nucl Med 2003;44(11):1789–1796.

93. Minotti AJ, Shah L, Keller K. Positron emission tomography/computed tomography fusion imaging in brown adipose tissue. Clin Nucl Med 2004;29(1):5–11.

94. Hany TF, Gharehpapagh E, Kamel EM, et al. Brown adipose tissue: a factor to consider in symmetrical tracer uptake in the neck and upper chest region. Eur J Nucl Med Mol Imaging 2002;29:1393–1398.

95. Cohade C, Osman M, Pannu HK, et al. Uptake in supraclavicular area fat ("USA-Fat"): description on 18F-FDG-PET/CT. J Nucl Med 2003;44: 170–176.

96. Tatsumi M, Engles JM, Ishimori T, et al. Intense (18)F-FDG uptake in brown fat can be reduced pharmacologically. J Nucl Med 2004;45(7):1189–1193.

97. Gelfand MJ, O'Hara SM, Curtwright LA, MacLean JR. Pre-medication to limit brown adipose tissue uptake of (F-18) FDG on PET body imaging. Pediatr Radiol 2005;4(suppl 1):S54.

98. Bar-Sever Z, Keidar Z, Ben Arush M, et al. The incremental value of PET/CT over stand-alone PET in pediatric malignancies. Presented at the 51st annual meeting of the Society of Nuclear Medicine 2004: 379.

99. Shaefer N, et al. Non Hodgkin's lymphoma and Hodgkin's disease: coregistrated FDG PET and CT at staging and restaging. Do we need contrast enhanced CT? Radiology 2004;232:823–829.

100. Antoch G, Freudenberg LS, Beyer T, et al. To enhance or not to enhance? 18FDG and CT contrast agent in dual modality 18FDG PET/CT. J Nucl Med 2004;45:56S–65S.

101. Antoch G, Freudenberg LS, Stattaus J, et al. Whole-body positron emission tomography-CT: optimized CT using oral and IV contrast materials. AJR 2002;179:1555–1560.

102. Tatsumi M, Miller JH, Whal RL. (F-18) FDG-PET/CT in pediatric lymphoma: comparison with contrast enhanced CT. Presented at the 51st annual meeting of the Society of Nuclear Medicine 2004:1107.

103. Sugawara Y, Fisher SJ, Zasadny KR, et al. Preclinical and clinical studies of bone marrow uptake of fluorine-1–fluorodeoxyglucose with or without granulocyte colony-stimulating factor during chemotherapy. J Clin Oncol 1998;16:173–180.

104. Hollinger EF, Alibazoglu H, Ali A, et al. Hematopoietic cytokine-mediated FDG uptake simulates the appearance of diffuse metastatic disease on whole-body PET imaging. Clin Nucl Med 1998;23:93–98.

105. Brink I, Reinhardt MJ, Hoegerle S, et al. Increased metabolic activity in the thymus gland studied with 18F-FDG-PET: age dependency and frequency after chemotherapy. J Nucl Med 2001;42:591–595.

106. Bujenovic S, Mannting F, Chakrabarti R, et al. Artifactual 2-deoxy-2-((18)F)fluoro-D-deoxyglucose localization surrounding metallic objects in a PET/CT scanner using CT-based attenuation correction. Mol Imaging Biol 2003;5:20–22.

107. Valk PE, Budinger TF, Levin VA, et al. PET of malignant cerebral tumors after interstitial brachytherapy. Demonstration of metabolic activity and correlation with clinical outcome. J Neurosurg 1988;69:830–838.

108. Di Chiro G, Oldfield E, Wright DC, et al. Cerebral necrosis after radiotherapy and/or intraarterial chemotherapy for brain tumors: PET and neuropathologic studies. AJR 1988;150:189–197.

109. Glantz MJ, Hoffman JM, Coleman RE, et al. Identification of early recurrence of primary central nervous system tumors by (18F)fluorodeoxyglucose positron emission tomograph. Ann Neurol 1991;29:347–355.

110. Bruggers CS, Friedman HS, Fuller GN, et al. Comparison of serial PET and MRI scans in a pediatric patient with a brainstem glioma. Med Pediatr Oncol 1993;21(4):301–306.

111. Molloy PT, Belasco J, Ngo K, et al. The role of FDG-PET imaging in the clinical management of pediatric brain tumors. J Nucl Med 1999;40:129P.

112. Holthof VA, Herholz K, Berthold F, et al. In vivo metabolism of childhood posterior fossa tumors and primitive neuroectodermal tumors before and after treatment. Cancer 1993;1394–1403.

113. Hoffman JM, Hanson MW, Friedman HS, et al. FDGPET in pediatric posterior fossa brain tumors. J Comput Assist Tomogr 1992;16:62–68.

114. Pirotte B, Goldman S, Salzberg S, et al. Combined positron emission tomography and magnetic resonance imaging for the planning of stereotactic brain biopsies in children: experience in 9 cases. Pediatr Neurosurg 2003;38(3):146–155.

115. Kaplan AM, Bandy DJ, Manwaring KH, et al. Functional brain mapping using positron emission tomography scanning in preoperative neurosurgical planning for pediatric brain tumors. J Neurosurg 1999;91:797–803.

116. Molloy PT, Defeo R, Hunter J, et al. Excellent correlation of FDG-PET imaging with clinical outcome in patients with neurofibromatosis type I and low grade astrocytomas. J Nucl Med 1999;40:129P.

117. Jadvar H, Alavi A, Mavi A, Shulkin BL. PET imaging in pediatric diseases. Radiol Clin North Am 2005;43:135–152.

118. Inoue T, Shibasaki T, Oriuchi N, et al. 18F-alpha-methyl tyrosine PET studies in patients with brain tumors. J Nucl Med 1999;40:399–405.

119. Utriainen M, Metsahonkala L, Salmi TT, et al. Metabolic characterization of childhood brain tumors: comparison of 18F-fluorodeoxyglucose and 11C-methionine positron emission tomography. Cancer 2002;95:1376–1386.

120. Vander Borght T, Pauwels S, Lambotte L, et al. Brain tumor imaging with PET and 2-(carbon-11)thymidine. J Nucl Med 1994;35:974–982.

121. Weckesser M, Langen KJ, Rickert CH, et al. Initial experiences with O-(2-(18F)-fluorethyl)-L-tyrosine PET in the evaluation of primary bone tumors. Presented at the 51st annual meeting of the Society of Nuclear Medicine Meeting 2004:513.

122. Philip I, Shun A, McCowage G, Howman-Giles R. Positron emission tomography in recurrent hepatoblastoma. Pediatr Surg Int 2005;21(5):341–345.

123. Barrington SF, Carr R. Staging of Burkitt's lymphoma and response to treatment monitored by PET scanning. Clin Oncol 1995;7:334–335.

124. Bangerter M, Moog F, Buchmann I, et al. Whole-body 2–(18F)-fluoro-2-deoxy-D-glucose positron emission tomography (FDG-PET) for accurate staging of Hodgkin's disease. Ann Oncol 1998;9:1117–1122.

125. Jerusalem G, Warland V, Najjar F, et al. Whole-body 18F-FDG-PET for the evaluation of patients with Hodgkin's disease and non-Hodgkin's lymphoma. Nucl Med Commun 1999;20:13–20.

126. Leskinen-Kallio S, Ruotsalainen U, Nagren K, et al. Uptake of carbon-11-methionine and fluorodeoxyglucose in non-Hodgkin's lymphoma: a PET study. J Nucl Med 1991;32:1211–1218.

127. Moog F, Bangerter M, Kotzerke J, et al. 18-F-fluorodeoxyglucose positron emission tomography as a new approach to detect lymphomatous bone marrow. J Clin Oncol 1998;16:603–609.

128. Moog F, Bangerter M, Diederichs CG, et al. Extranodal malignant lymphoma: detection with FDG-PET versus CT. Radiology 1998;206:475–481.

129. Moog F, Bangerter M, Diederichs CG, et al. Lymphoma: role of whole-body 2-deoxy-2-(F-18)fluoro-D-glucose (FDG) PET in nodal staging. Radiology 1997;203:795–800.

130. Okada J, Yoshikawa K, Imazeki K, et al. The use of FDG-PET in the detection and management of malignant lymphoma: correlation of uptake with prognosis. J Nucl Med 1991;32:686–691.

131. Okada J, Yoshikawa K, Itami M, et al. Positron emission tomography using fluorine-18–fluorodeoxyglucose in malignant lymphoma: a comparison with proliferative activity. J Nucl Med 1992;33:325–329.

132. Rodriguez M, Rehn S, Ahlstrom H, et al. Predicting malignancy grade with PET in non-Hodgkin's lymphoma. J Nucl Med 1995;36:1790–1796.

133. Newman JS, Francis IR, Kaminski MS, et al. Imaging of lymphoma with PET with 2-(F-18)-fluoro-2-deoxy-D-glucose: correlation with CT. Radiology 1994;190:111–116.

134. de Wit M, Bumann D, Beyer W, et al. Whole-body positron emission tomography (PET) for diagnosis of residual mass in patients with lymphoma. Ann Oncol 1997;8(suppl 1):57–60.

135. Cremerius U, Fabry U, Neuerburg J, et al. Positron emission tomography with 18-F-FDG to detect residual disease after therapy for malignant lymphoma. Nucl Med Commun 1998;19:1055–1063.

136. Hoh CK, Glaspy J, Rosen P, et al. Whole-body FDGPET imaging for staging of Hodgkin's disease and lymphoma. J Nucl Med 1997;38:343–348.

137. Romer W, Hanauske AR, Ziegler S, et al. Positron emission tomography in non-Hodgkin's lymphoma: assessment of chemotherapy with fluorodeoxyglucose. Blood 1998;91:4464–4471.

138. Stumpe KD, Urbinelli M, Steinert HC, et al. Whole-body positron emission tomography using fluorodeoxyglucose for staging of lymphoma: effectiveness and comparison with computed tomography. Eur J Nucl Med 1998;25:721–728.

139. Lapela M, Leskinen S, Minn HR, et al. Increased glucose metabolism in untreated non-Hodgkin's lymphoma: a study with positron emission tomography and fluorine-18-fluorodeoxyglucose. Blood 1995;86:3522–3527.

140. Carr R, Barrington SF, Madan B, et al. Detection of lymphoma in bone marrow by whole-body positron emission tomography. Blood 1998;91:3340–3346.

141. Segall GM. FDG-PET imaging in patients with lymphoma: a clinical perspective. J Nucl Med 2001;42(4):609–610.

142. Moody R, Shulkin B, Yanik G, et al. PET FDG imaging in pediatric lymphomas. J Nucl Med 2001;42(5 suppl):39P.

143. Kostakoglu L, Leonard JP, Coleman M, et al. Comparison of FDG-PET and Ga-67 SPECT in the staging of lymphoma. Cancer 2002;94(4):879–888.

144. Lin PC, Chu J, Pocock N. F-18 fluorodeoxyglucose imaging with coincidence dual-head gamma camera (hybrid FDG-PET) for staging of lymphoma: comparison with Ga-67 scintigraphy. J Nucl Med 2000;41(5 suppl):118P.

145. Tomas MB, Manalili E, Leonidas JC, et al. F-18 FDG imaging of lymphoma in children using a hybrid pet system: comparison with Ga-67. J Nucl Med 2000;41(5 suppl):96P.

146. Tatsumi M, Kitayama H, Sugahara H, et al. Whole-body hybrid PET with 18F-FDG in the staging of non-Hodgkin's lymphoma. J Nucl Med 2001;42(4):601–608.

147. Körholz D, Kluge R, Wickmann L, et al. Importance of F18-fluorodeoxy-D-2-glucose positron emission tomography (FDG-PET) for staging and therapy control of Hodgkin's lymphoma in childhood and adolescence—consequences for the GPOH-HD 2003 protocol. Onkologie 2003;26:489–493.

148. Klein M, Fox M, Kopelewitz B, et al. Role of FDG PET in the follow up of pediatric lymphoma. Presented at the 51st annual meeting of the Society of Nuclear Medicine 2004:378.

149. Tatsumi M, Miller JH, Wahl RL. Initial assessment of the role of FDG PET in pediatric malignancies. Presented at the 51st annual meeting of the Society of Nuclear Medicine 2004:383.

150. Hudson MM, Krasin MJ, Kaste SC. PET imaging in pediatric Hodgkin's lymphoma. Pediatr Radiol 2004;34:190–198.

151. Krasin MJ, Hudson MM, Kaste SC. Positron emission tomography in pediatric radiation oncology: integration in the treatment-planning process. Pediatr Radiol 2004;34:214–221.

152. Franzius C, Schober O. Assessment of therapy response by FDG-PET in pediatric patients. Q J Nucl Med 2003;47(1):41–45.
153. Kahkonen M, Metsahonkala L, Minn H, et al. Cerebral glucose metabolism in survivors of childhood acute lymphoblastic leukemia. Cancer 2000;88:693–700.
154. Briganti V, Sestini R, Orlando C, et al. Imaging of somatostatin receptors by indium-111-pentetreotide correlates with quantitative determination of somatostatin receptor type 2 gene expression in neuroblastoma tumor. Clin Cancer Res 1997;3:2385–2391.
155. Shulkin BL, Hutchinson RJ, Castle VP, et al. Neuroblastoma: positron emission tomography with 2- (fluorine-18)-fluoro-2-deoxy-D-glucose compared with metaiodobenzylguanidine scintigraphy. Radiology 1996; 199:743–750.
156. Kushner BH, Yeung HW, Larson SM, et al. Extending positron emission tomography scan utility to high risk neuroblastoma: fluorine-18 fluorodeoxyglucose positron emission tomography as sole imaging modality in follow-up of patients. J Clin Oncol 2001;19:3397–3405.
157. Shulkin BL, Wieland DM, Castle VP, et al. Carbon-11 epinephrine PET imaging of neuroblastoma. J Nucl Med 1999;40:129P.
158. Vaidyanathan G, Affleck DJ, Zalutsky MR. Validation of 4-(fluorine-18) fluoro-3-iodobenzylguanidine as a positron-emitting analog of MIBG. J Nucl Med 1995;36:644–650.
159. Ott RJ, Tait D, Flower MA, et al. Treatment planning for 131I-mIBG radiotherapy of neural crest tumors using 124I-mIBG positron emission tomography. Br J Radiol 1992;65:787–791.
160. Shulkin BL, Chang E, Strouse PJ, et al. PET FDG studies of Wilms' tumors. J Pediatr Hematol Oncol 1997;19:334–338.
161. Frouge C, Vanel D, Coffre C, et al. The role of magnetic resonance imaging in the evaluation of Ewing sarcoma—a report of 27 cases. Skeletal Radiol 1988;17:387–392.
162. MacVicar AD, Olliff JFC, Pringle J, et al. Ewing sarcoma: MR imaging of chemotherapy-induced changes with histologic correlation. Radiology 1992;184:859–864.
163. Lemmi MA, Fletcher BD, Marina NM, et al. Use of MR imaging to assess results of chemotherapy for Ewing sarcoma. AJR 1990;155:343–346.
164. Erlemann R, Sciuk J, Bosse A, et al. Response of osteosarcoma and Ewing sarcoma to preoperative chemotherapy: assessment with dynamic and static MR imaging and skeletal scintigraphy. Radiology 1990;175:791–796.
165. Holscher HC, Bloem JL, Vanel D, et al. Osteosarcoma: chemotherapy-induced changes at MR imaging. Radiology 1992;182:839–844.
166. Lawrence JA, Babyn PS, Chan HS, et al. Extremity osteosarcoma in childhood: prognostic value of radiologic imaging. Radiology 1993;189:43–47.
167. Watanabe H, Shinozaki T, Yanagawa T, et al. Glucose metabolic analysis of musculoskeletal tumours using 18fluorine-FDG PET as an aid to preoperative planning. J Bone Joint Surg Br 2000;82:760–767.
168. Wu H, Dimitrakopoulou-Strauss A, Heichel TO, et al. Quantitative evaluation of skeletal tumours with dynamic FDG PET: SUV in comparison to Patlak analysis. Eur J Nucl Med 2001;28:704–710.
169. Daldrup-Link HE, Franzius C, et al. Whole-body MR imaging for detection of bone metastases in children and young adults: comparison with skeletal scintigraphy and FDG PET. AJR 2001;177:229–236.

170. Franzius C, Daldrup-Link HE, Sciuk J, et al. FDG-PET for detection of pulmonary metastases from malignant primary bone tumors: comparison with spiral CT. Ann Oncol 2001;12:479–486.

171. Franzius C, Sciuk J, Daldrup-Link HE, et al. FDG-PET for detection of osseous metastases from malignant primary bone tumours: comparison with bone scintigraphy. Eur J Nucl Med 2000;27:1305–1311.

172. Franzius C, Daldrup-Link HE, Wagner-Bohn A, et al. FDG-PET for detection of recurrences from malignant primary bone tumors: comparison with conventional imaging. Ann Oncol 2002;13:157–160.

173. Lenzo NP, Shulkin B, Castle VP, et al. FDG-PET in childhood soft tissue sarcoma. J Nucl Med 2000;41(5 suppl):96P.

174. Abdel-Dayem HM. The role of nuclear medicine in primary bone and soft tissue tumors. Semin Nucl Med 1997;27:355–363.

175. Shulkin BL, Mitchell DS, Ungar DR, et al. Neoplasms in a pediatric population: 2-(F-18)-fluoro-2-deoxy-D-glucose PET studies. Radiology 1995; 194:495–500.

176. Hawkins DS, Rajendran JG, Conrad III EU, et al. Evaluation of chemotherapy response in pediatric bone sarcomas by (F-18)-fluorodeoxy-D-glucose positron emission tomography. Cancer 2002;94:3277–3284.

177. Even-Sapir E, Metser U, Flusser G, et al. Assessment of malignant skeletal disease: initial experience with 18F-fluoride PET/CT and comparison between 18F-fluoride PET and 18F-fluoride PET/CT. J Nucl Med 2004; 45:272–278.

178. Franzius C, Hotfilder M, Hermann S, et al. Feasibility of high resolution animal PET of Ewing tumors and their metastasis in a NOD/SCID mouse model. Presented at the 51st annual meeting of the Society of Nuclear Medicine 2004:382.

179. Ben Arush MW, Israel O, Kedar Z, et al. Detection of isolated distant metastasis in soft tissue sarcoma by fluorodeoxyglucose positron emission tomography: case report. Pediatr Hematol Oncol 2001;18(4):295–298.

180. Lucas JD, O'Doherty MJ, Cronin BF, et al. Prospective evaluation of soft tissue masses and sarcomas using fluorodeoxyglucose positron emission tomography. Br J Surg 1999;86:550–556.

181. Lucas JD, O'Doherty MJ, Wong JC, et al. Evaluation of fluorodeoxyglucose positron emission tomography in the management of soft-tissue sarcomas. J Bone Joint Surg Br 1998;80:441–447.

182. Bredella MA, Caputo GR, Steinbach LS. Value of FDG positron emission tomography in conjunction with MR imaging for evaluating therapy response in patients with musculoskeletal sarcomas. AJR 2002;179: 1145–1150.

183. Pacak K, Eisenhofer G, Carrasquillo JA, et al. 18-6-(18F)fluorodopamine positron emission tomographic (PET) scanning for diagnostic localization of pheochromocytoma. Hypertension 2001;38:6–8.

184. Sabbaga CC, Avilla SG. Schulz C, et al. Adrenocortical carcinoma in children: clinical aspects and prognosis. J Pediatr Surg 1993;28:841–843.

185. Evans HL, Vassilopoulou-Sellin R. Adrenal cortical neoplasms. A study of 56 cases. Am J Clin Pathol 1996;105:76–86.

186. Maurea S, Mainolfi C, Wang H, et al. Positron emission tomography (PET) with fludeoxyglucose F 18 in the study of adrenal masses: comparison of benign and malignant lesions. Radiol Med 1996;92:782–787.

187. Boland GW, Goldberg MA, Lee MJ, et al. Indeterminate adrenal mass in patients with cancer: evaluation at PET with 2-(F-18)-fluoro-2–deoxy-glucose. Radiology 1995;194:131–134.

188. Kreissig R, Amthauer H, Krude H, et al. The use of FDG-PET and CT for the staging of adrenocortical carcinoma in children. Pediatr Radiol 2000; 30:306.

189. Philip I, Shun A, McCowage G, Howman-Giles R. Positron emission tomography in recurrent hepatoblastoma. Pediatr Surg Int 2005;21(5): 341–345.

Section 5

Imaging Atlas

29

PET–Computed Tomography Atlas

M. Beth McCarville

Fluorine-18-fluorodeoxyglucose (FDG) positron emission tomography (PET) is a functional imaging modality that capitalizes on the fact that pathologic processes are generally highly metabolically active and accumulate more glucose (and FDG) than normal tissue. However, sites of normal metabolic activity can also demonstrate intense FDG uptake and can sometimes be difficult to distinguish from disease activity. Fusion imaging modalities that acquire both functional and correlative anatomic imaging provide an important advantage over PET alone because they allow the accurate anatomic localization of sites of increased FDG activity (1–5). In this chapter, normal sites of FDG activity are correlated with computed tomography (CT) anatomy in images obtained during PET-CT scanning. Examples of pathologic FDG activity are included to illustrate the unique value of this fusion imaging modality in distinguishing normal from pathologic activity.

Head and Neck

Identifying normal FDG activity in the head and neck, as elsewhere in the body, is aided by its bilaterally symmetric distribution. Because the brain is exclusively dependent on glucose metabolism, it accumulates intense FDG activity. Accumulation is greatest in the cerebral cortex, basal ganglia, thalamus, and cerebellum (Figs. 29.1 and 29.2). Intense activity is sometimes present, not only in the brain, but also in the ocular muscles and optic nerves (Fig. 29.2). Because FDG is known to accumulate in saliva (6,7), minimal to moderate activity may be present in the salivary and parotid glands (Fig. 29.3). Fluorodeoxyglucose uptake also occurs in the lymphatic tissues of the pharynx, specifically within the Waldeyer ring, which consists of the nasopharyngeal, palatine, and lingual tonsils (Fig. 29.3). In patients who are tense, FDG activity may be very prominent in the neck muscles secondary to contraction-induced metabolic activity. Fluorodeoxyglucose activity in the normal thyroid gland is usually absent or minimal but can be prominent. Intrinsic laryngeal muscles of phonation can exhibit intense FDG activity

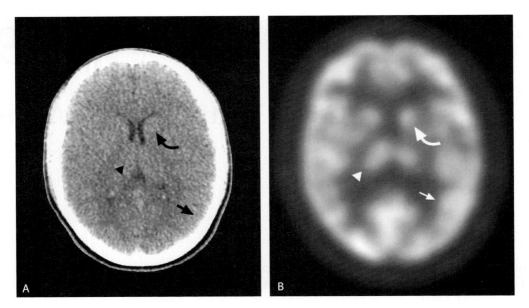

Figure 29.1. A,B: Axial positron emission tomography–computed tomography (PET-CT) images show fluorodeoxyglucose (FDG) activity in normal cerebral cortex (arrows), head of caudate (curved arrows), and thalami (arrowheads).

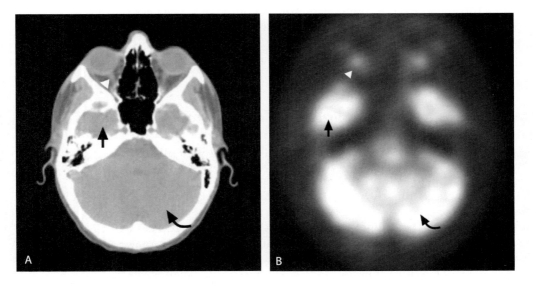

Figure 29.2. A,B: Axial PET-CT images show FDG activity in normal optic nerves (arrowheads), temporal lobes (straight arrows), and cerebellum (curved arrows).

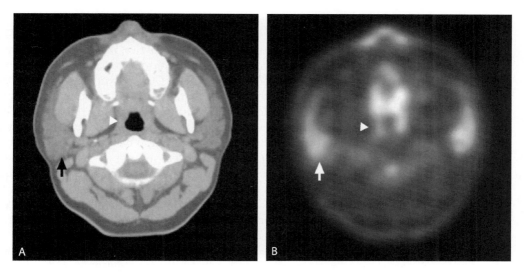

Figure 29.3. A,B: Axial PET-CT images show FDG uptake in a normal Waldeyer ring (arrowheads) and normal parotid glands (arrows).

especially in patients who engage in speech activity immediately before or after the injection of FDG (Fig. 29.4) (7–9). To reduce such activity, patients should be encouraged to remain silent beginning 15 minutes prior to radioisotope injection until the imaging session is complete.

Chest

Intense FDG activity is often present within brown adipose tissue in the supraclavicular regions, axilla, and paraspinal regions of the posterior mediastinum. The primary function of brown adipose tissue is

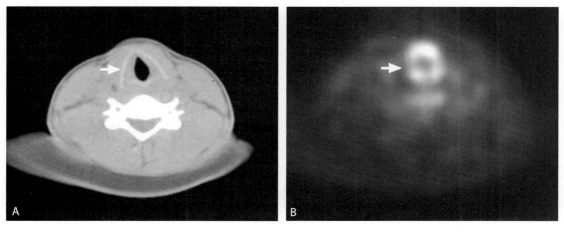

Figure 29.4. A,B: Axial PET-CT images show normal FDG activity in the perilaryngeal tissues (arrows) often seen in patients who have engaged in speech after FDG injection.

the production of heat. Brown fat differs from other tissues by the presence of an uncoupling protein within its mitochondria. This protein leads to a markedly reduced production of adenosine triphosphate (ATP) while increasing the oxidation of fatty acids to a maximal rate, resulting in the production of heat. During stimulated thermogenesis, glucose prevents this highly metabolic brown fat from becoming ATP-deprived by providing ATP through anaerobic glycolysis (10). Thermogenesis, therefore, leads to an accumulation of glucose and FDG within brown fat. Brown fat is known to be particularly metabolically active in pediatric patients, females, and persons with a low body mass index (10–12). Positron emission tomography–CT is especially useful in localizing sites of intense FDG activity in the supraclavicular regions because the CT will demonstrate either the absence (in the case of brown fat) or the presence of a soft tissue mass in the area of increased activity (Figs. 29.5 and 29.6).

The thymus is located in the anterior mediastinum and extends from the thoracic inlet to the heart. Normal thymic FDG activity is homogeneous and may be minimal, moderate, or more intense than the mediastinal blood pool (Fig. 29.7). On CT the thymus has a quadrilateral-shaped configuration with homogeneous density. In

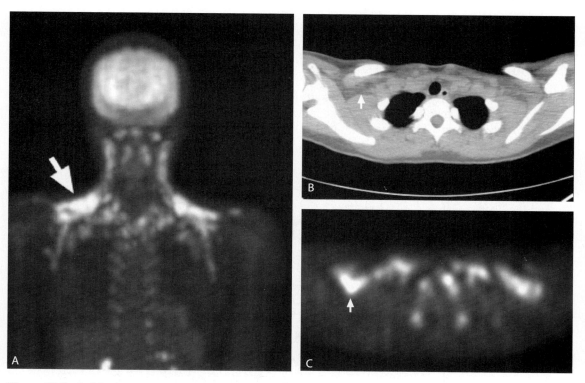

Figure 29.5. A: Maximum intensity projection (MIP) image showing intense, symmetric activity in the supraclavicular regions (arrow). B,C: Axial PET-CT images allow localization of this activity to supraclavicular brown fat (arrows). This finding is common in pediatric patients.

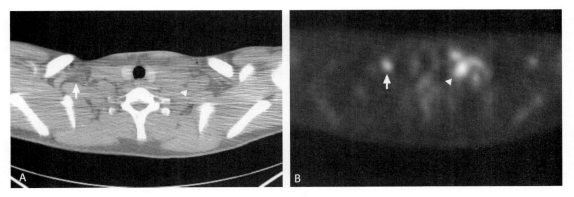

Figure 29.6. A 26-year-old woman with non-Hodgkin's lymphoma. A,B: Axial PET-CT images show FDG activity in both supraclavicular brown fat (arrows) and pathologic supraclavicular nodes (arrowheads). This example illustrates the value of PET-CT in identifying adenopathy that may be difficult to distinguish from physiologic brown fat activity on PET alone.

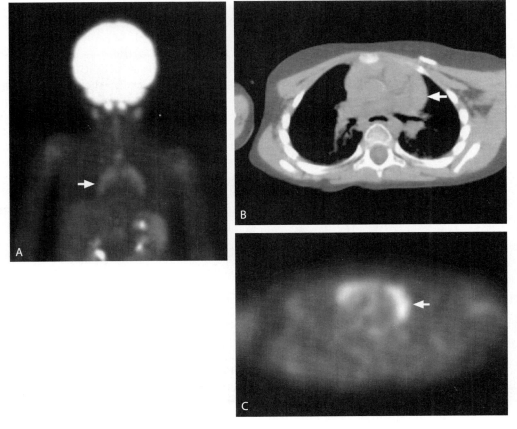

Figure 29.7. A: MIP anterior PET image shows normal thymic contour and FDG activity (arrow) in a 3-year-old girl. B,C: Axial PET-CT images allow localization of activity to the thymus (arrows).

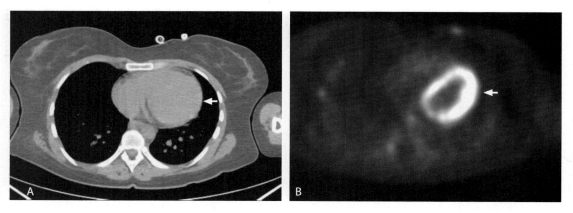

Figure 29.8. A,B: Axial PET-CT images show typical intense FDG activity in a normal left ventricular myocardium (arrows).

early childhood, the lateral margins are slightly convex outward until adolescence when the thymus begins to involute and becomes more triangular in appearance. The normal thymus should have smooth margins and should never be nodular or lobulated (13). At about 1 hour after injection of FDG, blood pool activity in the mediastinum is moderate whereas lung activity is low. The heart has variable FDG avidity, usually with intense activity seen in the left ventricular myocardium (Fig. 29.8). Activity in the myocardium is dependent on serum insulin levels. When insulin levels are high, such as following a meal, the myocardium shifts from the metabolism of free-fatty acids to the glycolytic pathway, resulting in intense myocardial FDG activity (14,15). Fasting for 4 to 6 hours before the administration of FDG reduces both serum glucose and insulin availability, leading to decreased myocardial FDG activity. Minimal to moderate FDG activity may be present within the distal esophagus due to gastroesophageal reflux, muscle contraction, or inflammation (8,15).

Abdomen and Pelvis

Fusion imaging is especially helpful in the abdomen and pelvis because sites of FDG activity can be difficult to localize accurately on PET alone, and sites that demonstrate abnormal FDG uptake may be overlooked on CT alone when the abnormality is subtle or unexpected (Fig. 29.9). In the upper abdomen, the cruces of the diaphragms and accessory muscles of respiration may demonstrate intense FDG activity, particularly in patients with increased work of breathing (Fig. 29.10) (8). There may be intense activity in the region of the adrenal glands within normal retroperitoneal brown fat. Liver activity is usually patchy but uniform in distribution without focal areas of intense activity. Splenic

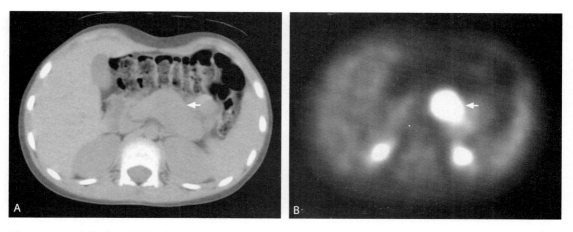

Figure 29.9. A,B: Axial PET-CT images show intense FDG activity within a metastatic deposit in the pancreas (arrows) of a 10-year-old girl with widely metastatic rhabdomyosarcoma. This pancreatic deposit was not clinically suspected and was overlooked on a CT scan performed 2 days earlier.

uptake is generally uniform and equal to or less than that of the liver (Figs. 29.10, 29.11, and 29.12).

Fluorodeoxyglucose activity in the bowel is commonly seen but poorly understood. Postulated causes of bowel activity include smooth muscle contraction, metabolically active mucosa, uptake in lymphoid tissue, swallowed secretions containing FDG, and colonic microbial uptake (15–17). The stomach usually shows minimal to moderate activity within the fundus, although occasionally intense activity is seen

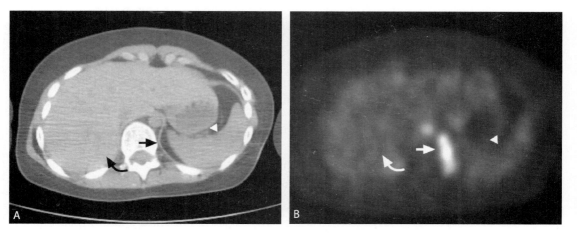

Figure 29.10. A,B: Axial PET-CT images show normal FDG activity in the crus of the left diaphragm (straight arrows) and normal, homogeneous FDG uptake within the liver (curved arrows) and spleen (arrowheads). The spleen usually shows activity that is equal to or less than that of the liver.

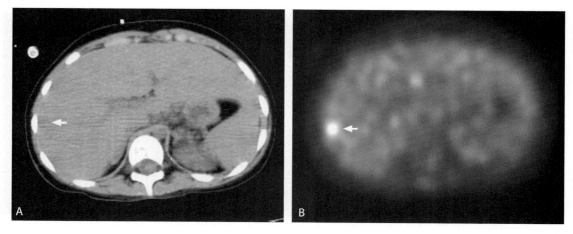

Figure 29.11. A,B: Axial PET-CT images show a focal area of abnormal activity that localizes to the liver (arrows). This was proven by biopsy to be metastatic Hodgkin's lymphoma in this 12-year-old girl with ataxia-telangiectasia and Hodgkin's lymphoma.

(Fig. 29.13). In these instances, correlating with CT imaging is useful in excluding obvious abnormalities within the stomach wall or to localize the activity to adjacent soft tissue abnormalities, such as adenopathy or pancreatic neoplasms. The degree of FDG activity in the small bowel and colon may be minimal, moderate, or intense and can be focal or diffuse (Fig. 29.14). Fluorodeoxyglucose activity in the small bowel and colon is often increased in patients who have fasted and is often most pronounced in the region of the cecum and right colon (15). The value of PET imaging in colorectal cancer is well established; however,

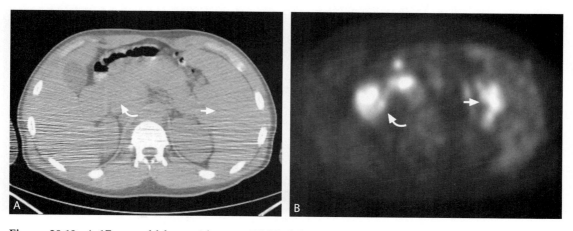

Figure 29.12. A 17-year-old boy with stage IV Hodgkin's disease. A,B: Axial PET-CT images show abnormal FDG activity in the spleen and nodes in the splenic hilum (straight arrows) and porta hepatis (curved arrows), consistent with lymphomatous involvement. Note that splenic activity is greater than the normal liver.

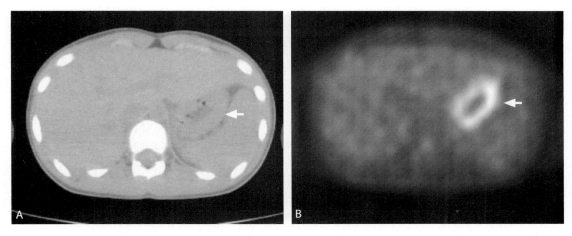

Figure 29.13. A,B: Axial PET-CT images show moderate FDG activity in the wall of a normal stomach (arrows). Normal gastric FDG activity can vary from minimal to intense.

without correlative CT imaging, the findings of bowel activity on PET alone can be misleading. Computed tomography is useful in localizing the activity to the bowel and may demonstrate underlying bowel pathology such as a focal mass or an apple core lesion (Fig. 29.15). Even so, evaluation of the bowel by CT performed as part of a standard PET-CT scan may be limited by the lack of oral or intravenous contrast material. If bowel pathology is a specific concern, the use of contrast agents may enhance lesion conspicuity.

Fluorodeoxyglucose also accumulates in the glomerular filtrate but, unlike glucose, it is not resorbed in the renal tubules. This results in the intense accumulation of FDG in the renal collecting systems, ureters, and bladder (Fig. 29.16). The value of PET in evaluating the

Figure 29.14. MIP anterior image showing normal colonic activity (arrows).

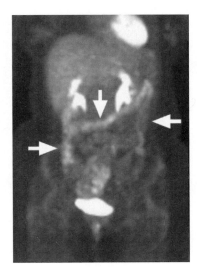

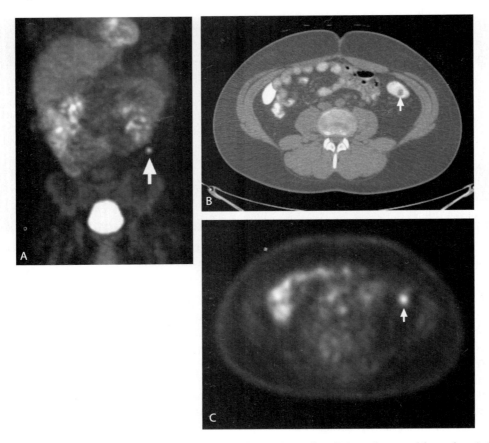

Figure 29.15. This example illustrates the value of PET-CT in localizing abnormal bowel activity. A: MIP anterior image shows a small focus of intense activity in the left abdomen (arrow) in this 19-year-old man with previously treated neuroendocrine tumor. B,C: Axial PET-CT images localize the activity to a small colonic filling defect that was biopsied and found to be an adenomatous polyp.

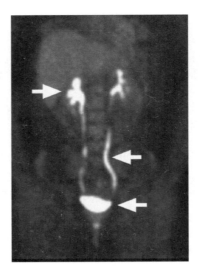

Figure 29.16. MIP anterior image of the abdomen shows the normal distribution of FDG activity in the kidneys (arrow), ureters (arrow), and urinary bladder (arrow).

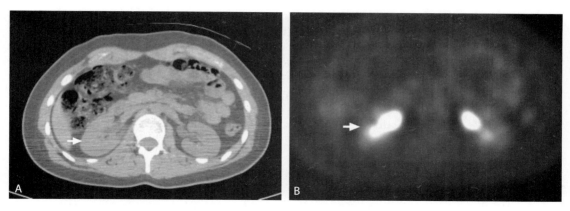

Figure 29.17. A,B: Axial PET-CT images show the normally intense activity seen in the kidneys (arrows) due to the accumulation of FDG in the glomerular filtrate.

kidneys is limited by the intense activity normally present within the renal collecting systems, which may obscure underlying abnormalities (Fig. 29.17). However, correlative PET-CT imaging may improve lesion conspicuity and localization of renal tumors. Intense FDG activity within the ureters is a common finding due to pooling of the radiotracer in the recumbent patient (8). Correlation with CT imaging allows distinction of the normal ureter from abnormal adjacent structures.

Within the female pelvis, intense FDG activity may be present in normal ovaries and uteri, depending on the phase of the patient's menstrual cycle (18). Positron emission tomography–CT is extremely useful in localizing FDG activity to these structures (Fig. 29.18). Activity within normal ovaries may not be bilaterally symmetric because the

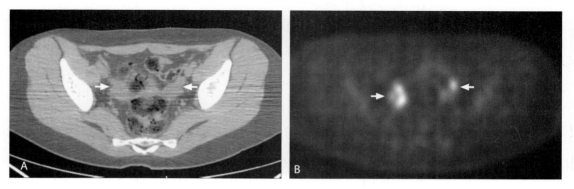

Figure 29.18. A,B: Axial PET-CT images show FDG activity within normal ovaries (arrows) in this 17-year-old girl who was in remission from stage IIA Hodgkin's disease. The degree of FDG uptake in the ovaries and uterus varies with menstrual phase. Normal ovarian activity may be asymmetric, as in this case.

ovary containing the dominant follicle may be more physiologically active than the contralateral ovary. Correlation with the patients' clinical history is useful in ruling out malignancy as an underlying cause of FDG uptake in the uterus and ovaries. In equivocal cases, follow-up PET-CT should show resolution or a diminution of FDG activity when the etiology is physiologic in nature (18). Within the male pelvis, activity in the normal testes can vary from minimal to intense, but should be bilaterally symmetric (Fig. 29.19).

Musculoskeletal

Increased uptake of glucose into skeletal muscle is known to occur during muscle exercise (19). Likewise, the uptake of glucose, and hence FDG, into skeletal muscle is increased when muscle is electrically stimulated to undergo isometric contraction (19,20). The mechanism of glucose uptake into muscle is poorly understood, but it is distinct from the regulation of glucose metabolism by insulin. Increased blood flow and the translocation of glucose from the intracellular pool to the sarcolemmal membrane and activation of the protein carriers GLUT-1 and GLUT-4, in response to calcium released from the sarcoplasmic reticulum during muscle stimulation, may be responsible (19). When PET imaging reveals muscle FDG activity that is bilaterally symmetric (Fig. 29.20), it is likely due to increased glucose metabolism secondary to voluntary muscle contraction. Symmetric uptake of FDG in the neck and paravertebral muscles can be caused merely by patient anxiety. Administration of the muscle relaxant and anxiolytic agent diazepam has been effective in abolishing the high muscle FDG uptake seen in some patients (19). Asymmetric muscle activity can be due to the sequelae of local treatments such as surgery or radiation therapy or can be seen in a recently exercised muscle, even if the activity occurred prior to the

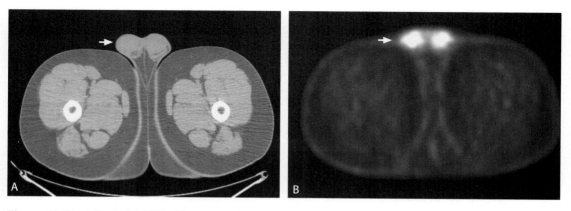

Figure 29.19. A,B: Axial PET-CT images show bilaterally symmetric and intense activity in normal testes in this 19-year-old boy. The degree of FDG activity in normal testes can vary from minimal to intense but should be symmetric.

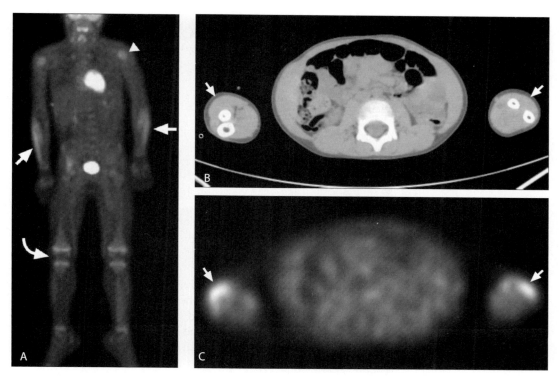

Figure 29.20. Three-year-old boy with previously treated rhabdomyosarcoma of the left lower leg. A: MIP anterior image of the body shows symmetric activity in the forearm muscles (arrows). Note also the appearance of the normal bone marrow with increased activity in the growing physes of the proximal humeri (arrowhead), knees (curved arrow), and distal tibiae. The distribution of bone marrow activity depends on patient age. Younger children have relatively more metabolically active marrow than older children. Normal marrow activity is generally equal to or less than the liver. B,C: Axial PET-CT images localize the forearm activity to the forearm muscles (arrows). Such activity can be seen in tense patients or may be related to physical activity.

injection of FDG (Fig. 29.21) (15). When FDG muscle activity is not bilaterally symmetric, the correlative anatomic information provided by CT is extremely useful in elucidating the underlying cause of the abnormality particularly when an intra- or perimuscular mass is present.

Interpretation of the PET appearance of normal bone marrow in children requires knowledge of the age-dependent conversion patterns from hematopoietic to fatty marrow (21–24). Younger children have relatively more metabolically active and FDG-avid hematopoietic marrow within long bones than older children whose marrow has undergone fatty conversion. Intense FDG activity may be present in the physes of growing children (Fig. 29.20). Fluorodeoxyglucose uptake in normal bone marrow is generally less than or equal to that of the liver (Fig. 29.20). Diffuse and symmetric increased FDG bone marrow activity is often seen in patients receiving granulocyte colony-stimulating factor (G-CSF) (Fig. 29.22) (25). Occasionally, focal areas of increased FDG activity are present within the vertebral bodies that can be difficult to

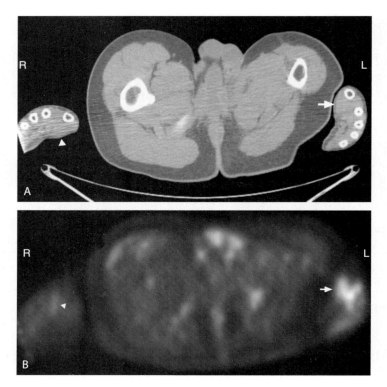

Figure 29.21. A 14-year-old boy with metastatic osteosarcoma. A,B: Axial PET-CT images show increased activity in the thenar muscles of the left hand (arrows) relative to the right (arrowheads). This was felt to be related to the physical activity of this patient, who had exercised the left hand while playing a video game prior to FDG injection.

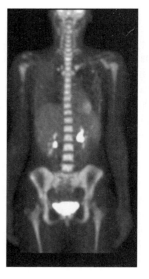

Figure 29.22. An 18-year-old woman under treatment for rhabdomyosarcoma who had recently received granulocyte colony-stimulating factor (G-CSF). MIP anterior image shows marrow activity that is diffusely increased relative to the liver. This pattern of marrow activity is commonly seen in patients receiving G-CSF.

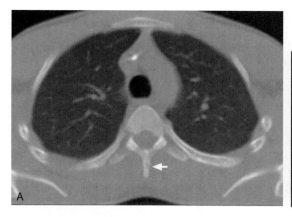
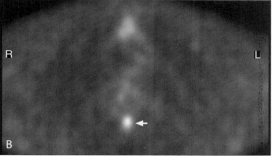

Figure 29.23. This example illustrates the value of correlative PET-CT imaging in determining the cause of abnormal activity in the spine in this 19-year-old man with previously treated osteosarcoma. A,B: Axial PET-CT images localize a focus of abnormal activity to the spinous process of a thoracic verte-bra (arrow). Utilizing a bone window, the CT image demonstrates a lucent line (arrowhead). This patient was involved in a motor vehicle accident several months before this scan, with injury to this area, although no fracture was diagnosed at that time. This activity resolved on subsequent PET-CT imaging and was felt to be due to fracture.

distinguish from a pathologic process. Generally, a repeating pattern of patchy increased activity throughout the spine can be seen on the sagittal or coronal images that is characteristic of physiologic uptake. When increased bone marrow activity is solitary or nonuniformly distributed, other causes, such as infection, metastatic disease, or primary bone malignancies, should be considered. Correlative CT imaging, utilizing a bone window, may reveal an underlying destructive process, fracture, or other pathology (Fig. 29.23).

References

1. Kluetz PG, Meltzer CC, Villemagne VL, et al. Combined PET/CT imaging in oncology. Impact on patient management. Clin Positron Imaging 2000;3: 223–230.
2. Eubank WB, Mankoff DA, Schmiedl UP, et al. Imaging of oncologic patients: benefit of combined CT and FDG PET in the diagnosis of malignancy. AJR 1998;171:1103–1110.
3. Charron M, Beyer T, Bohnen NN, et al. Image analysis in patients with cancer studied with a combined PET and CT scanner. Clin Nucl Med 2000; 25:905–910.
4. Bar-Shalom R, Yefremov N, Guralnik L, et al. Clinical performance of PET/CT in evaluation of cancer: additional value for diagnostic imaging and patient management. J Nucl Med 2003;44:1200–1209.
5. Townsend DW, Beyer T. A combined PET/CT scanner: the path to true image fusion. Br J Radiol 2002;75(Spec No.):S24–S30.
6. Stahl A, Dzewas B, Schwaiger M, et al. Excretion of FDG into saliva and its significance for PET imaging. Nuklearmedizin 2002;41:214–216.
7. Goerres GW, Von Schulthess GK, Hany TF. Positron emission tomography and PET CT of the head and neck: FDG uptake in normal anatomy, in

benign lesions, and in changes resulting from treatment. AJR 2002;179: 1337–1343.

8. Kostakoglu L, Hardoff R, Mirtcheva R, et al. PET-CT fusion imaging in differentiating physiologic from pathologic FDG uptake. Radiographics 2004;24:1411–1431.

9. Zhu Z, Chou C, Yen TC, et al. Elevated F-18 FDG uptake in laryngeal muscles mimicking thyroid cancer metastases. Clin Nucl Med 2001;26: 689–691.

10. Himms-Hagen J. Brown adipose tissue thermogenesis: interdisciplinary studies. FASEB J 1990;4:2890–2898.

11. Hany TF, Gharehpapagh E, Kamel EM, et al. Brown adipose tissue: a factor to consider in symmetrical tracer uptake in the neck and upper chest region. Eur J Nucl Med Mol Imaging 2002;29:1393–1398.

12. Cohade C, Osman M, Pannu HK, et al. Uptake in supraclavicular area fat ("USA-Fat"): description on 18F-FDG PET/CT. J Nucl Med 2003;44: 170–176.

13. Hedlund GL, Kirks DR. Respiratory system. In: Kirks DR, ed. Practical Pediatric Imaging, 2nd ed. Cincinnati: Little, Brown, 1991:517–707.

14. Gordon BA, Flanagan FL, Dehdashti F. Whole-body positron emission tomography: normal variations, pitfalls, and technical considerations. AJR 1997;169:1675–1680.

15. Shreve PD, Anzai Y, Wahl RL. Pitfalls in oncologic diagnosis with FDG PET imaging: physiologic and benign variants. Radiographics 1999;19:61–77.

16. Kostakoglu L, Wong JC, Barrington SF, et al. Speech-related visualization of laryngeal muscles with fluorine-18-FDG. J Nucl Med 1996;37:1771–1773.

17. Tatlidil R, Jadvar H, Bading JR, et al. Incidental colonic fluorodeoxyglucose uptake: correlation with colonoscopic and histopathologic findings. Radiology 2002;224:783–787.

18. Chander S, Meltzer CC, McCook BM. Physiologic uterine uptake of FDG during menstruation demonstrated with serial combined positron emission tomography and computed tomography. Clin Nucl Med 2002; 27:22–24.

19. Barrington SF, Maisey MN. Skeletal muscle uptake of fluorine-18-FDG: effect of oral diazepam. J Nucl Med 1996;37:1127–1129.

20. Mossberg KA, Mommessin JI, Taegtmeyer H. Skeletal muscle glucose uptake during short-term contractile activity in vivo: effect of prior contractions. Metabolism 1993;42:1609–1616.

21. Daldrup-Link HE, Franzius C, Link TM, et al. Whole-body MR imaging for detection of bone metastases in children and young adults: comparison with skeletal scintigraphy and FDG PET. AJR 2001;177:229–236.

22. Babyn PS, Ranson M, McCarville ME. Normal bone marrow. In: Mirowitz SA, Jaramillo D, eds. MRI Clinics. Philadelphia: WB Saunders, 1998: 473–495.

23. Moore SG, Dawson KL. Red and yellow marrow in the femur: age-related changes in appearance at MR imaging. Radiology 1990;175:219–223.

24. Ricci C, Cova M, Kang YS, et al. Normal age-related patterns of cellular and fatty bone marrow distribution in the axial skeleton: MR imaging study. Radiology 1990;177:83–88.

25. Sugawara Y, Fisher SJ, Zasadny KR, et al. Preclinical and clinical studies of bone marrow uptake of fluorine-1-fluorodeoxyglucose with or without granulocyte colony-stimulating factor during chemotherapy. J Clin Oncol 1998;16:173–180.

30

Common Artifacts on PET Imaging

Peeyush Bhargava and Martin Charron

Whole-body positron emission tomography (PET) with fluoro-deoxyglucose (FDG) is fast becoming the standard of care in management of a variety of malignant and nonmalignant conditions. Two excellent reviews by Rohren et al. (1) and Kostakoglu et al. (2) describe the clinical applications of PET in oncology in adult patients. As more experience is gained in the pediatric population, indications for pediatric FDG-PET imaging are emerging (3–5).

As with any other nuclear imaging modality, it is very important to recognize artifacts while reading the whole-body FDG-PET images for the subsequent correct management of patients. Recognition of artifacts improves the sensitivity and specificity of the study tremendously and reduces the need for further evaluation with other radiologic tests. This chapter discusses the normal biodistribution of FDG in pediatric patients, common artifacts seen on whole-body FDG-PET images, common causes of false-positive and false-negative findings, and recognition of artifacts.

Scanning Protocol

Performing FDG-PET studies on pediatric patients presents a special challenge. The issues that require consideration specifically in the pediatric population include intravenous access, sedation, fasting, consent, and urinary tract activity. These technical issues specific to pediatric PET imaging have been dealt with in recent articles (6–8). Procedure guidelines and patient preparation techniques for the adult FDG-PET imaging have been published in the literature (9–11). Institutions performing PET studies on pediatric patients are recommended to consult these reports and to develop their own protocols.

Essentially, patient preparation is the same for pediatric patients as for adults. Typically after an overnight fast (or fasting for 6 to 8 hours), fluorine-18 (^{18}F)-FDG is injected intravenously, and after waiting for an uptake period of around an hour (with minimal physical activity), multiple bed positions emissions scans are acquired on a dedicated whole-body scanner from the base of skull to the level of thighs. The blood glucose level is usually checked by finger-stick method at the time of radiotracer injection. Paying careful attention to injection and scanning protocol is very important in acquiring and interpreting good-quality images and avoiding artifacts. Images are reconstructed using an iterative reconstruction algorithm, and attenuation correction is applied. When using a PET–computed tomography (CT) scanner, CT data can be used for attenuation correction and the scan can be acquired in a shorter period of time. Getting a good history from the patient or parents and making sure that recent CT or magnetic resonance imaging (MRI) films are available for correlation at the time of reading PET studies is a prerequisite for avoiding common pitfalls.

Reviewing PET Studies

Positron emission tomography images are always reviewed on a computer monitor. This provides the ease of toggling between the different set of images and different cross sections and changing the intensity. Raw projection image (or the rotating image) can also be reviewed. We strongly discourage reading PET images from films and recommend review of cross-sectional images in gray scale. After some experience, readers develop their own style of reviewing images. In our default display, the rotating attenuation corrected image is seen on the left side of the window, and different cross sections (coronal, transaxial, and sagittal) are on the right. We review the coronal images first (from anterior to posterior), then confirm our findings on other cross sections, and, if needed, review the non–attenuation-corrected images. The non–attenuation-corrected images show intense uptake in the superficial structures and photopenia in the region of deeper structures. They can be differentiated from attenuation-corrected images by intense uptake in skin and in the superficial aspect of the right lobe of liver and by scattered activity in the lungs (Fig. 30.1). The reconstructed transmission image may also be used on occasion as a guide to anatomy. We feel that anatomy of FDG distribution is best appreciated in coronal views, but we have noticed that radiology residents and radiologists prefer looking at transaxial images. It is very important to know the transaxial and sagittal anatomy also, especially for direct comparison of PET images to CT or MRI films. It is also good to know all available options for image manipulation. For example, in one option, a mouse click over any lesion seen on one cross-sectional slice brings up the corresponding slice on other cross-sectional images. Images are always read with attention to patient preparation, scanning protocol, indication, and detailed patient history and are compared to recent CT and MRI images, whenever available.

Asymmetric uptake should be viewed with suspicion, especially in the head and neck region. Active neoplastic lesions or malignant lesions are usually seen as foci of intense FDG activity (or abnormal focal hypermetabolism). The standard uptake value (SUV) of lesions should be measured and reported. An SUV value of more than 2.5 is

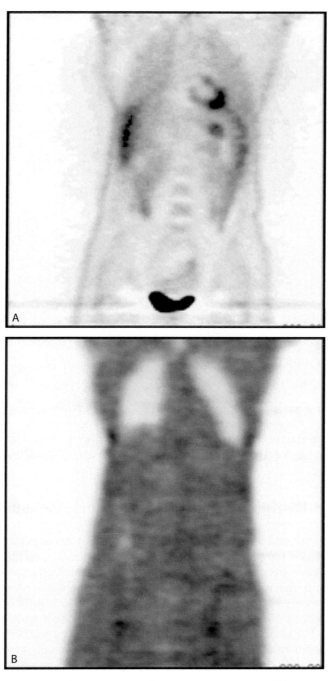

Figure 30.1. Coronal non–attenuation-corrected image (A), reconstructed transmission image (B), and attenuation-corrected image (C) from a whole-body positron emission tomography (PET) scan.

(Continued)

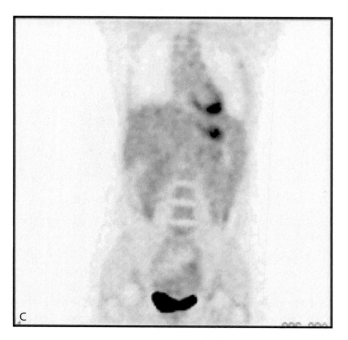

Figure 30.1. *Continued.*

likely to be consistent with malignancy. When evaluating lung nodules, activity is compared with mediastinal blood pool uptake and more active lesions are considered likely to be malignant. If adrenal nodules are more active than liver uptake, they are considered likely to be malignant.

Normal Distribution of FDG in Pediatric Patients

To recognize what is abnormal on PET images, it is very important to know the normal biodistribution of FDG and normal variants. Various articles have described in detail the normal distribution of FDG in adults and the artifacts and pitfalls that can be encountered while reading whole-body FDG-PET images (12–16). The normal distribution of FDG does not differ significantly between adult and pediatric patients. Some of the important differences seen on pediatric images are moderate to intense and symmetric uptake in the epiphysis of long bones, mild to moderate activity in the thymus (seen an inverted V-shaped structure in anterior mediastinum; Fig. 30.2), and changes in glucose metabolism in the brain in neonates.

After the age of 1 year, cerebral glucose metabolism is similar to that in adults. Otherwise, the biodistribution of FDG is similar in pediatric patients and adults, with intense activity seen in the cortex, basal ganglia, and cerebellum. White matter and ventricles are usually seen as photopenic defects. Extraocular muscle activity is generally seen as

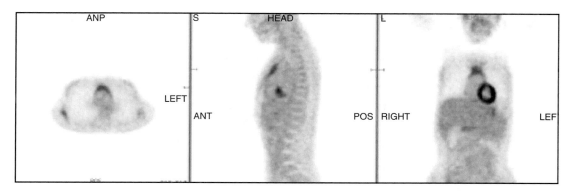

Figure 30.2. Characteristic inverted V-shaped uptake in thymus.

small foci of moderate to intense activity in orbital region. Mild to moderate activity can be seen in the spinal cord, especially proximally. Mild to moderate, variable, and symmetric activity is seen in the oropharynx, tonsils, and salivary glands. Moderate to intense activity is seen in the vocal cords (usually as an inverted U-shaped structure), especially if the patient is talking during the uptake period (Fig. 30.3).

Variable uptake can be seen in skeletal muscles depending on physical activity. Muscular uptake is usually mild to moderate in intensity, linear, and symmetric. Thyroid, airways, and esophagus are normally not seen on PET images. Diffuse uptake in thyroid could be from thyroiditis or Graves' disease (Fig. 30.4). Focal uptake in the thyroid should be viewed with suspicion and evaluated further. Physiologic uptake in brown fat can be seen in the neck, supraclavicular regions, axilla, mediastinum, and posterior intercostal regions as foci of

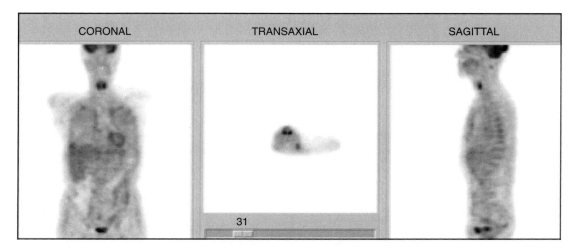

Figure 30.3. Physiologic uptake in vocal cords.

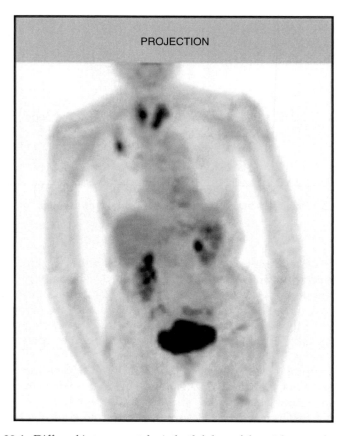

Figure 30.4. Diffused intense uptake in both lobes of thyroid, secondary to thyroiditis. A malignant lung nodule is seen in the right upper lobe.

moderate to intense uptake that are symmetric (Fig. 30.5). This finding was initially thought to be muscle uptake but is now believed to be related to thermoregulation. Lungs, cortices of long bones, and usually muscles also are seen as photopenic areas.

Mild mediastinal blood pool activity is usually seen as focal lesions in the lungs and hilum; those more intense than the mediastinal blood pool activity are considered suspect for neoplastic involvement. Walls of large vessels may be seen from inflammation in the atherosclerotic plaques. The diaphragm and intercostal and accessory muscles may be visualized in patients with respiratory distress (Fig. 30.6). Variable degree of uptake can be seen in myocardium depending on patient preparation, insulin, and blood glucose levels. Administration of insulin (or a recent meal) forces FDG (and glucose) to be taken up by myocardium, muscle, and fatty tissue. This is helpful in cardiac imaging. Minimal or no myocardial uptake is usually recommended for oncologic imaging, especially for evaluation of hilar nodes. Moderate and sometimes heterogeneous activity is seen in the liver. Normally, the spleen is smaller than the liver and less intense in uptake. A

Figure 30.5. A: Projection image of a patient with lymphoma showing symmetric foci in the supraclavicular region. Computed tomography (CT) correlation with transaxial image (B) shows uptake in a region of fat density (C).

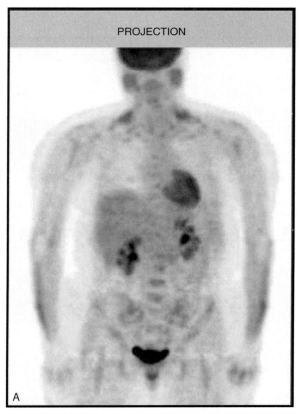

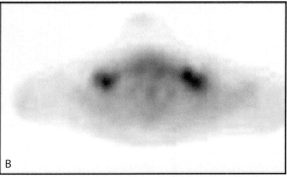

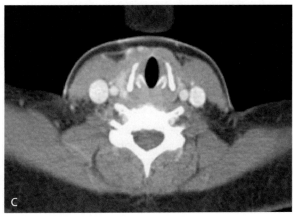

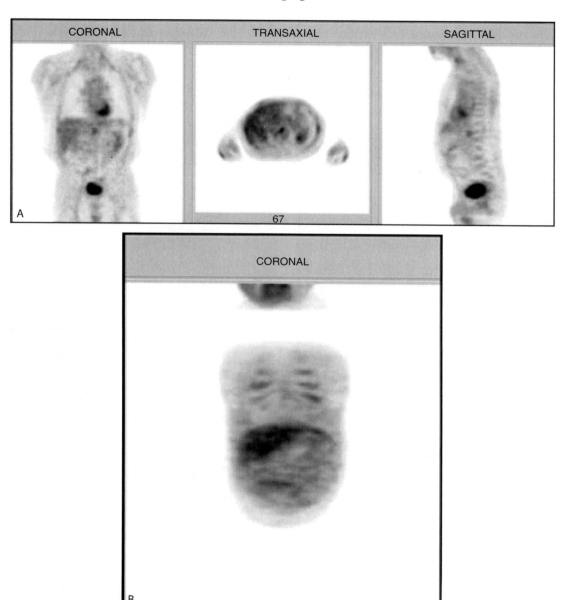

Figure 30.6. A: Image showing focal hypermetabolism in right diaphragmatic crus in a hyperventilating patient. B,C: Anterior and posterior coronal images showing uptake in intercostal muscles.

variable degree of uptake is seen in bowel. Usually the stomach wall and colonic activity is prominent. This physiologic uptake could be intense, but it is generally linear and diffuse. Focal uptake should be evaluated further by colonoscopy.

Mild physiologic uptake in bone marrow leads to faint visualization of vertebral bodies, the pelvis, and the proximal ends of humerus and femur. Increased uptake in bone marrow can be seen in anemia, rebound from chemotherapy, or from pharmacologic stimulation (therapy with colony-stimulating factors) (Fig. 30.7). Because FDG is excreted by the kidneys, mild to moderate activity is seen in the cortex, and intense activity can be seen in the pelvis, ureters, and urinary bladder. Focal stasis in the ureter and activity in bladder diverticulum can be confused with hypermetabolic adenopathy. A history should be obtained about any surgeries, such as renal transplant and diversion procedures. Reproductive structures in the pelvis are usually not visualized, but physiologic activity is frequently seen in the uterus as a focus superior to the bladder (Fig. 30.8). Mild to moderate and usually symmetric activity is seen in the testes. Fatty tissue is usually seen as photopenic areas in the subcutaneous region and in the abdomen.

Various interventions have been reported to reduce or eliminate some of these artifactual foci of FDG activity. Bowel cleansing or motility inhibitors can reduce activity in bowel loops. Diuretics and catheterization can wash out activity in the urinary tract. Oral diazepam has

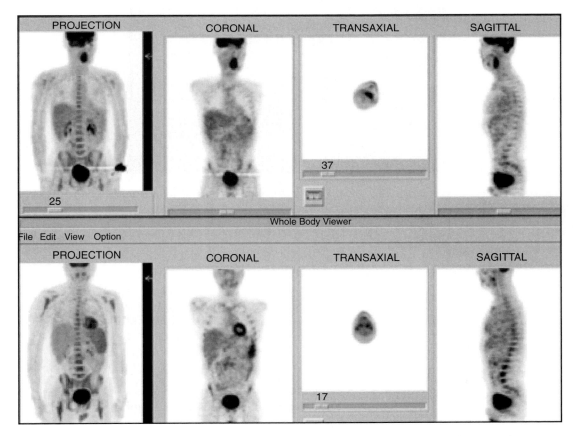

Figure 30.7. Upper row images (pretherapy scan) show uptake in tonsillar lymphoma and injection artifact at the level of the left wrist. Lower row images (posttherapy scan) show intense bone marrow and spleen activity secondary to chemotherapy.

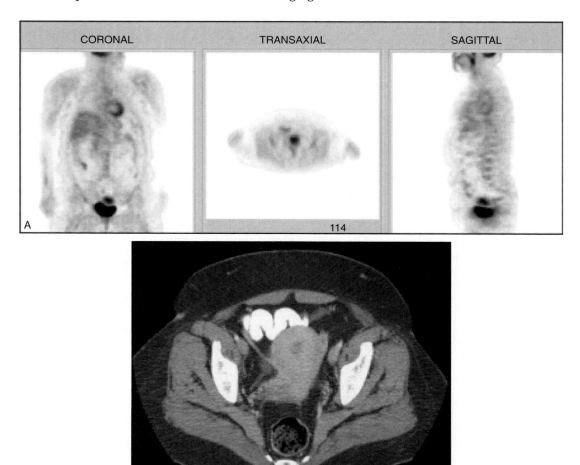

Figure 30.8. A: PET image showing a focus of intense uptake superior to the urinary bladder that corresponds to the uterus (menstruating) on CT scan image (B).

been shown to reduce muscle and fat uptake. We have found that these interventions require a lot of effort, interfere with day-to-day work flow, and do not provide much additional gain in clinical information. In the pediatric population, however, sedation and bladder catheterization may sometimes be required for patient immobilization and reduced risk of contamination.

Artifacts Related to Image Acquisition and Reconstruction

Whenever possible, whole-body images should be acquired with the patient's arms up. In patients with head and neck pathology, a second bed position should be acquired of the head and neck, with the arms down. When chest images are acquired with the arms down, focal skin-fold uptake in axilla can mimic hypermetabolic nodes. It is important that the patient stays still during the entire scan, as patient motion can give rise to artifacts (Fig. 30.9). These can be confirmed on non–attenuation-corrected images. If required, patients can be sedated by using IV medication or even general anesthesia.

Care should be taken during injection of FDG to avoid any tissue infiltration and to make sure that the injection is given in the arm opposite to the affected side. Dose infiltration is usually seen as a large focus of intense activity with surrounding streak photopenia (Fig. 30.7). Nodal uptake from infiltrated dose can be mistaken for neoplastic involvement. Dose infiltration also interferes with calculation of SUV value. Positron emission tomography images are reconstructed using iterative reconstruction algorithms as opposed to filtered back-projection.

Even with iterative reconstruction algorithms, photopenic areas are seen around the foci of intense uptake, such as the urinary bladder, or dose infiltration. This may interfere with evaluation of the pelvis. Attenuation correction can also create artifacts, especially in very obese patients and in using CT data for attenuation correction, especially

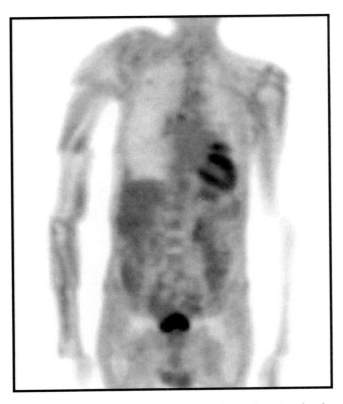

Figure 30.9. Coronal image at level of myocardium showing focal uptake in left perihilar region, an artifact from patient motion.

when using IV and oral contrasts. These can be avoided by the review of non–attenuation-corrected images.

Iatrogenic Artifacts

Oncologic patients presenting for PET imaging have elaborate histories complicated by medical and surgical procedures, which can alter the distribution of FDG (17). A careful history should be taken about various medical and surgical procedures, chemotherapy, and radiation therapy, with their respective dates. Information should be taken about the insertion of IV catheters (Fig. 30.10), ports (Fig. 30.11), tubes, and

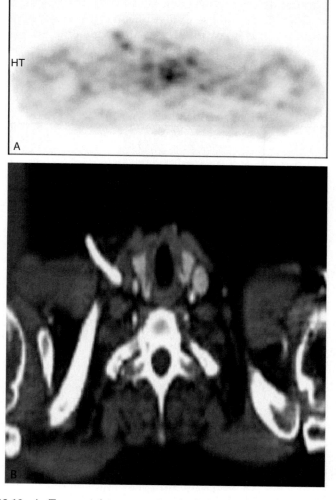

Figure 30.10. A: Transaxial image at level of shoulders showing focal hyper-metabolism in the right supraclavicular region corresponding to the insertion of a central venous catheter on CT scan (B).

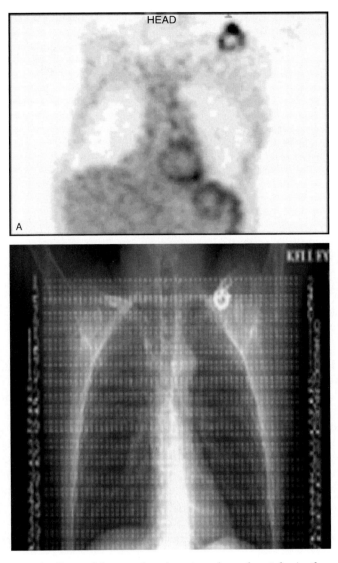

Figure 30.11. A: Coronal image showing ring-shaped uptake in the region of the left shoulder that corresponds to a chemotherapy port seen in the left anterior chest wall on a CT scan image (B).

ileostomies (Fig. 30.12). Inflammatory uptake may be seen in superficial surgical wounds for 4 to 6 weeks. Sites of surgery and biopsies usually fill with serous hypometabolic fluid in the next few days and may be seen on PET scan as ring-shaped foci, with surrounding inflammation (Fig. 30.13). False-positive findings can be seen from inflammation secondary to radiation.

Postradiation changes can persist for 4 to 6 months. Radiation to marrow causes replacement with fatty tissue, which is seen on PET as

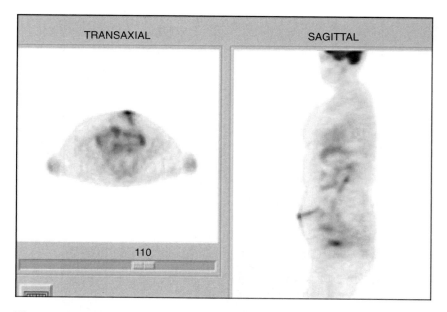

Figure 30.12. PET images showing focal uptake in the right lower quadrant of the abdomen from an ileostomy.

a photopenic area (Fig. 30.14). Radiation-induced pneumonitis, esophagitis, myositis, or vasculitis can also be visualized on PET (18). Radiation-induced changes can be recognized by the geographic pattern of lesions, in the shape of a radiation port (Fig. 30.15). Chemotherapy is also known to change the biodistribution of FDG. The reason for this is not entirely known, but posttherapy images frequently show increased uptake in the myocardium, small and large bowel loops, and, to some extent, the liver and spleen. Rebound bone marrow activity is seen as diffuse and moderate to intense uptake. This can be difficult to distinguish from bone metastasis.

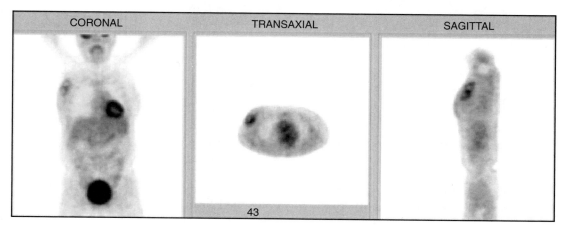

Figure 30.13. Two, small, ring-shaped foci seen in the region of the right breast in a patient who recently had biopsy of tumor and resection of axillary lymph node.

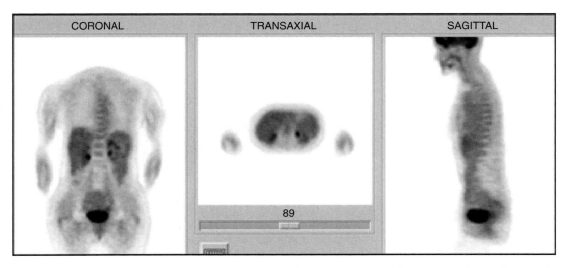

Figure 30.14. PET images of a patient with a history of radiation to the abdomen, showing a photopenic defect in the region of lumbar vertebral bodies.

A prosthesis of any kind, if large enough, is generally seen as a photopenic defect on PET imaging. If the prosthesis is recently placed, inflammatory uptake can be seen around it, which may last for 4 to 6 weeks. Nonspecific activity is known to persist around a hip prosthesis for years (Fig. 30.16).

Increased uptake in the thymus can be seen secondary to chemotherapy, stem cell transplantation, radiotherapy, or iodine-131 therapies. Acute changes in blood glucose levels can also affect the distribution of FDG. The administration of insulin or glucose or a recent meal can

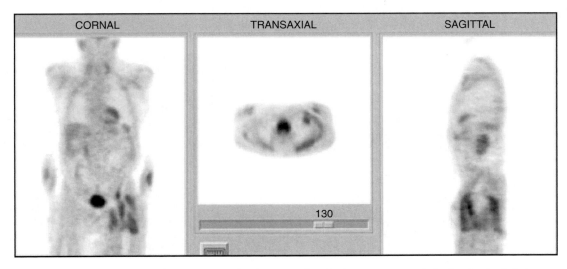

Figure 30.15. PET images of a patient with a history of radiation to metastatic lesion in the left femur. Increased uptake in pattern of geographic radiation port is suggestive of myositis and vasculitis.

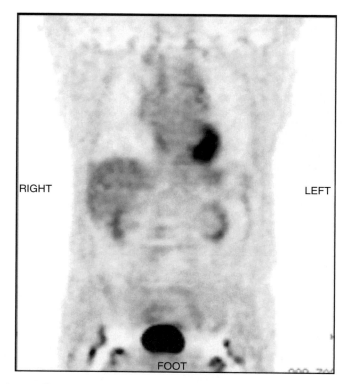

Figure 30.16. Coronal image of a patient showing nonspecific activity around hip prostheses.

cause increased uptake in skeletal muscles, myocardium, and fatty tissue. Acute intravascular thrombosis elicits an inflammatory response that can be seen as a focus of increased FDG activity. As the thrombus becomes chronic and gets replaced by scar tissue, the focus becomes photopenic (Fig. 30.17). Catheter-related focal FDG activity can be from intravascular thrombosis or infection (Fig. 30.18) (19).

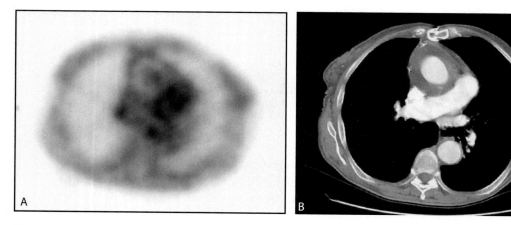

Figure 30.17. A: Transaxial chest image showing a ring-shaped photopenic defect in the anterior mediastinum that corresponds to a chronic thrombus post-repair of an ascending aortic aneurysm (B).

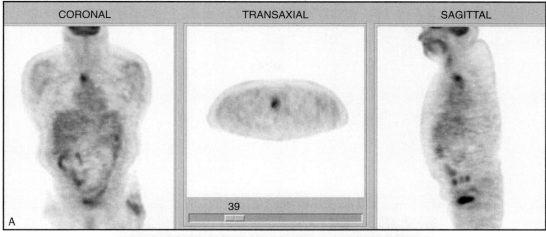

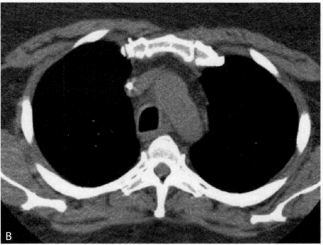

Figure 30.18. A: PET images showing focal intense uptake in right paratracheal region corresponding to a catheter in the superior vena cava (B).

Common Causes of False-Positive Findings

Fluorodeoxyglucose as a tracer is not specific to tumors or malignancies; increased FDG activity can also be seen in inflammatory and infectious lesions. Inflammatory cells also show increased glucose metabolism. False-positive findings from these foci of inflammation or infection are an important cause of low specificity of PET studies (Fig. 30.19) (20). Dual time point imaging has been advocated to recognize these false-positive findings with some success. This technique is useful in the evaluation of solitary pulmonary nodules. It has been shown that FDG uptake in neoplastic lesion increases over a period of

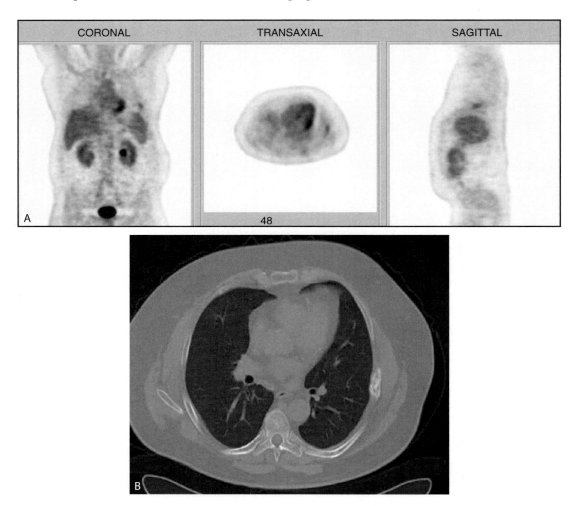

Figure 30.19. A: PET images of a patient with lung nodule showing focal hypermetabolism in peripheral lower left lateral lung/chest wall that corresponds to a healing rib fracture on CT scan (B).

time and that of benign lesion decreases. Therefore, a second acquisition 2 hours after FDG injection may be helpful in differentiating the two. Benign tumors and second primaries are also an important cause of false-positive or incidental findings on PET scans (21). These should be pursued further by obtaining a more complete history from the patient or referring physician, comparing PET images to other radiologic imaging, and by evaluating further. An exhaustive list of benign causes of FDG uptake on whole-body FDG imaging can be found in the article by Bakheet and Powe (22).

Common Causes of False-Negative Findings

Fluorodeoxyglucose-PET is known to be limited in evaluation of low-grade malignancies such as low-grade lymphomas, bronchoalveolar cancers, and carcinoids. Micrometastases in lymph nodes are usually missed on PET scans. Also, with PET imaging, confident evaluation is not possible of lesions smaller than 1 cm in size on anatomic imaging. Hyperglycemia (by competition between blood glucose and the injected FDG) is also known to be a cause of false-negative PET findings.

Common Causes of Photopenic Defects

Frequently, photopenic foci or larger areas are seen on PET images. These can result from hypometabolic structures (white matter and ventricles, fatty tissue, resting skeletal muscle, cortical bone), benign cavities (stomach, bowel, lungs, gall bladder), benign effusions (pleural and pericardial effusions, ascites, hydrocele), postsurgical collections (hematoma, seroma), benign cysts (renal, hepatic cysts), prostheses (breast, hip, and knee prostheses, chemotherapy ports), malignant collections (tumor necrosis), acquisition artifacts (around kidneys and bladder activity), posttherapy changes (scar tissue post–chemo/radiation and bone marrow replacement after radiation), or other causes (chronic thrombi, crossed cerebellar diaschisis, or calcified uterine fibroids). It is important to recognize these artifacts and to correlate them with anatomic imaging. Large tumors frequently show central necrosis that is seen on PET imaging as a photopenic defect, with the lesion itself seen as a ring-shaped focus with hypermetabolic margins. The gallbladder may be seen as a photopenic defect, and inflammation of its walls may cause increased FDG uptake (Fig. 30.20).

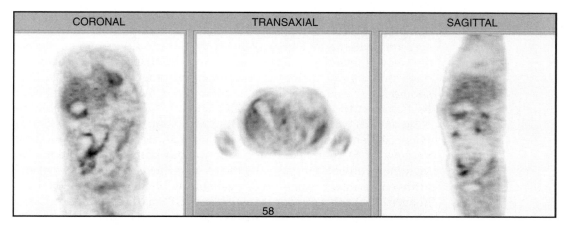

Figure 30.20. PET images of a patient with chronic cholecystitis showing a photopenic defect in the region of the gallbladder and increased uptake in the gallbladder wall.

PET-CT Artifacts

The new imaging technology of acquiring PET and CT images in one machine at the same time, using CT data for attenuation correction, has many advantages but also has its share of artifacts and pitfalls (23–25). These artifacts can be divided into three groups: attenuation-correction artifacts, motion artifacts, and CT truncation artifacts. Because of differences in energy and the way photons are attenuated by the body tissues, when CT transmission data are used for attenuation correction, FDG–avid false-positive findings are seen in the region of metallic implants, IV and oral contrast media, and other radiodense areas. These false-positive findings can be recognized by reviewing the non–attenuation-corrected images and by the presence of beam-hardening artifact on CT images. They can be avoided by not using IV contrast, by using water-based oral contrast, or by using a low-dose CT for attenuation correction and acquiring a separate contrast-enhanced diagnostic CT scan. Motion artifact may result when there is patient or organ motion between the PET scan and the CT scan. This can cause misregistration in the regions of the diaphragm, head and neck, and extremities. Some of this can be avoided by having patients hold their breath at the end of normal expiration during CT scanning, breathe normally during PET acquisition, and lying still during the scan. Computed tomography truncation artifacts can be avoided by having the patient place both arms up during PET and CT acquisition.

Recognizing Artifacts

It is impossible to list all possible false-positive and false-negative findings that can be seen on PET images. Experience is the best way to recognize pitfalls and artifacts while reading these studies. The artifacts discussed in this chapter are from the authors' experience of reading PET studies predominantly in adult patients, but they give a comprehensive idea of possible artifacts and their patterns that may be seen on pediatric PET images. Every reader should develop a consistent way of reviewing images and should correlate images with a thorough and careful history and findings on other imaging tests. One should know as much as possible about the patient. The reader should be conversant in cross-sectional anatomy and should be able to compare PET images directly to CT or MRI images whenever available. He or she should be well versed in normal distribution and normal variants of FDG uptake. Information about patient preparation, the imaging protocol, the patient's blood sugar level, and the site of the intravenous injection should be available at the time of review of these images. Positron emission tomography–CT has been proposed as a way to avoid some of these artifacts and pitfalls. Recognizing these artifacts increases the sensitivity and specificity of a scan, reduces the number of equivocal findings, and prevents unnecessary additional workup.

References

1. Rohren EM, Turkington TG, Coleman RE. Clinical applications of PET in oncology. Radiology 2004;231(2):305–332.
2. Kostakoglu L, Agress H Jr, Goldsmith SJ. Clinical role of FDG-PET in evaluation of cancer patients. Radiographics 2003;23(2):315–340.
3. Jadvar H, Alavi A, Mavi A, el al. PET in pediatric diseases. Radiol Clin North Am 2005;43(1):135–152.
4. Hahn K, Pfluger T. Has PET become an important clinical tool in paediatric imaging? Eur J Nucl Med Mol Imaging 2004;31(5):615–621.
5. Shulkin BL. PET imaging in pediatric oncology. Pediatr Radiol 2004;34(3):199–204.
6. Foehrenbach H, Edeline V, Bonardel G, et al. Technique and indications in pediatric oncology. Positron emission tomography with 18F-fluorodeoxyglucose. Arch Pediatr 2004;11(4):378–382.
7. Roberts EG, Shulkin BL. Technical issues in performing PET studies in pediatric patients. J Nucl Med Technol 2004;32(1):5–9.
8. Borgwardt L, Larsen HJ, Pedersen K, et al. Practical use and implementation of PET in children in a hospital PET centre. Eur J Nucl Med Mol Imaging 2003;30(10):1389–1397.
9. Bombardieri E, Aktolun C, Baum RP, et al. FDG-PET: procedure guidelines for tumour imaging. Eur J Nucl Med Mol Imaging 2003;30(12):BP115–124.
10. Hamblen SM, Lowe VJ. Clinical 18F-FDG oncology patient preparation techniques. J Nucl Med Technol 2003;31(1):3–7.
11. Schelbert HR, Hoh CK, Royal HD, et al. Procedure guideline for tumor imaging using fluorine-18-FDG. Society of Nuclear Medicine. J Nucl Med 1998;39(7):1302–1305.
12. El-Haddad G, Alavi A, Mavi A, et al. Normal variants in [18F]-fluorodeoxyglucose PET imaging. Radiol Clin North Am 2004;42(6):1063–1081.
13. Cook GJ, Wegner EA, Fogelman I. Pitfalls and artifacts in 18FDG-PET and PET/CT oncologic imaging. Semin Nucl Med 2004;34(2):122–133.
14. Gordon BA, Flanagan FL, Dehdashti F. Whole-body positron emission tomography: normal variations, pitfalls, and technical considerations. AJR 1997;169(6):1675–1680.
15. Cook GJ, Fogelman I, Maisey MN. Normal physiological and benign pathological variants of 18–fluoro-2–deoxyglucose positron-emission tomography scanning: potential for error in interpretation. Semin Nucl Med 1996;26(4):308–314.
16. Engel H, Steinert H, Buck A, et al. Whole-body PET: physiological and artifactual FDG accumulations. J Nucl Med 1996;37(3):441–446.
17. Bhargava P, Zhuang H, Kumar R, et al. Iatrogenic artifacts on whole-body F-18 FDG-PET imaging. Clin Nucl Med 2004;29(7):429–439.
18. Bhargava P, Reich P, Alavi A, et al. Radiation-induced esophagitis on FDG-PET imaging. Clin Nucl Med 2003;28(10):849–850.
19. Bhargava P, Kumar R, Zhuang H, et al. Catheter-related focal FDG activity on whole body PET imaging. Clin Nucl Med 2004;29(4):238–242.
20. Strauss LG. Fluorine-18 deoxyglucose and false-positive results: a major problem in the diagnostics of oncological patients. Eur J Nucl Med 1996;23(10):1409–1415.
21. Agress H Jr, Cooper BZ. Detection of clinically unexpected malignant and premalignant tumors with whole-body FDG-PET: histopathologic comparison. Radiology 2004;230(2):417–422.

22. Bakheet SM, Powe J. Benign causes of 18-FDG uptake on whole body imaging. Semin Nucl Med 1998;28(4):352–358.
23. Kostakoglu L, Hardoff R, Mirtcheva R, et al. PET-CT fusion imaging in differentiating physiologic from pathologic FDG uptake. Radiographics 2004;24(5):1411–1431.
24. Kapoor V, McCook BM, Torok FS. An introduction to PET-CT imaging. Radiographics 2004;24(2):523–543.
25. Schoder H, Erdi YE, Larson SM, et al. PET/CT: a new imaging technology in nuclear medicine. Eur J Nucl Med Mol Imaging 2003;30(10):1419–1437.

Index